Transcultural Concepts in Nursing Care

NINTH EDITION

Joyceen S. Boyle, PhD, RN, FTNSS, FAAN

Adjunct Professor of Nursing
College of Nursing
University of Arizona
Tucson, Arizona
Adjunct Professor of Nursing
College of Nursing
Augusta University
Augusta, Georgia

John W. Collins, PhD, MS, RN, FTNSS

Dean and Associate Professor
School of Nursing and Health Sciences
Rochester University
Rochester Hills, Michigan

Patti Ludwig-Beymer, PhD, RN, CTN-A, NEA-BC, CPPS, FTNSS, FAAN

Associate Professor and Nurse Executive
 Concentration Coordinator
College of Nursing
Purdue University Northwest
Hammond, Indiana

Margaret M. Andrews, PhD, RN, FTNSS, FAAN

Founding Dean and Professor Emerita
School of Nursing
University of Michigan–Flint
Flint, Michigan

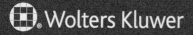 Wolters Kluwer

Philadelphia • Baltimore • New York • London
Buenos Aires • Hong Kong • Sydney • Tokyo

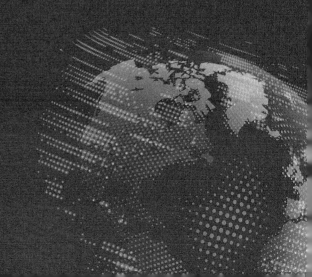

Vice President and Publisher: Julie K. Stegman
Manager, Nursing Education and Practice Content: Jamie Blum
Senior Acquisitions Editor: Susan Hartman
Development Editor: Phoebe Jordan-Reilly
Editorial Coordinator: Anju Radhakrishnan
Editorial Assistant: Devika Kishore
Marketing Manager: Wendy Mears
Production Project Manager: Kirstin Johnson
Manager, Graphic Arts & Design: Stephen Druding
Art Director, Illustration: Jennifer Clements
Manufacturing Coordinator: Margie Orzech
Prepress Vendor: Straive

Ninth edition

Cataloging-in-Publication Data available on request from the Publisher

ISBN: 978-1-9752-2296-3

MPP1123

Contributors to the Ninth Edition

Margaret M. Andrews, PhD, RN, FTNSS, FAAN
Founding Dean and Professor Emerita
School of Nursing
University of Michigan–Flint
Flint, Michigan

Martha B. Baird, PhD, RN, FTNSS
Clinical Assistant Professor
School of Nursing
University of Kansas Medical Center
Kansas City, Kansas

Heather M. Bowers, MSN, RN
Clinical Assistant Professor
College of Nursing
Purdue University Northwest
Hammond, Indiana

Joyceen S. Boyle, PhD, RN, FTNSS, FAAN
Adjunct Professor of Nursing
College of Nursing
University of Arizona
Tucson, Arizona
Adjunct Professor of Nursing
College of Nursing
Augusta University
Augusta, Georgia

John W. Collins, PhD, MS, RN, FTNSS
Dean and Associate Professor
School of Nursing and Health Sciences
Rochester University
Rochester Hills, Michigan

Melva Craft-Blacksheare, DNP, CNM, RN
Associate Professor
School of Nursing
University of Michigan–Flint
Flint, Michigan

Marilyn K. Eipperle, DNP, RN, FNP-BC, CTN-A
Nursing Faculty Lecturer II
School of Nursing
University of Michigan–Flint
Flint, Michigan

Mary Lou Clark Fornehed, PhD, RN
Assistant Professor
School of Nursing
Tennessee Technological University
Cookeville, Tennessee

Linda Sue Hammonds, DNP, RN
Associate Professor
Community Mental Health
University of South Alabama
Mobile, Alabama

Patti Ludwig-Beymer, PhD, RN, CTN-A, NEA-BC, CPPS, FTNSS, FAAN
Associate Professor and Nurse Executive
Concentration Coordinator
College of Nursing
Purdue University Northwest
Hammond, Indiana

Sandra J. Mixer, PhD, RN, FTNSS, CTN-A
Associate Professor Emerita
College of Nursing
University of Tennessee
Knoxville, Tennessee

Dula F. Pacquiao, EdD, MA, RN, FTNSS
Professor Emerita
School of Nursing
Rutgers, The State University of
    New Jersey
Newark, New Jersey

Julia L. Rogers, DNP, APRN, CNS, FNP-BC, FAANP
Assistant Professor
College of Nursing
Purdue University Northwest
Hammond, Indiana
Family Nurse Practitioner
Northwest Health Pulmonary and Critical Care
Valparaiso, Indiana

Karina E. Strange, PhD, BSN, BA, RN
Assistant Professor
School of Nursing
Duquesne University
Pittsburgh, Pennsylvania

Foreword

I am pleased for the opportunity to write the Foreword once again, this time, for the ninth edition of the *Transcultural Concepts in Nursing Care* book by Drs. Joyceen S. Boyle, John Collins, Patti Ludwig-Beymer, and Margaret M. Andrews. Each one of these authors has followed in the footsteps of the founder of transcultural nursing, the late Dr. Madeleine Leininger, a giant in the area of the relevance of culture, caring, health, and nursing; Dr. Leininger paved the way for what is now known in academic, political, and social/public arenas as DEI—diversity, equity, and inclusion—in the United States and around the world; however, her views included caring and the transcendent. Drs. Boyle and Andrews saw the need to advance transcultural concepts in nursing care and wrote the first edition of this book, along with chapter contributions written by other authors, in 1989. Subsequent editions of this book have provided the foundation to study transcultural concepts related to diverse cultures of individuals, groups, and communities and are used extensively in Schools of Nursing across the United States and in other nations. The first author, Dr. Joyceen Boyle, was mentored by the renowned nurse–anthropologist, Dr. JoAnn Glittenberg Hinrichs. Joyceen and I were classmates and privileged to be in the first transcultural nursing PhD program under the leadership of Dean Leininger at the University of Utah, College of Nursing in 1977. We were challenged by Dr. Leininger to study the substantive cultural, nursing, and caring knowledge to cocreate new knowledge-models and theories through research for the development of the discipline and profession of transcultural nursing. In 2023, the University of Utah, College of Nursing celebrated its 75th anniversary, and in 2024, the Transcultural Nursing Society celebrates 50 years since its inception, showing the world how outstanding transcultural nursing graduates, like Drs. Boyle, Andrews, Ludwig-Beymer, and Collins, mentored by Dr. Andrews, have sought to change the world of national and international transcultural nursing practice by means of their scholarship in the provision of culturally competent care. The chapters in this book, now in its ninth edition, reveal this scholarship by continuing to illuminate the application of the authors' **Transcultural Interprofessional Practice (TIP) Theory and Model** introduced in the seventh edition. The TIP Model captures and communicates the widest range of the rich foundational knowledge of cultural and transcultural nursing knowledge for diverse populations, such as addressing multicultural and population health across the lifespan, including the health of indigenous groups, palliative and end-of-life care, seeking person/patient/client-centered contributions to transcultural nursing assessments, transcultural maternal–child care, pursuing cultural understanding of mental healthcare, creating culturally competent healthcare organizations, addressing environmental science and social justice, identification and assessment of transcultural religious, ethical and moral foundations, animal contributions, and furthering global health via cognizance of the United Nations sustainable development goals and many others. The world of transcultural nursing practice has been changed by the authors' creation, communication, and dissemination of their **TIP** Model, which is more critical than ever, now that attention to cultural illness and health, cultural competence, and interprofessionalism are advancing as the norm in contemporary nursing education, research, and practice, especially in the United States. Their book meets the new essentials and current directives of the American Association of

Colleges of Nursing (AACN, 2021), the National League for Nursing (NLN), and the American Nurses Association (ANA) and other organizations for preparation of nurses in transcultural nursing to provide evidence-based culturally competent care to people.

I would like to share the significance of each editor's illustrious career, especially as writers and editors of this text, which has contributed to the remarkable evolution of transcultural nursing. Dr. Joyceen Boyle conducted research on maternal and child health in a "squatter" or marginal settlement in Guatemala in the early 1980s in the middle of a 36-year civil war or "armed conflict." This experience set the stage for further research and activism focusing on the myriad of relationships between social equity and health, and concern for migrants/asylum-seekers at the southern border of the United States. Joyceen also conducted research with Salvadorans in Utah who had fled violence from that country. She helped many members from this research sample to obtain U.S. citizenship owing in large part to the signed human assurance forms proving their residence in the country for the allotted number of years. Joyceen also served as a consultant to the College of Nursing at the University of Baghdad before the highly contested Desert Storm and later Iraqi wars. Her efforts helped to preserve academic nursing education with direct communication with the late President Saddam Hussein. Cultural considerations, and caring behaviors, as well as human rights and migrant health led to her many years of work with Amnesty International. In 2019, she received the first Asylum Casework Award from Amnesty International, USA. Her concentration on human rights became the bedrock of Dr. Boyle's public service and contributed to the development and evolution of her role as a global transcultural nurse. Major contributions of her career were educating undergraduate and graduate nursing students in community health and transcultural nursing, 14 years of which were spent teaching undergraduate nursing students at the University of Utah. Joyceen followed her faculty position in Utah with faculty positions at the Medical College of Georgia and the University of Arizona, researching continuously and publishing widely. While working at the Medical College of Georgia, Joyceen formed a Qualitative Research Group with three of her graduate students. For 12 years, they collected data and published extensively about African American mothers who provided care to adult children with HIV/AIDS. She served as the first President of the Transcultural Nursing Society. Dr. Boyle furthered the commitment to humane and scientific knowledge-development by describing, explaining, and interpreting transcultural nursing, which acknowledged diverse cultures, kinship systems, ideologies, history, and geopolitical environments of many nation states to provide theory-guided, culturally congruent care.

Dr. John Collins joined the team of editors of this text in the eighth edition and continues as a coeditor on the ninth edition. Following his PhD in transcultural nursing under the leadership of Drs. Margaret Andrews and Marilyn McFarland, John served as Project Director of the Health Resources and Services Administration (HRSA) funded Veteran Bachelor of Science in Nursing (BSN) Program at the University of Michigan, Flint. He identified and educated others about the unique culture of persons transitioning from military service (active duty) to veteran status, increased opportunities for veteran nursing education, and made available important cultural information for the profession of nursing within the Veterans Administration. As a retired USAF Colonel and veteran myself, and a contributor to another HRSA grant for Veteran BSN education in primary care at Florida Atlantic University, I appreciated sharing over the years with John about his commitment for veterans and their families. Dr. Collins is now a nursing administrator, the Dean of the School of Nursing, at Rochester University, Michigan. As a university leader and educator, he is devoted to an emphasis on student and faculty transcultural awareness, spiritual underpinnings, and the provision of culturally competent care to people of all cultures and ages. John's ethnonursing research has focused on using

Leininger's culture care theory as the organizing framework for a federal project on cultural competence. He is dedicated to continued research and teaching on cultural competence in nursing and healthcare, and addressing cultural aspects of end-of-life advanced care planning responding to the needs of culturally diverse persons, especially African Americans. Dr. Collins previously served on Wolters Kluwer's PrepU editorial board as a Bias Editor. His research with transcultural nursing collaborators on advanced care planning of African Americans is published in the *Journal of Transcultural Nursing*. Currently, as a Fellow of the Transcultural Nursing Society, Transcultural Nursing Scholars' group (FTNSS), he serves as Treasurer.

Dr. Patti Ludwig-Beymer, a transcultural nurse executive and nursing educator, is another esteemed editor of this ninth edition. She was influenced early in her career by an introduction to anthropology, followed by conference attendance at Duquesne University with key nursing leaders, Watson and Leininger. What she discovered as the missing link in nursing was culture. She hurried to the University of Utah in 1981 for her PhD but discovered that Dr. Leininger had moved on to the research scientist role at Wayne State University. Dr. Leininger, however, was never far from any nurse interested in the study of transcultural nursing. Patti was greatly supported through prayer and loving kindness by Dr. Leininger as she was pursuing motherhood, which unfolded for Patti with the birth of her daughter, Theresa. At the University of Utah, Patti discovered that she was a PhD classmate of Dr. Margaret Andrews and had the distinct honor to be educated by Dr. Joyceen Boyle, and the coeditors of this book, the contents of which were discussed among these authors and a few others in the early 1980s. Patti used Leininger's "Culture Care Diversity and Universality Theory" in many of her professional endeavors in nursing education, administrative nursing, parish nursing, and staff nursing. She also contributed faithfully to the Transcultural Nursing Society in many leadership roles and for many years was dedicated to

the TCN Scholars' selection committee. Upon nursing in a large Chicago hospital, Patti became more aware of health disparities and the need for population health. She, with colleagues in the Chicago suburbs, established a Hispanic Community Center, named Genesis Center for Health and Empowerment for the community to address the Social (and Cultural) Determinants of Health. With her commitment to transcultural nursing practice, Patti led interprofessional teams to improve and provide culturally congruent care for persons with diabetes, asthma, and heart failure, and established key initiatives to improve immunizations and care for newborns, children, and adults. With this experience, Patti began to focus on creating culturally competent, complex healthcare organizations and has published widely on this subject. As an executive, she has always been guided in her practice by Transcultural Nursing, recognizing its impact on quality patient care and the care provided to nurses and other clinicians. As a faculty member, Dr. Ludwig-Beymer teaches executive nursing students. Major concepts and theories, including the **TIP** Theory and Model essential to effective nursing practice, organizational culture, and population health, guide her teaching.

Joining Drs. Boyle, Collins, and Ludwig-Beymer for the ninth edition is Dr. Margaret (Marge) Andrews. Marge did not participate actively in the writing of the ninth edition; however, because of her past significant contributions as a coeditor of *Transcultural Concepts in Nursing Care*, she is included among the lead editors listed on this edition. Dr. Andrews, who with Dr. Boyle and a select group of scholars, is the original creator of the dynamics of the text and a central coauthor of the first through eighth editions of the book, and the Transcultural Interprofessional theory and TIP Model. As an early transcultural/multicultural sage, Dr. Andrews was a resolute international academic scholar and Pediatric Nurse Practitioner clinician working for 3 years in West Africa in the Igbo-dominated East Central State of Nigeria. Her early childhood experience under the care and love of her parents, and her African experience gave her a profound understanding of spiritual and religious healing, which too were the impetus to pursue additional education in transcultural nursing. As a mentee of Dr. Leininger's theoretical foundations and exploration in transcultural nursing, a committed PhD and student of Dr. Boyle, followed by faculty leadership and Deanship roles at the University of Michigan, Flint, and the Transcultural Nursing Society, she exemplified a national and international commitment to developing cultural competence for persons of diverse cultures *and* nursing's professional transcultural capabilities. As an educator, Dr. Andrews focused on the workforce of nurses, preparing students, faculty, clinicians, and administrators to be thoroughly educated and clinically prepared to deliver high quality, accessible, theoretical, and evidence-based transcultural care to people of diverse backgrounds around the world. She was a great mentor and support to Drs. Marilyn McFarland and Hiba Wehbe-Alamah on her faculty, who continued the publication of Leininger's Transcultural Nursing book after Leininger's death in 2012. Dr. Andrews had a particular interest in the academic success of students from diverse and traditionally underrepresented populations. Her scholarly work addresses those issues as Editor of the *Online Journal of Cultural Competence in Nursing and Healthcare* (http://www.ojccnh.org) and in other publications and presentations. Her publications not only point to the scholarship presented in this book but also the development of a core curriculum for transcultural nursing that highlights the provision of culturally competent care based upon knowledge and skill of understanding cultural illness and health across the lifespan. Dr. Andrews is now retired from her illustrious career as Dean of the School of Nursing at the University of Michigan, Flint, where she led faculty and students to be successful in transcultural nursing academics, research, administration, and practice, fulfilling the mission of Dr. Leininger, that "...the professional nurse scientist and humanist is to discover, know, and creatively use culturally based care knowledge with its fullest meanings, expressions,

symbols, and functions for healing, and to promote or maintain well-being (or health) with people of diverse cultures in the world" (Leininger, 1991, p. 73).

The chapters in this ninth edition address the historical and current trends in transcultural knowledge for national and international communities, innovative approaches in primary and preventive care, organizational cultures, interprofessional care, and immigrant and refugee care with a focus on public health and policy. As mentioned, a most essential element of this book is the Andrews/Boyle Transcultural Interprofessional Practice (TIP) Model, a transcultural nursing/healthcare theory and model that speaks to the need for a conceptual framework to guide transcultural nursing education, research, administration, and practice. I recently was present at the International Council of Nurses (ICN) Congress in Montreal, Canada, attended by almost 7,000 nurses. It focused on leadership in nursing, the workforce, and the ongoing global nurse shortage, advanced practice nursing and primary care, digital technology, strengthening health systems, communicable diseases and international health, nursing policy and global health. Although it was international, in my view what was missing from a *theoretical* perspective were transcultural nursing and caring paradigms, which would have synthesized important concepts for the international practice of nursing. Although falling short of transcultural nursing theories, the Congress helped me realize once more the creativity of Madeleine Leininger and what an effective mentor she was. The motto articulated at the outset of the initiation of the Transcultural Nursing Society that "the cultural needs of people in the world would be met by nurses prepared in transcultural nursing" sparked deep thoughts within me at this latest 2023 international conference of the need to continue to create and publish transcultural nursing theory, which is more critical than ever. The authors' theory and TIP Model illuminate transcultural communication, teamwork, collaboration, and culturally competent skills. As an interprofessional and person-centered theory,

TIP also emphasizes the contributions of persons (patients/clients) who are being served transculturally to participate in *sharing their views of their own cultural care practices with the healthcare team.* We know that there are few care plans used in nursing within healthcare organizations that include the patient's *own* views of their health and their cultural care practices. In a culturally diverse world and as the need for transcultural nursing becomes even more relevant, the reinforcement of theories, or the emergence of new transcultural nursing theories, will continue to improve the practice of person-centered care and ultimately enhance the discipline of transcultural nursing and contribute to the legacy created by Leininger in the 1950s.

As we witness rapid changes in science, technology and artificial intelligence (AI) and robotics, genetics, genomics, population healthcare, economics, geopolitics, transportation, demographics, migration and immigration, refugee challenges, religious ideologies, wars, and global issues including DEI, human rights, and social justice, nurses are challenged to understand new ways of engaging with persons and professional colleagues transculturally. In complexity sciences and the generation of enormous quantities of research of every affiliation and diverse philosophical, political, technological, and religious perspective, we can see the interconnectedness of everything in the universe and the necessity for discernment and evaluation of what is really happening in the world. Theoretical and experiential cultural knowledge about our responsibilities to one another and the world community is thus growing and impacts the need for intense communication to examine and solve problems both locally and globally. Continuing to identify relevant issues to promote health, human safety, and improve the quality of life of all people is a major goal of thoughtful transcultural healthcare professionals. These developments have shaped Boyle, Collins, Ludwig-Beymer, and Andrews' paradigmatic, theoretical and practical thinking in the ninth edition. Their interest in addressing the historical and ideological challenges throughout the

lifespan of the interconnectedness of all through their Transcultural Interprofessional Practice Model (TIP Theory) illuminates the necessity for increased collaboration and communication with all healthcare professionals *and* politicians who are serving diverse citizens, including indigenous peoples, to address the complexity of the age. Additionally, migration with multiple languages represented, the developments of innovative approaches to learning, AI, robotics, and the digital age in general challenge all transcultural nurses to appreciate the *meaning* of transculturality or interculturality in the provision of culturally congruent, safe, and competent care. The key concepts identified in the TIP Model are *context, the interprofessional healthcare team, communication, and the problem-solving process.* The cultural *context* (health-related beliefs and practices that weave together environmental, economic, social, religious, moral, legal, political, educational, biophysical, genetic, and technological factors) encourage transcultural nurses and the interprofessional healthcare team (nurses, physicians, social workers, therapists, pharmacists, clients, and others) to become more aware of the meaning of *cross-cultural communication* among clients, families, families of choice, significant others, "folk" and traditional healers, and religious and spiritual healers and members of organizations to facilitate solving problems in a complex world. The problem-solving steps in this text include comprehensive holistic patient/client assessment, mutual goal setting, planning, implementation of the plan of action and interventions, and evaluation of the plan for effectiveness to achieve the stated goals and desired outcomes; providing culturally congruent and competent care; delivering quality care that is safe and affordable; and ensuring that the care is evidence-based with best practices.

As I reflect on the work of my colleagues, Joyceen Boyle, John Collins, Patti Ludwig-Beymer, and Margaret Andrews, not only within the pages of this book, but also, what each of them has accomplished over many years as innovators, leaders, teachers, researchers, classroom, and online educators, what comes to mind is their *deep dedication and devotion* to the discipline and profession of Transcultural Nursing. Through their intellectual astuteness and creative actions, they are role models and mentors to students and other leaders who can enlighten and broaden transcultural care knowledge worldwide. They are committed to the primary goal of transcultural nursing to facilitate culturally congruent knowledge and care so that people of the world are understood, and their healthcare needs can be met within the dynamics of their cultures and global cultural understanding. A ninth edition of a book attests to the fact that students, faculty, and other practitioners will find within its pages relevant and challenging information and a theory and model to learn about and apply to diverse culture groups, know how to relate to and serve them, conduct research, and facilitate the solving of problems. Today *interprofessional collaboration and communication* are the key to change and effective transcultural care. The authors have captured that essence in their Transcultural Interprofessional Practice (TIP) Theory and Model presented in this work.

I wholeheartedly endorse this new edition. I am most proud to call these authors not only my colleagues but also my friends as they move forward in the evolution of what can be termed authentic transcultural nursing by means of collaboration and interprofessionalism. Nursing students, faculty, other healthcare professionals, and practitioners of every healthcare and anthropological/sociological discipline will be stimulated by the theory and the content expressed by the authors and the many contributors in this new edition to improve the health of and help people of diverse cultures worldwide.

Leininger, M. (Ed.). (1991). *Culture care diversity & universality: A theory of nursing.* National League for Nursing Press.

With gratitude and caring thoughts,

Marilyn A. Ray, RN, PhD, CTN-A, SfAA, FAAN, FESPCH (Hon), FNAP, HSGAHN, FTNSS, Hon. LLD
Colonel (Retired), United States Air Force, Nurse Corps
Professor Emeritus, and Adjunct Professor, Aging and Caring Science Program Specialist
The Christine E. Lynn College of Nursing
Florida Atlantic University
Boca Raton, Florida

Preface

Nurses are accustomed to completing patient assessments and performing complete head-to-toe assessments on every assigned patient on every shift while working at inpatient clinical facilities. Assessments are also completed multiple times within a given shift to assess possible changes in cardiac, respiratory, neurologic, endocrine, and other bodily systems impacted by both chronic and acute disease. However, as a discipline, we have only minimally embraced the tenets of cultural assessment and the concepts provided in this text. To properly provide Culturally Competent Care, we must seek to better understand the values, beliefs, and lifeways of the patients and their families who we serve, as well as the physiologic assessment findings. To that end, given the large number of cultures and subcultures in the world, it is impossible for nurses to know everything about them all; however, it is possible for nurses to develop excellent cultural assessment and cross-cultural communication skills and to follow a systematic, orderly process for the delivery of culturally competent care.

The Andrews/Boyle Transcultural Interprofessional Practice (TIP) Model, which we introduced in the seventh edition of *Transcultural Concepts in Nursing Care*, has been well received at national and international conferences and by readers. Chapters 1 and 2 emphasize the need for effective communication, efficient client- and patient-centered teamwork, teambuilding, and collaboration among members of the interprofessional healthcare team.

The TIP Model has a theoretical foundation in transcultural nursing that fosters communication and collaboration between and among all members of the team and enables multiple team members to manage complex, frequently multifaceted transcultural care issues, moral and ethical dilemmas, challenges, and care-related problems in a collegial, respectful, synergistic manner. The process used in the TIP Model is an adaptation and application of the classic scientific problem-solving method. The model has application in the care of people from different national origins, ethnicities, races, socioeconomic backgrounds, religions, genders, marital statuses, sexual orientations, ages, abilities/disabilities, sizes, veteran status, and other characteristics used to compare one group of people to another.

The Commission on Collegiate Nursing Education (CCNE), the American Association of Colleges of Nursing's (AACN) Essentials of Baccalaureate Education for Professional Nursing Practice (revised and adopted in 2021), Accreditation Commission for Education in Nursing, most state boards of nursing, and other accrediting and certification bodies require or strongly encourage the inclusion of cultural aspects of care in nursing curricula. This, of course, underscores the importance of the purpose, goal, and objectives for *Transcultural Concepts in Nursing Care*, ninth edition.

Purpose: To contribute to the development of theoretically based transcultural nursing knowledge and the advancement of transcultural nursing practice.

Goal: To increase the delivery of culturally competent care to individuals, families, groups, communities, and institutions.

Objectives:

1. To apply a transcultural nursing framework to guide nursing practice in diverse healthcare settings across the lifespan.
2. To analyze major concerns and issues encountered by nurses in providing transcultural nursing care to individuals, families, groups, communities, and institutions.

3. To expand the theoretical basis for using concepts from the natural and behavioral sciences and from the humanities to provide culturally competent nursing care.

4. To provide a contemporary approach to transcultural nursing that includes effective cross-cultural communication, team work, and interprofessional collaborative practice.

The editors and chapter authors share a commitment to:

- Foster the development and maintenance of a disciplinary knowledge base and expertise in culturally competent care that positively impacts nurses' clinical judgment.
- Synthesize existing theoretical and research knowledge regarding nursing care of different ethnic/minority/marginalized and other disenfranchised populations.
- Identify and describe evidence-based practice and best practices in the care of diverse individuals, families, groups, communities, and institutions.
- Create an interdisciplinary and interprofessional knowledge base that reflects heterogeneous healthcare practices within various cultural groups.
- Identify, describe, and examine methods, theories, and frameworks appropriate for developing knowledge that will improve health and nursing care to minority, underserved, underrepresented, disenfranchised, and marginalized populations.

Recognizing Individual Differences and Acculturation

We believe that it is tremendously important to recognize the myriad of health-related values, beliefs, and lifeways that exist within population categories. For example, differences are rarely recognized among people who identify themselves as Hispanic/Latino yet this group includes people from along the United States–Mexico border, Mexican Americans, Puerto Ricans, Guatemalans, Cubans (such as those living in "little Havana" in Miami), as well as other Central and South American countries. These individuals may share some similarities (e.g., speaking Spanish) but also have distinct cultural differences. It should be noted that people from Spain do not necessarily culturally self-identify with individuals from the cultural groups previously cited; rather, they take pride in being Spanish and speaking Castilian Spanish, the term for the dialects from the northern half of Spain. This brief explanation demonstrates the necessity of cultural assessment with individual patients and their families; assumptions beyond holding knowledge (basic tenets generally held by members of a cultural group) can result in gross misunderstandings by healthcare professionals and may estrange the patient–nurse relationship.

We would also like to comment briefly on the terms *minority* and *ethnic minorities*. These terms are perceived by some to be offensive because they may connote inferiority and marginalization. Although we have used these terms occasionally, we prefer to make reference to a specific culture or subculture whenever possible. We refer to categorizations according to race, ethnicity, religion, or a combination, such as ethnoreligion, but we make every effort to avoid using any label in a pejorative manner. We do believe, however, that occasionally the concepts or terms *minority* or *ethnicity* are limiting, not only for those to whom the label may apply but also for nursing theory and practice. We believe the concept of *culture* is richer and has more theoretical usefulness and that *diverse cultures* is a descriptor of the uniqueness and individuality within the breadth and scope of both cultural universality and distinctiveness. In addition, we believe and espouse that all individuals have cultural attributes while not all are from a minority group or claim a particular ethnicity. Look no further than the familial food traditions and the manner of celebration of a holiday to begin to identify the cultural distinctions of your own family and those of your parents and grandparents. Further, many cultures today draw characteristics from several previously distinctive culture groups, due to population migration, intermarriage among individuals from different cultures, and the impact of changing family dynamics.

Critical Thinking Linked to Delivering Culturally Competent Care

We believe that nurses' critical thinking, cultural assessment, and clinical judgment and problem-solving abilities will provide the necessary knowledge and skills on which to base transcultural nursing care. Using this approach, we believe that nurses will be able to provide culturally competent and contextually meaningful care for clients from a wide variety of cultural backgrounds, rather than simply memorizing the esoteric health beliefs and practices of any specific cultural group. Culturally competent nurses must acquire the skills needed to assess clients from virtually any and all groups they encounter throughout their professional life and to provide culturally competent and contextually meaningful care for clients—individuals, groups, families, communities, and institutions.

Many educational programs in nursing are now teaching transcultural nursing content across the curriculum. We suggest that *Transcultural Concepts in Nursing Care* be used by faculty members to integrate transcultural content across the curriculum in the following manner:

- Chapters 1, 2, 3, and 4 should be used in the first clinical courses when students are learning how to conduct health histories, health assessments, and physical examinations.
- Chapters 5, 6, 7, and 8 include nursing care across the lifespan and are particularly useful in courses that focus on the nursing care of:
  o The childbearing family
  o Children
  o Adults and older adults

- Chapter 9 examines approaches for creating and maintaining culturally competent healthcare organizations, including the need to understand and address population health. The chapter is useful in courses that focus on nursing leadership and management.
- Chapters 10 and Chapters 11 align with mental health nursing and family and community nursing in the appropriate specialty nursing courses. Chapter 11 also has new information about Emergency and Disaster Planning, for individuals and communities.
- Chapter 12 explores the interconnections between religion, culture, and nursing, including health-related beliefs and practices of selected religions.
- Chapter 13 focuses on competence in ethical decision-making and includes updates on ethical implications for population health.

New to the Ninth Edition

All content in this edition was reviewed and updated to capture the nature of the changing healthcare delivery system, new research studies and theoretical advances, emphasis on effective communication, teamwork and collaboration, and to explain how nurses and other healthcare providers can use culturally competent skills to improve the care of clients, families, groups, and communities. In writing the ninth edition, we have been impressed with the developments in the field of transcultural nursing and included appropriate current trends and issues. The Andrews/Boyle Transcultural Interprofessional Practice Model provides a contemporary framework for putting the client or patient first and expanding the traditional notion of those who should be included as members of the healthcare team. While credentialed healers such as nurses, physicians, pharmacists, social workers, interpreters, and therapists remain key to health, wellness, and healing, the team also includes others whom the clients or patients believe contribute to their care, such as folk, indigenous, spiritual, and religious healers. This expansion of the team membership requires openness by credentialed healers to those with different scopes of practices, health belief systems, and healing practices. Clients or patients should always be included as integral members of the healthcare team as their understanding, acceptance, and cooperation are essential to the delivery of culturally competent healthcare. Similarly, the conceptualization of family and/or significant other has expanded to include the needs of those with diverse sexual orientations and gender identities (LGBTQ+), reflecting changing norms in some cultures, societies, and nations. Lastly, the Andrews/Boyle TIP Practice Model includes service animals, pets, and other sentient beings that clients and patients find therapeutic and might request as part of their plan of care.

New Contributors

We welcome Dr. Patti Ludwig-Beymer as a contributing editor to the book. Dr. Ludwig-Beymer was part of the original group that conceptualized this book and has been a chapter contributor for all eight previous editions of *Transcultural Concepts in Nursing Care*. Dr. Ludwig-Beymer is a long-standing Transcultural Nursing Society colleague and friend from Purdue University Northwest College of Nursing in Hammond, Indiana, where she is currently Associate Professor and Coordinator of the Nurse Executive MSN Concentration. Dr. Ludwig-Beymer earned a diploma in nursing from Mercy Hospital School of Nursing, a BSN and MSEd from Duquesne University, and a PhD in nursing from University of Utah. Dr. Ludwig-Beymer has published in the areas of transcultural nursing, population health, and organizational culture and has a rich history in both clinical nursing roles and as a nursing educator.

We are pleased to welcome Dr. Julia Rogers, contributing author for the newly revised Chapter 3, Cultural Competence in the History and Physical Examination. Dr. Rogers received her associate and baccalaureate degrees in nursing from Purdue North Central and her MSN and Doctor of Nursing Practice degrees from Valparaiso University. She is a Family Nurse Practitioner and is an Associate Professor at Purdue University Northwest in Hammond, Indiana. Her research interests include pathophysiology, culture, 3D visualization for nursing education, and enculturation of new faculty. She has authored and presented on an array of topics for both nurse educators and nurse practitioners.

We are very pleased that Ms. Heather Bowers has joined us as the contributing author of Chapter 6, Transcultural Perspectives in the Nursing Care of Children. Ms. Bowers is a Clinical Assistant Professor at Purdue University Northwest College of Nursing, where her teaching focuses on pediatrics, community health, and drug dosage calculation. Ms. Bowers earned a BSN from Bethel College, her MSN from Indiana Wesleyan University, and is a PhD candidate at Liberty University. Her research interests include health and education disparities, nursing education, and nursing faculty satisfaction and retention. Ms. Bowers has an extensive clinical background providing care for marginalized pediatric populations, and she is passionate about health equity and social justice.

Drs. Mary Lou Fornehed, Katrina Strange, and Sandra Mixer are new chapter contributors and collaborated to write Chapter 8, Transcultural Perspectives in the Care of Older Adults. Dr. Fornehed is Associate Professor of Nursing at Tennessee Technological University, Cookeville, Tennessee, and graduated with a PhD and postmasters in nursing education in 2017 from the University of Tennessee, Knoxville, Tennessee. Her research focus has been palliative and end-of-life care within the older adult, adult, and pediatric populations. Dr. Fornehed is an Acute Care Nurse Practitioner and has been caring for adults and older adult patients with acute and chronic problems, for 26 years.

Dr. Strange recently earned her PhD in Nursing at the University of Tennessee, Knoxville, Tennessee, and recently began her position as an

Assistant Professor at the Duquesne University School of Nursing. Before becoming a nurse, Dr. Strange earned a BA in Cultural and Linguistic Anthropology at Vassar College and has served in the U.S. Peace Corps, AmeriCorps, and Nurse Corps. These service experiences inspired her interests in transcultural nursing and community health. Dr. Strange has practiced in federally qualified and nonprofit clinics, where she has provided care and advocacy for vulnerable populations experiencing health disparities. Her research interests include faith influences on the health of older adults and the improvement of community health nursing education.

Dr. Sandra J. Mixer is Associate Professor Emerita in the College of Nursing at the University of Tennessee, Knoxville, Tennessee, and is a longtime Transcultural Nursing Society (TCNS) colleague and collaborator, and has served in many leadership positions within the organization. She earned her PhD in nursing education/transcultural nursing cognate from the University of Northern Colorado. Dr. Mixer's scholarship uses the framework of culture care and academic–community–practice partnerships to improve the health of vulnerable populations, enhance quality of life, foster dignified death, and develop healthcare providers' cultural competency. Dr. Mixer has led interdisciplinary partnerships in urban and rural areas with faith and community leaders, residents, and practice partners. Her research has been supported by several grants, including a $2.6 million HRSA award to transform RN roles in community-based integrated primary care settings caring for underserved populations.

Finally, we welcome Dr. Linda Sue Hammonds, contributing author of Chapter 10, Transcultural Perspectives in Mental Health Nursing. Dr. Hammonds is an Associate Professor and Doctor of Nursing Practice Coordinator at the University of South Alabama. Dr. Hammonds earned a MSN and Family Nurse Practitioner from East Caroline University, and her DNP with a Psych Mental Health Nurse Practitioner from the University of South Alabama. Dr. Hammonds has published in the areas of adult and pediatric mental disorders, abuse and neglect of vulnerable populations, and multiple transcultural nursing topics.

Chapter Pedagogy

Learning Activities

All of the chapters include review questions and learning activities to promote critical thinking and improve clinical judgment. In addition, learning objectives and key terms are included at the beginning of each chapter to help readers understand the purpose and intent of the content.

Evidence-Based Practice Features

Current research studies related to the content of the chapter are presented as Evidence-Based Practice boxes. We have included a section in each box describing clinical implications of the research.

Case Studies

Case studies, when used, are based often on the authors' actual clinical experiences and research findings and are presented to make conceptual linkages to illustrate how concepts are applied in healthcare settings. Case studies are oriented to assist the reader to begin to develop cultural competence with selected cultures.

Text Organization

Part One: Foundations of Transcultural Nursing

This first section focuses on the foundational aspects of transcultural nursing. The development of transcultural nursing frameworks that include concepts from the natural and behavioral sciences is described as they apply to nursing practice. Because nursing perspectives are used to organize the content in *Transcultural Concepts in Nursing Care*, the reader will not find a chapter purporting to describe the nursing care of a specific cultural group. Instead, the nursing needs of culturally diverse groups are used to illustrate cultural concepts used in nursing practice. As the reader will learn throughout the text, distinct nursing care of diverse cultures is always based on the cultural assessment of the individual patient and their values, beliefs, and lifeways. Chapter 1 provides an overview of the theoretical foundations of transcultural nursing, and Chapter 2 introduces key concepts associated with cultural competence using the Andrews/Boyle Transcultural Interprofessional Practice Model as the organizing framework. In Chapter 3, we discuss the domains of cultural knowledge that are important in cultural assessment and describe how this cultural information can be incorporated into all aspects of care. Chapter 4 provides a summary of the major cultural belief systems embraced by people of the world with special emphasis on their health-related and culturally based values, attitudes, beliefs, and practices.

Part Two: Lifespan

Chapters 5, 6, 7, and 8 use a developmental framework to discuss transcultural concepts across the lifespan. The care of childbearing people and their families, children, adolescents, middle-aged adults, and older adults is examined, and information about cultural groups is used to illustrate common transcultural nursing issues, trends, and concerns. Chapter 7, "Transcultural Perspectives in the Nursing Care of Adults," is the collaborative effort of Drs. Boyle and Collins. Originally developed and written by Drs. Boyle and Baird, the ninth edition content has been updated with new references, new insights, and more contemporary examples.

Part Three: Healthcare Settings

In the third section of the text (Chapters 9, 10, and 11), we explore the components of cultural competence in mental health and in family and community healthcare settings, including emergency and disaster planning. We also examine cultural competence in healthcare organizations, cultural diversity in the healthcare workforce, and population health, three very critical and current topics of concern. The clinical application of concepts throughout this section uses situations commonly encountered by nurses and describes how transcultural nursing principles can be applied in diverse settings. The chapters in this section are intended to illustrate the application of transcultural nursing knowledge to nursing practice using the lens of *communities and organizations* rather than *individual patients and families*.

Part Four: Other Considerations in Culturally Competent Care

In the fourth section of the text, Chapters 12 and 13, we examine selected contemporary issues and challenges that face nursing and healthcare. In the updated and revised Chapter 12, we review major religious traditions of the United States, the changing demographic of religious beliefs in many parts of the world, and the interrelationships among religion, culture, and nursing. Recognizing the numerous moral and ethical challenges in contemporary healthcare as well as within transcultural nursing, Chapter 13 has added information regarding the ever-increasing perspective of population health and discusses cultural competence in ethical and moral dilemmas from a transcultural perspective.

Resources for Instructors

Tools to assist you with teaching your course are available upon adoption of this text on at https://thePoint.lww.com/Andrews9e.

- The **Test Generator** offers a bank of NCLEX-style questions to help you assess your students' understanding of the course material.
- **PowerPoint Presentations** provide an easy way for you to integrate the textbook with your students' classroom experience, either via slide shows or handouts.
- **Case Studies** bring the content to life through real-world situations with scenarios

that can be used in class activities or group assignments.

- **Assignments** and **Discussion Topics** help you enhance your lessons and assignments by structuring student learning and evaluating understanding.

Resources for Students

An exciting set of resources is available on to help students review material and become even more familiar with vital concepts. Students can access all these resources at https://thePoint.lww.com/Andrews9e using the codes printed in the front of their text.

- **Online Student Review Questions** help students master important concepts and practice for exams.
- **Journal Articles** corresponding to book chapters offer access to current research available in Wolters Kluwer journals.

Lippincott® CoursePoint

The same trusted solution, innovation, and unmatched support that you have come to expect from *Lippincott CoursePoint* is now enhanced with more engaging learning tools and deeper analytics to help prepare students for practice. This powerfully integrated, digital learning solution combines learning tools, real-time data, and the most trusted nursing education content on the market to make curriculum-wide learning more efficient and to meet students where they're at in their learning. And now, it's easier than ever for instructors and students to use, giving them everything they need for course and curriculum success!

Lippincott CoursePoint includes the following:

- Engaging course content provides a variety of learning tools to engage students of all learning styles.
- Interactive learning activities help students learn the critical thinking and clinical judgment skills needed to help them become practice-ready nurses.

- Unparalleled reporting provides in-depth dashboards with several data points to track student progress and help identify strengths and weaknesses.
- Unmatched support includes training coaches, product trainers, and nursing education consultants to help educators and students implement CoursePoint with ease.

Building Clinical Judgment Skills

Nursing students are required to obtain nursing knowledge and apply foundational nursing processes to practice effective clinical judgment. Being able to apply clinical judgment in practice is critical for patient safety and optimizing outcomes. The content provided in this text includes features, such as Case Studies, Evidence-Based Practice Boxes, Critical Thinking Activities, and Review Questions, that strengthen students' clinical judgment skills by giving them opportunities to apply knowledge and practice critical thinking. Additionally, accompanying products CoursePoint and Lippincott NCLEX-RN PassPoint provide an adaptive experience that allows students to build confidence by answering questions like those found on the Next Generation NCLEX (NGN) examination.

Inclusive Language

A note about the language used in this book: Wolters Kluwer recognizes that people have a diverse range of identities, and we are committed to using inclusive and nonbiased language in our content. In line with the principles of nursing, we strive not to define people by their diagnoses, but to recognize their personhood first and foremost, using as much as possible the language diverse groups use to define themselves, and including only information that is relevant to nursing care.

We strive to better address the unique perspectives, complex challenges, and lived experiences of diverse populations traditionally underrepresented in health literature. When describing or referencing populations discussed in research studies, we will adhere to the identities presented in those studies to maintain fidelity to the evidence presented by the study investigators. We follow best practices of language set forth by the *Publication Manual of the American Psychological Association*, seventh edition, but acknowledge that language evolves rapidly, and we will update the language used in future editions of this book as necessary.

Acknowledgments

We are very pleased to acknowledge the support and good wishes of our friends, families, and colleagues in making the ninth edition of *Transcultural Concepts in Nursing Care* possible. It has been a long journey since several of us sat around a conference table as doctoral students and decided to publish a textbook about transcultural nursing. We appreciate the help of many nursing faculty members, practitioners, and our students who have offered helpful comments and suggestions. It has been very gratifying to call on new colleagues for help and advice in this addition, including writing new or different chapters for us. We want to acknowledge our colleague and dear friend, Dr. Margaret M. Andrews, who, although not actively involved in this edition, was happy to provide advice and counsel from afar.

We would like to gratefully acknowledge and thank Phoebe Jordan-Reilly, Developmental Editor at Wolters Kluwer, for her insightful, constructive, and helpful recommendations. We are most appreciative of the time she spent reviewing and re-reviewing the chapters and appendices. We also thank Susan Hartman, Senior Editor at Wolters Kluwer for her professionalism and interest and help throughout this project. There were numerous others at Wolters Kluwer who were very active behind the scenes and helped to bring this text to publication. We thank all of them.

We deeply appreciate all of friends and professional colleagues who wrote encouraging e-mails and texts, or phoned to express their interest and encouragement. We thank those members of the Transcultural Nursing Society who came to our discussion sessions at the annual conferences to tell us how they used our textbook and expressed interest and encouragement. We thank those many unknown colleagues who purchased and used our book. We especially thank our students over the years, several of whom have participated in the various editions of this textbook.

With this ninth edition, we are pleased to acknowledge our chapter authors who have been an integral part of this project. The profession and practice of nursing is changing rapidly, and we appreciate their professional expertise and clinical skills. We believe that transcultural nursing—nursing care that is culturally competent and consistent with the cultural beliefs and practices of clients from diverse backgrounds—will provide the knowledge and clinical skills to meet the healthcare challenges of the future.

Joyceen S. Boyle, PhD, RN, FTNSS, FAAN
John W. Collins, PhD, RN, FTNSS
Patti Ludwig-Beymer, PhD, RN, FTNSS, FAAN
Margaret M. Andrews, PhD, RN, FTNSS, FAAN

Contents

PART THREE Healthcare Systems 223

PART FOUR Other Considerations in Culturally Competent Care 307

Foundations
of Transcultural Nursing

Theoretical Foundations of Transcultural Nursing

Chapter 1

• Margaret M. Andrews and Joyceen S. Boyle

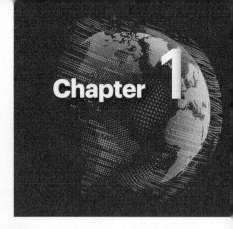

Key Terms

Anthropology
Assessment
Assumptions
Chronemics
Communication
Core Curriculum
Cross-cultural communication
Cultural competence
Cultural context
Culture-specific
Culture-universal
Culturally congruent nursing
  care

Culture
Ethnicity
Ethnonursing research
Evaluation
Evidence-based practice
Hijab
Implementation
Interprofessional collaboration
Interprofessional healthcare
  team
Language
Modesty
Monochronic culture
Mutual goal setting
Nonverbal communication

Paralanguage
Personal space
Planning
Polychronic culture
Problem-solving process
Proxemics
Race
Subculture
Transcultural Interprofessional
  Practice (TIP) Model
Transcultural nursing
Transcultural nursing
  certification
Verbal communication

Learning Objectives

1. Explore the historical and theoretical foundations of transcultural nursing.
2. Critically examine the relevance of transcultural nursing in addressing contemporary issues and trends in nursing.
3. Analyze Madeleine Leininger's contributions to the creation and development of transcultural nursing as a theory- and evidence-based formal area of study and practice within the nursing profession.
4. Critically examine the contributions of selected transcultural scholars to the advancement of transcultural nursing theory and practice.
5. Discuss key components of the Andrews/Boyle Transcultural Interprofessional Practice (TIP) Model.

Introduction

In her classic, groundbreaking book titled *Nursing and Anthropology: Two Worlds to Blend*, Leininger (1970) analyzed the ways in which the fields of anthropology and nursing are interwoven and interconnected (cf. Brink, 1976; McKenna, 1985). Leininger used the term **transcultural nursing** (TCN) to describe the blending of nursing and anthropology into an area of specialization within the discipline of nursing. Using the concepts of culture and care, Leininger established TCN as a theory- and evidence-based formal area of study and practice within nursing that focuses on people's culturally based beliefs, attitudes, values, behaviors, and practices related to health, illness, healing, and human caring (Leininger, 1991, 1995; Leininger & McFarland, 2002, 2006; McFarland & Wehbe-Alamah, 2016a, 2018).

TCN is sometimes used interchangeably with cross-cultural, intercultural, and multicultural nursing. The goal of TCN is to develop a scientific and humanistic body of knowledge to provide culture-specific and culture-universal nursing care practices for individuals, families, groups, communities, and institutions of similar and diverse cultures. **Culture-specific** refers to particular values, beliefs, and patterns of behavior that tend to be special or unique to a group and that do not tend to be shared with members of other cultures. **Culture-universal** refers to the commonly shared values, norms of behavior, and life patterns that are similarly held among cultures about human behavior and lifestyles (Leininger, 1978, 1991, 1995; Leininger & McFarland, 2002, 2006; McFarland & Wehbe-Alamah, 2016a, 2018). For example, although the need for food is a culture-universal, there are culture-specifics that determine what items are considered to be edible; methods used to prepare and eat meals; rules concerning who eats with whom, the frequency of meals, and gender- and age-related rules governing who eats first and last at mealtime; and the amount of food that individuals are expected to consume.

Given that culture is the central focus of anthropology and TCN, we begin this chapter by introducing, defining, and describing the concept of culture. We'll then discuss the historical and theoretical foundations of TCN, including its relevance in contemporary nursing practice and the significant contributions of Leininger and other TCN scholars, leaders, and clinicians to the global advancement of TCN research, theory, education, and clinical practice. In the remainder of the chapter, we examine the Andrews/Boyle Transcultural Interprofessional Practice (TIP) Model as a framework for delivering client-centered, high-quality nursing and healthcare that are culturally congruent and competent, safe, affordable, and accessible to people from diverse backgrounds across the lifespan. The term client is used throughout the book because nursing concerns not only the care of people who are ill but also those who strive for optimum health and wellness in their lives.

Anthropology and Culture

To understand the history and foundations of TCN, we begin by providing a brief overview of **anthropology**, an academic discipline that is concerned with the scientific study of humans, past and present. Anthropology builds on knowledge from the physical, biologic, and social sciences as well as the humanities. A central concern of anthropologists is the application of knowledge to the solution of human problems. Historically, anthropologists have focused their education on one of four areas: sociocultural anthropology, biologic/physical anthropology, archaeology, and linguistics. Anthropologists often integrate the perspectives of several of these areas into their research, teaching, and professional lives (American Anthropological Association, 2018; Council on Nursing and Anthropology, 2018). One of the central concepts that anthropologists study is **culture**. A complicated, multifaceted concept, culture has literally hundreds of definitions. The earliest recorded definition comes from a 19th-century British pioneer in the field of anthropology named Edward Tylor, who defined culture as the complex whole that includes knowledge, beliefs, art, morals, law, customs, and any other capabilities and habits acquired by members of a society (Tylor, 1871). Influenced by her formal academic preparation in anthropology, Leininger defines culture as the "learned, shared, and transmitted values, beliefs, norms, and lifeways of a particular group of people that guide thinking, decisions, and actions in a patterned way.... Culture is the blueprint that provides the broadest and most comprehensive means to know, explain, and predict people's lifeways over time and in different geographic locations" (McFarland & Wehbe-Alamah, 2016a, p. 10).

Culture influences a person's definition of health and illness, including when it is appropriate to self-treat and when the illness is sufficiently serious to seek assistance from one or more healers outside of the immediate family. The choice of healer and length of time a person is allowed to recover, after the birth of a baby or following the onset of an illness, are culturally determined. How a person behaves during an illness and the help rendered by others in facilitating healing also are culturally determined. Culture determines who is permitted, or expected, to care for someone who is ill. Similarly, culture determines when a person is declared well and when they are healthy enough to resume activities of daily living and/or return to work. When someone is dying, culture often determines where, how, and with whom the person will spend their final hours, days, or weeks. Although the term culture sometimes connotes a person's racial or ethnic background, there are also many other examples of *nonethnic cultures*, such as those based on *socioeconomic status*, for example, the culture of poverty or affluence and the culture of people experiencing homelessness; *ability or disability*, such as the culture of those who are deaf or hard-of-hearing and the culture of those who are blind or visually impaired; *sexual orientation and gender identity*, such as the lesbian, gay, bisexual, transgender, and queer (LGBTQ) cultures; *age*, such as the culture of adolescence and the culture of older adults; and *occupational* or *professional* cultures, such as nursing (see Fig. 1-1), medicine, and other professions in

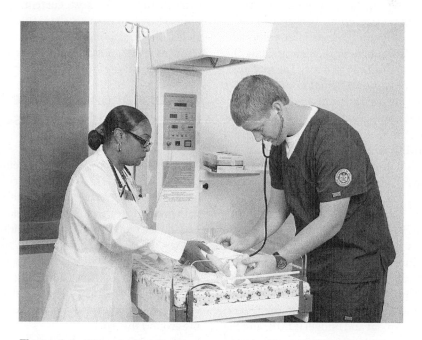

Figure 1-1. The profession of nursing is an example of a nonethnic occupational culture. The faculty member on the left is transmitting the requisite knowledge and skills from one generation to the next by mentoring the nursing student on the right.

healthcare, the military, business, education, and related fields.

In a classic study of culture by the anthropologist Edward Hall (1984), three levels of culture are identified: primary, secondary, and tertiary. The *primary level* of culture refers to the implicit rules known and followed by members of the group, but seldom stated or made explicit, to outsiders. The *secondary level* refers to underlying rules and **assumptions** that are known to members of the group but rarely shared with outsiders. The primary and secondary levels are the most deeply rooted and most difficult to change. The *tertiary level* refers to the explicit or public face that is visible to outsiders, including dress, rituals, cuisine, and festivals.

The term **subculture** refers to groups that have values and norms that are distinct from those held by the majority within a wider society. Members of subcultures have their own unique shared set of customs, attitudes, and values, often accompanied by group-specific language, jargon, and/or slang that sets them apart from others. A subculture can be organized around a common activity, occupation, age, ethnic background, race, religion, or any other unifying social condition. In the United States, subcultures might include the various racial and ethnic groups. For example, Hispanic is a *panethnic* designation that includes many subcultures consisting of people who self-identify with Mexican, Cuban, Puerto Rican, and/ or other groups that often share Spanish language and culture (Morris, 2015).

Ethnicity is defined as the perception of oneself and a sense of belonging to a particular ethnic group or groups. It can also mean a feeling that one does not belong to any group because of multiethnicity. Ethnicity is not equivalent to race, which is a biologic identification. Rather, ethnicity includes commitment to and involvement in cultural customs and rituals (Douglas et al., 2018). In the United States, ethnicity and race are defined and numbers tracked by the federal Office of Management and Budget (OMB) and the U.S. Census Bureau; they provide standardized categories, which are used in the collection of census information on racial and ethnic populations and are also often used by biomedical researchers. The following ethnic and racial categories were used to collect data in the 2020 census: White, Black or African American, American Indian or Alaska Native, Asian, Native Hawaiian or other Pacific Island, or some other race (U.S. Census Bureau, 2021). The Census Bureau also classifies Americans as "Hispanic or Latino" and "not Hispanic or Latino," which identifies Hispanic and Latino Americans as a racially diverse *ethnicity* (U.S. Census Bureau, 2021).

In the traditional anthropologic and biologic systems of classification, **race** refers to a group of people who share genetically transmitted traits such as skin color, hair texture, and eye shape or color. Races are arbitrary classifications that lack definitional clarity because all cultures have their own ways of categorizing or classifying their members. (Some define race as a geographically and genetically distinct population, whereas others suggest that racial categories are socially constructed.) The most current scientific data indicate that all humans share the same 99.9% of genes; the remaining 0.1% accounts for the differences in humans (National Human Genome Research Institute, 2022).

Historical and Theoretical Foundations of Transcultural Nursing

More than 70 years ago, Madeleine Leininger (1925–2012; see Fig. 1-2) noted cultural differences between nurses and families of children with mental health needs. This clinical nursing experience piqued her interest in cultural anthropology. As a doctoral student in anthropology, she conducted field research on the care practices of people in Papua New Guinea and subsequently studied cultural similarities and differences in the culture care perceptions and expressions of people around the world.

At the same time that Leininger (Leininger, 1978, 1991, 1995, 1997, 1999; Leininger &

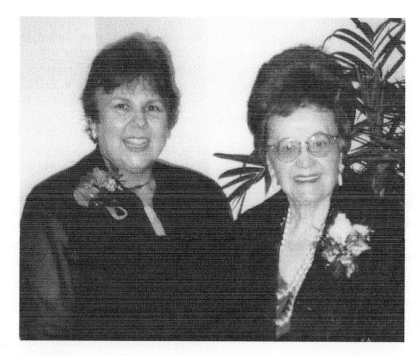

Figure 1-2. Author, Dr. Margaret M. Andrews (*left*), and Transcultural Nursing Foundress, Dr. Madeleine Leininger (*right*), at a meeting of the American Academy of Nursing.

McFarland, 2002, 2006; McFarland & Wehbe-Alamah, 2016a, 2018) was establishing TCN, other anthropologists, nurse–anthropologists, and nurses who were studying, teaching, and writing about ethnicity, race, diversity, and/ or culture in nursing used terms such as cross-cultural nursing, *ethnic nursing care* (Orque et al., 1983), or referred to *caring for people of color* (Branch & Paxton, 1976). The term *transcultural nursing* is used in this book, in recognition of the historical, research, and theoretical contributions of Leininger (1978), who used this term in her research and other scholarly works.

Leininger cites eight factors that influenced her to establish TCN as a framework for addressing 20th-century societal and healthcare challenges and issues, all of which remain relevant today:

1. A marked increase in the migration of people within and between countries worldwide

2. A rise in multicultural identities, with people expecting their cultural beliefs, values, and ways of life to be understood and respected by nurses and other healthcare providers

3. An increase in healthcare providers' and patients' use of technologies that connect people globally and simultaneously may become the source of conflict with the cultural values, beliefs, and practices of some of the people receiving care

4. Global cultural conflicts, clashes, and violence that impact healthcare as more cultures interact with one another

5. An increase in the number of people traveling and working in different parts of the world

6. An increase in legal actions resulting from cultural conflict, negligence, ignorance, and the imposition of healthcare practices

7. A rise in awareness of gender issues, with growing demands on healthcare systems to meet the gender- and age-specific needs of adults and children

8. An increased demand for community- and culturally based healthcare services in diverse environmental contexts (Leininger, 1995; McFarland & Wehbe-Alamah, 2018)

TCN exists today as an evidence-based, dynamic area of specialization within the nursing profession because of the visionary leadership of its founder, Madeleine Leininger, and many other nurses committed to the provision of care that is consistent with and "fits" the cultural beliefs and practices of those receiving it. The following section explores the contributions of Leininger and then examines the ways in which other nursing scholars contributed to the development and advancement of TCN theory, research, practice, education, and administration globally.

Leininger's Contributions to Transcultural Nursing

Leininger's Theory of Culture Care Diversity and Universality describes, explains, and predicts nursing similarities and differences in care and caring in human cultures (Leininger, 1991; McFarland & Wehbe-Alamah, 2016a, 2016b, 2018). Leininger uses concepts such as worldview, social and cultural structure, language, ethnohistory, environmental context, and folk and professional healing systems to provide a comprehensive and holistic view of factors that influence culture care. Culturally based care factors are recognized as major influences on human experiences related to well-being, health, illness, disability, and death. After conducting a comprehensive cultural assessment based on the preceding factors, the three modes of nursing decisions and actions—culture care preservation and/or maintenance, culture care accommodation and/or negotiation, and culture care repatterning and/or restructuring—are

used to provide culturally congruent nursing care (Leininger, 1991, 1995; Leininger & McFarland, 2002, 2006; McFarland & Wehbe-Alamah, 2018). **Culturally congruent nursing care** "refers to those cognitively based assistive, supportive, facilitative, or enabling acts or decisions that are mostly tailor-made to fit with an individual's, group's or institution's cultural values, beliefs, and lifeways in order to provide meaningful, beneficial, satisfying care that leads to health and well-being" (Leininger, 1991, p. 47). Cultural congruence is central to Leininger's Theory of Culture Care Diversity and Universality.

Among the strengths of Leininger's theory is its flexibility for use with individuals, families, groups, communities, and institutions in diverse health systems. To help develop, test, and organize the emerging body of knowledge in TCN, Leininger recognized that it would be necessary to have a specific conceptual framework from which various theoretical statements are developed. Figure 1-3 depicts components of the Theory of Culture Care Diversity and Universality, provides a visual representation of the components of Leininger's Sunrise Enabler to Discover Culture Care, and illustrates the interrelationships among the components. As the world of nursing and healthcare has become increasingly multicultural, the theory's relevance has increased as well.

While creating TCN as a respected and recognized nursing specialty and developing her theory, Leininger also had the foresight to establish the Transcultural Nursing Society (TCNS), generate the *TCNS Newsletter*, and create the *Journal of Transcultural Nursing* (JTN), for which she served as the founding editor. The TCNS holds regional and annual conferences, disseminates the newsletter, and collaborates with Sage Publishing to produce six issues per year of the *Journal of Transcultural Nursing*, all of which provide forums for the exchange of TCN knowledge, research, and evidence-based best practices relative to the provision of culturally congruent and culturally competent nursing and healthcare. To integrate TCN into

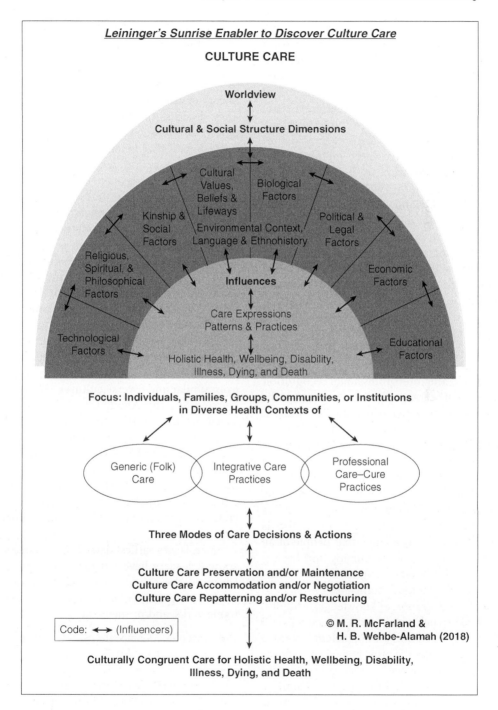

Figure 1-3. Leininger's Sunrise Enabler to Discover Culture Care. (Source: Used with permission McFarland, M. R. & Wehbe-Alamah, H. B. (2018). *Transcultural nursing concepts, theories, research, & practice* (4th ed.). McGraw-Hill Education. ISBN: 978-0-07-184113-9.)

the curricula of schools of nursing, Leininger established the first master's and doctoral programs in nursing with a theoretical and research focus in TCN and provided exemplars for TCN courses and curricula suitable for all levels of nursing education (undergraduate and graduate) through her lectures, publications, and consultations. Leininger also created a new qualitative research method called **ethnonursing research** to investigate phenomena of interest in TCN (Leininger, 1995; Leininger & McFarland, 2002, 2006; McFarland et al., 2012; McFarland & Wehbe-Alamah, 2016a, 2018). Hundreds of studies have been conducted using ethnonursing research, which is the first research methodology developed by a nurse for use in studying topics relevant to nursing. Ray and colleagues studied caring, complexity science, and transcultural caring dynamics in nursing and healthcare (Davidson et al., 2011; Ray, 2016; Ray & Turkel, 2014). Leininger's contributions to TCN rapidly gained global and interprofessional recognition as many healthcare professionals from medicine, physical therapy, occupational therapy, social work, and related disciplines learned about the Theory of Culture Care Diversity and Universality and either adopted or adapted it to fit their respective disciplines.

As nursing and healthcare have become increasingly multicultural and diverse, TCN's relevance has increased as well. There also is heightened societal awareness that people of all cultures deserve to receive nursing and healthcare that are culturally congruent and culturally competent. **Cultural competence** refers to the complex integration of knowledge, attitudes, values, beliefs, behaviors, skills, practices, and cross-cultural encounters that include effective communication and the provision of safe, affordable, quality, accessible, evidence-based, and efficacious nursing care for individuals, families, groups, and communities of diverse and similar cultural backgrounds. Cultural competence is discussed in detail in Chapter 2.

Advancements in Transcultural Nursing

McFarland and Wehbe-Alamah (2019) have provided a historical perspective of Leininger's Theory of Culture Care Diversity and Universality. They describe the theory's purpose, the goals, tenets, assumptions, and major core constructs. They suggest that Leininger's work will be used to guide future research for evidence-based nursing practice, develop nursing courses and curricula to prepare culturally competent nurses, and inform public policy regarding social justice and health equity. The mandate of transcultural nursing is to support equitable and accessible transculturally based healthcare worldwide.

In addition to Leininger, many other TCN scholars and leaders around the world have made, and continue to make, significant contributions to the body of transcultural knowledge, research, theory, and **evidence-based practices** that guide nurses in the delivery of culturally congruent and culturally competent care for people from similar and diverse cultures (Transcultural Nursing Society: About Us, 2022b). Evidence-based practice in TCN refers to a process that quickly incorporates best research practices into clinical practice. While the authors of this textbook have chosen to emphasize the research and theory generated by Leininger, there are many different ways to conceptualize TCN and deliver culturally congruent and culturally competent nursing care.

Since TCN's earliest days, TCN nursing scholars and leaders have enhanced, expanded, and advanced the specialty through their research, teaching, publications, conceptual models, frameworks, and/or theories:

- Josepha Campinha-Bacote (Campinha-Bacote, 2011, 2015)
- Marilyn Douglas, Dula Pacquiao, and Larry Purnell (Douglas et al., 2018)
- Geri-Ann Galanti (Galanti, 2014)
- Joyce Newman Giger (Giger, 2017)
- Marianne Jeffreys (Jeffreys, 2016)

- Larry Purnell (Purnell, 2013, 2014; Purnell & Fenkl, 2018)
- Marilyn Ray (Ray, 2016; Ray & Turkel, 2014)
- Priscilla Sagar (Sagar, 2012, 2014)
- Rachel Spector (Spector, 2017)

The Core Curriculum

In collaboration with a group of other TCN scholars and experts globally, the editor and associate editor of the JTN published the **Core Curriculum** in Transcultural Nursing and Health Care to "establish a core base of knowledge that supports TCN practice" (Douglas & Pacquiao, 2010, p. S5). The Core Curriculum marks the culmination of many years of research and theory development in TCN and draws on knowledge and research from the natural, social, and behavioral sciences; philosophy, theology, and religious studies; history; the fine arts; and applied or professional disciplines such as medicine, social work, education, and other fields. The Core Curriculum clearly identifies, delineates, and authoritatively establishes the core of knowledge that supports TCN practice.

The Core Curriculum includes the following:

- Contributions by many of the foremost experts in TCN from around the world who provide concrete and specific curricular outline for TCN.
- A comprehensive compendium that contains an overview of the key knowledge, research, evidence, and general content areas that collectively form the foundation for TCN practice.
- Content on subjects such as global health; comparative systems of healthcare delivery; cross-cultural communication; culturally based health and illness beliefs and practices across the lifespan; culturally based healing and care modalities; cultural health assessment; educational issues for students, organizational staff, patients, and communities; organizational cultural competency; research methodologies for investigating

cultural phenomena and evaluating interventions; and professional roles and attributes of the transcultural nurse.

- Content that will prepare nurses to take one or both of the examinations leading to **transcultural nursing certification**: basic certification in transcultural nursing (CTN-B) and advanced certification in transcultural nursing (CTN-A). Both exams are offered by the TCNS's Certification Commission (Transcultural Nursing Society, 2022a) and appear on the list of Magnet national certifications for inclusion on the Demographic Data Collection Tool. See Sagar (2015) for additional information about certification in TCN and/or visit the Transcultural Nursing Society website for an application (TCNS, 2022a).

The Core Curriculum also is used in colleges of nursing, hospitals, health departments, and other healthcare organizations to determine the key content to be included in seminars, workshops, conferences, and credit-bearing and continuing professional development courses on TCN and cultural competency. Those interested in cultural competence, multiculturalism, diversity, and related topics from multiple disciplines will also find valuable information in the Core Curriculum. As scientific, technological, and discipline-specific advances are made in TCN, the Core Curriculum will be updated and refined.

The coauthors of this book contributed to the Core Curriculum, as did many of the chapter contributors; therefore, the key concepts contained in the Core Curriculum also are found in this book.

Andrews/Boyle Transcultural Interprofessional Practice Model

Conceptual frameworks, theoretical models, and theories in nursing are structured ideas about human beings and their health. Models enable nurses and other healthcare team members to organize and understand what happens in practice, critically analyze situations for clinical decision-making, develop a plan of care, propose appropriate nursing interventions, predict the outcomes from the care, and evaluate the effectiveness of the care provided (Alligood, 2014). Fawcett (2016) stated that a conceptual model is the starting point and serves as a guide for all nursing activities.

Goals, Assumptions, and Components of the Model

The goals of the Andrews/Boyle **Transcultural Interprofessional Practice (TIP) Model** are to:

- Provide a systematic, logical, orderly, scientific process for delivering culturally congruent, culturally competent, safe, affordable, accessible, and quality care to people from diverse backgrounds across the lifespan.
- Facilitate the delivery of nursing and healthcare that is beneficial, meaningful, relevant, culturally congruent, culturally competent, and consistent with the cultural beliefs and practices of clients from diverse backgrounds.
- Provide a conceptual framework to guide nurses in the delivery of culturally congruent and competent care that is theoretically sound, is evidence-based, and utilizes best professional practices.

Fundamental assumptions underlying the TIP Model include those related to TCN (Box 1-1), humans (Box 1-2), and **cross-cultural communication** between and among team members (Box 1-3). These assumptions are ideas that are formed or taken for granted as having veracity without proof or evidence. Assumptions are useful in providing a basis for action and in creating "what-if..." scenarios to simulate possible situations until such time as there is proof or evidence available to corroborate or refute the assumption.

The TIP Model consists of the following interconnected and interrelated components:

1. The context from which people's health-related values, attitudes, beliefs, and practices emerge
2. The interprofessional healthcare team
3. Communication
4. The problem-solving process

Cultural Context

Derived from the Latin word *contexere* (*con-* meaning together and *texere* meaning to weave or braid), the term context refers to the conditions, circumstances, and/or situations that exist when and where something happens, thereby providing meaning to what transpired. In the TIP Model, the following factors contribute to the **cultural context** of human experiences and need to be assessed, interpreted, examined, and evaluated when clients interact with nurses and other members of the interprofessional healthcare team: environmental, social, economic, religious, philosophical, moral, legal, political, educational, biologic (genetic/inherited factors), and technological. In TCN, culture is the lens through which nurses see the world, their clients, and other members of the team. When culture is interwoven with the other factors (see Fig. 1-4), it forms the health-related cultural values, attitudes, beliefs, and practices of humans worldwide, including clients and other members of the team.

Interprofessional Healthcare Team

The transcultural **interprofessional healthcare team** has at its core the *client*, who is the team's raison d'être (reason for being). In addition to the client, the team may have one or more of the following members:

- The *clients' families* and *others significant in their lives*, including a legally appointed *guardian* who might not be genetically related

BOX 1-1   Assumptions About Transcultural Nursing

- Transcultural nursing is a theoretical and evidence-based formal area of study and practice within professional nursing that focuses on people's culturally based beliefs, attitudes, values, behaviors, and practices related to wellness, health, birth, illness, healing, dying, and death.
- Transcultural nursing requires that nurses engage in an ongoing process of constructively critical, reflective self-assessment that enables them to identify their own culturally based values, attitudes, beliefs, behaviors, biases, stereotypes, prejudices, and practices.
- Transcultural nursing knowledge is interconnected with the knowledge, research, and scholarship of other disciplines in the natural sciences (e.g., biology, chemistry, physics), social and behavioral sciences (e.g., anthropology, sociology, psychology, economics, political science), professional disciplines (e.g., medicine, pharmacy, social work, education), and the humanities (e.g., music, art, history, languages, philosophy, theater).
- Transcultural nursing practice encompasses autonomous and collaborative care of individuals of all ages across the lifespan regardless of health status, condition, or ability.
- Transcultural nursing engages nurses in the care of families, groups, populations, and communities globally.
- Transcultural nursing includes the promotion of health, the prevention of disease, and the care of people who are sick, ill, disabled, and dying from diverse cultures across the lifespan from birth to old age.
- Transcultural nursing roles include advocacy, research, health policy development, health systems leadership, management, education, clinical practice, and consultation.

- Transcultural nursing practice requires that nurses establish and maintain a caring, empathetic, therapeutic relationship with clients and a collaborative, collegial relationship with other members of the interprofessional healthcare team.
- Transcultural nursing assessment is facilitated when the nurse's communications are client-centered and focused on establishing and maintaining a therapeutic nurse–client relationship.
- Transcultural nursing practice requires that nurses be aware of changes in the world that influence and challenge their knowledge of the unfolding meaning of diversity and the need for the delivery of nursing and healthcare that is respectful and responsive to individual needs and differences of the people and communities served.
- Transcultural nursing practice encompasses autonomous and collaborative care of individuals of all ages, families, groups, and communities, sick or well and in all settings.
- Transcultural nursing practice requires that nurses establish and maintain a caring, empathetic, therapeutic relationship with clients; formally educated and/or licensed credentialed healers, such as registered nurses, licensed physicians, and other health professionals; and folk, traditional, religious, spiritual, and other healers who are identified by clients as significant to their health and well-being.
- In transcultural nursing practice, the nurse's communications are oriented and focused on what is best for the client's health, well-being, recovery, or peaceful death.
- Transcultural nursing practice requires that nurses be respectful and responsive to individual needs and differences of the people and communities served.

BOX 1-2   Assumptions About Humans

- Humans are complex biologic, cultural, psychosocial, spiritual beings who experience health and illness along a continuum throughout the span of their lives from birth to death.
- All humans have the right to safe, accessible, and affordable nursing and healthcare, regardless of national origin, race, ethnicity, gender, age, socioeconomic background, religion, sexual orientation, size, and related characteristics.
- Each person deserves to be respected by nurses and other members of the healthcare team, regardless of socioeconomic background, religion, gender, or race.
- As people from different racial, ethnic, and cultural backgrounds travel and comingle with those having backgrounds that differ from their own, the likelihood of intermarriage and offspring of mixed racial and ethnic heritage increases.
- Regardless of their national origin or current citizenship, humans around the world share culture-universal needs for food, shelter, safety, and love; seek well-being and health; and endeavor to avoid, alleviate, or eliminate the pain and suffering associated with disease, illness, dying, and death.
- Although humans have common culture-universal needs, they also have culture-specific needs that are interconnected with their health-related values, attitudes, beliefs, and practices.
- In times of health and illness, humans seek the therapeutic (beneficial) assistance of various types of healers to promote health and well-being, prevent disease, and recover from illness or injury.
- Humans seek therapeutic interventions from family and significant others; credentialed or licensed healthcare providers; folk, traditional, indigenous, religious, and/or spiritual healers; and companion or therapy animals and pets as they perceive appropriate for their condition, situation, or problem.
- Interventions are judged to have a therapeutic effect when they result in a desirable and beneficial outcome, whether the outcome was expected, unexpected, or even an unintended consequence of the intervention.

BOX 1-3   Assumptions About Effective Communication

- Effective communication begins with an assessment of the client's ability to read, write, speak, and comprehend messages.
- Effective communication in contemporary society sometimes requires literacy in the use of computers, smartphones, and numerous technology-assisted medical or health devices.
- Effective communication includes the ability to convey sincere interest in others, patience, and willingness to intervene or begin again when misunderstandings occur.
- To provide safe, quality, affordable, accessible, efficacious, culturally congruent, and culturally competent nursing and healthcare, members of the interprofessional healthcare team must communicate effectively.
- Communication occurs verbally, nonverbally, in writing, and in combination with technology.
- Communication should be appropriate for the client's age, gender, health status, health literacy, and related factors.
- When nurses communicate with others from cultural and linguistic backgrounds different from their own, the probability of miscommunication increases significantly.
- In promoting effective cross-cultural communication with clients from diverse backgrounds, nurses should avoid technical jargon, slang, colloquial expressions, abbreviations, and excessive use of medical terminology.

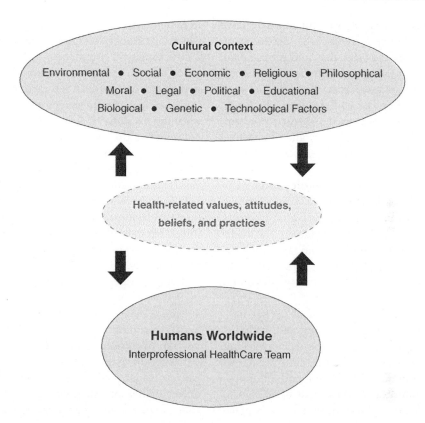

Figure 1-4. Influence of cultural context on health values, beliefs, and practices of the interprofessional healthcare team. (© Margaret M. Andrews.)

- *Credentialed health professionals* such as nurses; physicians; physical, occupational, respiratory, music, art, dance, recreational, and other therapists; social workers; health navigators; public and community health workers; and related professionals with formal academic preparation, licensure, and/or certification
- *Indigenous or traditional healers*—unlicensed individuals who learn healing arts and practices through study, observation, apprenticeship, and imitation and sometimes by inheriting healing powers, for example, herbalists, curanderos, medicine people, Amish brauchers, bonesetters, lay midwives, sabadors, and healers with related names
- *Religious or spiritual healers*—clergy or lay members of religious groups who heal through prayer, religious or spiritual rituals, faith healing practices, and related actions or interventions, for example, priests, priestesses, elders, rabbis, imams, monks, Christian Science practitioners, and others believed to have healing powers derived from faith, spiritual powers, or religion
- *Others* identified by clients as significant to their health, well-being, or healing such as companion animals or pets as culturally appropriate

The World Health Organization defines **interprofessional collaboration** as multiple health workers from different professional backgrounds working together with patients, families, caregivers, and communities to deliver the highest quality of care (World Health Organization, 2010).

In collaboration with leaders in nursing, dentistry, and other healthcare fields, the Institute of Medicine (2011) advocates that interprofessional collaboration be integrated into the curricula of health professions programs, building on recommendations from its earlier report, *To Err Is Human*, which focuses on the threat to patient safety caused by human error and ineffective interprofessional communication (Institute of Medicine, 1999).

To be successful in interprofessional collaboration, the following core competencies are required: values and ethics related to interprofessional practice, knowledge of the roles of team members, and a team approach to healthcare (Fulmer & Gaines, 2014; Institute of Medicine, 1999, 2011; Interprofessional Education Collaborative Expert Panel, 2011). Interprofessional collaboration is a partnership that starts with the client and includes all involved healthcare providers working together to deliver client- and family-centered care. Trust must be established, and an appreciation of each other's roles must be gained in order for effective collaboration to take place (Interprofessional Education Collaborative Expert Panel, 2016). Health professionals must recognize their own individual scope of practice and skill set and have an awareness of and appreciation for other health professionals' capacity to contribute to the delivery of care to clients in order to achieve optimal health outcomes. Working as a member of an interprofessional team requires communication, cooperation, and collaboration (Fulmer & Gaines, 2014; Institute of Medicine, 2011; Interprofessional Education Collaborative Expert Panel, 2011; Interprofessional Education Collaborative, 2016).

Communication

Derived from the Latin verb *communicare*, meaning to share, **communication** refers to the meaningful exchange of information between one or more participants. The information exchanged may be conveyed through ideas, feelings, intentions, attitudes, expectations, perceptions, instructions, or commands. Communication is an organized, patterned system of behavior that makes all nurse–client interactions possible. It is the exchange of messages and the creation of meaning (Munoz & Luckman, 2008). Because communication and culture are acquired simultaneously, they are integrally linked. Figure 1-5 illustrates the ways in which communication, cultural context, and health-related values, attitudes, beliefs, and practices of members of the interprofessional healthcare team are interconnected and interrelated. In effective communication, there is mutual understanding of the meaning attached to the messages.

Being respectful and polite, using language that is understood by other(s), and speaking clearly will facilitate verbal (or spoken) communication. Barriers to effective **verbal communication** occur when participants are using different languages; when technical terms, abbreviations, idioms, colloquialisms, or regional expressions are used; or when the tone of voice conveys a message that is inconsistent with the words spoken (e.g., a client in the postanesthesia care unit following major surgery verbally denies having pain, but the nurse observes that the client has clenched teeth, taut muscles, pursed lips, and a wrinkled brow, all of which are nonverbal indicators of pain). Whereas **language** refers to what is said, **paralanguage** refers to *how it is said* and relates to all aspects of the voice that are not part of the verbal message. Paralanguage may modify or nuance meaning or convey emotion through rhythm, pitch, stress, volume, speed, hesitations, or intonation. For example, consider the sentence, "I would like to help you." By placing emphasis on the words *I, like, help,* and *you* in four different sentences, the meaning of the sentence changes significantly. **Nonverbal communication** refers to how people convey meaning without words using facial expressions, gestures, posture (body language), and the physical distance between the communicators (proxemics).

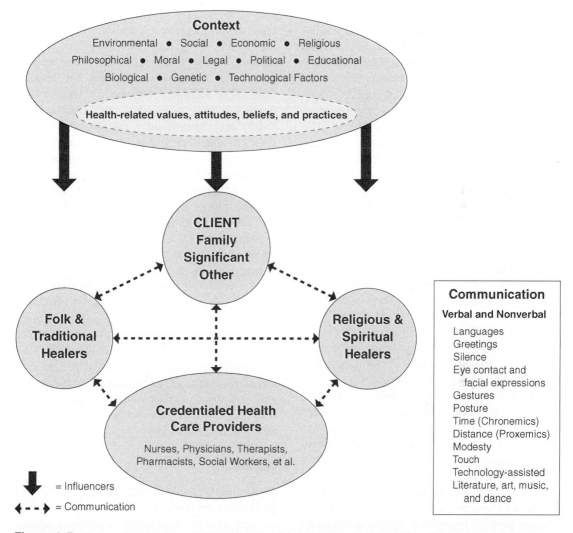

Figure 1-5. Cross-cultural communication among members of the interprofessional healthcare team—clients, family, significant others, credentialed health professionals, and traditional, religious, and spiritual healers. (© Margaret M. Andrews.)

The many nuances of verbal and nonverbal communication are interconnected, interwoven, interrelated, and often embedded in one another. Aspects of communication that are of particular importance for the transcultural nurse include language, the use of interpreters, greetings, silence, eye contact and facial expressions, gestures, posture, chronemics (time), proxemics, modesty, touch, technology-assisted communication, and literature, art, music, and dance.

Language

It is estimated that more than 7,000 languages are spoken throughout the world. Approximately 21.5% of persons living in the United States speak a language other than English at home, and 8.2% reported that they speak English "less than very well." Spanish is the second most commonly spoken language in the United States, spoken by 37 million people aged 5 years and older.

Nine percent of those individuals who speak Spanish indicated that they did not speak English at all. After English (230.9 million speakers) and Spanish (37.5 million), Chinese (2.8 million) was the language most spoken at home (U.S. Census Bureau, 2020). More than 350 languages are spoken in U.S. homes including languages such as Pennsylvania Dutch, Yiddish, and Navajo (U.S. Census Bureau, 2021). Language is one of the primary ways that culture is transmitted from one generation to the next.

Interpreters

One of the greatest challenges in cross-cultural communication for nurses occurs when the nurse and client speak different languages. After assessing the language skills of the client who speaks a different language from the nurse, the nurse may be in one of two situations: either struggling to communicate effectively through an interpreter or communicating effectively when there is no interpreter. Box 1-4 provides recommendations for overcoming language barriers.

Even a person from another culture or country who has a basic command of the language spoken by the majority of nurses and other health professionals may need an interpreter when faced with the anxiety-provoking situation of entering a hospital, encountering an unfamiliar symptom, or discussing a sensitive topic such as birth control or gynecologic or urologic concerns. A trained medical interpreter knows interpreting techniques, has knowledge of medical terminology, and understands patients' rights. The trained interpreter is also knowledgeable about cultural beliefs and health practices. This person can help bridge the cultural gap and can give advice concerning the cultural appropriateness of nursing and medical recommendations.

Although the nurse is in charge of the focus and flow of the interview, the interpreter should be viewed as an important member of the healthcare team. It can be tempting to ask a relative, a friend, or even another client to interpret because this person is readily available and likely is willing to help. However, this violates confidentiality for the client, who may not want personal information shared. Furthermore, the friend or relative, though fluent in ordinary language usage, is likely to be unfamiliar with medical terminology, hospital or clinic procedures, and healthcare ethics. In ideal circumstances, ask the interpreter to meet the client beforehand to establish rapport and obtain basic descriptive information about the client such as age, occupation, educational level, and attitude toward healthcare. This eases the interpreter and client into the relationship and allows clients to talk about aspects of their lives that are relatively nonthreatening.

When using an interpreter, expect that the interaction with the client will require more time than is needed if the nurse and client speak the same language. It will be necessary to organize nursing care so that the most important interactions or procedures are accomplished first before the client becomes fatigued. In the absence of an interpreter, try using electronic devices with translation software and other applications that may be helpful in effectively communicating and delivering care for people who speak a language different from the nurse.

Greetings

Some cultures value formal greetings at the start of the day or whenever the first encounter of the day occurs—a practice found even among close family members. When communicating with people from cultures that tend to be more formal, it is important to call a person by their title, such as Mr., Mrs., Ms., Dr., Reverend, and related greetings as a sign of respect, and until such time as the individual gives permission to address them less formally. The recommended best practice at the time the nurse initially meets a client or new member of the healthcare team is to state their own name and then ask the client or team member by what name they prefer to be called.

BOX 1-4   Overcoming Language Barriers

Using an Interpreter

- Before locating an interpreter, determine the language the client speaks at home; it may be different from the language spoken publicly (e.g., French is sometimes spoken by well-educated and high-income members of certain Asian or Middle Eastern cultures).
- After assessing client's health literacy, use electronic devices such as cell phones, tablets, and laptop computers to connect client with web-based translation programs.
- Avoid interpreters from a rival tribe, state, region, or nation.
- Be aware of gender differences between interpreter and client. In general, the same gender is preferred.
- Be aware of age differences between interpreter and client. In general, an older, more mature interpreter is preferred to a younger, less experienced one.
- Be aware of socioeconomic differences between interpreter and client.
- Ask the interpreter to translate as closely to verbatim as possible.
- Expect an interpreter who is not a relative to seek compensation for services rendered.

Recommendations for Institutions

- Keep pace with assistive equipment and technology for people who are deaf, hard-of-hearing, blind, visually impaired, and/or disabled.
- Maintain a computerized list of interpreters, including those certified in sign language, who may be contacted as needed.
- Network with area hospitals, colleges, universities, and other organizations that may serve as resources.

What to Do When There Is No Interpreter

- Be polite and formal.
- Greet the person using the last or complete name. Gesture to yourself and say your name. Offer a handshake or nod. Smile.

- Proceed in an unhurried manner. Pay attention to any effort by the patient or family to communicate.
- Speak in a low, moderate voice. Avoid talking loudly. There is often a tendency to raise the volume and pitch of one's voice when the listener appears not to understand, but this may lead the listener to perceive that the nurse is shouting and/or angry.
- Use any words known in the patient's language.
- Use simple words, such as *pain* instead of *discomfort*. Avoid medical jargon, idioms, and slang. Avoid using contractions. Use nouns repeatedly instead of pronouns. For example, do *not* say, "He has been taking his medicine, hasn't he?" Do say, "Does Juan take medicine?"
- Pantomime words and simple actions while verbalizing them.
- Give instructions in the proper sequence. For example, do *not* say, "Before you rinse the bottle, sterilize it." Do say, "First, wash the bottle. Second, rinse the bottle."
- Discuss one topic at a time. Avoid using conjunctions. For example, do *not* say, "Are you cold and in pain?" Do say, "Are you cold [while pantomiming]?" "Are you in pain?"
- Validate whether the client understands by having them repeat instructions, demonstrate the procedure, or act out the meaning.
- Write out several short sentences in English and determine the person's ability to read them.
- Try a third language. Many Southeast Asians speak French. Europeans often know three or four languages. Numerous Americans speak Spanish.
- Ask if a family member or friend of the same gender could serve as an interpreter.
- Use online translation program for the appropriate languages, contact hospitals for a list of interpreters, and use both formal and informal networking to locate a suitable interpreter.

Adapted from Andrews, M. (2000). Transcultural considerations in health assessment. In C. Jarvis (Ed.), *Physical examination and health assessment* (p. 69). W.B. Saunders.

Silence

Wide cultural variations exist in the interpretation of silence. Some individuals find silence extremely uncomfortable and make every effort to fill conversational lags with words. By contrast, many Native Americans consider silence essential to understanding and respecting the other person. A pause following a question signifies that what has been asked is important enough to be given thoughtful consideration. In traditional Chinese and Japanese cultures, silence may mean that the speaker wishes the listener to consider the content of what has been said before continuing. Other cultural meanings of silence may be found. Persons from Middle Eastern cultures may use silence out of respect for another's privacy, whereas people of French, Spanish, and Russian descent may interpret it as a sign of agreement. Japanese or Chinese cultures often use silence to demonstrate respect for elders. Among some African Americans, silence is used in response to a question perceived as inappropriate.

Eye Contact and Facial Expressions

Eye contact and facial expressions are the most prominent forms of nonverbal communication. Eye contact is a key factor in setting the tone of the communication between two people and differs greatly between cultures and countries. In American, Canadian, Western European, and Australian cultures, eye contact is interpreted similarly: conveying interest, active engagement with the other person, forthrightness, and honesty. People who avoid eye contact when speaking are viewed negatively and may be perceived as withholding information and/or lacking in confidence. In some Asian, African, and Middle Eastern cultures and in certain Native American nations, direct eye contact may be seen as disrespectful, a sign of aggression, or a sign that the other person's authority is being challenged. In some cultures, staring at someone for a prolonged period of time communicates that the person doing the staring has a sexual interest in the other person. People who make eye contact, but only briefly, are viewed as respectful and courteous. In some Native American cultures, the person might look at the floor while someone in a position of authority is speaking as a sign of respect and interest. Among some African American and White American cultures, *occulistics* (eye rolling) takes place when someone speaks or behaves in a manner that is regarded as inappropriate.

Strongly influenced by a person's cultural background, facial expressions include *affective displays* that reveal emotions, such as happiness through a smile or sadness through crying, and various other nonverbal gestures that may be perceived as appropriate or inappropriate according to the person's age and gender. These nonverbal expressions are often unintentional and can conflict with what is being said verbally.

Gestures

Gestures that serve the same function as words are referred to as *emblems.* Examples of emblems include signals that mean okay, the "thumbs-up" gesture, the "come here" hand movement, or the hand gesture used when hitchhiking. Gestures that accompany words to illustrate a verbal message are known as *illustrators.* Illustrators mimic the spoken word, such as pointing to the right or left while verbally saying the words right or left. *Regulators* convey meaning through gestures such as raising one's hand before verbally asking a question. Regulators also include head nodding and short sounds such as "uh huh" or "Hmmmm" and other expressions of interest or boredom. Without feedback, some people find it difficult to carry on a conversation. *Adaptors* are nonverbal behavior that either satisfy some physical need such as scratching or adjusting eyeglasses or represent a psychological need such as biting fingernails when nervous, yawning when bored, or clenching a fist when angry. The use of adaptors occurs more frequently in private gatherings rather than in public places (Galvin et al., 1988). All of the nonverbal communication previously described varies widely cross-culturally and cross-nationally.

Posture

Posture reflects people's emotions, attitudes, and intentions. Posture may be open or closed and is believed to convey an individual's degree of confidence, status, or receptivity to another person. An open posture is characterized by hands apart or comfortably placed on the arms of a chair while directly facing the person speaking. The person often leans forward, toward the speaker. Open posture communicates interest in someone and a readiness to listen. Someone seated in a closed posture might have their arms folded and legs crossed or be positioned at a slight angle from the person with whom they are interacting. The person may also allow their eyes to dart quickly from one spot to another in an unfocused, distracted manner. Closed posture usually conveys lack of interest or discomfort.

Chronemics

There are cultural variations in how people understand and use time. **Chronemics** is the study of the use of time in nonverbal communication. The manner in which a person perceives and values time, structures time, and reacts to time contributes to the context of communication. Social scientists have discovered that individuals are divided in two major groups in the ways they approach time: monochronic or polychronic. In **monochronic cultures**, such as many groups in the United States, Northern Europe, Israel, and much of Australia, time is seen as a commodity, and people tend to use expressions such as "waste time" or "lose time" or "time is money." Given that time is so highly valued, showing up late, especially for a meeting or a dinner, is usually perceived as very disrespectful to the individuals who are made to "waste their time" waiting (Lombardo, n.d.). A monochronic culture functions on clock time. People tend to focus on one thing at a time and usually prefer to complete objectives in a systematic way. In a meeting, for example, it is considered culturally appropriate to follow the predetermined agenda and avoid straying from the agenda by talking about unrelated topics (Rutledge, 2013).

People in **polychronic cultures**, such as some groups in Southern Europe, Latin America, Africa, and the Middle East, take a very different view of time. People from these cultures often believe that time cannot be controlled and that it is flexible. Days are planned based on events rather than the clock. For many people in these cultures, when one event is finished, it is time to start the next, regardless of what time it is. In a polychronic culture, following an agenda might not be very important. Instead, many tasks, such as building relationships, negotiating, and/or problem-solving, can be accomplished at the same time. In parts of Asia, such as Japan, China, and Taiwan, people tend to arrive a little early. In many parts of Europe, the northeast and western areas of the United States, Canada, Israel, and Australia, people tend to arrive precisely on time and may perceive it as an inconvenience to others if they arrive too early. In many parts of Latin and Central America, and Arabic-speaking areas in the Middle East, people tend to be more flexible in their notion of arrival times and may show up significantly later than the mutually agreed-upon time. Among certain Native American groups, an appointment or event begins "when everyone arrives," and there is considerable tolerance for those who show up after the appointed time. However, these examples are stereotypes, and not all members of a culture or subculture will perceive time in the same manner.

Proxemics

Another form of nonverbal communication is manifested in closeness and **personal space**. The study of space and how differences in that space can make people feel more relaxed or more anxious is referred to as **proxemics**, a term that was coined in the 1950s by the anthropologist and cross-cultural researcher Edward T. Hall. Distances have been identified based on the relationship between or among the people involved (Hall, 1984, 1990):

1. *Intimate space* (touching to 1 foot) is typically reserved for whispering and embracing;

however, nurses and other healthcare providers sometimes need to enter this intimate space when providing care for clients.

2. *Personal space* (ranges from 2 to 4 ft) is used among family and friends or to separate people waiting in line, for example, at the drug store or ATM.
3. *Social space* (4 to 10 ft) is used for communication among business or work associates and to separate strangers, such as those taking a course on natural childbirth.
4. *Public space* (12 to 25 ft) is the distance maintained between a speaker and the audience.

Cultural and ethnic variations occur in proxemics. For example, when having a conversation, with persons from Arabic speaking countries of the Middle East, France, and Latin America, people generally prefer to stand closer to one another than those from Canadian, American, and British cultures, who also tend to feel more uncomfortable when they must sit or stand close to one another (Munoz & Luckman, 2008). There are also important factors related to age and sex to consider in cross-cultural communication. In general, clients are likely to prefer a nurse or other healthcare provider of the *same sex*, particularly when care requires entering their personal space and/or touching the client. Similarly, the same sex may be preferred when the health history and/or physical examination includes the reproductive organs. In some ethnic and religious groups, it may be inappropriate or forbidden for healthcare providers of a different sex to shake hands, provide care, or otherwise touch the client. For example, observant Muslim women are not permitted to shake hands with male physicians, nurses, or other health professionals. As a sign of respect to the man, some Muslim women will place one or both arms over their chest and slightly bow their head. Whenever an observant Muslim is having a conversation with a person of another sex, a third person needs to be present to avoid the appearance of impropriety. Among some people from Chinese, Japanese, or other Asian cultures, there

may be both sex and age factors to be considered in cross-cultural communication.

Modesty

Modesty is a form of mixed nonverbal and verbal communication that refers to reserve or propriety in speech, dress, or behavior. It conveys a message that is intended to avoid encouraging sexual attention or attraction in others (aside from a person's spouse). In cultures that have been studied by anthropologists or transcultural nurses, people have cultural beliefs about modesty and rules concerning which behavior and dress are appropriate in various situations and circumstances. The following are examples of groups that have required rules or optional guidelines pertaining to modesty.

Traditional Muslim women beyond the age of puberty wear a headscarf to cover their head and hair as a sign of modesty and religious faith. The word **hijab** describes the act of covering up generally but is sometimes used to describe the headscarves worn by Muslim women (Fig. 1-6). These scarves come in many styles and colors and have different names around the world, such as *niqab, al-mira, shayla, khimar, chador,* and *burka.* The type of hijab most commonly worn in the United States, Canada, Australia, and Western Europe covers the head and neck but leaves the face clear. In various parts of the Arab world, cultural expectations for women may include covering the head, face, neck, or entire body in order to conform to certain standards of modesty established by various Islamic denominations and groups. The *burka* is the most concealing of all Islamic coverings. It is a one-piece veil that conceals the face and body, often leaving just a mesh screen to see through. There are differences between modesty at home and modesty in public. At home, Muslim women typically do not wear veils, scarves, or other coverings in the presence of male family members such as their fathers, husbands, sons, and other male or female relatives.

Women from observant Orthodox and Hasidic Judaism, Amish, Mennonite, and some

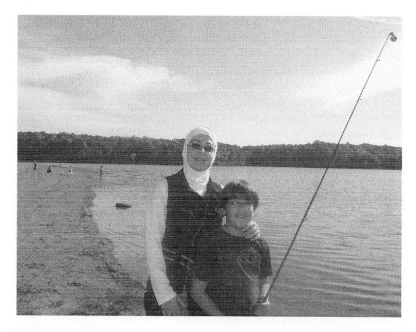

Figure 1-6. When in public places, some Muslim women wear a headscarf (hijab) to cover their hair, head, and neck, as a sign of modesty and religious faith.

conservative Catholic background cover their heads, arms, and/or legs as a cultural and/or religious expression of modesty and often as a sign of their affiliation with a particular religious order within Catholicism. The Hebrew word *tznius* or *tzniut* means modesty. It is generally used in reference to women and also relates to humility and general conduct, especially between men and women. Hasidic, Sikh, and Amish men often cover their heads and/or wear clothing that conveys modesty. For Buddhists, modesty is the quality of being unpretentious about one's virtues or achievements. The most important thing is not what type of clothes an individual wears or their color but the quality of their hearts. Buddhist monks have modesty guidelines pertaining to the way they wear their robes, never allowing skin to show on both sides of the body.

The Church of Jesus Christ of Latter-Day Saints (LDS) has issued official statements on modesty and dress for its members. Modesty is an attitude of propriety and decency in dress, grooming, language, and behavior. Clothing such as "short shorts" and short skirts, shirts that do not cover the stomach, and clothing that does not cover the shoulders or is low cut in the front or the back are discouraged, as are tattoos and body piercings. Members are also encouraged to avoid extremes in clothing or hairstyles. Most LDS members do not wear sleeveless shirts or blouses or shorts that fail to reach the knee. Women do not wear pants or slacks to religious services, and all members attend services well-groomed and well-dressed (Allred, 2020).

All cultures have rules, often unwritten, concerning who may touch whom, where, when, how, for what reason, and for how long. In general, it is best for nurses to refrain from touching clients or coworkers of any gender unless necessary for the accomplishment of a job-related task, such as the provision of safe client care. Typically, people from Chinese and Japanese cultures are not as overtly demonstrative of affection or as tactile as those from European American, Hispanic, or African American cultures. Generally, they refrain from public embraces, kissing, loud talking, laughter, and boisterous behavior in public.

Affection is expressed in a more reserved manner, usually in private rather than public places. In some instances, nurses and other members of the healthcare team from cultures that differ from the client's may send unintended messages through their use of touch. Special attention to relationships between different genders and to the age of the client is warranted in nurse–client interactions and especially when it is necessary to touch members of another gender.

Technology-Assisted Communication

Communication sometimes uses a combination of verbal, nonverbal, and written signals. With innovations in healthcare devices and software, technological advances are changing how care is delivered and the nature of the nursing profession. One of the major challenges of technology from a transcultural perspective is the gap between the regions and nations that have greater resources than others. While some strides are being made, it will still be many years before technological capabilities are mobilized in ways that benefit people globally by enhancing safe, quality, accessible, affordable, evidence-based, culturally congruent, and culturally competent nursing and healthcare. This is a matter of social justice that will be addressed as an integral component of TCN in Chapter 13.

Although linguists have known that language changes over time, the digital language is changing faster than any other language in recorded history. By 2018, people worldwide were sending 180 billion texts per month. Ninety-five percent of all adults in the United States own a smartphone—94% of White adults, 98% of African American adults, and 97% of Hispanic adults (Pew Internet Research Center, 2018). In many healthcare agencies, nurses are given smartphones, pagers, tablets, and other technology-assisted devices for job-related activities to improve patient outcomes. While these digital shortcuts may be expedient and timesaving, nurses and other members of the healthcare team need to communicate in multiple ways, balancing face-to-face and digital interactions. It is important for the nurse to identify the client's preferred mode for communication as an integral component of the overall assessment of communication used by the client, their family, and significant others.

Literature, Art, Music, and Dance

The literature, art, music, and dance of various cultural groups communicate to the world the cherished values, beliefs, history, traditions, and contributions of people from nations, tribes, and population groups. The creative products, in the form of books, poems, artwork, music, and dance, describe the social climate of the day; portray religious, racial, gender, political, class, and other perspectives; and serve as unique historical documents and artifacts to help people better see, hear, know, understand, and appreciate the richness of the world's diverse cultures as they are communicated through the literary works, artistic and musical creations, and dance of people from cultures around the world.

Problem-Solving Process

The TIP Model is intended to guide members of the interprofessional healthcare team in determining what decisions, actions, and interventions the client needs to achieve an optimal state of well-being and health. As indicated in Figure 1-7, the model helps nurses to conceptualize the care of people from diverse backgrounds in a logical, orderly, systematic, scientific five-step **problem-solving process**:

1. A comprehensive cultural **assessment**. The cultural assessment includes a self-assessment and a holistic assessment of the client that includes a health history and physical examination (Chapter 3 provides an in-depth discussion of these topics, and the Assessment Guides in Appendices A, B, C, and D offer further specific details).

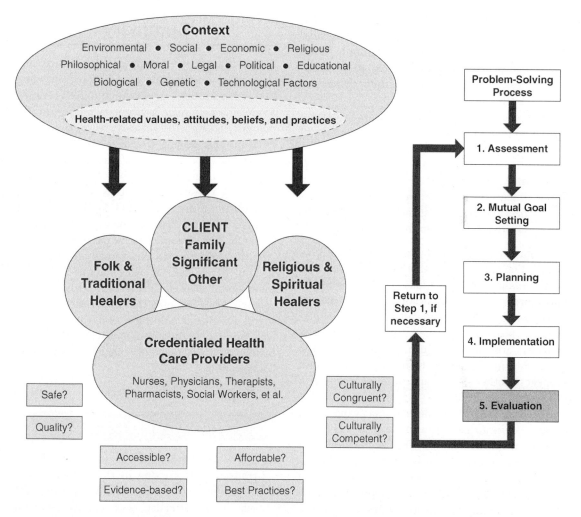

Figure 1-7. The five-step problem-solving process is a key part of the Transcultural Interprofessional Practice (TIP) Model. This client-centered model also includes the context from which people's health-related values, attitudes, beliefs, and practices emerge; the interprofessional healthcare team; and communication. (© Margaret M. Andrews.)

2. **Mutual goal setting** that takes into account the perspectives of each member of the healthcare team—the client, the client's family and significant others, and all those who are coparticipants with the client in the decision-making and goal-setting processes including credentialed health professionals and folk, traditional, indigenous, religious, and/or spiritual healers.

3. **Planning** care that includes input from and dialogue with members of the interprofessional healthcare team.

4. **Implementation** of the care plan through a wide range of actions and interventions.

5. **Evaluation** of the care plan from multiple, diverse perspectives to determine the degree to which the plan:

a. Is effective in achieving the intended goal(s)
b. Provides care that is *culturally congruent* with and fits the client's culturally based beliefs and practices related to wellness, health, illness, disease, healing, dying, and death
c. Reflects the delivery of *culturally competent* care by nurses and other members of the interprofessional team
d. Provides *quality* care that is *safe, affordable,* and *accessible*
e. Integrates *research, evidence-based practice, and best practices* (Melnyk & Fineout-Overholt, 2023) into the care

Data from the formal evaluation of the plan guide the nurses and other team members in determining if modifications or changes to the plan are necessary to accomplish the mutual goal(s) in Step 2 or if new goals need to be discussed, proposed, planned, and established. If changes are needed, return to assessment, the first step in the problem-solving process, and repeat the other steps as appropriate until each of the mutual goals is met.

As indicated in Benner's classic work titled *From Novice to Expert*, a nurse passes through levels of proficiency in the acquisition and development of problem-solving skills: novice, advanced beginner, competent, proficient, and expert (Benner, 1984). The development of proficiency in using the previously described problem-solving process requires time and repeated simulated and/or in situ clinical experiences. As Benner aptly observes, the process leading to proficiency as an expert takes place gradually and seldom follows a direct pathway from novice to expert; rather, a nurse passes through the intermediate stages, sometimes regressing to an earlier stage of competence, other times catapulting to a more advanced stage (Benner, 1984; Benner et al., 2010). The process of developing competence in clinical problem-solving is uneven and nonlinear, as is the process of developing cultural competence, a topic that is discussed in the next chapter.

Summary

In this chapter, we examined the historical and theoretical foundations of TCN and its close ties with anthropology. In the mid-20th century, Madeleine Leininger, a visionary nurse–anthropologist, created the infrastructure to support, develop, and expand TCN by establishing the TCNS, the JTN, and graduate programs in TCN at schools of nursing and by creating the ethnonursing research method. We also explored the contributions of selected TCN leaders and scholars to the advancement of TCN practice, research, and theory. Lastly, we described the TIP Model that serves as a framework for nurses seeking to collaborate with clients and other members of the healthcare team in the delivery of quality nursing care that is beneficial, meaningful, relevant, culturally congruent, culturally competent, and consistent with the cultural beliefs and practices of clients from diverse backgrounds.

REVIEW QUESTIONS

1. When Dr. Madeleine Leininger established transcultural nursing in the middle of the 20th century, she identified eight reasons why this specialty was needed. Review the reasons and discuss the relevance of these reasons in contemporary nursing and healthcare.
2. In your own words, describe the meaning of culture and its relationship to nursing.
3. Identify at least five nonethnic cultures and describe the characteristics of each.
4. Describe the composition of the interprofessional healthcare team in the Transcultural Interprofessional Practice (TIP) Model and identify factors that facilitate effective communication between and among team members.
5. Identify six examples of nonverbal communication and briefly describe each one.

6. In the Transcultural Interprofessional Practice Model, what criteria are used to determine the effectiveness of the plan of care in meeting mutual goals established by the patient and other members of the interprofessional healthcare team?

CRITICAL THINKING ACTIVITIES

1. Visit the TCNS's official website (https://tcns.org):
   a. Briefly summarize the information you find at the website.
   b. Critically evaluate the strengths and limitations of this information source and the data available. What else would you like to know about transcultural nursing that is not available on this website?
   c. Critically reflect on the information about transcultural nursing that you've learned and indicate how it will help you to provide nursing care for people from cultures that differ from your own.
   d. Search for other websites on transcultural nursing. What are the similarities and differences in the perspectives on transcultural nursing presented by the TCNS and other websites? How is it helpful or unhelpful to review different viewpoints on the same subject?

2. Using the keyword transcultural nursing, search for online resources that were posted during the last 2 years. Visit the website of the Transcultural Nursing Society. Focus on a specific cultural group and review the articles published in *The Journal of Transcultural Nursing* during the past year.
   a. How many references did you find?
   b. Did they contain information that you believe would be useful in clinical practice?

3. Conduct an electronic search for websites about modesty among observant Muslims and Orthodox and Hasidic Jewish people:
   a. Evaluate the credibility, accuracy, veracity, and currency of each website and the information available on the topic.
   b. Compare and contrast the beliefs and practices of each group, paying special attention to those that are gender-specific.
   c. What are the clinical implications of this information?

4. Maria Rodriguez is a 61-year-old woman who self-identifies as Mexican American. She reads, writes, and speaks Spanish; it is her primary language. Although she speaks English well enough to manage activities of daily living, she has difficulty reading and comprehending medical documents in English. Maria is scheduled to be discharged from the hospital on her 3rd day postoperatively following a below-the-knee amputation of her right leg. She is diagnosed with peripheral vascular disease, diabetes mellitus, obesity, and hypertension. Maria lives alone in a two-story single dwelling. Her son, age 30, is on active military duty. Her 21-year-old daughter is 8 months pregnant and lives out of state. Unable to manage her care at home, Maria is unhappy that she will need to be discharged to a rehabilitation center for the next several weeks. She tells the nurse manager that she is severely depressed and is considering suicide. Using the Transcultural Interprofessional Practice (TIP) Model as a guiding framework, analyze the case and develop a plan of care for Maria.

REFERENCES

Alligood, M. R. (2014). *Nursing theory: Utilization and application* (5th ed.). Mosby-Elsevier.

Allred, S. H. (2020). *Modesty: A timeless principle for all*. The Church of Jesus Christ of Latter-Day Saints. https://abn.churchofjesuschrist.org/study/liahona/2009/07/modesty-a-timeless-principle-for-all?lang=eng&adobe_mc_ref=https://www.churchofjesuschrist.org/study/liahona/2009/07/modesty-a-timeless-principle-for-all?lang=

American Anthropological Association. (2018). *What is anthropology?* https://www.americananthro.org/AdvanceYourCareer/Content.aspx?ItemNumber=2150&navItemNumber=740

Benner, P. (1984). *From novice to expert: Excellence and power in clinical nursing practice.* Addison-Wesley. https://doi.org/10.1002/nur.4770080119

Benner, P., Sutphen, M., Leonard, V., & Day, L. (2010). *Educating nurses: A call for a radical transformation.* Jossey-Bass.

Branch, M. F., & Paxton, P. P. (Eds.). (1976). *Providing safe nursing care for ethnic people of color.* Appleton-Century-Crofts.

Brink, P. J. (1976). *Transcultural nursing care.* Prentice-Hall, Inc.

Campinha-Bacote, J. (2011). Delivering patient-centered care in the midst of cultural conflict: The role of cultural competence. *Online Journal of Issues in Nursing, 16*(2), 5. https://doi.org/10.3912/OJIN.Vol16No02Man05

Campinha-Bacote, J. (2015). *A biblically based model of cultural competence in the delivery of healthcare services.* Transcultural C.A.R.E Associates. http://transculturalcare.net/a-biblically-based-model-of-cultural-competence/

Council on Nursing and Anthropology. (2018). https://www.conaa.org/index.php/about-us/what-is-conaa

Davidson, A., Ray, M., & Turkel, M. (Eds.). (2011). *Nursing, caring, and complexity science: For human-environment well-being.* Springer Publishing Company. https://doi.101891/9780826125880

Douglas, M. K., & Pacquiao, D. F. (Eds.). (2010). Core curriculum in transcultural nursing and health care. *Journal of Transcultural Nursing, 21*(Suppl. 1), 53S–136S.

Douglas, M., Pacquiao, D., & Purnell, L. (Eds.). (2018). *Global applications of culturally competent health care: Guidelines for practice.* Springer International Publishing AG part of Springer Nature. https://doi.org/10.1007/978-3-319-69332-3

Fawcett, J. (2016). *Applying Conceptual Models of Nursing.* Springer Publishing Company. https://doi.org/org/10.1891/9780826180063.0001

Fulmer, T., & Gaines, M. (Eds.). (2014). Conference conclusions and recommendations. In G. E. Thibault, T. Fulmer, & M. Gaines (Eds.). *Partnering with patients, families, and communities to link interprofessional practice and education: Proceedings of a conference sponsored by the Josiah Macy Foundation, Arlington, VA, 3–6 April* (pp. 27–45). Josiah Macy Foundation.

Galanti, G. A. (2014). *Cultural sensitivity: A pocket guide for health care professionals.* University of Pennsylvania Press.

Galvin, M., Prescott, D., & Huseman, R. C. (1988). *Business communication: Strategies and skills.* Holt, Rinehart, & Winston.

Giger, J. N. (2017). *Transcultural nursing: Assessment and intervention* (7th ed.). Mosby/Elsevier.

Hall, E. T. (1984). *The dance of life: The other dimension of time.* Anchor Press/Doubleday.

Hall, E. T. (1990). *Distance: The hidden dimension.* Anchor Press/Doubleday.

Institute of Medicine. (1999). *To err is human.* The National Academies Press. https://doi.org/10.17226/9728

Institute of Medicine. (2011). *The future of nursing: Leading change, advancing health.* The National Academies Press. https://doi.org/10.17226/12956

Interprofessional Education Collaborative Expert Panel. (2011). *Core competencies for interprofessional collaborative practice: Report of an expert panel.* Washington, DC.

Interprofessional Education Collaborative. (2016). *Core competencies for interprofessional collaborative practice: 2016 update.* https://nebula.wsimg.com/

Jeffreys, M. R. (2016). *Teaching cultural competence in nursing and health care: Inquiry, action and innovation* (3rd ed.). Springer Publishing. https://doi.org/10.1891/9780826119971

Leininger, M. M. (1970). *Nursing and anthropology: Two worlds to blend.* John Wiley & Sons.

Leininger, M. M. (1978). *Transcultural nursing: Concepts, theories and practices.* John Wiley & Sons.

Leininger, M. M. (1991). *Culture care diversity and universality: A theory of nursing.* National League for Nursing.

Leininger, M. M. (1995). *Transcultural nursing: Concepts, theories, research and practices.* McGraw-Hill.

Leininger, M. M. (1997). Future directions in transcultural nursing in the 21st century. *International Nursing Review, 44*(1), 19–23. https://pubmed.ncbi.nlm.nih.gov/9034876/

Leininger, M. M. (1999). What is transcultural nursing and culturally competent care? *Journal of Transcultural Nursing, 10*(1), 9. doi:10.1177/104365969901000105

Leininger, M. M., & McFarland, M. R. (2002). *Transcultural nursing: Concepts, theories and practices.* McGraw-Hill.

Leininger, M. M., & McFarland, M. R. (2006). *Culture care diversity and universality: A worldwide theory for nursing* (2nd ed.). Jones & Bartlett Publishers.

Lombardo, J. (n.d.). *Monochronic and polychronic cultures: Definitions and communication styles.* Study.com. http://education-portal.com/academy/lesson/monochronic-vs-polychronic-cultures-definitions-communication-styles.html

McFarland, M. R., Mixer, S. J., Webhe-Alamah, H., & Burk, R. (2012). Ethnonursing: A qualitative research method for all disciplines. *International Journal of Qualitative Methods, 11*(3), 259–279. https://doi.org/10.1177/160940691201100306

McFarland, M. R., & Wehbe-Alamah, H. B. (2016a). *Leininger's culture care diversity and universality: A worldwide theory of nursing* (3rd ed.). Jones & Bartlett Learning. https://doi.org/10.1177/1043659619867

McFarland, M. R., & Wehbe-Alamah, H. B. (2016b). The theory of culture care diversity and universality. In M. R. McFarland & H. B. Wehbe-Alamah (Eds.), *Leininger's culture care diversity and universality: A worldwide nursing theory* (pp. 1–34). Jones and Bartlett Learning. https://doi.org/10.1177/1043659619867

McFarland, M. R., & Wehbe-Alamah, H. B. (2018). *Transcultural nursing: Concepts, theories, research, and practices* (4th ed.). McGraw-Hill, Medical Publishing Division.

McFarland, M. R., & Wehbe-Alamah, H. B. (2019). Leininger's theory of culture care diversity and universality: An overview with a historical retrospective and a view toward the future. *Journal of Transcultural Nursing, 30*(6), 540–557. https://doi:10.1177/1043659619867134

McKenna, M. (1985). Anthropology and nursing: The interaction between two fields of inquiry. *Western Journal of Nursing Research, 6*(4), 423–431.

Melnyk, B. M., & Fineout-Overholt, E. (2023). *Evidence-based practice in nursing and healthcare* (5th ed.). Wolters Kluwer.

Morris, E. (2015). An examination of subculture as a theoretical social construct through an ethnonursing study of urban African American adolescent gang members. In M. R. McFarland & H. B. Wehbe-Alamah (Eds.), *Leininger's culture care diversity and universality: A worldwide nursing theory* (pp. 255–286). Jones and Bartlett Learning. https://doi.org/10.1177/1043659619867

Munoz, C., & Luckman, J. (2008). *Transcultural communication in nursing* (2nd ed.). Delmar Learning.

National Human Genome Research Institute. (2022). https://www.genome.gov/about-genomics/educational-resources/fact-sheets/human-genome-project

Orque, M. S., Bloch, B., & Monrroy, L. S. (1983). *Ethnic nursing care.* C.V. Mosby.

Pew Internet Research Center. (2018). *Mobile technology fact sheet.* http://www.pewinternet.org/fact-sheet/mobile

Purnell, L. (2013). *Transcultural health care: A culturally competent approach* (4th ed.). F.A. Davis Company.

Purnell, L. (2014). *Guide to culturally competent health care.* F.A. Davis Company.

Purnell, L., & Fenkl, E. (2018). *Guide to culturally competent health care.* F.A. Davis Company. https://doi.org/10.1007/978-3-030=51399-3

Ray, M. (2016). *Transcultural caring dynamics in nursing and health care.* F.A Davis Company. .

Ray, M., & Turkel, M. (2014). Caring as emancipatory nursing praxis: The theory of relational caring complexity. *Advances in Nursing Science, 37*(2), 132–146.

Rutledge, B. (2013). Cultural differences—Monochronic vs polychronic. *The Articulate CEO.* https://hearticulate-ceo.typepad.com/my-blog/2011/08/cultural-differences-monochronic-versus-polychronic.html

Sagar, P. L. (2012). *Transcultural nursing theory and models: Application in nursing education, practice, and administration.* Springer Publishing Company.

Sagar, P. L. (2014). *Transcultural nursing education strategies.* Springer Publishing Company.

Sagar, P. L. (2015). Transcultural nursing certification: Its role in nursing education, practice, and administration. In M. R. McFarland & H. B. Wehbe-Alamah (Eds.), *Leininger's culture care diversity and universality: A worldwide theory of nursing* (3rd ed., pp. 579–592). Jones & Bartlett Learning. https://doi.org/10.1177/1043659619867

Spector, R. E. (2017). *Cultural diversity in health and illness* (9th ed.). Pearson.

Transcultural Nursing Society (TCNS). (2022a). *Transcultural nursing certification.* https://tcns.org/tcncertification/

Transcultural Nursing Society (TCNS). (2022b). *About Us.* tcns.org/abouttcns/

Tylor, E. B. (1871). *Primitive culture* (Vols. 1 and 2). Murray.

U.S. Census Bureau. (2020). *Measuring Racial and Ethnic Diversity for the 2020 Census.* https://www.census.gov/newsroom/blogs/random-samplings/2021/08/measuring-racial-ethnic-diversity-2020-census.html

U.S. Census Bureau. (2021). *Guidance on the presentation and comparison of race and Hispanic origin data.* https://www.census.gov/topics/population/hispanic-origin/about/comparing-race-and-hispanic-origin.html

World Health Organization (WHO). (2010). *Framework for action on interprofessional education and collaborative practice.*

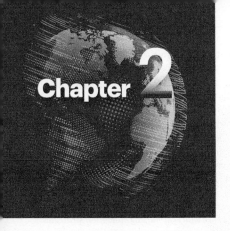

Chapter 2

Culturally Competent Nursing Care

• Patti Ludwig-Beymer and Margaret M. Andrews

Key Terms

Cross-cultural communication
Cultural assessment
Cultural baggage
Cultural competence
Cultural humility
Cultural imposition
Cultural self-assessment
Cultural stereotype
Culture of the deaf
Disabling hearing loss
Discrimination
Diversity

Emic
Emigrate
Ethnocentrism
Etic
Folk healer
Hard-of-hearing
Health tourism
Immigrant
Immigrate
Implicit bias
Individual cultural competence
Interprofessional collaborative
   practice

Language access services (LAS)
Microaggression
Organizational cultural
   competence
Population health
Prejudice
Racism
Refugee
Self-location
Social determinants of health
Social justice
Traditional healer
Vulnerable populations

Learning Objectives

1. Critically analyze the complex integration of knowledge, attitudes, and skills needed to deliver culturally competent nursing care.
2. Describe strategies used to build individual cultural competence.
3. Evaluate guidelines for the practice of culturally competent nursing care.
4. Use a transcultural interprofessional framework for the delivery of culturally congruent and culturally competent nursing care for clients with special needs.

Introduction

In this chapter, we provide an overview of the rationale for cultural competence in the delivery of nursing care and describe individual and organizational cultural competence, topics that will be discussed throughout the remainder of the book. We analyze cultural self-assessment, a valuable exercise that enables nurses to gain insights into their own unconscious cultural attitudes (biases, cultural stereotypes, implicit bias, prejudice, and tendencies to discriminate against people who are different from themselves). We discuss the need for cultural knowledge about other ethnic and nonethnic groups and psychomotor skills that are required for the delivery of culturally congruent and competent nursing care. We examine the use of the problem-solving process—assessment, mutual goal setting, planning, implementation, and evaluation—in the delivery of culturally congruent and competent care for clients from diverse backgrounds. We explore the roles and responsibilities of nurses and other members of the interprofessional healthcare team in the delivery of culturally competent care and the need for effective cross-cultural communication. We analyze the importance of assessing the cultural context and social determinants of health that influence the delivery of culturally competent care for clients from diverse cultures, for example, environmental, social, economic, religious, philosophical, moral, legal, political, educational, biologic, and technological factors. By introducing national and global guidelines for the delivery of culturally competent nursing care and identifying cultural assessment instruments, we provide nurses with tools to guide them in the delivery of care that is culturally acceptable and congruent with the client's beliefs and practices; culturally competent, affordable, and accessible; and rooted in state of the science research, evidence, and best practices. Lastly, we examine clients with special needs including those at high risk for health disparities, those who are deaf, and those with communication and language needs.

Rationale for Culturally Competent Care

Multiple factors are converging at this time in history to heighten societal awareness of cultural similarities and differences among people. There is growing awareness of social injustice for people from diverse backgrounds and the moral imperative to safeguard the civil and healthcare rights of vulnerable populations. **Vulnerable populations** are groups that have experienced social or economic obstacles in accessing the healthcare system because of ethnic, cultural, geographic (rural and urban settings), or health characteristics, such as disabilities or multiple chronic conditions (Douglas et al., 2018; Pacquiao & Douglas, 2019).

Immigrants move from one country or region to another for economic, political, religious, social, and personal reasons. The verb **emigrate** means to leave one country or region to settle in another; **immigrate** means to enter another country or region for the purpose of living there. People *emigrate from* one country or region and *immigrate to* a different nation or region.

In the United States, for example, 44.9 million people (13.6% of the population) are "foreign born," a term used by the Census Bureau in reference to anyone who is not a U.S. citizen at birth, including those who eventually become citizens through naturalization (U.S. Census Bureau, 2023). Additionally, an estimated 10.5 to 12 million people from other countries are living in the United States without documentation (Kamarak & Stenglein, 2019). In many countries, such as the European Union, national borders have become increasingly porous and fluid, enabling people to move more freely from one country or region to another.

Nurses respond to global healthcare caused by natural and human-made disasters and infectious disease epidemics. Nurses provide care to **refugees** (people who flee their country of origin for fear of persecution based on ethnicity, race, religion, political opinion, or related reasons) and other casualties of civil unrest or war in politically unstable parts of the world. **Health tourism** allows patients from other countries to obtain more affordable care services or receive specialized care that is unavailable in their own country. In all of these situations, nurses are expected to demonstrate effective **cross-cultural communication** and deliver culturally congruent and culturally competent nursing care to people from diverse countries and cultures.

Technological advances in science, engineering, transportation, communication, information and computer sciences, healthcare, and health profession education result in increased electronic and face-to-face communications between nurses and people from diverse backgrounds. Population demographics, healthcare standards, laws, and regulations make cultural competence integral to nursing practice, education, research, administration, and interprofessional collaborations.

Interprofessional collaborative practice refers to multiple health providers from different professional backgrounds working together with patients, families, caregivers, and communities to deliver the highest quality care (Moss et al., 2016). Interprofessional teams have a collective identity and shared responsibility for a client or group of clients. Culturally competent care is a component of interprofessional collaborative practice (Moss et al., 2016; National Academies of Sciences, Engineering, and Medicine, 2021), involving clients and their families; credentialed or licensed health professionals; folk or traditional healers from various philosophical perspectives, such as herbalists, medicine men or women, and others; and religious and spiritual leaders, such as rabbis, imams, priests, elders, monks, and other religious representatives or clergy, all of whom are integral members of the interprofessional team. The religious and spiritual healers are especially helpful when the client is discerning which decision or action in health-related matters is best, especially when there are moral, ethical, or spiritual considerations involved (see Chapter 12, Religion, Faith, Culture, and Nursing, and Chapter 13, Health Equity, Social Justice, and Cultural Competence).

Guidelines for the Practice of Culturally Competent Nursing Care

Guidelines developed by a task force consisting of members of the American Academy of Nursing (AAN) Expert Panel on Global Nursing and Health and the Transcultural Nursing Society (TCNS) have been endorsed by the International Council of Nurses. Intended to present universally accepted guidelines that can be embraced by nurses around the world, the 10 items listed in Table 2-1 provide a useful framework for implementing culturally competent care. The guidelines include knowledge of culture, education, and training in culturally competent care, critical reflection, cross-cultural communication, culturally competent practice, cultural competence in systems and organizations, patient advocacy and empowerment, multicultural workforce, cross-cultural leadership, and evidence-based practice and research. The guidelines have their foundation in principles of **social justice**, such as the belief that everyone is entitled to fair and equal opportunities for healthcare and to have their dignity protected. The guidelines and accompanying descriptions are intended to serve as a resource for nurses in clinical practice, administration, research, and education (Douglas et al., 2018).

Definitions and Categories of Cultural Competence

Cultural competence has been defined in a variety of ways. In a comprehensive concept analysis, Sharifi et al. (2019) emphasized that cultural competency is a dynamic process and identified six defining attributes of cultural competence: cultural awareness, cultural knowledge, cultural sensitivity, cultural skill, cultural proficiency, and dynamicity. The Agency for Healthcare Research and Quality (2019) defined cultural competence as a set of congruent behaviors, attitudes, and policies that enables effective interactions in a cross-cultural framework. The Centers for Disease

Table 2-1	Guidelines for the Practice of Culturally Competent Nursing Care
Guideline	**Description**
1. Knowledge of cultures	Nurses shall gain an understanding of the perspectives, traditions, values, practices, and family systems of culturally diverse individuals, families, communities, and populations they care for, as well as knowledge of the complex variables that affect the achievement of health and well-being.
2. Education and training in culturally competent care	Nurses shall be educationally prepared to provide culturally congruent healthcare. Knowledge and skills necessary for assuring that nursing care is culturally congruent shall be included in global healthcare agendas that mandate formal education and clinical training as well as required ongoing, continuing education for all practicing nurses.
3. Critical reflection	Nurses shall engage in critical reflection of their own values, beliefs, and cultural heritage in order to have an awareness of how these qualities and issues can impact culturally congruent nursing care.
4. Cross-cultural communication	Nurses shall use culturally competent verbal and nonverbal communication skills to identify client's values, beliefs, practices, perceptions, and unique healthcare needs.
5. Culturally competent practice	Nurses shall utilize cross-cultural knowledge and culturally sensitive skills in implementing culturally congruent nursing care.
6. Cultural competence in healthcare systems and organizations	Healthcare organizations should provide the structure and resources necessary to evaluate and meet the cultural and language needs of their diverse clients.
7. Patient advocacy and empowerment	Nurses shall recognize the effect of healthcare policies, delivery systems, and resources on their patient populations and shall empower and advocate for their patients as indicated. Nurses shall advocate for the inclusion of their patient's cultural beliefs and practices in all dimensions of their healthcare.
8. Multicultural workforce	Nurses shall actively engage in the effort to ensure a multicultural workforce in healthcare settings. One measure to achieve a multicultural workforce is through strengthening of recruitment and retention efforts in the hospitals, clinics, and academic settings.
9. Cross-cultural leadership	Nurses shall have the ability to influence individuals, groups, and systems to achieve outcomes of culturally competent care for diverse populations. Nurses shall have the knowledge and skills to work with public and private organizations, professional associations, and communities to establish policies and guidelines for comprehensive implementation and evaluation of culturally competent care.
10. Evidence-based practice and research	Nurses shall base their practice on interventions that have been systematically tested and shown to be the most effective for the culturally diverse populations that they serve. In areas where there is a lack of evidence of efficacy, nurse researchers shall investigate and test interventions that may be the most effective in reducing the disparities in health outcomes.

Source: Douglas, M. K., Rosenkoetter, M., Pacquiao, D. F., Callister, L. C., Hattar-Pollara, M., Lauderdale, J., Milstead, J., Nardi, D., Purnell, L. (2014). Guidelines for implementing culturally competent nursing care. *Journal of Transcultural Nursing, 25*(2), 110–129. Reprinted with permission from Sage Publications, Inc.

Control and Prevention (CDC, n.d.) refers to an ability to interact effectively with people of different cultures. Further, the CDC (2021) differentiates between cultural competence, awareness, knowledge, and sensitivity. They emphasize that cultural competence involves effectively operating in different cultural contexts and altering practices to reach a variety of cultural groups.

Cultural awareness, knowledge, and sensitivity do not include these actions.

There is general consensus that cultural competence can be divided into two major categories: (1) **individual cultural competence**, which refers to the care provided for an individual client by one or more nurses, physicians, social workers, and/or other healthcare, education, or social service professionals, and (2) **organizational cultural competence**, which focuses on the organizational leadership, collective competencies of the members of an organization, and their effectiveness in meeting the diverse needs of their clients, patients, staff, and community (CDC, 2021; Douglas, 2018) (see Chapter 9, Creating Culturally Competent Healthcare Organizations).

Before nurses can provide culturally competent care for individual clients or contribute to organizational cultural competence, they need to engage in a cultural self-assessment to identify their cultural baggage. **Cultural baggage** refers to the tendency for a person's own culture to be foremost in their assumptions, thoughts, words, and behavior. People are seldom consciously aware that culture influences their worldview and interactions with others.

Cultural Self-Assessment

The purpose of the **cultural self-assessment** is for nurses to critically reflect on their own culturally based attitudes, values, beliefs, and practices and gain insight into, and awareness of, the ways in which their background and lived experiences have shaped and informed the people they have become. Cultural critical self-reflection is an ongoing process whereby nurses continuously review their thoughts, feelings, and beliefs about others with backgrounds different from their own and their professional, moral, and ethical obligation to care for all without bias or prejudice (Purnell & Fenkl, 2018). Cultural humility is an important part of this process. **Cultural humility** incorporates a lifelong commitment to self-evaluation and self-critique. With cultural humility, the individual

minimizes power imbalances and develops mutually beneficial partnerships with communities for individuals and defined populations (Foronda, 2020).

The nurse's cultural self-assessment is a personal and professional journey that emphasizes strengths and areas for continued growth, thereby enabling nurses to set goals for overcoming barriers to the delivery of culturally congruent and competent nursing care. Part of the cultural self-assessment process includes nurses' awareness of their human tendencies toward implicit bias, ethnocentrism, cultural imposition, cultural stereotyping, prejudice, and discrimination. **Implicit (or unconscious) bias** is the unconscious collection of stereotypes and attitudes we develop toward groups of people. These are developed early in life and are shaped by family beliefs, media messages, institutional policies, and other factors. Implicit biases affect our interactions and may result in treatment disparities (Edgoose et al., 2019).

The term **ethnocentrism** refers to the human tendency to view one's own group as the center of and superior to all other groups. People born into a particular culture grow up absorbing and learning the values and behaviors of the culture, and they develop a worldview that considers their culture to be the norm. Other cultures that differ from that norm are viewed as inferior. Ethnocentrism may lead to pride, vanity, belief in the superiority of one's own group over all others, contempt for outsiders, and cultural imposition. Table 2-2 identifies other examples of "-isms"—preconceived, unfavorable judgments about people based on personal characteristics of another. "-Isms" are derived from cultural baggage, biases, stereotypes, prejudice, and/or discrimination related to someone with a background that differs from one's own. **Racism**, the belief that one's own race is superior and has the right to dominate others, has a profound impact on the body's stress management system. Exposure to racism results in activation of the stress response system and is considered a risk factor for many conditions, including cardiovascular disease, obesity, diabetes, depression, cognitive impairment, and

Characteristic	Type of -Ism
Race	Racism
Ethnicity	Ethnocentrism
National origin	Nationalism
Socioeconomic class	Classism
Gender	Sexism
Sexual orientation	Homophobism
Disability	Ableism
Religion	Islamism (political ideology associated with some denominations of Islam) Anti-Semitism (anti-Jewish) Anti-(name of religion), e.g., anti-Mormonism
Political opinion	Anti-(name of ideology), e.g., anticapitalism, anticommunism
Size	Sizeism

Table 2-2 | Selected Examples of "-Isms" Based on Preconceptions About Others

both inflammatory and autoimmune disorders (American Psychological Association, 2023). See Evidence-Based Practice 2-1 for a discussion of the effects of racism on African Americans' health.

Cultural imposition is the tendency of a person or group to impose their values, beliefs, and practices onto others. **Cultural stereotype** refers to a preconceived, fixed perception or impression of someone from a particular cultural group without meeting the person. The perception generally has little or no basis in fact but nonetheless is perpetuated by individuals who are unwilling to re-examine or change their perceptions even when faced with new evidence that disproves their position. Cultural stereotypes fail to recognize individual differences, group changes that occur over time, and personal preferences. Ethnocentrism, cultural imposition, and cultural stereotypes are barriers to effective cross-cultural communication and the provision of culturally competent care.

Prejudice refers to inaccurate perceptions of others or preconceived judgments about people based on ethnicity, race, national origin, gender, sexual orientation, social class, size, disability, religion, language, political opinion, geographic location, living environment, substance use,

incarceration, profession, or related personal characteristics (CDC, n.d.).

Whereas prejudice concerns perceptions and attitudes, **discrimination** refers to the *act* or behavior of setting one individual or group apart from another, thereby treating one person or group differently from other people or groups. In the context of civil rights law, *unlawful* discrimination refers to unfair or unequal treatment of an individual or group based on age, disability, ethnicity, gender, marital status, national origin, race, religion, and sexual orientation (Titles I and V of the Americans with Disabilities Act of 1990; Title VII of the Civil Rights Act of 1964 [Public Law 88–352]).

Microaggression is a less overt act that expresses prejudice toward a member of a marginalized group. Microaggression may be subtle and unconscious and may manifest as an offhand comment, a joke, or an insult. While the speaker may not have intended to offend, the comment or action reminds the receiving person that they are not fully accepted or trusted. The term was created by psychiatrist Chester Pierce in the 1970s to describe the subtle insults he observed by White students to African American students (Psychology Today, n.d.).

Effects of Racism on the Health and Well-Being of African Americans

The complex interrelationships among genetics, racism, and social determinants of health (environment, neighborhood, lifestyle, stress, employment, etc.) are being studied by multidisciplinary teams comprised of biologists, geneticists, physicians, nurses, ethicists, and social and behavioral scientists (Pacquiao & Douglas, 2019).

Racism and the resulting social exclusion trigger stress-related biologic mechanisms in African Americans. Exposure to racism increases sympathetic nervous system activation and affects the *HPA (hypothalamus, pituitary, and adrenal) axis*, a neuroendocrine system that controls reactions to stress. The HPS axis regulates many body processes, including digestion, the immune system, mood and emotions, sexuality, and energy storage and expenditure. Consequently, racism is associated with morbidities including low birth weight, hypertension, abdominal obesity, and cardiovascular disease even when there is no socioeconomic hardship among affected African Americans.

Racism impacts the ability of individuals, families, and communities to access healthcare and often results in the following:

- Fewer diagnostic and treatment options (e.g., cardiac catheterizations)
- Less follow-up or referral appointments for post-operative community services after discharge
- Increased presence of epinephrine, resulting in increased heart rate and blood pressure
- Higher mortality rates for African American men with cardiovascular disease

Due to the presence of epinephrine, both blood pressure and heart rate are raised significantly; therefore, racism influences the prevalence of hypertension through stress exposure, prolonged elevation of blood pressure, strain on the myocardium and left ventricle, and hypertrophy as a compensatory mechanism to offset the increased vascular resistance produced by hypertension. The process of sustained sympathetic activation eventually causes heart failure. Renal failure may result when the kidneys respond to hypertension. When a person experiences racism on a daily basis, the stress response becomes overwhelmed, and the adrenal system is no longer able to maintain homeostasis. Chronic adrenal fatigue often leads to depression, obesity, hypertension, diabetes, cancer, ulcers, allergies, eczema, autoimmune diseases, headaches, and liver disease.

Clinical Implications

Nurses need to position themselves strategically to bring about change in the healthcare system by acting as patient advocates, addressing racism for individual clients, and acting collectively as members of the nursing profession to rid the system of racism through systemic changes. Strategies for action include the following:

- Acknowledging the ways in which nurses' own race, culture, class, gender, socioeconomic background, and other social identities influence their beliefs, attitudes, and the care provided to patients from similar and different racial and ethnic backgrounds
- Addressing how inequities intersect and overlap to deepen disadvantage and how advocacy by nurses can bring about change
- Providing leadership in analyzing organizational approaches to racial diversity and workplace policies to foster inclusiveness, equity, and justice in health systems
- Conducting research on populations experiencing racism in their daily lives and within the healthcare system
- Ensuring that people from a variety of racial backgrounds are represented in investigations and on research councils that review proposals and allocate funds for nursing and healthcare research

References: Goosby, B. J., Cheadle, J. E., & Colter, M. (2018). Stress-related biosocial mechanisms of discrimination and African American Health Inequities. *Annual Review of Sociology*, 44(1), 319–340; Hill, L. K., Hoggard, L. S., Richmond, A. S., Gray, D. L., Williams, D. P., & Thayer, J. F. (2017). Examining the association between perceived discrimination and heart rate variability in African Americans. *Cultural Diversity and Ethnic Minority Psychology*, 23(1), 5–14; World Health Organization. (2018). Fact sheet. *Deafness and hearing loss*. http://www.who.int/en/news-room/fact-sheets/detail/deafness-and-hearing-loss

By engaging in cultural humility while demonstrating genuine interest in and curiosity about the client's cultural beliefs and practices, nurses learn to develop their cultural competency and learn to put aside their own ethnocentric or biased tendencies. Box 2-1 contains a cultural self-assessment tool that enables nurses to gain insights into how they relate to people grouped into five categories based on race/ethnicity, social issues/problems, religious differences, physical and emotional disabilities, and political perspectives. After completing and scoring the cultural self-assessment contained in Box 2-1, continue to the next section, which focuses on the cultural assessment of clients.

Cultural Assessment of Clients

The Andrews/Boyle Transcultural Interprofessional Practice Model (Andrews & Boyle, 2019) provides a client-centered, logical, and systematic process for delivering safe, culturally congruent, and competent care to people from diverse backgrounds. The foundation for culturally competent and culturally congruent nursing care is the **cultural assessment**, a term that refers to the collection of data about the client's health state. There are two major categories of data: *subjective data* (i.e., what clients say about themselves during the admission or intake interview) and *objective data* (i.e., what health professionals observe about clients during the physical examination through observation, percussion, palpation, and auscultation). See Chapter 3, Cultural Competence in Health History and Assessment, for an in-depth discussion of cultural competence in the health history and physical examination.

When conducting a comprehensive cultural assessment of clients, nurses need to be able to successfully form, foster, and sustain relationships with people who come from a cultural background that is different from the nurse's, thus making it necessary to quickly establish rapport with the client. The ability to see the situation from the client's point of view is known as an **emic** or insider's perspective; looking at the situation from an outsider's vantage point is known as an **etic** perspective.

The ability to successfully form, foster, and sustain relationships with members of a culture that differ from one's own requires effective cross-cultural communication. Understanding social, moral, and legal contexts is based on knowledge of many factors, such as the other person's values, perceptions, attitudes, manners, social structure, decision-making practices, and verbal and nonverbal communication within the group.

Knowledge about a client's family and kinship structure helps nurses to ascertain the values, decision-making patterns, and overall communication within the household. It is necessary to identify the significant others whom clients perceive to be important in their care and who may be responsible for decision-making that affects their healthcare. For example, for many clients, familism—which emphasizes interdependence over independence, affiliation over confrontation, and cooperation over competition—may dictate that important decisions affecting the client be made by the family, not the individual alone. When working with clients from cultural groups that value cohesion, interdependence, and collectivism, nurses may perceive the family as being overly involved and usurping the autonomy of both the client and the nurse. At the same time, clients are likely to perceive the involvement of family as a source of mutual support, security, comfort, and fulfillment.

The family is the basic social unit in which children are raised and where they learn culturally based values, beliefs, and practices about health and illnesses. Relationships that may seem obvious sometimes warrant further exploration when the nurse interacts with clients from culturally diverse backgrounds. Terms must always be clarified. For example, most European Americans define siblings as two persons with the same mother, the same father, the same mother and father, or the same adoptive parents. In some Asian cultures, a sibling relationship is defined as any infant breastfed by the same person. In other cultures, certain kinship patterns, such as maternal first cousins, are defined as sibling relationships. In some African cultures, anyone from the same village or town may be called brother or sister.

BOX 2-1	How Do You Relate to Various Groups of People in Society?

Described below are different levels of response you might have toward a person.

Levels of Response

1. *Greet*: I feel I can *greet* this person warmly and welcome them sincerely.
2. *Accept*: I feel I can honestly *accept* this person as they are and be comfortable enough to listen to their problems.
3. *Help*: I feel I would genuinely try to *help* this person with their problems as they might relate to or arise from the label–stereotype given to them.
4. *Background*: I feel I have the *background* of knowledge and/or experience to be able to help this person.
5. *Advocate*: I feel I could honestly be an *advocate* for this person.

Scoring Guide: The following is a list of individuals. The 32 types of individuals can be grouped into five categories: ethnicity and/or race, social/moral/legal, spiritual and/or lifestyle choice, current physical and/or mental health status, and political viewpoint. Read down the list and place a check mark next to anyone you would **not** "greet" or would hesitate to "greet." Then, move to response level 2, "accept," and follow the same procedure. Continue through response level 5. Try to respond honestly, not as you think that might be socially or professionally desirable. Your answers are only for your personal use in understanding your initial reactions to different people. If you have a concentration of checks within a specific category of individuals or at specific levels, this may indicate a conflict that could hinder you from rendering effective professional help.

Level of Response	1	2	3	4	5
Individual	Would not Greet	Would not Accept	Would not Help	No Background	Could not Advocate for
Ethnicity and/or race					
Haitian or Haitian American	☐	☐	☐	☐	☐
Mexican or Mexican American	☐	☐	☐	☐	☐
Navajo	☐	☐	☐	☐	☐
Iraqi or Iraqi American	☐	☐	☐	☐	☐
Chinese exchange student	☐	☐	☐	☐	☐
Irish or Irish American	☐	☐	☐	☐	☐
Social/moral/legal					
Reformed criminal	☐	☐	☐	☐	☐
Sex worker	☐	☐	☐	☐	☐
Unmarried pregnant teenager	☐	☐	☐	☐	☐
Computer hacker or pirate	☐	☐	☐	☐	☐
Shoplifter	☐	☐	☐	☐	☐
Spiritual practice, lifestyle choice, and/or identity					
Observant Jewish person	☐	☐	☐	☐	☐

BOX 2-1	How Do You Relate to Various Groups of People in Society? (continued)

Level of Response	1	2	3	4	5
Individual	Would not Greet	Would not Accept	Would not Help	No Background	Could not Advocate for
Practicing Roman Catholic	☐	☐	☐	☐	☐
Transgender person	☐	☐	☐	☐	☐
Practicing Muslim	☐	☐	☐	☐	☐
Atheist	☐	☐	☐	☐	☐
Vegan/vegetarian	☐	☐	☐	☐	☐
Member of Jehovah's Witnesses	☐	☐	☐	☐	☐
Amish person	☐	☐	☐	☐	☐
Current physical and/or mental health status					
Person with obesity or overweight	☐	☐	☐	☐	☐
Older adult with Alzheimer disease	☐	☐	☐	☐	☐
Person in a wheelchair	☐	☐	☐	☐	☐
Person who is HIV positive	☐	☐	☐	☐	☐
Person with cancer	☐	☐	☐	☐	☐
Person with anorexia or bulimia	☐	☐	☐	☐	☐
Person who smokes cigarettes	☐	☐	☐	☐	☐
Person with an opioid dependency	☐	☐	☐	☐	☐
Political viewpoint					
Neo-Nazi activist	☐	☐	☐	☐	☐
Member of a worker's union	☐	☐	☐	☐	☐
Feminist	☐	☐	☐	☐	☐
Socialized healthcare proponent	☐	☐	☐	☐	☐
Ku Klux Klansman	☐	☐	☐	☐	☐

Adapted from Randall-David, E. (1989). Assessing your own cultural heritage. In *Strategies for working with culturally diverse communities and clients* (1st ed., pp. 7–9). Association for the Care of Children's Health. https://archive.org/details/strategiesforwor00rand

Among some Hispanic groups, female members of the nuclear or extended family such as sisters and aunts are primary providers of care for infants and children. In some African American families, the grandmother may be the decision maker and primary caretaker of children. To provide culturally congruent and competent care, nurses must identify and effectively communicate with the appropriate decision maker(s).

When making health-related decisions, some clients may seek assistance from other members of the family. In some cultures, a relative (e.g., parent, grandparent, eldest son, or eldest brother) may be expected to make decisions about important health-related matters. For example, in Japan, it is the obligation and duty of the eldest son and his spouse to assume primary responsibility for aging parents and to make healthcare decisions for them. Among the Amish, the entire community is affected by the illness of a member and pays for healthcare from a common fund. The Amish join together to meet the needs of both the sick person and their family throughout the illness, and the roles of dozens of people in the community are likely to be affected by the illness of a single member. The individual value orientation concerning relationships is predominant among the dominant cultural majority in North America. Although members of the immediate family may participate to varying degrees, decision-making about health and illness is often an individual matter. Nurses should ascertain the identity of all key participants in the decision-making process; sometimes, decisions are made after consultation with family members, but the individual is the primary decision maker.

Individual Cultural Competence

Individual cultural competence is a complex integration of knowledge, attitudes, values, beliefs, behaviors, skills, practices, and cross-cultural nurse–client interactions that include effective communication and the provision of safe, high quality, affordable, accessible, evidence-based, acceptable, and efficacious nursing care for clients from diverse backgrounds. The term diverse or **diversity** refers to clients' uniqueness in the dimensions of race; ethnicity; national origin; socioeconomic background; age; gender; sexual orientation; philosophical and religious ideology; lifestyle; level of education; literacy; marital status; physical, emotional, and psychological ability; political ideology; size; and other characteristics used to compare or categorize people (Kroeber, 2018).

Although the connotation of diversity is generally positive, it is sometimes argued that the term diversity is itself an ethnocentric term because it focuses on how different the other person is from *me*, rather than how different *I* am from *the other person*. In using the term *cultural diversity*, the White panethnic group frequently is viewed as the norm against which the differences in everyone else (ethnocentrically referred to as non-Whites) are measured or compared. It is important for the nurse to realize this and avoid the tendency to consider White as the norm.

Cultural competence is not an end point but a dynamic, ongoing, lifelong, developmental process that requires self-reflection, intrinsic motivation, and commitment by the nurse to value, respect, and refrain from judging the beliefs, language, interpersonal styles, behaviors, and culturally based health-related practices of individuals, families, and communities receiving services as well as the professional and auxiliary staff who are providing such services (Kroeber, 2018). Strategies for continuing to grow in cultural competence are presented in Box 2-2. Culturally competent nursing and healthcare require effective cross-cultural communication and a diverse workforce and are provided in a variety of social, cultural, economic, environmental, and other contexts across the lifespan. Scholars and professional groups representing nursing, medicine, psychology, social work, physical therapy, education, anthropology, and many other disciplines have written about cultural competence; diversity, equity, and inclusion; and social determinants of health (The American Medical Association, 2023; Montgomery, 2019; National Academies of Sciences, Engineering, and Medicine, 2021; Purnell & Fenkl, 2018; McFarland & Wehbe-Alamah, 2018).

Given the large number of cultures and subcultures in the world, it's impossible for nurses to know everything about them all; however, it is possible for nurses to develop excellent cultural assessment and cross-cultural communication skills and to follow a systematic, orderly process for the delivery of culturally competent care. Nurses are encouraged to study in depth the top two or three cultural groups that they

BOX 2-2 | Strategies for Continued Growth in Cultural Competence

- Reflect on your own values and beliefs.
- Be aware of the privileges that you bring to an encounter. These privileges may be related to race, ethnicity, gender, age, education, socioeconomic status, or other variables.
- Recognize and mitigate the implicit bias within yourself.
- Read books written by authors from backgrounds different from yours—both nonfiction and fiction.
- Attend plays and movies about people from diverse backgrounds.
- Visit art, dance, music, and other events featuring artists from diverse backgrounds.
- Review history, considering how Indigenous Peoples and enslaved people were marginalized.

- Identify historical and existing policies and practices that continue to marginalize groups.
- Connect with people from different backgrounds; listen to learn and understand.
- Support colleagues who have different backgrounds from you; help them belong to the team.
- Watch for and respond to prejudice, microaggressions, and discrimination.
- Call out racism, sexism, and other "-isms" when you encounter them.
- Consider participating in or initiating a health equity journal club.
- Advocate for diversity, equity, and inclusion and health equity.
- Reflect on how each experience above has changed how you think and act.

encounter most frequently in their clinical practice and develop the affective (feelings or emotions), cognitive (conscious mental activities such as thinking), and psychomotor (combined thinking and motor) skills necessary to deliver culturally competent nursing care. As new groups move into a geographic area, nurses need to update their knowledge and skills in order to be responsive to the changing demographics. Keeping pace with client diversity is challenging and complex and needs to become an integral component of the nurse's continuing professional development. Professional organizations, employer-sponsored in-service programs, and web-based resources provide nurses with valuable sources of information on culturally based health beliefs and practices of clients from diverse backgrounds.

Chapter 1 provides the TIP Model for problem-solving, useful for delivering culturally congruent and competent nursing care for individual clients. Clients (the individual, their family, and significant others) are at the center and are the focus of the interprofessional healthcare team (which includes credentialed and/or licensed health professionals and folk, traditional, religious, and spiritual healers).

Step 1 of the process is assessment—of both the nurse and the client. This begins with nurses' *self-assessment* of their attitudes, values, and beliefs about people from backgrounds that differ from their own; their *knowledge* of their own **self-location** (cultural, gender, class, and other social self-identities) compared to those of clients and other team members; and the *psychomotor skills* needed for the delivery of culturally congruent and competent care (see Box 2-3). The self-assessment includes self-reflection and reflexivity (analysis of cause–effect relationships) for the purpose of uncovering the nurse's implicit biases, cultural stereotypes, prejudices, and discriminatory behaviors. Nurses then have the opportunity to change, or rectify, affective, cognitive, or psychomotor deficits by reframing their attitude toward certain individuals and groups from diverse backgrounds, learning more about the cultures and subcultures most frequently encountered in their clinical practice, and developing psychomotor skills that enhance their ability to use and their clinical skills to deliver culturally congruent and competent nursing care.

BOX 2-3	Selected Examples of Psychomotor Skills Useful in Transcultural Nursing

Assessment

- Techniques for assessing biocultural variations in health and illness, for example, assessing cyanosis, jaundice, anemia, and related clinical manifestations of disease in clients with darkly-pigmented skin, differentiating between congenital dermal melanocytosis and ecchymoses (bruises)
- Measurement of head circumference and fontanelles in infants using techniques not in violation of taboos for selected cultural groups
- Growth and development monitoring for children of Asian heritage using culturally appropriate growth grids
- Cultural modification of the Denver II and other developmental tests used for children
- Conducting culturally appropriate obstetric and gynecologic examinations of people from various cultural backgrounds

Communication

- Speaking and writing the language(s) used by clients
- Using alternative methods of communicating with non–English-speaking clients and families when no interpreter is available

(e.g., pantomime, e-translators for smartphones, tablets, and other devices)

Hygiene

- Skin care for people of various racial/ethnic backgrounds
- Hair care for people of various racial/ethnic backgrounds, for example, care of African American clients' hair

Activities of Daily Living

- Assisting Chinese American clients to regain the use of chopsticks as part of rehabilitation regimen after a stroke
- Assisting Amish clients who are paralyzed with dressing when buttons and pins are used
- Assisting West African clients who use "chewing sticks" for oral hygiene

Religion

- Emergency baptism and anointing of the sick for Roman Catholics
- Care before and after ritual circumcision by *mohel* (performed 8 days after the birth of a male Jewish infant)

The comprehensive cultural assessment of the client and their family and significant others (people, companion animals, and pets) (Fig. 2-1) requires nurses to gather subjective and objective data through the health history and the physical examination (see Chapter 3, Cultural Competence in Health History and Assessment). The nurse should consider the influence of the following factors: environmental, social, economic, religious, philosophical, moral, legal, political, educational, biological (genetic and acquired diseases, conditions, disorders, injuries, and illnesses), and technological (McFarland & Wehbe-Alamah, 2018). In addition, the nurse may have professional and organizational cultures that influence the

nurse–patient interaction, such as hospital or agency policies that determine visiting hours or laws governing the nurse's scope of practice and professional responsibilities within a particular jurisdiction or setting. The influence of cultural and health belief systems (on the nurse and the client) must also be considered in relation to disease causation, healing modalities, and choice of healer(s). See Chapter 4, Influence of Cultural and Health Belief Systems on Healthcare Practices, for detailed information.

In Steps 2 to 4, the nurse collaborates with the client, the client's family and significant others, and members of the healthcare team (credentialed, folk, traditional, religious, and spiritual healers).

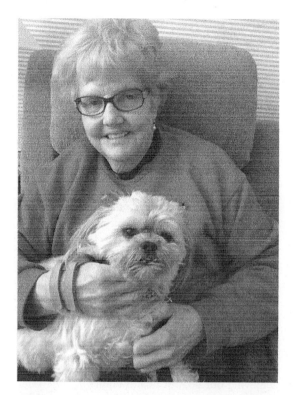

Figure 2-1. During visiting hours, this pet is a frequent companion to a patient recovering from knee replacement surgery in a rehabilitation facility with a pet-friendly policy.

The terms folk healer and traditional healer sometimes are used interchangeably. **Folk healers** typically learn healing practices through an apprenticeship with someone experienced in folk healing. Folk healers primarily use herbal remedies, foods, and inanimate objects in a therapeutic manner. **Traditional or indigenous healers** often are divinely chosen and/or learn the art of healing by applying knowledge, skills, and practices based on experiences indigenous to their culture, for example, Native American medicine men/women and shamans. The focus of most traditional and indigenous healers is on establishing and restoring balance and harmony in the body–mind–spirit through the use of spiritual healing interventions, such as praying, chanting, drumming, dancing, participating in sweat lodge rituals, and storytelling. The definition and scope of practice of religious and spiritual healers vary widely, but these healers

often help clients analyze complex health-related decisions involving moral and/or ethical issues (see Chapter 12, Religion, Faith, Culture, and Nursing, and Chapter 13, Health Equity, Social Justice, and Cultural Competence). All healers whom the client wants to be involved in care should be included in Steps 2 to 5 to the extent feasible.

In *Step 2*, mutual goals are set, and objectives are established to meet the goals and desired health outcomes.

In *Step 3*, the plan of care is developed using approaches that are client centered and culturally congruent with the client's socioeconomic, philosophical, and religious beliefs, resources, and practices. Members of the healthcare team assume roles and responsibilities according to their educational background, clinical knowledge, and skills. For credentialed or licensed members of the team such as nurses; physicians; physical, occupational, and respiratory therapists; social workers; and similar health professions, roles, responsibilities, and scope of practice are delineated by ministries of health, provincial or state health professions licensing, and/or registration boards. In most instances, the credentialed or licensed healer has formal academic preparation and has passed an examination that tested knowledge and skills deemed necessary for clinical practice.

In *Step 4*, decisions, actions, treatments, and interventions that are congruent with the patient's health-related cultural beliefs and practices are implemented by those team members who are best prepared to assist the client. In some instances, there is overlapping of scope of practice, roles, and responsibilities between and among team members (Fig. 2-2). Client-centered interprofessional team conferences are usually helpful in sorting out roles and responsibilities of team members when there is lack of clarity about who will deliver a particular service.

Lastly, in *Step 5*, the client and members of the healthcare team collaboratively evaluate the care plan and its objectives to determine if the care is safe; culturally acceptable, congruent, and competent; affordable; accessible; of high quality; and based on research, scientific evidence, and/or best

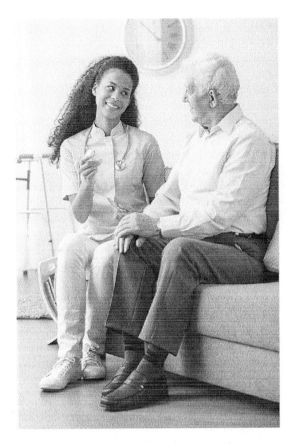

Figure 2-2. Effective cross-cultural communication is vital to the establishment of a strong nurse–client relationship. It is important to understand both verbal and nonverbal cues when communicating with people from different cultural backgrounds. (Photographee.eu/Shutterstock.com)

practices. If modifications or changes are needed, the nurse should return to previous steps and repeat the process. Throughout the five steps, the nurse behaves in an empathetic, compassionate, caring manner that matches, "fits," and is consistent with the client's cultural beliefs and practices.

Individual cultural competence, as described in this chapter, is necessary for the achievement of organizational cultural competence. Organizational cultural competence is discussed in detail in Chapter 9, Creating Culturally Competent Healthcare Organizations. Appendix C contains the Andrews/Boyle Transcultural Nursing Assessment Guide for Healthcare Organizations and Facilities.

Clients With Special Needs

In the remainder of this chapter, we discuss the delivery of culturally competent nursing care for three groups of clients with special needs: those at high risk for health inequities and health disparities, those who are deaf, and those with communication and special language needs.

Health Disparities

Health disparities are preventable differences in the burden of disease, injury, violence, or in opportunities to achieve optimal health. Health disparities exist in all age groups (U.S. Department of Health and Human Services, Centers for Disease Control and Prevention, 2023). These differences can affect **population health**, determining how frequently a disease affects a group, how many people get sick, or how often the disease causes death.

Social determinants of health (SDOH) influence health disparities and prevent us from achieving our goal of health equity. SDOH refer to the conditions in the environments in which people are born, live, learn, work, play, worship, and age (U.S. Department of Health and Human Services, Centers for Disease Control and Prevention, 2023). SDOH affect a wide range of health, functioning, and quality-of-life outcomes and risks. For example, in the early days of the COVID-19 pandemic, deaths were more common in Black and Hispanic individuals because of living and working conditions. Later, deaths were more common in individuals of any race or ethnicity who refused COVID-19 vaccinations.

Many different populations are affected by disparities. These include the following:

- Certain racial and ethnic groups
- Residents of rural areas
- Women, children, and older adults
- Persons with disabilities
- Other special populations such as those who are deaf and those who have difficulty hearing and those who are blind and visually impaired

In the United States, health disparities are a well-known problem among panethnic groups, particularly African Americans, Asian Americans, Native Americans, and Latinos. When examining health disparities within countries and globally, the World Health Organization uses the term health inequities (World Health Organization, 2021).

Recently, there have been substantial improvements in healthcare quality for Black, Hispanic, and American Indian and Alaska Native communities in the United States. However, these improvements have not eliminated disparities when compared to health outcomes for White Americans, and significant disparities in all domains of healthcare quality persist (Agency for Healthcare Research and Quality, 2022). In addition, these groups are less likely to receive routine medical procedures. Disparities in healthcare exist even when controlling for gender, condition, age, and socioeconomic status (Mandal, 2018; Purnell & Fenkl, 2018). The U.S. Department of Health, Health Resources and Services Administration identifies culturally competent nursing care as an effective approach in reducing and eliminating health disparities and inequities in high-risk populations such as Black Americans, Latinos, and American Indians. Studies demonstrate that these groups have a higher prevalence of chronic conditions, along with higher rates of mortality and poorer health outcomes when compared with counterparts in the general population. For example, the overall infant mortality rate in the United States has declined dramatically over the past several decades, from a rate of 55.7 per 1,000 live births in 1935 to 5.8 in 2017. However, the racial disparity remains; the mortality rate for Black infants was 10.8 per 1,000 live births, 2.2 times higher than the mortality rate of 4.8 for White infants (U.S. Department of Health and Human Services, Health Resources and Services Administration, Office of Health Equity, 2020).

Understanding health disparities is essential for achieving health equity and improving population health. These improvements require a concerted effort by healthcare organizations and by other sectors of society, including those responsible for air quality, education, employment, healthy food and water, housing, transportation, and others. As culturally competent individuals, nurses should be aware of these barriers to health equity Throughout the remaining chapters of the book, we will discuss interventions and strategies for reducing health disparities and inequities through the delivery of culturally congruent and culturally competent nursing and healthcare for people from diverse backgrounds across the lifespan.

Although nurses tend to think about clients from racially and ethnically diverse backgrounds, when discussing culturally competent nursing care, there are many people who self-identify with *nonethnic cultures* or with more than one culture or subculture. Some examples include groups based on disability, geographic location (such as rural settings), incarceration, living conditions (such as the population of people experiencing homelessness), sexual orientation and gender identity (LGBTQ+ communities), spiritual beliefs, and substance use disorder. While we cannot discuss each nonethnic culture, the **culture of the deaf** is provided as an example.

Culture of the Deaf

More than 5% of the world's population (466 million adults and 34 million children) experience disabling hearing loss (World Health Organization, 2018b). **Disabling hearing loss** is defined as the loss of greater than 40 decibels in the better ear in adults and the loss of greater than 30 decibels in the better ear in children. Disabling hearing loss means that a client has very little or no hearing, which has consequences for interpersonal communication, psychosocial well-being, quality of life, and economic independence. Hearing loss may affect one or both ears, can be congenital or acquired, and occurs on a continuum from mild to severe. Hearing loss leads to difficulty in hearing conversational speech or loud sounds. Clients who are **hard-of-hearing** usually communicate through spoken language and can benefit from hearing aids, captioning, and assistive listening devices (National Institute on Deafness and Other Communication Disorders, 2018; World Health Organization, 2018a).

If hearing loss develops in childhood, it impedes speech and language development and, in severe cases, requires special education. In adulthood, disabling hearing loss can lead to embarrassment, loneliness, social isolation, stigmatization, prejudice, abuse, mental health problems such as depression, difficulties in interpersonal relationships with partners and children, restricted career choices, occupational stress, and lower earnings when compared with counterparts who do not have disabling hearing loss. Approximately one third of people over 65 years of age are affected by disabling hearing loss. The prevalence in this age group is greatest in South Asia, Asia Pacific, and sub-Saharan Africa (World Health Organization, 2018b).

There are known practices to reduce deafness related to infections, prenatal care, and exposure to loud noises, as outlined in Box 2-4. In addition, some clients with congenital deafness or others with significant hearing losses may benefit from cochlear implants, but the decision to have a cochlear implant is interconnected with an animated debate within and between members of the deaf culture and members of the culture of medicine concerning the appropriateness of cochlear implants. The fundamental issues underlying the debate relate to philosophical beliefs about deafness and the concept of deaf culture.

From an emic perspective, many deaf people see their bodies as well, whole, and nonimpaired, and they self-identify as members of a linguistic minority, not with the culture of disability (Leigh & Andrews, 2017; Mandal, 2018). As members of a cultural minority, some deaf people perceive themselves as being on a journey of cultural awareness, one of several stages on the way to achieving a positive sense of self- and deaf identity. On the other hand, others who are deaf advocate reframing the concept of a deaf culture and conceptualizing it as the deaf experience based on values stemming from a visual orientation. Recognizing that the literature and the arts provide forums for cultural awareness, appreciation, and expression of ideas and feelings, there are a growing number of deaf people using

---

BOX 2-4 Prevention of Deafness

Fifty percent of all cases of hearing loss can be prevented through primary prevention. Strategies for prevention include the following:

- Immunizing children against childhood diseases, including measles, meningitis, rubella, and mumps
- Immunizing female adolescents and adults of reproductive age against rubella before pregnancy
- Screening for and treating syphilis and other infections in pregnant people
- Improving antenatal and perinatal care, including promotion of safe childbirth
- Avoiding the use of ototoxic drugs, unless prescribed and monitored by a qualified physician, nurse practitioner, or other healthcare providers
- Referring infants with high-risk factors (such as those with a family history of deafness and those born with low birth weight, birth asphyxia, jaundice, or meningitis) for early assessment of hearing, prompt diagnosis, and appropriate management, as required
- Reducing exposure (both occupational and recreational) to loud noises by creating awareness, using personal protective devices, and developing and implementing suitable legislation

Data from World Health Organization. (2018b). *Deafness prevention.* https://www.who.int/deafness/en/

these media to communicate their experiences with one another and with hearing members of society.

From an etic (outsider's) perspective, some members of the hearing society emphasize the differences between deaf and hearing communities, placing unwanted, unwarranted, and unnecessary limitations on deaf people's lives and capabilities. In the biologic sciences, for example, the bodies of hearing people historically have been constructed with a normative bias. In other words, the body that hears is the normative prototype. Some physicians engage in the cultural imposition of medical and surgical interventions on members of the deaf culture through eugenics (a science that tries to improve the human race by controlling which people become parents), genetic engineering, and insistence that deaf people should use hearing aids, agree to cochlear implant surgery, and embrace other technologies that profoundly change their lives and their culture.

Box 2-5 uses the framework of the five-step process for delivering culturally congruent and competent nursing care for people who self-identify as members of the deaf culture, beginning with a cultural assessment of self and the client, mutual goal setting, planning, implementation, and evaluation.

There are hundreds of sign language dialects in use around the world. Each culture has developed its own form of sign language to be compatible with the language spoken in that country. In the United States, an estimated 500,000 people communicate by using American Sign Language (ASL), including many who are deaf and hard-of-hearing and family members, friends, or teachers of people who are hard-of-hearing (Harrington, 2016). An ASL interpreter is often helpful in avoiding communication difficulty when caring for someone who is deaf or hard-of-hearing. Signaling and assistive listening devices, alerting devices, telecommunication devices for the deaf (TDD), and telephone amplifiers might also help promote effective communication and facilitate the provision of culturally competent care in home, community, hospital, and other settings.

Additionally, nurses will encounter clients who are of "dual minority," for example, both Black and deaf, LGBTQ+ and deaf, Native American and deaf, and many other combinations of two or more cultures. Providing care for individuals with multiple vulnerabilities is complicated. As with other groups, nurses must recognize their own biases. In addition, they should realize that the dual minorities can be fluid based on the situation. For example, an African American who is deaf may be more focused on race in some situations and in hearing loss in others. However, the effect on prejudice and discrimination is cumulative and may impact the individual's ability to access resources.

Communication and Language Assistance

With growing concerns about racial, ethnic, and language disparities in health and healthcare and the need for healthcare systems to accommodate increasingly diverse patient populations, **language access services (LAS)** have become a matter of increasing national importance. In 2019, about 20% of the U.S. population speaks a language other than English at home (U.S. Census Bureau, 2022), and 10.4% of public school students has limited English proficiency (National Center for Education Statistics, 2022).

It is essential that we provide healthcare information in a language understood by the client. Research suggests that the use of interpreter services is associated with shorter perioperative lengths of stay (de Crescenzo et al., 2022) and may reduce diagnostic errors, missed screenings, harmful medication interactions, healthcare-associated infections, adverse birth outcomes, and inappropriate care transitions (Agency for Healthcare Research and Quality, 2019). To assist, the Office of Minority Health (2021) created the National Standards for Culturally and Linguistically Appropriate Services in Health and Health Care (the National CLAS Standards). CLAS require that clients be asked to identify their preferred language for healthcare discussions and

BOX 2-5 Culturally Congruent and Competent Care for Deaf Clients

1. **Cultural Assessment**
   - **Self-Assessment**
     - o What is your attitude toward people who are deaf?
     - o Do you think of people who are deaf as able-bodied or disabled?
     - o How do you feel about those who use hearing aids and other assistive devices for hearing?
     - o How do you assess your self-location with regard to culture, gender, class, age, and other self-identities compared to the client's background?
     - o What do you know about deafness, for example, causes, categories or types, and assistive devices?
     - o Do you know anyone who is deaf?
       - ◻ If so, how do you feel about the interactions you had with this person(s)?

   - **Client Assessment**
     Health History (Subjective Data)—See Appendix A, *Andrews/Boyle Transcultural Nursing Assessment Guide for Individuals and Families,* for questions you might want to pose in the following categories:
     - o Cultural affiliations or self-identities associated with deafness?
     - o Client's preferred method for communication?
       - ◻ Sign language?
       - ◻ Written communication?
       - ◻ Verbal communication?

     - ◻ Are any assistive devices needed for effective communication?
     - ◻ Has exclusion from communication significantly impacted everyday life?
     - o Is there any evidence of feelings of loneliness, isolation, and frustration, particularly for older adults with hearing loss?
     - o Cultural sanctions and restrictions?
     - o Economic or financial concerns?
     - o Adults with hearing loss have a much higher unemployment rate and earn less than counterparts who have hearing. Is the client employed?
     - o Education and health literacy levels?
     - o In resource-limited countries, children with hearing loss and deafness rarely receive any schooling. What is the educational and health literacy level of the client? Improving access to education and vocational rehabilitation services and raising awareness, especially among employers, would decrease unemployment rates among adults with hearing loss.
     - o Health-related beliefs and practices?
     - o Kinship and social support network?
     - o Nutrition and diet?
     - o Religion and spirituality?
     - o Value orientation of the client, including their perspective on culturally acceptable interventions to improve hearing?
   - **Physical Examination (Objective Data)**: See Chapter 3, *Cultural Competence in Health History and Assessment.*

2. **Mutual Goal Setting**
3. **Care Planning**
4. **Implementation of Care Plan**
5. **Evaluation of Care**

In collaboration with client's family; significant others; credentialed, licensed members of the healthcare team (e.g., audiologist, speech-language pathologist); and folk, traditional, religious, and/or spiritual healers

   - Culturally acceptable, congruent, and competent?
   - Affordable?
   - Accessible?
   - Quality?
   - Evidence based?
   - Best practices?

be informed about the availability of assistance in their preferred language. Healthcare organizations and providers that receive federal financial assistance without providing free language assistance services could be in violation of Title VI of the Civil Rights Act of 1964 and its implementation regulations. Additional details on CLAS Standards are presented in Chapter 9.

Summary

In this chapter, the reader was introduced to individual cultural competence and provided with the knowledge and skills needed to deliver culturally congruent and competent nursing care to individual clients from diverse cultures. Nurses are encouraged to think about the delivery of care as a five-step process consisting of:

1. Self-assessment of the nurse's own attitudes, knowledge, and skills and a cultural assessment of clients from diverse backgrounds by gathering subjective and objective data using the health history and physical examination
2. Mutual goal setting in collaboration with the client and other members of the interprofessional healthcare team (family, significant others, credentialed, licensed, folk, traditional, religious, and/or spiritual healers)
3. Development of the plan of care in collaboration with the client and support systems
4. Implementation of the care plan in collaboration with the client and support systems
5. Evaluation of the plan for client acceptance, cultural congruence, affordability, accessibility, and use of research and other evidence

When necessary, the steps in the process are repeated. Interprofessional collaboration with the client and members of the healthcare team is integral to the provision of culturally congruent and competent nursing care. Lastly, we examined clients with special needs including those at high risk for health disparities, those who are deaf, and those with communication and language needs.

REVIEW QUESTIONS

1. Explain the importance of developing and continuing to enhance cultural competence as a nurse.
2. Describe the five steps in the process for delivering culturally congruent and competent care for clients from diverse backgrounds.
3. In your own words, define the following terms: cultural baggage, cultural imposition, ethnocentrism, implicit bias, prejudice, microaggression, and discrimination.
4. Identify key strategies to assist clients with communication and language needs.

CRITICAL THINKING ACTIVITIES

1. After critically analyzing the definitions of cultural competence presented in the chapter, craft a definition of the term in your own words.

2. In discussions of culturally competent nursing care, the culture of the deaf and hard-of-hearing is sometimes overlooked because it is categorized as a nonethnic culture. Search the internet for information on the culture of the deaf. What cultural characteristics do deaf people have in common with members of other cultural groups? If a client is both deaf and self-identifies as a member of another ethnic or nonethnic culture, how does this influence your ability to deliver culturally congruent and culturally competent nursing care?

3. To provide culturally competent nursing care, you should engage in a cultural self-assessment. Answer the questions in Box 2-1: How Do You Relate to Various Groups of People in Society? Score your answers using the guide provided. What did you learn about yourself? How would you approach learning more about the health-related beliefs and practices of groups for which you need more

background knowledge? What resources might you use in your search for information?

4. At the request of the Bureau of Primary Health Care, Health Resources and Services Administration, U.S. Department of Health and Human Services, staff at the National Center for Cultural Competence (NCCC) developed the *Cultural Competence Health Practitioner Assessment* (available online at https://multiculturalmentalhealth.ca/training/self-assessment/#:~:text=The%20Cultural%20Competence%20Health%20Practitioner%20Assessment%20%28CCHPA%29%20is,skill%20level%20for%20each%20of%20the%20six%20subscales). Visit the NCCC website and complete this assessment.

5. Mary Johnson is a new graduate nurse working in the postanesthesia care unit (PACU). When Mrs. Li, a recent immigrant from China, arrives in the PACU following a major bowel resection for cancer, Mary assesses Mrs. Li for pain. Mary notes that Mrs. Li is not complaining about pain, is lying quietly in her bed, and has a stoic facial expression. Mary comments to another nurse that "all Chinese patients seem to do just fine without postoperative pain medications. I'm not going to administer any analgesics unless she asks me for something." Do you agree with Nurse Johnson's assessment of Mrs. Li's pain? What nonverbal manifestations of pain would you assess? How would you reply to Nurse Johnson's statement that she doesn't intend to administer any pain medication?

REFERENCES

Agency for Healthcare Research and Quality. (2022). *2021 National Healthcare Quality and Disparities Report.* https://www.ahrq.gov/research/findings/nhqrdr/nhqdr21/index.html

Agency for Healthcare Research and Quality. (2019). *Cultural competence and patient safety.* https://psnet.ahrq.gov/perspective/cultural-competence-and-patient-safety

American Medical Association. (2023). https://www.ama-assn.org/

American Psychological Association. (2023). *Fact sheet: Health disparities and stress.* https://www.apa.org/topics/racism-bias-discrimination/health-disparities-stress

Andrews, M. M., & Boyle, J. S. (2019). The Andrews/Boyle Transcultural Interprofessional Practice (TIP) model. *Journal of Transcultural Nursing, 30*(4), 323–303.

Centers for Disease Control. (n.d.) *Cultural and diversity considerations.* https://view.officeapps.live.com/op/view.aspx?src=https%3A%2F%2Fwww.cdc.gov%2Ftb%2Feducation%2Fskillscourse%2Fday2%2Fcultural_and_diversity_considerations%2Fday-2-cultural-and-diversity-considerations_final.pptx&wdOrigin=BROWSELINK

Centers for Disease Control and Prevention. (2021). *Cultural competence in health and human services.* https://npin.cdc.gov/pages/cultural-competence

de Crescenzo, C., Chen, Y-W., Adler, J., Zorigtbaatar, A., Kirwan, C., Maurer, L. R., Chang, D. C., & Heidi, Y. (2022). Increasing frequency of interpreting services is associated with shorter peri-operative length of stay. *Journal of Surgical Research, 270*, 178–186.

Douglas, M. K. (2018). Building an organizational environment of cultural competence. In M. K. Douglas, D. F. Pacquiao, & L. Prunell (Eds.), *Global applications of culturally competent health care: Guidelines for practice* (pp. 203–313). Springer International Publishing.

Douglas, M. K., Pacquiao, D. F., & Purnell, L. (2018). *Global applications of culturally competent health care: Guidelines for practice.* Springer International Publishing.

Edgoose, J., Quigue, M., & Sidhar, K. (2019). How to identify, understand, and unlearn implicit bias in patient care. *Family Practice Management, 26*(4), 29–33.

Foronda, C. (2020). A theory of cultural humility. *Journal of Transcultural Nursing, 31*(1), 7–12. https://doi.org/10.1177/1043659619875184

Harrington, T. (2016). *Sign language: Ranking and number of users.* Gallaudet University. http://libguides.gallaudet.edu/content.php?pid=114804&sid=991835

Kamarak, E., & Stenglein, C. (2019). *How many undocumented immigrants are in the United States and who are they?* Brookings. https://www.brookings.edu/policy2020/votervital/how-many-undocumented-immigrants-are-in-the-united-states-and-who-are-they/#:~:text=Estimates%20of%20the%20number%20of%20undocumented%20immigrants%20living,to%20less%20than%20half%20of%20the%20undocumented%20population

Kroeber, A. L. (2018). *Culture: A critical review of concepts and definitions.* Forgotten Books. http://www.forgottenbooks.com

Leigh, I. W., & Andrews, J. F. (2017). *Deaf people and society: Psychological, sociological and educational perspectives* (2nd ed.). Routledge.

Mandal, A. (2018). *What are health disparities?* News-Medical. https://www.news-medical.net/health/What-are-Health-Disparities.aspx

McFarland, M. R., & Wehbe-Alamah, H. B. (2018). *Transcultural nursing: Concepts, theories, research, and practices* (4th ed.). McGraw-Hill, Medical Publishing Division.

Montgomery, M. (2019). *Language, media, and culture: The key concepts*. Routledge.

Moss, E., Seifert, C. P., & O'Sullivan, A. (2016). Registered nurses as interprofessional collaborative partners: Creating value-based outcomes. *The Online Journal of Issues in Nursing, 21*(3), 4. https://doi.org/10.3912/OJIN.Vol21No03Man04

National Academies of Sciences, Engineering, and Medicine. (2021). *The future of nursing 2020-2030: Charting a path to achieve health equity*. The National Academies Press. https://doi.org10.17226/25982

National Center for Education Statistics. (2022). English learners in public schools. *Condition of education*. https://nces.ed.gov/programs/coe/indicator/cgf.

National Institute on Deafness and Other Communication Disorders. (2018). *Age-related hearing loss*. https://www.nidcd.nih.gov/health/age-related-hearing-loss

Pacquiao, D. F., & Douglas, M. (2019). *Social pathways to health vulnerability: Implications for health professionals*. Springer International Publishing AG, part of Springer Nature.

Psychology Today. (n.d.) *Microaggression*. https://www.psychologytoday.com/us/basics/microaggression

Purnell, L., & Fenkl, E. (2018). *Guide to culturally competent health care*. F.A. Davis.

Sharifi, N., Adib-Hajbaghery, M., & Najafi, M. (2019). Cultural competence in nursing: A concept analysis. *International Journal of Nursing Studies, 99*:103386. doi:10.1016/j.ijnurstu.2019.103386.

Title VII of the Civil Rights Act of 1964 (Public Law 88–352). http://www.eeoc.gov/laws/statutes/ada.cfmwww.eeoc.gov/laws/statutes/titlevii.cfm

Titles I and V of the Americans with Disabilities Act of 1990 (Pub. L. 101–336) (ADA). http://www.eeoc.gov/laws/statutes/ada.cfm

U.S. Census Bureau. (2023). *Measuring America's people, places, and economy*. https://www.census.gov/

U.S. Census Bureau. (2022). *Nearly 68 million people spoke a language other than English at home in 2019*. https://www.census.gov/library/stories/2022/12/languages-we-speak-in-united-states.html

U.S. Department of Health and Human Services, Centers for Disease Control and Prevention. (2023). *Social determinants of health*. https://www.cdc.gov/publichealthgateway/sdoh/index.html

U.S. Department of Health and Human Services, Health Resources and Services Administration, Office of Health Equity. (2020). *Health Equity Report 2019-2020: Special Feature on Housing and Health Inequalities*. https://www.hrsa.gov/sites/default/files/hrsa/about/organization/bureaus/ohe/hrsa-health-equity-report.pdf

U.S. Department of Health and Human Service, Office of Minority Health. (2021). *Think cultural health: The national CLAS standards*. https://minorityhealth.hhs.gov/omh/browse.aspx?lvl=2&lvlid=53

World Health Organization. (2021). *Health Equity*. https://www.who.int/health-topics/health-equity#tab=tab_1

World Health Organization. (2018a). *Social determinants of health: key concepts*. http://www.who.int/social_determinants/thecommission/finalreport/key_concepts/en/

World Health Organization. (2018b). *Deafness and hearing loss*. http://www.who.int/news-room/fact-sheets/detail/deafness-and-hearing-loss

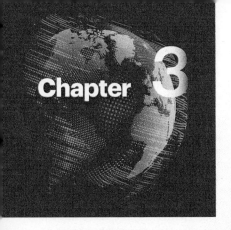

Chapter 3

Cultural Competence in Health History and Assessment

• Julia L. Rogers and Margaret M. Andrews

Key Terms

Addison disease
Albinism
Clinical decision-making
Congenital dermal
    melanocytosis
Cultural assessment
Cultural care accommodation
    or negotiation
Cultural care preservation or
    maintenance
Cultural care repatterning or
    restructuring

Cultural competence
Cultural humility
Cultural norms
Cyanosis
Diversity
Ecchymoses
Epigenetics
Equity
Erythema
Ethnohistory
Evaluation
Genetics
Genome

Genomics
Jaundice
Oral hyperpigmentation
Pain
Pallor
Petechiae
Pharmacogenomics
Presbycusis
Social determinants of health
Uremia
Vitiligo

Learning Objectives

1. Explore the process and content needed for a culturally competent health assessment of clients.
2. Identify the impact of social determinants of health on health and illness.
3. Integrate genetic and genomic components associated with perpetuating health disparities when presented from a racial or cultural lens.
4. Critically review transcultural perspectives in the health history and physical examination.

Introduction

In this chapter, we provide information for nurses to customize and tailor health assessments for all clients. A definition and description of the cultural assessment is provided. Transcultural perspectives on the health history, the physical examination, clinical decision-making, and interventions are described.

An individual's health history includes reason for seeking care, biographic and genetic data, medications, history of present illness, past health, family and social history, cultural perspectives, and the five **social determinants of health**: environment, education access, access to quality healthcare, economics, and social and community context. After conducting a thorough health history, a physical assessment is completed.

The health history and physical examination are interconnected and interrelated. For example, the nurse may hear audible wheezing as the client verbally reports having increased shortness of breath during the history of illness. The nurse gathers additional data during the physical examination by first inspecting the client for clinical manifestations of cyanosis, nasal flaring, and intercostal retraction; palpating for symmetry, synchrony, and volume of each breath; auscultating for adventitious sounds; and percussing to determine resonance. Based on the findings of the physical examination, the nurse might ask additional questions, such as the length of time the client has experienced the symptoms and family history of respiratory disease. The nurse may pursue additional assessment related to the respiratory and cardiovascular systems.

In the physical examination, the nurse compares and contrasts typical and atypical variations, general appearance, skin, sweat glands, head (hair, eyes, ears, nose, mouth), mammary plexus, and the musculoskeletal system. Lastly, transcultural perspectives in **clinical decision-making** and interventions are explored. After completing a comprehensive cultural assessment through the health history, physical examination, and analysis of laboratory test results, the next steps are to analyze the information, set mutual goals with the client, develop a mutually accepted plan of care, confer with and make referrals to other members of the interprofessional healthcare team as needed, and implement a comprehensive healthcare plan.

Cultural Assessment

With more than 334 million people, the United States is the third most populous nation in the world, behind China and India (U.S. Census Bureau, 2020b). The U.S. population is more diverse than ever before. The 2017 U.S. National Population Projections explored changes in the age, race, and ethnic composition of the population. By the year 2050, it is estimated that nearly 50% of the U.S. population will be composed of people from diverse backgrounds. Hispanic and Asian populations are expected to double between now and 2050 and are followed in growth by Black Americans, Native Americans, Native Hawaiians, and other Pacific Islanders (U.S. Census Bureau, 2017). The population of people who are two or more races is projected to be the fastest-growing group over the next several decades, growing by 200% by 2060 (Vespa et al., 2020). With this growing **diversity** comes the need for nurses to be culturally competent and develop knowledge and skills in cultural assessment. During their professional careers, nurses will need the skill set to assess clients and families with cultural humility to ensure an empowering and inclusive environment. Other diversities include age, biology, disability status, sex, gender identity, geographical, language, religious, sexual orientation, spiritual, socioeconomic status, and other sociological characteristics.

Cultural assessment, or *culturologic assessment*, refers to a systematic, comprehensive examination of individuals, families, groups, and communities regarding their health-related cultural beliefs, values, and practices. Although the focus in this chapter is on the individual client, there are some instances in which clients' families and others in close contact may need to be involved, for example, when the cultural assessment reveals the presence of a genetic, infectious, or communicable disorder. Cultural assessments form the foundation for the clients' plan of care, providing valuable data for setting mutual goals, planning care, intervening, and evaluating the care. The goal of the cultural assessment is to determine the nursing and healthcare needs of people and intervene in ways that are culturally acceptable, congruent, safe, affordable, accessible, high quality, and based on current research, evidence, and best practices (McFarland & Wehbe-Alamah, 2018). Campinha-Bacote (2018) coined the term *cultural competemility* to describe the synergistic relationship between cultural competence and cultural humility. **Cultural competence** includes five components: cultural awareness, cultural skills, cultural knowledge, cultural encounter, and cultural desire, all of which are infused through **cultural humility** (Campinha-Bacote, 2013; O'Brien et al., 2021; Prosen, 2015; Repo et al., 2017).

Cultural assessments tend to be broad and comprehensive, given that they deal with cultural values, belief systems, and lifeways. It is sometimes necessary to conduct an abbreviated assessment when time is limited, the client's reason for seeking care is urgent or time sensitive, the client is unable to provide all the necessary data, or other circumstances require a shorter, more focused assessment. The cultural assessment consists of both *process* and *content*. *Process* refers to how to approach the client, consideration of verbal and nonverbal communication, and the sequence and order in which data are gathered. The *content* of the cultural assessment consists of the actual data categories in which information about clients is gathered. Nurses are required to complete assessments before and/or at the time of admission to healthcare facilities, when opening home healthcare cases, and prior to many types of medical and surgical procedures. Depending on the circumstances, assessments may be very brief, or they may be detailed and in-depth. Ideally, the cultural assessment is integrated into the overall

assessment of the client, family, and significant others. It is usually impractical to expect that nurses will have the time to conduct a separate cultural assessment, so questions aimed at gathering cultural data should be integrated into the overall assessment using the format provided by healthcare facilities, agencies, or organization for their admissions or intake assessment.

Appendix A is the Andrews and Boyle Transcultural Nursing Assessment Guide for Individuals and Families for use when initially assessing clients, for example, when conducting an admission assessment or opening a case in home healthcare or ambulatory settings. The major categories in this guide include cultural affiliations, values orientation, communication, health-related beliefs and practices, nutrition, socioeconomic considerations, organizations providing cultural support, education, religion, cultural aspects of disease incidence, genetic variations, and developmental considerations across the lifespan. Appendix B is the Andrews and Boyle Transcultural Nursing Assessment Guide for Groups and Communities. The major categories in this guide include family and kinship systems, social life and networks, political or government systems, language and traditions, worldview, values, norms, religious beliefs and practices, health beliefs and practices, and healthcare systems.

Transcultural Perspectives on the Health History

The purpose of the health history is to gather *subjective data*—a term that refers to information provided by the primary source such as the client or family of the client. The health history provides a comprehensive overview of a client's past and present health, and it examines the manner in which the person interacts with the environment. The health history enables the nurse to assess health strengths, including cultural beliefs and practices that might influence the nurse's ability to provide culturally competent nursing care. The history is combined with the *objective data*—a term that refers to measurable data. The objective data are derived from the physical examination and the laboratory results. The subjective and objective data gathered are used to form a diagnosis about the health status of a person.

For the well client, the history is used to assess lifestyle, which includes activity, exercise, diet, and related personal behaviors and choices that nurses may gather to identify potential risk factors for disease. The history should include an assessment of social determinants of health by asking about the client's environment, education access, access to quality healthcare, economics, and social and community context. For the ill client, the health history includes a chronologic record of the health problem(s). For both well and ill clients, the health history is a screening tool for abnormal symptoms, health problems, and concerns. The health history also provides valuable information about the social determinants of the client's health, coping strategies, and health-related behaviors and responses used previously by clients and family members.

In many healthcare settings, the client is expected to fill out a printed history form or checklist. From a transcultural perspective, this approach has both positive and negative aspects. On the positive side, this approach provides the client with ample time to recall details such as relevant family history and the dates of health-related events such as surgical procedures and illnesses. It is expedient for nurses because it takes less time to review a form or a checklist than to elicit the information in a face-to-face or telephone interview.

However, this approach has limitations. First, the form is likely to be in English. Those whose primary language is not English might find the form difficult or impossible to complete accurately. Although some healthcare facilities provide forms translated into Spanish, French, or other languages, translating forms can be costly and is not always effective. In some instances, the literal translation of medical terms is not possible. Slightly over 8% of the U.S. population has a non-English language preference (U.S. Census Bureau, 2020a). In some instances, clients might be unable

to read or write in any language; thus, an assessment of the client's literacy level should precede the use of printed history forms or checklists. During the history intake, the nurse should ask what language the individual is most comfortable speaking and reading (Tosun et al., 2021).

In other instances, the symptom or disease is not recognized in the culture with which the client identifies. For example, in asking about symptoms of depression, there might be many factors that influence the client's interpretation of the question. If healthcare providers fail to understand the cultural meaning of the symptoms, unnecessary, invasive, and costly tests might be performed to rule out disease.

Although there is wide variation in health history formats, most contain the following categories: *biographic data, reason for seeking care, review of medications and allergies, past history, present health or history of present illness, family and social history,* and *review of systems. Genetic data* are also important for the transcultural nurse to consider as part of the health history. This chapter will not provide a comprehensive overview of these categories but will present them as they relate to providing culturally congruent and culturally competent nursing care.

Biographic Data

Although the biographic information (e.g., name, address, phone, age, gender, preferred language) might seem straightforward, several cultural variations in recording age are important to note. Having an accurate age has many clinical implications, including assessing developmental milestones and determining appropriate medication dosages, and certain legal implications as well. For many reasons, age may not be reported correctly. Some clients may not wish to report their correct age; other clients may not know or be able to provide a specific age in the way healthcare providers may expect it.

Documenting the appropriate gender is imperative to be inclusive of clients who are not cisgender. A client's assigned sex at birth may be different from current gender identity; therefore, both must be documented so the nurse can assess and deliver appropriate care to the client (Thompson et al., 2021). Data on sex assigned at birth are also useful for clinical decision-making.

Other areas that nurses should assess are the client's self-reported cultural affiliation and ancestry or **ethnohistory**. Knowledge of the client's ethnohistory is important in determining risk factors for genetic and acquired diseases and in understanding the client's cultural heritage. In addition to the standard descriptive information about clients, it is necessary to record who has furnished the data. Though this is usually the client, the source might also be a relative, guardian, or friend. Documentation should include whether an interpreter is used and indicate the interpreter's relationship to the client.

Genetic Data

Genetics is a branch of biology that studies heredity and the variations of inherited characteristics. This area continues to be a rapidly evolving science; genetics exerts a significant influence on the health of people from cultures around the world. Whereas genetics scrutinizes the functioning and composition of a specific gene, **genomics** addresses all genes and their interrelationship to identify their combined influence on the growth and development of the organism. The Human Genome Project, which concluded in 2003, revealed there are around 20,500 human genes, which is a surprising revelation as it was once estimated there were more than 50,000 human genes. An error in one of these genes can potentially lead to a recognizable genetic disease in a human (National Institute of Health, 2022a; Rogers, 2023). A **genome** is an organism's complete set of DNA, including all of its genes. Each genome contains all of the information needed to build and maintain that organism. In humans, a copy of the entire genome—more than three billion DNA base pairs—is contained in all cells that have a nucleus. Genetic mapping is continuing at a rapid rate, and these numbers and discoveries

are constantly being updated. **Epigenetics** is the study of how genes are influenced by forces such as the environment, obesity, or medication. For example, although the children in Figure 3-1 are twins, epigenetic modifications can cause individuals with the same DNA sequences to have different disease profiles (Rogers, 2023). As a result of epigenetic research, the critical role played by external forces is better understood and can now be integrated into client assessment and care. Previously, it was believed that health disparities were only linked to genetics, diet, and exercise. It is now understood that biases based on race, ethnicity, culture, or social determinants of health can have serious ramifications on a person's health and outcome. There is considerable evidence now that chronic stress from living with poverty and discrimination damages the body on a cellular level, leading to serious health problems over time. The term often used for this stress is "weathering." Geronimus, who coined the term,

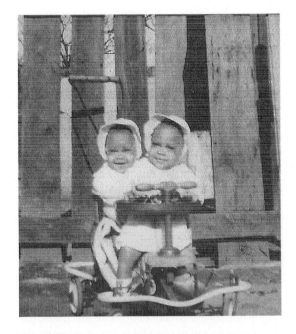

Figure 3-1. Due to diet, environment, and lifestyle, these identical twins have different disease profiles as they have matured into adulthood; however, both became registered nurses and nursing faculty.

reports weathering as wearing down the body's systems. It is not just about race, ethnicity, and culture, but how social and economic stressors are linked to biologic changes that cause disease (Geronimus, 2023).

While each person has approximately 20,500 genes, any two individuals share 99.9% of their DNA sequence, reflecting that the diversity among individuals accounts for approximately 0.1% of the DNA (National Institute of Health, 2022a, b; Rogers, 2023). Although humans are more alike than different, the growing inventory of human genetic variation helps explain why susceptibility to common diseases differs among individual clients and populations. It is not inherent differences but the combinations of multiple genetic variants and epigenetics that influence disease susceptibility, disease course, and response to treatment including response to certain medications (Rogers, 2023). These genetic variations provide the knowledge that healthcare professionals need to safely administer medications and counsel clients regarding the risk and prevention of disease. This discussion provides a foundation in genetic and genomic science to ensure that the nursing assessment is customized according to each client's unique background and current care needs.

Certain diseases affect different groups of people at different rates, resulting in some clients being considered at higher risk than others for these diseases. A complex interplay of environmental and genetic factors determines a person's risk for any given disease. Health disparities do not cause a person's risk. Instead, the environmental factors lead to the health disparities. The addition of genetics and genomics to the traditional nursing assessment will inform and engage clients to make key decisions in their personal healthcare plan. Nurses should consider how the client will use genetic and genomic information along with potential racial, ethnic, and cultural factors to provide support if clients experience moral or ethical issues. Most hospitals have ethics committees, chaplains, pastoral teams, and other resources to assist clients facing religious, moral, and ethical dilemmas.

The nurse should avoid oversimplifying the relationship between race/ethnicity and genetics when communicating with clients and their families. Knowledge of ethnicity might prompt genetic testing or detailed family history taking in particular instances; however, the issues are often too complex for the nurse to make unqualified assertions to clients that they are "at risk" for a particular illness or unlikely to respond to therapies solely on the basis of their racial/ethnic background. In most instances, the full interprofessional healthcare team will be the best catalyst for client information and interventions.

The client's genetic makeup results in distinctive patterns of drug absorption, metabolism, excretion, and effectiveness. Knowledge of clients' individual genotypes guides pharmacologic treatment and allows customization of choice of drug and dosage to ensure a therapeutic response and avoid toxicity (Duarte & Cavallari, 2021). For example, Evidence-Based Practice 3-1 describes genetically linked differences that occur in the conversion of codeine to morphine for analgesia. Human genetic information is accumulating at a rapid pace, and almost 7,000 diseases can now be diagnosed by testing for specific mutations (National Center for Biotechnology Information, 2022; Rogers, 2023). Pharmacogenetics (PGx), the study of the role of inherited and acquired genetic variation in drug response, is an evolving field that facilitates the identification of biomarkers that can help health providers optimize drug selection, dose, and treatment duration as well as eliminate adverse drug reactions. If a genotype can be linked to disease outcomes, then this seems to be a way to personalize medical therapy and remove race as factor in treatment decisions. However, **pharmacogenomics** research continues to use race to stratify genetic risk because assumptions are made that categorize a race as having a higher prevalence of specific genes. Race is then used as measure in diagnosis and treatment of disease processes. Specialty areas of nephrology, cardiology, urology, and obstetrics often use "corrected" values for labs, risk scores, and physiologic calculations based on race (Goodman & Brett, 2021).

Variations in the Conversion of Codeine to Morphine for Analgesia

Pharmacogenomics can improve pain management by considering variations in pain perception, susceptibility to medications, and sensitivities to medicines related to genetic diversity. The CYP2D6 enzyme is an important gene in pharmacogenomics because CYP2D6 catalyzes the metabolism of a large number of clinically important drugs, including antidepressants, neuroleptics, antiarrhythmics, β-blockers, and opioids. In fact, CYP2D6 is responsible for the metabolism and elimination of approximately 25% of clinically used drugs. CYP2D6 is primarily expressed in the liver, therefore any medications that are metabolized in the liver may not be absorbed or able to break down if an individual is more susceptible or sensitive to a medication. The major determinant of CYP2D6 activity and expression in liver is genetics.

There is considerable variation in the efficiency and amount of CYP2D6 enzyme produced by individuals from different backgrounds. For drugs that are metabolized by CYP2D6, certain individuals eliminate the drugs quickly (ultrarapid metabolizers), while others eliminate them slowly. If a drug is metabolized too quickly, it may decrease the drug's efficacy. If the drug is metabolized too slowly, toxicity may result. CYP2D6 catalyzes the conversion of codeine to morphine. In some individuals, an active form of the CYP2D6 enzyme, which is necessary to convert codeine into its active metabolite, morphine, is missing. These individuals experience the side effects of morphine without pain relief. The reduced sensitivity to morphine may be due to decreased production of morphine-6-glucuronide.

Clinical Implications

Healthcare providers need to consider the possibility of metabolic genetic variations in any client who experiences toxicity or does not receive adequate analgesia from codeine or other opioid drugs (e.g., hydrocodone and oxycodone). It is important to observe clients for the following signs of toxicity:

- Bluish-colored fingernails and lips
- Slow and labored breathing, shallow breathing, and no breathing
- Cold, clammy skin
- Coma (decreased level of consciousness and lack of responsiveness)
- Confusion
- Dizziness
- Drowsiness
- Fatigue
- Light-headedness
- Low blood pressure
- Muscle twitches
- Pinpoint pupils
- Spasms of the stomach and intestines
- Weakness
- Weak pulse

Improved treatment regimens that factor in pharmacogenetic differences in patients may reduce the risk of opioid dependency and effectively treat pain.

References: Chaturvedi, R., Alexander, B., & A'Court, A. M. (2020). Genomics testing and personalized medicine in the preoperative setting: Can it change outcomes in postoperative pain management? *Best Practice and Research Clinical Anaesthesiology*, 34, 283–295; Cornett, E. M., Carroll, Turpin M. A., & Pinner, A. (2020) Pharmacogenomics of pain management: the impact of specific biological polymorphisms on drugs and metabolism. *Current Oncology Reports*, 22, 18; Dean, L., & Kane, M. (2012). Codeine therapy and CYP2D6 genotype. In Pratt, V. M., Scott, S. A., & Pirmohamed, M. (Eds.), *Pharmacogenomics in drug discovery and development: Methods in molecular biology* (Vol. 2547). Humana; Kaye, A. D., Garcia, A. J., & Hall, O. M. (2019). Update on the pharmacogenomics of pain management. *Pharmacogenomics and Personalized Medicine*, 12, 125–143; Sachtleben, E. P., Rooney, K., Haddad, H., Lassiegne, V. L., & Boudreaux, M. (2022). The role of pharmacogenomics in postoperative pain management. In Q. Yan (Ed.), *Pharmacogenomics in drug discovery and development. Methods in molecular biology* (Vol. 2547). Humana. https://doi.org/10.1007/978-1-0716-2573-6_18; Stoker, A. D., Rosenfeld, D. M., & Buras, M. R. (2019). Evaluation of clinical factors associated with adverse drug events in patients receiving sub-anesthetic ketamine infusions. *Journal of Pain Research 12*, 3413–3421; Tirona, R. G., & Kim, R. B. (2017). Introduction to clinical pharmacology. In D. Robertson & G. H. Williams (Eds.), *Clinical and translational science* (2nd ed., pp. 365–388). Elsevier.

This is seen in several clinical guidelines as well as recommendations for genetic screening prior to using certain drugs from the Food and Drug Administration (FDA). However, this reflects a flawed system. Embedding race into the basic data and decisions of healthcare propagates race-based medicine. Many race-adjusted algorithms guide decisions in ways that may direct more attention or resources away from members of racial and ethnic minorities (Vyas et al., 2020).

The following genetic screenings may be useful to clients, nurses, and other members of the healthcare team:

- *Drug efficacy or sensitivity*: Researchers have identified the HLA-B1502 allele that is associated with hypersensitivity reactions (toxic epidermal necrolysis and Stevens-Johnson syndrome) to the anticonvulsant and mood-stabilizing drug carbamazepine (Tegretol) in people of Asian descent (U.S. Food and Drug Administration, 2022). For other drugs such as warfarin (Coumadin) and clopidogrel (Plavix), genetic testing for variants in specific genes may be warranted to help guide the drug dosage.
- *Carrier screening*: Genetic tests can identify heterozygous carriers for many recessive diseases such as cystic fibrosis, sickle cell disease, and Tay-Sachs disease. A couple may wish to undergo carrier screening to help make reproductive decisions, especially in populations where specific diseases are relatively common, for example, Tay-Sachs disease in Ashkenazi Jewish populations and beta-thalassemia in Mediterranean populations.
- *Prenatal diagnostic tests*: Genetic testing is individualized and may be requested by parents-to-be or a healthcare provider based on medical and family history. Single gene tests look for changes in only one gene and is also used when there is a known genetic mutation in a family that causes a specific condition such as Duchenne muscular dystrophy or sickle cell disease. A panel genetic test is done to look for changes in multiple

genes and large-scale genetic or genomic testing looks at genes and DNA related to medical conditions (Centers for Disease Control and Prevention, 2022a; March of Dimes, 2020; National Center for Biotechnology Information, 2022; U.S. Department of Health and Human Services, 2023).

- *Cancer screening*: At nearly 50%, cancer is the largest therapeutic area of new FDA pharmacogenomics approvals. Among noncancer drugs, the average proportion of approved pharmacogenomics for other body systems was around 5% (neurology 9%; infectious disease 7.9%; psychiatry 5.6%; cardiology 4.5%; pulmonology and hematology 3.9% each, and gynecology, rheumatology, and urology near 2% each).

Review of Medications and Allergies

The review of medications includes all current prescription, over-the-counter, and home remedies, including herbs that a client might purchase or grow in a home garden. During the health history, document the name, dose, route of administration, schedule, frequency, purpose, and length of time that each medicine has been taken. Because of individual differences in clients' perceptions of what substances are considered medicines, it is important to ask about specific items by name. Inquire about vitamins, birth control pills, aspirin, antacids, herbs, teas, inhalants, poultices, vaginal and rectal suppositories, ointments, essential oils, and any other items taken by the client for therapeutic purposes. Be sure to gather data on the client's allergies to medicines and foods.

Table 3-1 provides an overview of commonly used herbs, their sources, uses, dosage, and warnings, such as contraindications (e.g., pregnancy, childhood, people with compromised immune systems) and interactions with prescription drugs. Many of the active ingredients in herbs or plant-derived drugs are unknown. These herbs and plant-derived drugs remain largely unregulated by government agencies, except for customs officials

Table 3-1 | Herbal Remedies

Aloe vera (Aloe vera, Aloe barbadensis, Aloe capensis)

Source	Leaf of *Aloe barbadensis*
Action	Topical analgesic, anti-inflammatory, antioxidant, and antifungal agent
Traditional uses	Applied as topical ointment for treatment of inflammation, minor burns, sunburn, cuts, bruises, and abrasions; administered orally as a laxative
Current uses	Promotes wound healing in soft tissue injuries and is used as a folk or traditional remedy for diabetes, asthma, epilepsy, and osteoarthritis *Aloe vera* gel, contained in the leaves of the plant, is found in skin products such as lotions and sunblocks Prevents wound pain by inhibiting the action of the pain-producing agent bradykinin
Dosage	Apply topically as needed; the FDA ruled that aloe is not safe as a stimulant laxative
Warnings	Pregnant people should avoid consumption of aloe vera Rarely, skin rash follows topical application Can cause hypokalemia, thyroid dysfunction, acute hepatitis, diarrhea, and abdominal cramps when taken orally and can decrease the absorption of many drugs

Chamomile (Matricaria recutita, Chamomilla recutita, Matricaria chamomilla)

Source	Aromatic herb
Action	Anti-inflammatory
Traditional uses	Used in ancient Egyptian and Greek medicine by crushing chamomile flowers to treat erythema and xerosis of the skin caused by harsh weather
Current uses	Stress, insomnia, anxiety, depression, glycemic control, muscle spasms, menstrual disorders, GI disorders, wounds, mucositis
Dosage	Used as a tea, made into topical creams, gels, or oils. Oral capsules
Warnings	Contraindicated in people who are allergic to ragweed, chrysanthemums, or members of the Compositae family and who have mugwort pollen allergies. May cause increased bleeding risk, hypersensitivity reactions including asthma, contact dermatitis, and anaphylaxis

Coenzyme Q10 (CoQ10) (2,3 dimethoxy-5 methyl-6-decaprenyl benzoquinone)

Source	Chemical made by the cells in the human body
Action	Antioxidant: cellular respiration and energy production
Traditional uses	CoQ10 has only been approved to use since 1976, initially in Japan, for heart failure
Current uses	Heart disease (coronary artery disease, congestive heart failure), hyperlipidemia, statin-induced myalgia, migraine prevention, Parkinson disease, and infertility
Dosage	Available in capsules, chewable tablets, liquid syrups, wafers, and IV
Warnings	Antagonizes effects of warfarin, increasing risk of blood clot, however it may also increase risk of bleeding when used with blood thinners. Safety during pregnancy and breast-feeding has not been established. Reduces effects of radiation therapy. Gastrointestinal side effects of abdominal pain, nausea, vomiting, diarrhea, loss of appetite, and insomnia

Echinacea (Echinacea angustifolia, E. pallida, E. purpurea)

Source	Member of the sunflower family, also known as purple coneflower
Action	Immunostimulant; Reduces cold symptoms
Traditional uses	Used to treat wounds and skin problems, such as acne or boils

Table 3-1	Herbal Remedies (continued)	

Current uses	Enhances the immune system to fight infection and to treat colds, rhinoviruses, upper respiratory infections, influenza, and wound healing. The parts of the plant above ground are used to make teas, juice, or extracts
Dosage	Follow directions on label, needed at onset of symptoms, usually taken for no longer than 2 weeks
Warnings	Contraindicated for pregnant or breast-feeding people, children, and those who are allergic to plants in the sunflower family, including ragweed, chrysanthemums, marigolds, and daisies. Not recommended for people with severely compromised immune systems such as those with cancer undergoing chemotherapy, HIV/AIDS, tuberculosis, or multiple sclerosis

Evening primrose oil (Oenothera biennis)

Source	Seeds of the wildflower evening primrose
Action	Anti-inflammatory, hypocholesterolemia effects, antihypertensive, immunostimulant, weight reduction
Traditional uses	Native to North and South America used as a folk remedy to treat eczema since the 1930s
Current uses	Believed to help inflammation, PMS, diabetes, eczema, fatigue, diabetic neuropathy, and rheumatoid arthritis
Dosage	Follow directions on label; will take at least 1 month to experience benefits
Warnings	Side effects include occasional reports of headache, nausea, and abdominal discomfort; not recommended for children or during pregnancy Some capsules may be altered with other types of oil such as soy or safflower

Feverfew (Tanacetum parthenium)

Source	Plant belonging to the daisy/sunflower family
Action	Parthenolide, a compound in feverfew blocks the formation of inflammatory proteins, preventing migraines
Traditional uses	Ancient Greece physicians used it to decrease fever, inflammation, and menstrual cramps
Current uses	Prevent migraines, arthritis, dysmenorrhea, psoriasis
Dosage	100–300 mg capsules up to four times per day
Warnings	Do not take if allergic to ragweed, chrysanthemums, marigolds, or other members of the Compositae family. Increases risk of bleeding. Side effects include GI upset, rash, mouth ulcerations if chewing fresh feverfew leaves.

Garlic (Allium sativum)

Source	Derived from the bulb or clove of the plant
Action	Antibacterial, antimicrobial, antiplatelet, and antihyperlipidemic activities
Traditional uses	Since 850 B.C. used for medicinal purposes. In many cultures, garlic was administered to provide strength and increase work capacity for laborers. Hippocrates has been documented to prescribe garlic for a variety of conditions. Garlic was given to the original Olympic athletes in Greece, as perhaps one of the earliest performance enhancing medications.
Current uses	Cardiovascular disease, hypercholesterolemia, hypertension, and infections
Dosage	Tablets 2,400 mg extract (liquid) orally daily, or 4 g (1–2 cloves) of raw garlic per day, or 300–2,400 mg daily garlic powder

(continued)

Table 3-1 | Herbal Remedies (continued)

Warnings	Increased bleeding risk, discontinue at least 7 days prior to surgery. May cause viral rebound in HIV, hepatotoxicity, headache, GI upset, diarrhea, hypoglycemia, changes in intestinal flora, and chemical burns of mucosa with consumption of crushed garlic. Interactions can occur with blood thinners, protease inhibitors, insulin, CYP450 substrates, and P-glycoprotein substrates

Ginger (Zingiber officinale)

Source	Native to Asia (China, Japan, India) Herb from the rhizome (underground stem) of the plant
Action	Antinausea, appetite stimulant
Traditional uses	Used in China for more than 2,500 years for medicinal purposes
Current uses	Currently is used to treat postsurgery nausea; nausea caused by motion, chemotherapy, and pregnancy; rheumatoid arthritis; osteoarthritis; and joint and muscle pain; appetite stimulant
Dosage	Boil 1-oz dried ginger root in 1 cup water for 15–20 minutes Follow label directions on ginger supplements
Warnings	Side effects may include increased bleeding and cholagogic effects Not recommended during pregnancy or lactation

Ginkgo (Ginkgo biloba)

Source	Extract from leaves of the ginkgo tree, one of the oldest types of trees in the world; is cultivated worldwide for its medicinal properties
Action	Antioxidant; improves blood circulation
Traditional uses	Used in Traditional Chinese Medicine for asthma, bronchitis, fatigue, circulatory disorders, sexual dysfunctions, and tinnitus
Current uses	Promotes vasodilation and improves memory, attention span, and mood in early stages of Alzheimer disease or dementia by improving oxygen metabolism in the brain; used to treat intermittent claudication, sexual dysfunction, multiple sclerosis, tinnitus, and other health conditions
Dosage	Available in tablets, capsules, teas, and occasionally skin products Follow labels on supplements
Warnings	Side effects may include headaches, diarrhea, nausea and vomiting, dizziness, hyponatremia, and bleeding Some people have reported allergic skin reactions Fresh ginkgo seeds can cause serious adverse reactions—including seizures and death Contraindicated for people who are pregnant or breast-feeding Contraindicated for persons with clotting disorders or those who are about to have surgery Not recommended for children

Ginseng (Panax quinquefolius [American], Panax ginseng [Asian])

Source	Dried root of several species of the genus *Panax* of the family Araliaceae
Action	Tonic
Traditional uses	Treatment of anemia, atherosclerosis, edema, ulcers, hypertension, influenza, colds, inflammation, and disorders of the immune system (American) Treatment of shock, diaphoresis, dyspnea, fever, thirst, irritability, diarrhea, vomiting, abdominal distention, anorexia, and impotence; considered a "heat-raising" tonic for the blood and circulatory system (Asian)

Table 3-1	Herbal Remedies (continued)
Current uses	Used to enhance sexual experience and treat impotence, though there is limited research to support this claim Also used to improve athletic performance, strength, and stamina, as well as to treat diabetes and cancer (American) Used to treat diabetes, cancer, hypertension, and HIV/AIDS and as an immunostimulant or to improve athletic performance (Asian) Improved sense of well-being (Asian)
Dosage	American: Follow directions on label Asian: 100 mg BID
Warnings	American: May cause dry mouth, tachycardia, insomnia, anxiety, breast tenderness, rashes, asthma attacks, and postmenopausal uterine hemorrhage Should be used with caution for the following conditions: pregnancy, insomnia, hay fever, fibrocystic breasts, asthma, emphysema, hypertension, clotting disorders, and diabetes Asian: same as American

Goldenseal (Hydrastis canadenisis)

Source	Derived from the root of the goldenseal plant
Action	Antioxidant
Traditional uses	North American botanical used by Native Americans for skin and eye irritations, fever, as a bitter tonic, and to improve digestive function
Current uses	Digestive disorders, spasms, and infections
Dosage	Capsule or tablet 250 mg–1 g three times daily, or 0.5–1 g dried rhizomes three times daily
Warnings	Contraindicated for pregnant or breast-feeding people; side effects include hypernatremia and photosensitivity; interactions may be seen when used with Metformin, Bosutinib, and CYP450 substrates

Melatonin (N-acetyl-methoxytryptamine)

Source	Produced endogenously in humans by pineal gland
Action	Controls the circadian rhythm and promotes sleep
Traditional uses	Free radical scavenger. Proposed initial function of melatonin was to detoxify free radicals generated during the processes of photosynthesis and metabolism
Current uses	Sleep disorders, insomnia, and jet lag. Helps with shift work disorder, seasonal affective disorder, and migraines. May reduce evening confusion and restlessness in people with Alzheimer disease
Dosage	Oral tablet or capsule 1–5 mg 30 minutes–1 hour before bedtime
Warnings	Do not use if diagnosed with autoimmune disease. Increases risk of bleeding and inhibits anticonvulsants. Increased blood pressure with concomitant nifedipine. Caution when used with diazepam and other CYP450 1A2 substrates. Adverse reactions include drowsiness, disorientation, tachycardia, pruritus, headache, dizziness, nausea, and hypothermia.

St. John's wort (Hypericum perforatum)

Source	Tea made from the leaves and flowering tops of the perennial *H. perforatum*, which is particularly abundant in late June, the feast of St. John the Baptist
Action	Antidepressant

(continued)

Table 3-1	Herbal Remedies (continued)
Traditional uses	Used first in ancient Greece and historically to treat insomnia, depression, lung and kidney ailments, mental disorders, and nerve pain. Also used to treat malaria, as a sedative, and topically for wounds, burns, and insect bites Also used by Native Americans to treat wounds, snakebites, and diarrhea
Current uses	Treatment of mild to moderate depression, anxiety, seasonal affective disorder, attention-deficit hyperactivity disorder, obsessive–compulsive disorders, and sleep disorders
Dosage	300 mg daily
Warnings	Fair-skinned people may experience photosensitivity Reduces effectiveness of some anticancer agents Can interact with antidepressants, birth control pills, cyclosporine, heart medications, HIV medications, anticoagulants, protease inhibitors, asthma drugs, and seizure control medications Clinical manifestations of depression should be considered seriously Encourage client to see a mental healthcare provider
Valerian (Valeriana officinalis)	
Source	Dried rhizome and roots of the tall perennial *V. officinalis*
Action	Mild tranquilizer and sedative
Traditional uses	Used as medicinal herb since Ancient Greece and Rome for insomnia, migraine, fatigue, and stomach cramps
Current uses	Used as a mild tranquilizer and sedative; relieves muscle spasms, anxiety, headaches, depression, premenstrual syndrome, and menopause Especially effective for insomniac persons and older adults
Dosage	Available in capsules, tablets, liquid extracts, and teas
Warnings	Reported side effects include headache, gastrointestinal upset, and dizziness Must not be taken in combination with other tranquilizers or sedatives Client should be cautioned against operating a motor vehicle after ingesting Should discontinue use at least 1 week before surgery because it may interact with anesthesia

Table based on data from Mayo Clinic. (2023). *Drugs and supplements*. https://www.mayoclinic.org/drugs-supplements; Memorial Sloan-Kettering Cancer Center. (2023). *About herbs, botanicals and other products*. http://www.mskcc.org/cancer-care/integrative-medicine/about-herbs-botanicals-other-products; National Center for Complementary and Integrative Health. (2023). *Herbs at a glance*. https://nccih.nih.gov/health/herbsataglance.htm; United States National Library of Medicine. (2022). *Herbs and supplements*. https://medlineplus.gov/druginfo/herb_All.html

who make efforts to control the flow of illegal drugs and the FDA's guidance information. FDA's guidance documents do not establish legally enforceable responsibilities related to herbs/botanicals; rather, they are the agencies' view on the topic and provide recommendations (U.S. Department of Health and Human Services, 2020).

Fresh or dried herbs are usually brewed into a tea, with the dosage adjusted according to the chronicity or acuteness of the illness, age, and size of the client. Traditional Chinese Medicine usually is used only as long as symptoms persist.

Some clients may extend this same logic to prescription medicines. For example, they might stop taking an antibiotic as soon as the symptoms subside instead of completing the course of treatment for the prescribed length of time. Be sure to consider the potential interaction of herbs with prescription medicines. The root of the shrub *ginseng*, for example, is widely used for the treatment of arthritis, back and leg pains, and sores. Because ginseng is known to potentiate the action of some antihypertensive drugs, nurses need to ask clients whether they are experiencing side effects or toxicity and should frequently monitor the client's blood pressure. It might be necessary to withhold doses of the prescribed antihypertensive medicine if the blood pressure is low or to ask the client to discontinue or reduce the strength of the ginseng. When assessing the client's use of non-Western medicine, nurses should be aware that some clients who use herbs topically do not consider them drugs; therefore, nurses might not know that the person is taking these medicines. Clients sometimes fail to disclose that they are taking herbs and plant-based medicines or using essential oils because they are concerned that their healthcare provider will disapprove. The National Center for Complementary and Integrative Health (2022) provides fact sheets with basic information about specific herbs or botanicals—common names, what the science says, potential side effects and cautions, and resources for more information.

For many years, people have attempted to identify plants, marine organisms, arthropods, animals, and minerals with healing properties. According to the World Health Organization (2023), the majority of the world depends on traditional medicine for healthcare needs, with around 88% of all countries estimated to use traditional medicine such as acupuncture, herbs, yoga, and indigenous therapy among others (WHO, 2023). Nearly 50% of Americans have reported using some form of complementary and alternative medicine; however, less than 40% of those disclosed the use to a healthcare provider (Falci et al., 2016; Ogbu et al., 2023). Treatment for respiratory problems, such as asthma, represents one of the largest medical applications of plant-derived drugs. In particular, nurses should be aware of the widespread use of plant-derived medications among clients and utilize this awareness when conducting a thorough health history.

Reason for Seeking Care

The *reason* or *reasons for seeking care* refers to a brief statement in the client's own words describing why they are visiting a healthcare provider. This part of the health history previously was called the *chief complaint*, a term that is now avoided because it focuses on illness rather than wellness and tends to label the person as a complainer. Not only does this terminology have a negative implication, but it also misdirects the focus of a clinical visit by suggesting to healthcare providers that patients typically arrive at a healthcare visit with a single issue they want to address. In reality, patients typically have multiple reasons for seeking care.

Symptoms are subjective and defined as phenomena experienced by an individual that signify a departure from normal function, sensation, or appearance. By comparison, *signs* are objective abnormalities that the examiner can detect on physical examination or through laboratory testing. As individuals experience symptoms, they may interpret them and react in ways that are congruent with their individual **cultural norms** or unconscious behavior patterns. Such behaviors are learned from parents, teachers, peers, and others whose values, attitudes, beliefs, and behaviors take place in the context of their own culture. Symptoms cannot be attributed to another person; rather, symptoms are perceived, recognized, labeled, reacted to, ritualized, and articulated in ways that make sense within the worldview of the person experiencing them. This perception, which may have multiple layers of context, must be considered in relation to other sociocultural factors and biologic knowledge (Foronda, 2020). The search for cultural meaning in understanding symptoms involves a translation process that includes the healthcare provider's and client's worldview. It is important to use the same terms for symptoms that the client uses. For example, if the client refers to "swelling" of the leg, nurses should refrain from medicalizing that to "edema." Nurses must be knowledgeable about the various dimensions of culture to provide culturally congruent and competent care (Leininger & McFarland, 2002, 2006; McFarland & Wehbe-Alamah, 2015). Nurses who are knowledgeable about cultural humility are better able to recognize explicit bias and minimize power differences, promote respect, be flexible, and focus on providing the best care for an ongoing life process (Foronda, 2020).

History of Present Illness

Obtaining the client's health history is an important component of the encounter. Personal health history is a narrative provided by the client, which may elicit vulnerability. The narrative history of a client's present illness includes responses to questions asked about their current condition, such as onset, location, quality, severity, duration, timing, context (i.e., what factors have aggravated or relieved the symptoms), and other associated symptoms. Nurses can reframe how questions are asked to place more emphasis on the possible structural drivers of the disease or condition (i.e., social inequities, social determinants of health, and living conditions) instead of merely focusing on the client's behavior as a cause. For example, a woman comes to the emergency department via an ambulance with a large open draining wound on her right breast. The nurse may ask, "Why did you wait so long to come in?" or "Why did you call an ambulance instead of driving yourself?" but these questions place the blame of her current illness on her behaviors. Instead, the nurse could ask, "Are there any healthcare providers near your home?" or "What forms of transportation are accessible to you?" These questions shift the narrative from the behavior of the individual to a health **equity** focus on the well-being of communities (Foronda, 2020).

Past Health

The past medical history can help narrow the differential diagnoses, making it a crucial part of any medical work-up. A comprehensive history assessment requires integrating physical, psychological, and socioeconomic factors. General past medical history should include allergies, medications, previous diagnoses, childhood diseases, past surgeries, and family and social history. It is important to maintain compassion for the individual and to preserve the embodied identity of each patient as they tell their life health story from their point of view. It is important to maintain compassion for the individual and to preserve the embodied identity of each patient as they tell their life health story from their point of view (Rogers, 2021).

Family and Social History

In this era of genetics and genomics, a comprehensive and accurate family history highlights diseases and disorders for which a client may be at increased risk. When conducting the family history, the nurse should include grandparents, parents, or siblings who have been diagnosed with genetic disorders. Because there are familial links to disease, it is essential for the nurse to ask about any family history of diabetes, premature coronary artery disease, or hypertension. If clients are aware that they are at increased risk for a certain condition, they may arrange with their healthcare provider to seek early screening and periodic surveillance. Providers need to discuss any barriers related to social determinants of health for the client that impact their well-being and health. For example, do they have safe housing, transportation, and/or a safe neighborhood where they can exercise regularly to maintain a healthy body mass index? Does the client have transportation to grocery stores with healthy foods to improve nutrition and decrease cardiovascular and diabetes risks?

In addition to diagramming a family tree to identify familial relationships and the presence of disease conditions among those related to the client, the nurse should assess the social history. It is important to obtain the client's lifestyle history, which includes nutrition, physical activity, tobacco use, alcohol consumption, sleep habits, stress management, and sexual history. See Appendix A for suggested interview topics aimed at eliciting information about family and social history. The nurse should also collect any information about the conditions in the environments where clients are born, live, learn, work, play, worship, and age that may affect their health, functioning, risks, and quality-of-life outcomes (Healthy People, 2030). According to *Healthy People 2030*, social determinants of health encompasses five domains: healthcare access and quality, education access and quality, social and community context, neighborhood environment, and economic stability. Social determinants of health may contribute to health disparities and inequities. For example, clients who don't have access to healthy foods because of lack of transportation to a grocery store are likely to have poor nutritional intake, which raises the risk of heart disease, diabetes, and obesity, leading to a lowered life expectancy (Healthy People, 2030). Creating social, physical, and economic environments that promote health and well-being are the overarching goals of *Healthy People 2030.*

Economic factors have been identified as causes of chronic work-related health problems, COVID-19, and less favorable outcomes among clients with cancer (Centers for Disease Control and Prevention, 2022b). Research confirmed that during the COVID-19 pandemic, there was a positive association between minoritized populations and COVID-19. There were significantly higher incidence and mortality rates within specific races, ethnicities, and lower income status (Liao & DeMaio, 2021). Evidence-Based Practice 3-2 summarizes the challenges in treating clients of different races,

---

Evidence-Based Practice 3-2

Considerations Related to Social Determinants of Health in Treating Clients With COVID-19

There were many challenges with the SARS-CoV-2 (COVID-19) pandemic, with one of the most concerning being the disproportionate morbidity and mortality in vulnerable populations. Those with COVID-19 who had limited access to care and therefore minimal treatment options were mainly based on social determinants of health. Factors affecting susceptibility to COVID included limited access to care, insecure housing, poverty, food insecurity, loss of employment, and social support networks. All these are collectively social determinants of health and are "circumstances…shaped by the distribution of money, power and resources at global, national and local levels" (World Health Organization, 2021). Disparities and inequalities were brought to the forefront during the pandemic and resulted in a deeper understanding of how social determinants of health impact the well-being of a client. This will allow healthcare providers to obtain a more thoughtful and impactful history and exam. Awareness of the underlying causes of poor health will help healthcare professionals and clients reach a collaborative plan of care that can assist in accessing support services, improve access, and partner with community resources (World Health Organization, 2021).

Clinical Implications

An integral part of caring for each person as an individual is making sure that the assessment and treatment of disease are individualized. Nurses have a key role to play in assisting clients from diverse backgrounds to effectively manage disease processes such as COVID-19. Nurses should continually work with the client and other health professionals to plan, implement, and evaluate interventions that are the most beneficial to that client, taking into consideration the individual experience of each client.

References: Fricke-Galindo, I., & Falfán-Valencia, R. (2021). Pharmacogenetics approach for the improvement of COVID-19 treatment. *Viruses, 13*(3), 413. https://doi.org/10.3390/v13030413; Goodman, C. W., & Brett, A. S. (2021). Race and pharmacogenomics—Personalized medicine or misguided practice? *JAMA, 325*(7), 625–626. https://doi.org/10.1001/jama.2020.25473; World Health Organization. (2021). *Social determinants of health.* https://www.who.int/health-topics/social-determinants-of-health

ethnicities, genders, and socioeconomic statuses with COVID-19.

Review of Systems

The purpose of the review of systems is threefold: (1) to evaluate the past and present health state of each body system, (2) to provide an opportunity for the client to report symptoms not previously stated, and (3) to evaluate health promotion practices.

Knowledge of current research on diseases prevalent in specific populations might be useful in asking appropriate questions in the review of systems. For example, if the nurse is gathering review of systems information from a client, it is useful to know that there is a statistically higher incidence of hypertension, sickle cell anemia, and type 2 diabetes in certain ethnic and racial groups. This will assist in customizing the review of systems questions and ensuring that symptoms of disease specific to the client's ethnic or racial heritage are included. For example, sickle cell anemia is a genetic condition more common among Black people in the United States, but it affects all races the same and occurs in individuals from other geographic regions. However, Black people may face unique challenges in receiving care for sickle cell disease due to disparities in the healthcare system (Askinazi, 2023; CDC, 2019; Haywood Jr et al., 2013; Kato et al., 2018; Meghani et al., 2012b). The questions posed by the healthcare provider often remind patients about healthcare concerns that they may not have thought about reporting in the history of present illness, or family and social history. Having a candid conversation about previous health concerns can elicit valuable information from the client (Phillips et al., 2017).

Physical Examination

There are a number of variants that nurses may encounter when conducting the physical examination of clients from different backgrounds. Accurate assessment and **evaluation** of clients

require knowledge of normal exam findings among healthy members of selected populations, as well as variations that occur during illness or within certain populations. For example, the characteristic "bulls-eye" rash indicative of Lyme disease has variable presentations on patients with light skin, brown skin, and black skin tones, leading to a high percentage of late or missed diagnoses (Figure 3-2).

When documenting the physical examination findings, it is important for nurses to include the skin color based on the Fitzpatrick classification of skin types I–VI or other phototype classification systems. During the physical examination, nurses need to maintain an environment that considers the client's possible difficulties in mobility, hearing, and vision. It is vital that all patients are approached with consideration. Clients are vulnerable during the physical examination due to the nature of an assessment, which requires the nurse to inspect, palpate, percuss, and auscultate multiple body systems and areas of the client's body (Rogers, 2021).

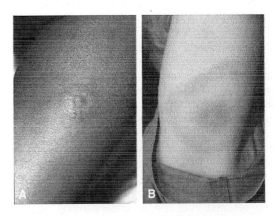

Figure 3-2. The characteristic Lyme disease "bulls-eye" rash can look significantly different depending on skin tone. A. Dark skin, B. Light skin. (Sources [*left–right*]: Reprinted from Bhate, C., & Schwartz, R. A. (2011). Lyme disease: Part I. Advances and perspectives. *Journal of the American Academy of Dermatology, 64*(4), 619–636. doi:10.1016/j.jaad.2010.03.046 with permission from Elsevier; CDC/James Gathany)

Vital Signs

There can be changes in vital signs in clients depending on history, sex, stress, comfort level with provider and healthcare system, and other factors (see Chapter 2, EBP 2-1).

Hypertension develops earlier in life for Black Americans, and the incidence is twice as high in Black Americans as it is in White Americans. In addition, Black Americans have the highest incidence of hypertension of anywhere in the world (American Heart Association, 2022). There is a higher prevalence of hypertension in individuals of African descent due to adverse social determinants of health, structural racism, and the downstream consequences of enslavement (Williamson, 2021). Furthermore, historical discrimination by healthcare professionals may diminish client–provider trust and contribute to less adherence to medications, vaccines, and medical follow-up. Uncontrolled hypertension over a period of time is a main reason for the higher incidence of cardiovascular disease, stroke, and kidney disease in Black Americans. Differences in the environment, health habits of White and Black individuals, and flawed studies and practices are among the potential causes. One such example is the estimated glomerular filtration rate (eGFR) in clients from African descent, which has led to a significant delay in treatment and increase in end-stage disease (Tsai et al., 2021). Other race-based protocols exist and are being challenged in a wide range of areas: body mass index risk for diabetes, fracture risk assessment score, pulmonary function test, urinary tract infection, atherosclerotic cardiovascular disease, and more. In contrast to a race-based approach, a race-conscious framework can promote antiracist practices, shifting focus from race to racism in all its forms (American Medical Association and Association of American Medical Colleges, 2021).

Assessment of Pain

Pain is the most frequent and compelling reason that people seek healthcare and is sometimes referred to as the fifth vital sign. A universally recognized phenomenon, the term pain is defined as an unpleasant sensory and emotional experience conveyed by the brain through sensory neurons arising from actual or potential tissue damage to the body. The American Academy of Pain Medicine classifies pain as **acute** or **chronic**. In *acute pain*, a direct, one-to-one relationship exists between an injury and pain, and the pain is frequently short-lived and self-limiting. Acute pain, however, can become persistent and intractable if the underlying cause continues for a prolonged period. *Chronic pain* is described as pain that persists greater than 3 months. Chronic pain is now considered the most frequent cause of disability in industrialized nations globally. As a multi–billion-dollar public health concern and major cause of disability, careful attention needs to be given to provision of culturally and linguistically appropriate care. Data show that in the United States, an estimated 50 million people experience chronic pain, at a cost of $635 billion in healthcare treatment and lost productivity (Dahlhamer, 2018; National Center for Complementary and Integrative Health, 2022). There is a higher prevalence of both chronic pain and high-impact chronic pain reported among women, older adults, previously but not currently employed adults, adults living in poverty, adults with public health insurance, and rural residents (Dahlhamer, 2018).

In terms of pain measurement, it is generally believed that humans experience similar sensation thresholds. However, pain perception thresholds, pain tolerance, and encouraged pain threshold vary considerably among individuals. *Sensation threshold* refers to the lowest stimulus that results in tingling or warmth. *Pain threshold* refers to the point at which the individual reports that a stimulus is painful. Cultural background has an effect on this measure of pain as well as on pain threshold, the point at which the individual reports that a stimulus is painful, and pain tolerance, the point at which the individual withdraws or asks to have the stimulus stopped (Gingras et al., 2023).

Research reveals that chronic disease, psychological distress, Medicaid insurance, lower education levels, and other social determinants of health are associated with higher incidences of severe pain (Gingras et al., 2023). Failure to adequately treat pain can lead to adverse outcomes, such as elevated heart rates postoperatively and increased risk of myocardial infarction, ischemic stroke, and hemorrhage resulting from elevated systemic vascular resistance and elevated levels of catecholamines. Other consequences of uncontrolled pain include reduced mobility, loss of strength, sleep disturbances, immune system impairment, increased susceptibility to disease, and medication dependence (Gingras et al., 2023).

The assessment of pain is complicated primarily because pain is an inherently subjective experience that necessitates the reliance on self-reporting, rather than objective measurements. Rating scales do not resolve uncertainties inherent in self-reporting methods. For example, self-report measures can be difficult to express for clients who speak a different language than their provider as well as for children and individuals with cognitive conditions. Therefore, the healthcare provider should assure appropriate steps taken to offer language assistance resources such as interpreters as essential collaborators (Ortega et al., 2022). Pain assessment is influenced by three factors: (1) client trust in provider, (2) the environmental context, and (3) the nurse's background and experience. Nurses and other healthcare providers sometimes project their own attitudes, beliefs, and opinions about pain onto their clients, a situation that encourages cultural stereotyping when assessing the client's self-reported level of pain (Meints et al., 2019).

Nurses and other healthcare providers are challenged to avoid bias when assessing pain and to take appropriate action commensurate with the level of self-reported pain. Research indicates that clients from racial minority groups are likely to be more active in their communications when the clinical encounter is race concordant, that is, when the healthcare provider is from the same racial group, and to be less active in their communications when the encounter is race discordant, that is, the healthcare provider is from a different racial group than the client (Poma, 2017). Studies of primary care physicians reveal that provider race bias exists, especially between White providers and Black or Hispanic clients (FitzGerald & Hurst, 2017; Meints et al., 2019).

Negative stereotypes have been documented for members of racial, gender, and ethnic groups who experience pain. For example, some primary care physicians underestimate pain intensity in Black clients compared to other sociodemographic groups, and Black and Hispanic clients are sometimes perceived as requiring more scrutiny for potential drug use and misuse, despite evidence to the contrary (Henschke et al., 2016; Kwok & Bhuvanakrishna, 2014; Meints et al., 2019; Tait & Chibnall, 2014). Black clients are more likely than non-Hispanic White clients to underreport pain in the clinical setting, especially in the presence of physicians who are perceived as having higher social status or are from a different racial background (Mack et al., 2018). There is extensive evidence that Black individuals and other racial-ethnic minorities lack trust in the healthcare system and in their physicians, nurse practitioners, and other health professionals with different cultural backgrounds from their own (Cuevas & O'Brien, 2017). This lack of trust stems from a long history of mistreatment from gruesome experiments such as forced sterilization and the infamous Tuskegee syphilis study (Rodriguez, 2023). Therefore, the client may fail to accurately report symptoms of pain, withhold information about the type and amount of medications they are using to control pain, and seek treatment outside Western medicine.

Factors contributing to racial and ethnic disparities in pain assessment include stereotypes and implicit biases of nurses and providers conducting the client assessment, nurse–client communication, the nurse's ability to empathize with clients from racial/ethnic groups different from their own, the client's educational and socioeconomic background, pain reporting skills, pain-coping ability, and level of trust in health-care providers. The client's perception of the seriousness of the cause of pain (e.g., pain caused by cancer) may also influence the client's experience of pain (Booker, 2016; Henschke et al., 2016).

Assessment of General Appearance

In assessing general appearance, survey the person's entire body. Note the general health state and any obvious physical characteristics and readily apparent biologic features unique to the individual. In assessing the client's general appearance, consider four areas: physical appearance, body structure, mobility, and behavior.

1. *Physical appearance* includes age, sex, level of consciousness, facial features, and skin color (evenness of color tone, pigmentation, intactness, and presence of lesions or other abnormalities).
2. *Body structure* includes stature, nutrition, symmetry, posture, position, and overall body build or contour.
3. *Mobility* includes gait and range of motion.
4. *Behavior* includes such variables as facial expression, mood and affect, fluency of speech, ability to communicate ideas, appropriateness of word choice, grooming, and attire or dress. For example, observant members of the following groups may wear culture-specific attire: Amish, Mennonites, Hasidic and Orthodox Jewish, and Muslims. Members of the Church of Jesus Christ of Latter-day Saints (LDS) (also known as Mormons) may wear undergarments that symbolize their temple covenants. Clients may want to leave the garments on during physical examinations. Nurses should respect the attire or clothing of all clients and those who ask to leave their garments on during the physical examination. In some instances, the client may not want nurses to handle their clothing.

In assessing a client's hygiene, it is useful to ask about typical bathing habits and customary use of various hygiene-related products. The level of self-care may suggest poor hygiene if unkempt and dirty. People in most cultures in the United States and Canada make a great effort to disguise their natural body odors by bathing frequently, or applying antiperspirants, colognes, and/or perfumes with scents that are deemed to be desirable (Mayo Clinic, 2021b). These practices may mask the symptoms of some diseases and infections. There are dozens of diseases associated with odors of the breath, skin, urine, stool, penis, and vagina (National Geographic, 2018).

During the assessment, the nurse should do the following:

- Note the nature of breath odor—sweet may suggest diabetic ketoacidosis (sickly sweet smell), alcoholism (acetone or vinegar), liver failure (a sweet smell), while an unpleasant or foul odor may suggest kidney failure (urine or fishlike breath due to ammonia) and infections of the mouth, nose, pharynx, or chest (putrid odor).
- Examine state of teeth and teeth hygiene and note whether the teeth are real or false—loose-fitting teeth may be responsible for mouth ulcers or decayed teeth, which may cause halitosis (bad breath odor).

Variations in Skin

An accurate and comprehensive examination of the skin of clients from diverse backgrounds requires knowledge of variations and skill in recognizing color changes, some of which might be subtle. Awareness of normal variations and the ability to recognize the unique clinical manifestations of disease are developed over time as the nurse gains experience with clients with various skin colors.

The assessment of a client's skin is subjective and is highly dependent on observational skill, the ability to recognize subtle color changes, and repeated exposure to individuals having various gradations of skin color. *Melanin* is responsible for the various colors and tones of skin observed in different people. Melanin protects the skin against harmful ultraviolet rays—a genetic advantage accounting for the lower incidence of skin cancer among darkly pigmented Black and Native American clients (Jarvis, 2016; Swope & Abdel-Malek, 2018).

Normal skin color ranges widely. Some healthcare practitioners have attempted to describe the variations by labeling their observations with some of the following adjectives: *copper, olive, tan*, and various shades of *brown* (*light, medium, and dark*). In observing pallor in clients, the term *ashen* is sometimes used. Skin color is one of the most important biological variations to assess in nursing care and of great clinical significance. The nurse's ability to establish a reliable description of baseline skin color and subsequently recognize when variations occur in an individual is of great importance, especially for clients whose health condition may be linked to changes in skin color (Slaught et al., 2022).

Congenital Dermal Melanocytosis (Formerly Known as Mongolian Spots)

Congenital dermal melanocytosis are irregular areas of deep blue pigmentation usually located in the sacral and gluteal areas but sometimes occurring on the abdomen, thighs, shoulders, or arms. Congenital dermal melanocytosis can be confused with bruises to the unfamiliar eye but are a normal variation in children of African, Asian, or Latin descent. Recognition of this normal variation is particularly important when dealing with children who might be erroneously identified as victims of child abuse, causing much anguish to the parents or guardians. During embryonic development, the melanocytes originate near the embryonic nervous system in the neural crest, then migrate into the fetal epidermis. Congenital dermal melanocytosis presents as areas of embryonic pigment that have been left behind in the epidermal layer during fetal development. The result looks like a bluish discoloration of the skin. The spots become lighter by adulthood, but usually remain visible. Congenital dermal melanocytosis is present in 90% of Black individuals, 80% of Asian and Native American individuals, and 9% of White individuals (Jarvis, 2016; Overfield, 2017).

Vitiligo

Vitiligo, an autoimmune condition in which the melanocytes become nonfunctional in some areas of the skin, is characterized by the appearance of unpigmented, patchy, white skin patches that are often symmetric bilaterally (Katz & Harris, 2021). Vitiligo affects an estimated two to five million Americans (Gandhi et al., 2022). There is no greater prevalence among dark-skinned individuals, although the disorder may cause greater psychosocial stress in some groups because it is more visible (Buttaro et al., 2016). Clients with vitiligo may still experience the social stigmas documented in ancient Indian and Buddhist writings, including the restriction of marriage (Katz & Harris, 2021). People with vitiligo also have a statistically increased incidence of other autoimmune disease (i.e., alopecia areata and type 1 diabetes mellitus) and have higher-than-normal risk for pernicious anemia and hyperthyroidism (Katz et al., 2021). These factors are believed to reflect an underlying genetic abnormality.

Hyperpigmentation

Other areas of the skin affected by hormones and, in some cases, differing for people from certain ethnic backgrounds are the sexual skin areas, such as the nipples, areola, scrotum, and labia majora. In general, these areas are darker than other parts of the skin in both adults and children, especially among clients with brown or black skin tones. When assessing these skin surfaces on darker-skinned clients, observe carefully for erythema, rashes, and other abnormalities because the darker color might mask their presence (Vashi et al., 2017).

Cyanosis

Cyanosis, a severe condition indicating a lack of oxygen in the blood, is the most difficult clinical sign to observe in people with darker-pigmented skin. For the client to manifest clinical evidence of cyanosis, the level of deoxygenated hemoglobin in the arteries is usually below 5 g/dL with an oxygen saturation below 85% (Overfield, 2017; Pahal

& Goyal, 2021). It is best to check the conjunctivae, oral mucosa, and nail beds rather than to rely on the assessment of the skin. The lips and tongue may be gray or white, whereas conjunctiva palms, soles, and nail beds will appear with a tinge of bluish color (Pusey-Reid et al., 2023; Rateau, 2022).

Given that most conditions causing cyanosis also cause decreased oxygenation of the brain, other clinical symptoms, such as changes in the level of consciousness, will be evident. Cyanosis usually is accompanied by increased respiratory rate, use of accessory muscles of respiration, nasal flaring, and other manifestations of respiratory distress (Rogers, 2023). Exercise caution when assessing persons of Mediterranean descent for cyanosis because their circumoral region is normally dark blue.

Jaundice

Jaundice is best observed by inspecting the sclera, by observing the area closest to the cornea, the oral mucosa, and hard palate for a yellow discoloration. When examining clients, exercise caution to avoid confusing other forms of pigmentation with jaundice. To distinguish between carotenemia and jaundice, it is necessary to inspect the posterior portion of the hard palate using bright daylight or good artificial lighting. Also, check the palms and soles for a yellow-orange color (Jarvis, 2016; Overfield, 2017; Pusey-Reid et al., 2023) and monitor for light- or clay-colored stools and dark golden urine as both often accompany jaundice.

Pallor

Assessing for **pallor** in clients with darker-pigmented skin can be difficult because the underlying red tones are absent. This is significant because these red tones are responsible for giving brown or black skin its luster. An individual with brown skin will manifest pallor with a more yellowish-brown color, and a person with black skin will appear ashen or gray (Pusey-Reid et al., 2023). Generalized pallor can be best observed in individuals with darker skin by inspecting the conjunctivae, mucous membranes, lips, and nail beds (Pusey-Reid et al., 2023; Rateau, 2022).

The palpebrae, conjunctivae, and nail beds are preferred sites for assessing the pallor of anemia. When inspecting the conjunctiva, lower the lid sufficiently to see the conjunctiva near the inner and outer canthi. The coloration is often lighter near the inner canthus.

In addition to changes seen on skin assessment, the pallor of impending shock is accompanied by other clinical manifestations, such as increasing pulse rate, oliguria, apprehension, and restlessness. Anemia, particularly chronic iron-deficiency anemia, might be manifested by the characteristic "spoon" nails, which have a concave shape. A lemon-yellow tint of the face and slightly yellow sclerae accompany pernicious anemia, which is also manifested by neurologic deficits and a red, painful tongue (Meiner & Yeager, 2019; Rogers, 2023). Fatigue, exertional dyspnea, tachycardia, dizziness, and impaired mental function accompany the most severe anemia (Jarvis, 2016; Overfield, 2017).

Erythema, Petechiae, and Ecchymoses

Skin pigmentation may mask visual appearance of **erythema** (redness) or ecchymosis (purplish hues) because the contrast between white and red or white and purple is more pronounced than it is when the skin color is darker (Black, 2018). Erythema is frequently associated with localized inflammation and is characterized by increased skin temperature. The degree of redness is determined by the quantity of blood in the subpapillary plexus, whereas the warmth of the skin is related to the rate of blood flow through the blood vessels. Nurses can compare and contrast affected and nonaffected areas of inflammation for increased warmth, skin color changes, and texture with palpation. During inspection, the nurse may observe differences around the inflamed area in shine, tautness, and pitting edema (Pusey-Reid et al., 2023). The dorsal surfaces of the fingers are the most sensitive to temperature sensations and should be used to assess for erythema. Skin areas with recently resolved inflammation appear darker than the patient's normal skin tone (Pusey-Reid et al., 2023).

The erythema associated with rashes is not always accompanied by noticeable increases in skin temperature. Macular, papular, and vesicular skin lesions are identified by a combination of palpation and inspection. In addition, it is important to listen to the client's description of symptoms. For example, persons with macular rashes will usually complain of itching, and evidence of scratching will be apparent. When the skin is only moderately pigmented, a macular rash might become recognizable when the skin is gently stretched. Stretching the skin decreases the normal red tone, thus providing more contrast and making the macules appear brighter. In some skin disorders with a generalized rash, the rash is most readily visible on the hard and soft palates.

Petechiae are best visualized in the areas of lighter melanization, such as the abdomen, buttocks, and volar surface of the forearm. Usually, the petechiae are found in clusters and consist of small, pinpoint spots that vary in color from red, brown, or purple (Mayo Clinic, 2021a). When the skin is darkly pigmented, petechiae are rarely visible on the skin. Most diseases that cause bleeding and the formation of microscopic emboli, such as thrombocytopenia, subacute bacterial endocarditis, and other septicemias, are characterized by petechiae in the mucous membranes and skin. Petechiae are most easily seen in the mouth, particularly the buccal mucosa, and in the conjunctiva of the eye (Pusey-Reid et al., 2023).

Ecchymoses areas appear darker than a person's usual skin tone. When differentiating petechiae and ecchymoses from erythema in the mucous membrane, pressure on the tissue will momentarily blanch erythema but not petechiae or ecchymoses (Black, 2018). Ecchymotic areas may be tender and easily palpable, depending on whether a hematoma is present (Pusey-Reid et al., 2023).

Addison Disease

A decrease in a client's cortisol and aldosterone levels is a characteristic of **Addison disease** along with an elevated adrenocorticotropic hormone (ACTH) level. The rise in ACTH causes lingual and buccal anomalies of melanocytes, which are responsible for hyperpigmentation. The intraoral pigmentation may be the only sign of Addison disease (Husebye et al., 2021). The nipples, areola, genitalia, perineum, and pressure points such as the axillae, elbow, inner thighs, and buttocks of pale skin may appear as bronze but is very difficult to recognize in people with darkly pigmented skin; therefore, other clinical manifestations of the disease and laboratory tests such as sodium, potassium, cortisol, and ACTH should be used to corroborate the skin changes (Jarvis, 2016; Vashi & Maibach, 2017). The clinical manifestations of Addison disease can include hypotension, loss of appetite, unintentional weight loss, chronic fatigue; nausea, vomiting; and abdominal, muscle, or joint pain (Husebye et al., 2021).

Uremia

Uremia is the illness accompanying kidney failure characterized by unexplained changes in extracellular volume, inorganic ion concentrations, or lack of known renal synthetic products. Uremic illness is largely due to the accumulation of organic waste products, not all identified, that are normally cleared by the kidneys (Rogers, 2023). Kidney failure causes retained urochrome pigments in the blood to turn a person with light skin and uremia gray or orange-green. In people with darkly pigmented skin, it may be difficult to visualize these skin color changes; therefore, skin manifestations of uremia are often masked (Goel et al., 2021). Kidney function tests (BUN, creatinine, and eGFR) are laboratory tests that can confirm the diagnosis. Clinical manifestations of uremia can corroborate a diagnosis of uremia. Findings include nausea, vomiting, fatigue, anorexia, weight loss, muscle cramps, pruritus, or changes in mental status.

Albinism

The term **albinism** refers to a group of inherited conditions. People with albinism have little or no pigment in their eyes, skin, or hair. They have inherited altered genes that do not make the usual amounts of the pigment melanin. One person in 18,000–20,000 in the United States has some type of albinism. In other parts of the world, the occurrence of albinism could be as high as 1 in 3,000 (National Organization for Albinism and Hypopigmentation, 2021). Albinism may affect people with any skin tone. Most children with albinism are born to parents who have typical hair and eye color for their ethnic backgrounds. Sometimes, people do not recognize that they have albinism. There are different types of albinism, and the amount of pigment in the eyes varies. Although some individuals with albinism have reddish or violet eyes, most have blue eyes, whereas others have hazel or brown eyes.

Vision problems are associated with all forms of albinism. People with albinism always have impaired vision (not correctable with eyeglasses) and many have low vision. Low vision refers to impaired vision in which there is a significant reduction in visual function that cannot be corrected by conventional glasses. With low vision, it may become hard or seem impossible to do normal tasks, yet this may be improved with special aids or devices to make the most out of the vision that is available (American Academy of Ophthalmology, 2021). The degree of vision impairment varies with the type of albinism. Many people with albinism are legally blind due to abnormal development of the retina and abnormal patterns of nerve connections between the eye and the brain. The presence of these eye problems defines the diagnosis of albinism. Therefore, the main test for albinism is an eye examination. People with albinism also need to take precautions to avoid damage to the skin caused by the sun, such as wearing sunscreen lotions, hats, and sun-protective clothing (American Academy of Ophthalmology, 2022; National Organization for Albinism and Hypopigmentation, 2021).

Normal Age-Related Skin Changes

Aging is accompanied by the growing presence of wrinkles in all people. Light skin shows the effects of sun damage more than dark skin, regardless of race or ethnicity, and the area of the skin that is exposed to the sun shows the effects of aging more than protected skin, such as those parts covered by clothing. Regardless of climate, dry skin is inevitable in individuals older than 70 years of age. Transepidermal water loss will result in a dry, tight, and often inflamed-looking appearance. It gives an impaired acid mantle and impaired immune response, impacting and compromising the skin's structural integrity. Examples of severe transepidermal water loss are eczema or psoriasis. These conditions occur when vital fluids evaporate, and the skin becomes very dry and inflamed. Restoring free water levels and thickening the matrix of the skin are an integral part of returning the skin back to a healthy functional state.

Moles occur when cells in the skin grow in a cluster instead of being spread throughout the skin. These cells are called melanocytes, and they make the pigment that gives skin its natural color. Moles may darken after exposure to the sun, during the teen years, and during pregnancy. Because the number of moles increases with age, they are thought to be the result of long-term exposure to the sun. People with lighter skin have more moles than those with darkly pigmented skin (Overfield, 2017). Most moles are benign; however, moles that are more likely to be cancer are those that look different than other existing moles or those that first appear after age 30. If nurses notice changes in a mole's color, height, size, or shape, they should consult with a dermatologist. Any client who has a mole that bleeds, oozes, itches, or becomes tender or painful should be referred immediately to a dermatologist (American Cancer Society, 2019; Jarvis, 2016).

The variability in appearance of aging skin can be associated with a client's ethnicity, skin type, environmental exposures, and genetics. Nurses and other healthcare providers must be astute in recognizing the difference in assessment techniques to make a thorough inspection, palpation, and assessment of the skin. Nurses will start to see more heterogeneous groups rather than homogenous groups in relation to the skin and the age-related skin changes as societies become more diverse in race, culture, and ethnicity (Vashi et al., 2016).

Variation in the Head

Nurses will notice marked, biocultural variations when examining the hair, eyes, ears, and mouths of clients from diverse backgrounds. The ability to distinguish typical variations from atypical ones could have serious implications as some variations are associated with systemic sometimes life-threatening conditions.

Hair

Perhaps one of the most obvious and widely variable cultural differences occurs with assessment of the hair, which varies widely in texture. It may be strong or very fragile and ranges from long and straight to short, spiraled, thick, silky, kinky, or absent.

Obtaining a baseline hair assessment is significant in the diagnosis and treatment of certain disease states. For example, a dermatologic condition known as alopecia areata causes patchy or complete baldness on the scalp, eyebrows, eyelashes, nose, ears, or anywhere hair grows. Clients with eating disorders or inadequate nutrition may have changes to hair pigment and hair texture (Zhang et al., 2023). Alopecia may occur in all nutritional disorders, but dyspigmentation typically appears in kwashiorkor, marasmus, and essential fatty acid deficiency. Certain endocrine and genetic disorders are also known to affect the amount, thickness, and texture of the client's hair (Vashi & Maibach, 2017).

Although gray hair correlates with age, there are ethnic differences in the rate of hair graying. In general, people from European descent gray faster than other ethnic groups, starting in their mid-30s. Among some Asian descendants, graying usually begins in late thirties and people of African descent start to gray in their mid-40s (Maymone et al., 2021; Park et al., 2018).

Eyes

There are differences in both the structure and color of the eyes in clients. Individual differences are evident in the palpebral fissures. Persons of Asian descent often have epicanthal eye folds, whereas the presence of narrowed palpebral fissures in non-Asian individuals might be diagnostic of a serious congenital anomaly known as Down syndrome or trisomy 21. Asian children with Down syndrome demonstrate incidence of epiblepharon, high rate of exotropia, and essentially no notable Brushfield spots, which contrast with the ocular findings in patients from European descent with Down syndrome. The overall incidence of ocular abnormalities in the Korean children with Down syndrome was 91% with upward slanting of the palpebral fissure being the most common ocular finding followed by epicanthus (Kim et al., 2002).

There is genetic variability in the color of the iris and in retinal pigmentation: darker irises are correlated with darker retinas. Clients with light retinas generally have better night vision but can experience pain in an environment that is too light. The majority of individuals from African and Asian descent have brown eyes, whereas many individuals of Scandinavian or Northern European descent have blue eyes (Overfield, 2017).

Ears

Ears come in a variety of sizes and shapes. Earlobes can be freestanding or attached to the face. Ceruminous glands are located in the external ear canal and are functional at birth. Cerumen (earwax) is genetically determined and comes in two major types, dry cerumen, which is gray and flaky and frequently forms a thin mass in the ear canal, and wet cerumen, which is dark brown and moist. The clinical significance of this occurs when examining or irrigating the ears; the presence and composition of cerumen are not related to poor hygiene, and flaky, dry cerumen should not be mistaken for the dry lesions of eczema. Therefore, nurses and healthcare providers need to be knowledgeable about which persons have a higher frequency of dry cerumen versus a higher frequency of wet cerumen to make an accurate assessment of the findings. Persons from Asian and Native American heritage have an 84% frequency of dry cerumen. Wet cerumen is found in 99% of African American individuals and 97% of White individuals (Overfield, 2017).

Hearing loss may be genetic, congenital, or acquired through aging, injury, infection, or accident. On rare occasions, hearing loss is caused by surgery when the excision of a brain tumor is necessary. Age-related hearing loss, or **presbycusis**, is the slow loss of hearing that occurs as people get older and the cilia (tiny hair cells) in the inner ear become damaged or die. The following factors that contribute to age-related hearing loss should be considered in the health history and physical examination: family history (age-related hearing loss tends to run in families), repeated exposure to loud noises, smoking (people who smoke are more likely to have hearing loss than those who do not), certain medical conditions (e.g., diabetes), and some prescription medicines (e.g., gentamicin). After age 40, people assigned male at birth have poorer hearing than people assigned female at birth. Black individuals have better hearing at high and low frequencies; White individuals have better hearing at middle frequencies. Melanin pigmentation is significantly more abundant in the cochlea of individuals from African descent than individuals from European descent.

Mouth

Oral hyperpigmentation can vary from genetic predispositions. Usually absent at birth, hyperpigmentation increases with age. Physiologic pigmentation presents clinically as macular pigmented areas of varying shapes and sizes in patients from many different ethnic backgrounds. It is seen more commonly in people with darker skin resulting from increased melanocytic activity and the development of post-inflammatory pigmentation in the oral cavity, which can be seen with chronic trauma or inflammatory conditions. Diagnosis of physiologic pigmentation is made with clinical examination and no treatment is needed (Rosebush et al., 2019).

Cleft uvula is a condition in which the uvula is split either completely or partially. Ethnic differences exist in the incidence of cleft lip and palate, with people of Asian descent having the highest incidence (0.82 to 4.04 per 1,000 live births), followed by people of European descent (0.9 to 2.69 per 1,000 live births), and people of African descent with the lowest incidence (0.18 to 1.67 per 1,000 live births (Vyas et al., 2020). The incidence of cleft lip and palate rises with increased parental age; older mothers with additional parity have an increased incidence of having children with cleft palate. Other factors include smoking, alcohol use, and environmental factors (Vyas et al., 2020).

Teeth

Dental caries or tooth decay is significant because there are known correlations between dental caries and other conditions such as cleft lip and palate, kidney failure, cystic fibrosis, immunosuppression, heart defects, low birth weight, seizures, maternal illness, and rickets (Kliegman et al., 2016). Untreated dental caries is highest in Black populations (39.6%), then in Latino or Hispanic and Mexican (29.4% and 30%), then White (22.6%), and lowest in Asian populations (14.7%; Centers for Disease Control and Prevention, 2022c). Dental care and periodontal disease are affected by adverse consequences of social determinants of health including access to care and health disparities. When obvious signs of periodontal disease are present, such as bleeding and edematous gums, a dental referral should be initiated.

Transcultural Perspectives in Clinical Decision-Making and Actions

After completing a comprehensive assessment, analyze the subjective and objective data. In order to help clients reach their highest level of wellness, Leininger suggests three major modalities to guide nursing decisions and actions when providing culturally congruent care that is beneficial, satisfying, and meaningful to clients— *cultural care preservation or maintenance*, *cultural care accommodation or negotiation*, and *cultural care repatterning or restructuring* (Leininger, 1991; Leininger & McFarland, 2002; McFarland & Wehbe-Alamah, 2015):

- Cultural care preservation or maintenance refers to those professional actions and decisions that help people of a particular culture to retain and/or preserve relevant care values so that they can maintain their well-being, recover from illness, or face disabilities and/or death (Leininger, 1991; Leininger & McFarland, 2002; McFarland & Wehbe-Alamah, 2015).
- Cultural care accommodation or negotiation refers to the healthcare provider and the client collaborating to create a shared plan of care that guides the client in reaching an optimum health outcome, while considering all aspects of that client (Leininger, 1991; Leininger & McFarland, 2002; McFarland & Wehbe-Alamah, 2015).
- Cultural care repatterning or restructuring refers to professional actions and decisions that help clients reorder, change, or greatly modify their lifeways for new, different, and beneficial healthcare patterns. This requires a trusting relationship between the client and the provider; the required changes are coestablished with the clients to allow them to achieve beneficial or healthier lifeways (Leininger, 1991; McFarland & Wehbe-Alamah, 2015).

Whether the nurse uses Leininger's three modes for decisions and actions or engages in other analytic processes, the next step in the process leading to culturally competent decision-making and actions is to set mutual goals with the client, develop a plan of care, confer with and make referrals to other members of the interprofessional healthcare team (when needed), and implement a plan of care, either alone or with others. This process, presented primarily from the nurse's vantage point, is based on the health histories and physical examinations by the nurse and other team members and focuses on the nurse–client interaction and those aspects of the care plan that fall within the scope of practice and responsibilities of professional nurses.

Credentialed or licensed health professionals (e.g., physicians, advanced practice nurses, pharmacists, social workers, dieticians, and physical, occupational, respiratory, and other therapists) have been educated to follow a similar process. Although some folk, traditional, religious, and spiritual healers may follow a comparable process, others might rely on a different approach, for example, reliance on subjective data from the client that are based on a spiritual assessment. Folk, traditional, religious, and spiritual healers may prefer to practice their healing interventions with the client in private and may or may not want to collaborate with other members of the team. Be mindful that the federal Health Insurance Portability and Accountability Act (HIPAA) regulations may prohibit the sharing of some information, especially when the client is too ill to provide informed consent to release medical information with family, friends, and healers without authorization.

Once the plan has been implemented, it should be evaluated in collaboration with the client, with the client's family and significant others, and with other credentialed, licensed, folk, traditional, religious, and spiritual healers who are members of the team. The evaluation includes a comprehensive analysis of the plan's effectiveness in meeting mutually established goals and desired outcomes. As illustrated in Figure 3-3, nurses collaborate with clients, physicians, and other members of the healthcare team to determine if the care delivered was culturally acceptable, congruent and competent, safe, affordable, accessible, high quality, and based on research, scientific evidence, and best professional practices. Establishing a trusting relationship is an important component of healthcare delivery. Gather additional subjective and objective data to determine the effectiveness of the intervention(s) and

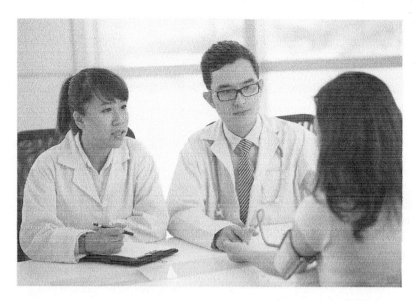

Figure 3-3. When conducting a comprehensive cultural assessment, the nurse collaborates with the client and physician as members of an interprofessional healthcare team. (Dragon Images/Shutterstock.com)

the client's overall satisfaction with care delivery and outcomes. Healthcare facilities, home and community health agencies, and related healthcare organizations usually have comprehensive evaluation processes and instruments that they administer to clients or patients and then subsequently review individually and in the aggregate for the purpose of improving the quality of care.

Summary

Many variations in health and illness are apparent in the health assessment and physical examination. For example, nurses will note differences based on the client's sex, age, ethnicity, and/or genetic makeup. In gathering subjective and objective assessment data, note individual differences in body measurements, pain perception, general appearance, and symptom manifestation. For example, in assessing the skin of lightly and darkly pigmented clients, there are notable differences in the manifestations of cyanosis, jaundice, pallor, erythema, petechiae, and ecchymoses. From the head to the toes, systematically use multiple techniques to gather data through observation, inspection, auscultation, palpation, and smell to conduct a comprehensive physical examination of the client. Upon completion of the health assessment and physical examination, analyze and synthesize subjective and objective findings from the assessment, review the results of laboratory tests, and collaborate with the client and other members of the healthcare team to develop mutual goals, make clinical decisions, plan care, implement the plan, and evaluate the care. After evaluating the care, it may be necessary to ask the client additional questions, conduct a more focused physical examination on a particular body system, and/or revise the plan of care to ensure that it provides safe, culturally acceptable, congruent, competent, affordable, accessible, high-quality care that is evidence based and reflects best professional practices.

REVIEW QUESTIONS

1. In your own words, describe the key components of a comprehensive cultural assessment.
2. Compare and contrast your approach to the assessment of light- and dark-skinned clients for cyanosis, jaundice, pallor, erythema, and petechiae.
3. Critically analyze the reasons for the current interest in herbal medicines by nurses, physicians, pharmacists, and other healthcare providers. How does knowledge of these medicines facilitate the nurse's ability to provide culturally competent and congruent nursing care?
4. If you are a student or nurse who is in a clinical practice setting with patients from diverse racial, ethnic, or cultural backgrounds, how will you use the information in this chapter to facilitate the collection of objective and subjective data in the health assessment and physical examination?

CRITICAL THINKING ACTIVITY

An Asian mother and Black father present to the pediatrician's office with their 14-year-old adolescent (C.J.) who identifies as male and was assigned female at birth. The nurse asks questions for the health history. The father reports the adolescent has been cutting his arms and burning himself with matches for the last 3 months. The mother reports she is concerned because C.J. is not eating and wants to stay in his bedroom after school. C.J. explains that he has been self-inflicting harm because of severe bullying at school. He reports he wishes he could just be left alone to be himself. He has burn and laceration areas on bilateral arms that the mother reports she thought were infected. Because of this, his parents want him to be examined. C.J. reports that no one understands, not even the doctors. He tells the nurse the last time he saw

the pediatrician was when he needed a school physical. He reports he felt ashamed when the pediatrician told him he had to check for a hernia and seemed surprised when he realized C.J. was assigned female at birth.

Questions:

1. What questions should the nurse ask the client and parents to determine the influence of culture as well as individual preferences?

2. How might skin assessments vary between individuals with different skin tones?

3. Explore three different strategies that would be helpful for the nurse in communicating with the parents of the child.

4. Discuss how the nurse can make the client feel more comfortable in order to elicit thorough responses and obtain an accurate and thorough health history and physical assessment on C.J.?

5. Reflect on your own bias regarding race, ethnicity, gender, age, and socioeconomic status. Describe why you feel that way and how you can overcome bias when caring for individuals.

REFERENCES

American Academy of Ophthalmology. (2021). *What is low vision?* https://www.aao.org/eye-health/diseases/low-vision
American Academy of Ophthalmology. (2022). *What is albinism?* https://www.aao.org/eye-health/diseases/albinism-diagnosis
American Cancer Society. (2019). *Signs and symptoms of basal and squamous cell skin cancers.* https://www.cancer.org/cancer/basal-and-squamous-cell-skin-cancer/detection-diagnosis-staging/signs-and-symptoms.html
American Heart Association. (2022). *High blood pressure among Black people.* https://www.heart.org/en/health-topics/high-blood-pressure/why-high-blood-pressure-is-a-silent-killer/high-blood-pressure-and-african-americans
American Medical Association and Association of American Medical Colleges. (2021). *Advancing Health Equity: Guide on Language, Narrative and Concepts.* Available at ama-assn.org/equity-guide

Askinazi, O. (2023). *Black people and sickle cell anemia: Your questions answered.* Healthline. https://www.healthline.com/health/sickle-cell-anemia-black-people#takeaway

Black, J. (2018). Using thermography to assess pressure injuries in patients with dark skin. *Nursing: September 2018, 48*(9), 60–61.

Booker, S. Q. (2016). African Americans' perceptions of pain and pain management: A systematic review. *Journal of Transcultural Nursing, 27*(1), 73–80. https://doi.org/10.1177/1043659614526250

Buttaro, T. M., Trybulski, J., Polgar Bailey, P., & Sandberg-Cook, J. (2016). *Primary care: A collaborative practice* (5th ed.). Elsevier.

Campinha-Bacote, J. (2013). *A biblically based model of cultural competence in the delivery of healthcare services: Seeing "Imago Dei"* (2nd ed.). Transcultural C.A.R.E. Associates.

Campinha-Bacote, J. (2018). Cultural competemility: A paradigm shift in the cultural competence versus cultural humility debate—Part I. *OJIN: The Online Journal of Issues in Nursing, 24*(1). https://doi.org/10.3912/OJIN.Vol24No01PPT20

Centers for Disease Control and Prevention. (2019). *Get screened to know your sickle cell status.* cdc.gov/ncbddd/sicklecell/documents/Factsheet_ScickleCell_Status.pdf

Centers for Disease Control and Prevention. (2022a). *Genetic testing.* http://www.cdc.gov/genomics/gtesting/index.htm

Centers for Disease Control and Prevention. (2022b). *Cigarette smoking and tobacco use among people of low socioeconomic status.* https://www.cdc.gov/tobacco/disparities/low-ses/index.htm

Centers for Disease Control and Prevention. (2022c). *Oral and dental health. Untreated dental caries, by selected characteristics: United States, selected years 1988–1994 through 2015–2018.* https://www.cdc.gov/nchs/fastats/dental.htm

Cuevas, A. G., & O'Brien, K. (2017). Racial centrality may be linked to mistrust in healthcare institutions for African Americans. *Journal of Health Psychology, 24*(14). https://doi.org/10.1177/1359105317715092Dahlhamer

Dahlhamer, J., Lucas, J., Zelaya, C., Nahin, R., Mackey, S., DeBar, L., Kerns, R., Von Korff, M., Porter, L., & Helmick, C. (2018). Prevalence of chronic pain and high-impact chronic pain among adults — United States, 2016. *MMWR. Morbidity and Mortality Weekly Report, 67,* 1001–1006. https://www.cdc.gov/mmwr/volumes/67/wr/mm6736a2.htm

Duarte, J. D., & Cavallari, L. H. (2021, September). Pharmacogenetics to guide cardiovascular drug therapy. *Nature Reviews Cardiology, 18*(9), 649–665.

Falci, L., Shi, Z., & Greenlee, H. (2016). Multiple chronic conditions and use of complementary and alternative medicine among US adults: Results from the 2012 National Health Interview Survey. *Preventing Chronic Disease, 13,* 150501. http://dx.doi.org/10.5888/pcd13.150501

FitzGerald, C., & Hurst, S. (2017). Implicit bias in healthcare professionals: A systematic review. *BMC Medical Ethics, 18,* 19. http://doi.org/10.1186/s12910-017-0179-8

Foronda, C. A. (2020). Theory of cultural humility. *Journal of Transcultural Nursing, 31*(1), 7–12. https://doi.org/10.1177/1043659619875184

Gandhi, K., Ezzedine, K., Anastassopoulos, K. P., Patel, R., Sikirica, V., Daniel, S. R., Napatalung, L., Yamaguchi, Y., Baik, R., & Pandya, A. G. (2022). Prevalence of Vitiligo among adults in the United States. *JAMA dermatology, 158*(1), 43–50. https://doi.org/10.1001/jamadermatol.2021.4724

Geronimus, A. T. (2023). *Weathering: The extraordinary stress of an ordinary life in an unjust society.* Little.

Gingras, F., Fiset, D., Plouffe-Demers, M. P., Deschênes, A., Cormier, S., Forget, H., & Blais, C. (2023). Pain in the eye of the beholder: Variations in pain visual representations as a function of face ethnicity and culture. *British Journal of Psychology, 114*(4), 621–637.

Goel, V., Sil, A., & Das, A. (2021). Cutaneous manifestations of chronic kidney disease, dialysis and post-renal transplant: A review. *Indian Journal of Dermatology, 66*(1), 3–11. https://doi.org/10.4103/ijd.IJD_502_20

Goodman, C. W., & Brett, A. S. (2021). Race and pharmacogenomics—Personalized medicine or misguided practice? *JAMA, 325*(7), 625–626. https://doi.org/10.1001/jama.2020.25473

Haywood Jr., C., Tanabe, P., Naik, R., Beach, M. C., & Lanzkron, S. (2013). The impact of race and disease on sickle cell patient wait times in the emergency department. *American Journal of Emergency Medicine, 31*(4), 651–656. https://doi.org/10.1016/j.ajem.2012.11.005

Henschke, N., Lorenz, E., Pokora, R., Michaleff, Z. A., Quartey, J., & Oliveira, V. C. (2016). Understanding cultural influences on back pain and back pain research. *Best Practice and Research Clinical Rheumatology, 30*(6), 1037–1049. https://doi.org/10.1016/j.berh.2017.08.004

Husebye, E. S., Pearce, S. H., Krone, N. P., & Kämpe, O. (2021). Adrenal insufficiency. *Lancet, 397,* 613–629.

Jarvis, C. (2016). *Physical examination and health assessment* (7th ed.). Elsevier/Saunders.

Kato, G., Piel, F., Reid, C., Gaston, M. H., Ohene-Frempong, K., Krishnamurti, L., Smith, W. R., Panepinto, J. A., Weatherall, D. J., Costa, F. F., & Vichinsky, E. P. (2018). Sickle cell disease. *Nature Reviews Disease Primers, 4,* 18010. https://doi.org/10.1038/nrdp.2018.10

Katz, E. L., & Harris, J. E. (2021, March 2). Translational research in Vitiligo. *Frontiers in Immunology, 12,* 624517.

Kim, J., Hwang, J. M., & Kim, H. (2002). Characteristic ocular findings in Asian children with Down syndrome. *Eye, 16,* 710–714. https://doi.org/10.1038/sj.eye.6700208

Kliegman, R. M., Stanton, B. F., Saint Geme, J. W., Schor, N. F., & Behrman, R. E. (2016). *Nelson's textbook of pediatrics* (20th ed.). Elsevier/Saunders.

Kwok, W., & Bhuvanakrishna, T. (2014). The relationship between ethnicity and the pain experience of cancer patients: A systematic review. *Indian Journal of Palliative Care, 20*(3), 194–200.

Leininger, M. M. (1991). *Culture care diversity and universality: A theory of nursing.* NLN Press.

Leininger, M. M., & McFarland, M. R. (2002). *Transcultural nursing: Concepts, theories, research and practices.* McGraw-Hill.

Leininger, M. M., & McFarland, M. R. (2006). *Culture care diversity and universality: A worldwide nursing theory.* Jones & Bartlett.

Liao, T. F., & De Maio, F. (2021). Association of social and economic inequality with coronavirus disease 2019 incidence and mortality across US counties. *JAMA Network Open, 4*(1), e2034578–e2034578.

Mack, D. S., Hunnicutt, J. N., Jesdale, B. M., & Lapane, K. L. (2018). Non-Hispanic Black-White disparities in pain and pain management among newly admitted nursing home residents with cancer. *Journal of Pain Research, 11*, 753–761. https://doi.org/10.2147/JPR.S158128

March of Dimes. (2020). *Prenatal tests.* https://www.marchofdimes.org/pregnancy/prenatal-tests.aspx

Mayo Clinic. (2021a). *Petechiae.* https://www.mayoclinic.org/symptoms/petechiae/basics/definition/sym-20050724

Mayo Clinic. (2021b). *Sweating and body odor.* https://www.mayoclinic.org/diseases-conditions/sweating-and-body-odor/symptoms-causes/syc-20353895

Maymone, M. B. C., Laughter, M., Pollock, S., Khan, I., Marques, T., Abdat, R., Goldberg, L. J., & Vashi, N. A. (2021). Hair aging in different races and ethnicities. *The Journal of Clinical and Aesthetic Dermatology, 14*(1), 38–44.

McFarland, M. R., & Wehbe-Alamah, H. B. (2015). *Leininger's culture care diversity and universality: A worldwide theory of nursing* (3rd ed.). Jones & Bartlett Learning.

McFarland, M. R., & Wehbe-Alamah, H. B. (2018). *Transcultural nursing: Concepts, theories, research, and practices* (4th ed.). McGraw-Hill, Medical Publishing Division.

Meghani, S., Byun, E., & Gallagher, R. (2012a). Time to take stock: A meta-analysis and systematic review of analgesic treatment disparities for pain in the United States. *Pain Medicine, 13*(2), 150–174. academic.oup.com/painmedicine/article/13/2/150/1935962

Meghani, S., Polomano, R. C., Tait, R. C., Vallerand, A. H., Anderson, K. O., & Gallagher, R. M. (2012b). Advancing a national agenda to eliminate disparity in pain care: Directions for health policy, education, practice and research. *Pain and Medicine, 13*(1), 5–28.

Meiner, S., & Yeager, J. J. (2019). *Gerontologic Nursing* (6th ed.). Elsevier.

Meints, S. M., Cortes, A., Morais, C. A., & Edwards, R. R. (2019, May). Racial and ethnic differences in the experience and treatment of noncancer pain. *Pain Management, 9*(3), 317–334.

National Center for Biotechnology Information. (2022). *Genetic testing registry.* https://www.ncbi.nlm.nih.gov/gtr/

National Center for Complementary and Integrative Health. (2022). *Herbs at a glance.* https://www.nccih.nih.gov/health/herbsataglance

National Institute of Health. (2022a). *Human genome project.* https://www.genome.gov/12011238/an-overview-of-the-human-genome-project/

National Institute of Health. (2022b). *X-linked congenital stationary night blindness.* https://ghr.nlm.nih.gov/condition/x-linked-congenital-stationary-night-blindness#statistics

National Organization for Albinism and Hypopigmentation (2021). Information for medical professionals. *Information Bulletin—What is Albinism.* https://www.albinism.org/medical/

National Geographic. (2018). *You can smell when someone's sick—Here's how.* https://news.nationalgeographic.com/2018/01/smell-sickness-parkinsons-disease-health-science/?user.testname=none

O'Brien, E. M., O'Donnell, C., Murphy, J., O'Brien, B., & Markey, K. (2021). Intercultural readiness of nursing students: An integrative review of evidence examining cultural competence educational interventions. *Nurse Education in Practice, 50*, 102966.

Ogbu, C. E., Oparanma, C., Ogbu, S. C., Ujah, O. I., Okoli, M. L., & Kirby, R. S. (2023). Trends in the use of complementary and alternative therapies among US adults with current asthma. *Epidemiologia, 4*(1), 94–105. https://doi.org/10.3390/epidemiologia4010010

Ortega, P., Shin, T. M., & Martínez, G. A. (2022). Rethinking the term "limited English proficiency" to improve language-appropriate healthcare for all. *Journal of Immigrant Minority Health, 24*, 799–805. https://doi.org/10.1007/s10903-021-01257-w

Overfield, T. (2017). *CRC revivals: Biologic variation in health and illness: Race, age and sex differences* (2nd ed.). CRC Press.

Pahal, P., Goyal, A., & Central and Peripheral Cyanosis. (2021, October 9). In: *StatPearls [Internet].* StatPearls Publishing.

Park, A. M., Khan, S., & Rawnsley, J. (2018). Hair biology: Growth and pigmentation. *Facial Plastic Surgery Clinics of North America, 26*(4), 415–424.

Phillips, A., Frank, A., Loftin, C., & Shepherd, S. (2017). A detailed review of systems: An educational feature. *The Journal for Nurse Practitioners, 13*(10), 681–686.

Poma, P. A. (2017). Race/ethnicity concordance between patients and physicians. *Journal of the National Medical Association, 109*(1), 6–8. http://dx.doi.org.libproxy.umflint.edu/10.1016/j.jnma.2016.12.002

Prosen, M. (2015). Introducing transcultural nursing education: Implementation of transcultural nursing in the postgraduate nursing curriculum. *Procedia: Social and Behavioral Sciences, 174*, 149–155. https://doi.org/10.1016/j.sbspro.2015.01.640

Pusey-Reid, E., Quinn, L., Samost, M., & Reidy, P. A. (2023). Skin assessment in patients with dark skin tone. *American Journal of Nursing 123*(3), 36-43. https://doi.org/10.1097/01.NAJ.0000921800.61980.7e

Rateau, M. R. (2022). Assessment: Integumentary system (p. 456). Assessment and Management of Clinical Problems, Single Volume.

Repo, H., Vahlberg, T., Salminen, L., Papadopoulos, I., & Leino-Kilpi, H. (2017). The cultural competence of graduating nursing students. *Journal of Transcultural Nursing, 28*(1), 98–107. https://doi.org/10.1177/1043659616632046

Rodriguez, T. (2023). Barriers to healthcare: A brief overview of healthcare stigmas among Black and Hispanic/Latino patients. *Nursing Made Incredibly Easy, 21*(3), 36–43.

Rogers, J. (2021). Understanding the most commonly billed diagnoses in primary care: General medical exam. *The Nurse Practitioner Journal, 46*(2), 35–43.

Rogers, J. (Ed.) (2023). *McCance and Huether's pathophysiology: The biologic basis for disease in adults and children* (9th ed.). C.V Mosby.

Rosebush, M. S., Briody, A. N., & Cordell, K. G. (2019). Black and brown: Non-neoplastic pigmentation of the oral mucosa. *Head and neck pathology, 13*(1), 47–55. https://doi.org/10.1007/s12105-018-0980-9

Slaught, C., Madu, P., Chang, A. Y., Williams, V. L., Kebaetse, M. B., Nkomazana, O., Molefe-Baikai, O. J., Bekele, N. A., Omech, B., Kellman, P. J., Krasne, S., & Kovarik, C. L. (2022 January–February). Novel education modules addressing the underrepresentation of skin of color in dermatology training. *Journal of Cutaneous Medicine and Surgery, 26*(1), 17–24.

Swope, V. B., & Abdel-Malek, Z. A. (2018, September). MC1R: Front and center in the bright side of dark Eumelanin and DNA repair. *International Journal of Molecular Science, 19*(9), 2667.

Tait, R. C., & Chibnall, J. T. (2014). Racial/ethnic disparities in the assessment and treatment of pain. *American Psychologist, 69*(2), 131–141.

Thompson, H. M., Kronk, C. A., Feasley, K., Pachwicewicz, P., & Karnik, N. S. (2021). Implementation of gender identity and assigned sex at birth data collection in electronic health records: Where are we now? *International Journal of Environmental Research and Public Health, 18*(12), 6599.

Tosun, B., Yava, A., Dirgar, E., Şahin, E. B., Yılmaz, E. B., Papp, K., et al. (2021). Addressing the effects of transcultural nursing education on nursing students' cultural competence: A systematic review. *Nurse Education in Practice, 55*, 103171.

Tsai, J. W., Cerdeña, J. P., Goedel, W. C., Asch, W. S., Grubbs, V., Mendu, M. L., & Kaufman, J. S. (2021). Evaluating the impact and rationale of race-specific estimations of kidney function: Estimations from U.S. NHANES, 2015-2018. *eClinical Medicine, 42*, 101197. https://doi.org/10.1016/j.eclinm.2021.101197

U.S. Census Bureau. (2017). *2017 National population projections tables.* https://www.census.gov/data/tables/2017/demo/popproj/2017-summary-tables.html

U.S. Census Bureau. (2020a). *People that speak English less than "very well" in the United States.*

U.S. Census Bureau. (2020b). https://www.census.gov/library/visualizations/interactive/people-that-speak-english-less-than-very-well.html

U.S. Department of Health and Human Services. (2020). *Botanical drug development guidance for industry.* Updated 5/7/2020. https://www.fda.gov/downloads/Drugs/Guidances/UCM458484.pdf

U.S. Department of Health and Human Services. (2023). *National Center on Birth Defects and Developmental Disabilities, Centers for Disease Control and Prevention.* https://www.cdc.gov/ncbddd/

U.S. Food and Drug Administration. (2022). *Table of pharmacogenomic biomarkers in drug labeling.* https://www.fda.gov/drugs/science-and-research-drugs/table-pharmacogenomic-biomarkers-drug-labeling

Vashi, N. A., De Castro Maymone, M. B., & Kundu, R. V. (2016). Aging differences in ethnic skin. *Journal of Clinical and Aesthetic Dermatology, 9*(1), 31–38. http://libproxy.umflint.edu/login?url=http://search.ebscohost.com/login.aspx?direct=true&db=a9h&AN=112227388&site=ehost-live&scope=site

Vashi, N. A., & Maibach, H. I. (2017). *Dermatoanthropology of ethnic skin and hair.* Springer International Publishing.

Vashi, N. A., Wirya, S. A., Inyang, M., & Kundu, R. V. (2017, April). Facial hyperpigmentation in skin of color: Special considerations and treatment. *American Journal of Clinical Dermatology, 18*(2), 215–230.

Vespa, J., Medina, L., & Armstrong, D. M. (2020). *Demographic turning points for the United States: Population projections for 2020 to 2060* (pp. 25–1144).

Vyas, D. A., Eisenstein, L. G., & Jones, D. S. (2020). Hidden in plain sight—Reconsidering the use of race correction in clinical algorithms. *New England Journal of Medicine, 383*(9), 874–882.

Williamson, L. (2021). *The link between structural racism, high blood pressure and Black people's health.* American Heart

Association. https://www.heart.org/en/news/2021/04/15/the-link-between-structural-racism-high-blood-pressure-and-black-peoples-health

World Health Organization. (2021). *Social determinants of health.* https://www.who.int/health-topics/social-determinants-of-health

World Health Organization. (2023). *WHO Global Centre for Traditional Medicine.* https://www.who.int/initiatives/who-global-centre-for-traditional-medicine

Zhang, D., Slaven, K., & Shields, B. E. (2023). Cutaneous signs of malnutrition secondary to eating disorders. *Cutis, 111*(5), 231–238.

Influence of Cultural and Health Belief Systems on Healthcare Practices

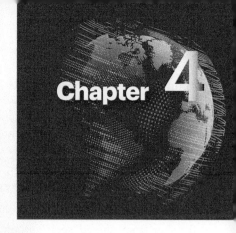

Chapter 4

• Marilyn K. Eipperle and Margaret M. Andrews

Key Terms

Allopathic medicine
Ayurvedic medicine
Complementary, integrative,
 and alternative health
Cultural belief systems
Cultural values and beliefs
Dietary supplements

Folk healers
Folk healing systems
Health behaviors
Health belief systems
Health literacy
Holistic paradigm
Illness behavior
Magico-religious paradigm
Naturopathy

Osteopathic medicine
Paradigm
Professional care systems
Scientific paradigm
Self-care
Sick role behavior
Traditional Chinese Medicine
Worldview

Learning Objectives

1. Describe the major belief systems of people from diverse cultures.
2. Compare and contrast professional healthcare and folk healing systems.
3. Identify major complementary and alternative healthcare therapies.
4. Describe cultural influences on illness symptoms and sick role behaviors.
5. Critically appraise the efficacy of selected traditional therapeutic approaches for health problems.

Introduction

In this chapter, we examine the major cultural belief systems embraced by people from diverse cultures and explore the characteristics of three of the most prevalent worldviews (or paradigms) related to health–illness beliefs: magico-religious, scientific/biomedical, and holistic. We explore self-care, integrative professional care, and folk (indigenous, traditional, generic, lay) care approaches along with their respective systems and healers. After analyzing

cultural values and beliefs and their influences on symptoms, sick roles, and illness behaviors, we examine selected complementary and alternative therapies used to treat acute and chronic physical and psychological illnesses and diseases.

Cultural Belief Systems

Cultural meanings and cultural belief systems develop from shared social group experiences and are expressed symbolically. The use of symbols to define, describe, and relate to the world around us is a basic characteristic of being human. One of the most common symbolism expressions is *metaphor*, wherein one aspect of life is connected to another through a shared symbol. For example, the phrase "what a tangled web we weave" expresses metaphorically the relationship between two normally disparate concepts—human deception and a spider's web. People often use metaphors as a way of thinking about and explaining life events.

People groups across time have attempted to explain the phenomena of *nature*. From each explanation emerged a common belief system. These explanations usually involved metaphoric imagery of magical, religious, natural/holistic, scientific, or biologic forms. These explanatory ranges were limited only by the human imagination.

The set of metaphoric explanations used by a group of people to explain life events and offer solutions to life mysteries can be described as its worldview or major paradigm. A **paradigm** is a universal interpretation of the world and its phenomena and encompasses the assumptions, premises, and linkages that bind together a prevailing interpretation of reality. Paradigms are slow to change and do so only if and when their explanatory power has been depleted.

Worldview reflects the total configuration of beliefs and practices and permeates every lifeway within a group culture. Members of a culture share a worldview without necessarily recognizing it as such. Group thought is patterned on or derives from this worldview because the culture

imparts a particular set of associated relational symbols used in thinking. Because these symbols are taken for granted, people typically do not question the cultural bias of their thoughts. Use of the term *American* by United States (U.S.) citizens as a referent only to themselves collectively reflects such an unconscious cultural bias. In reality, it is a generic term referring to all people in the Americas, which encompass the combined continental landmasses of North, Central, and South America, and islands located in the Western Hemisphere from Canada to Peru.

Another example of symbolism and worldview can be seen in the way nurses use terms such as *nursing care*, *health promotion*, *illness*, and *disease*. Nurses often take it for granted that all their clients define and relate to these concepts in the same way as themselves. This assumption reflects an unconscious belief that cultural symbols are shared by all and therefore do not require explanation within any given nurse–client context. Such assumptions account for many of the difficulties nurses encounter when communicating with clients and other nonmembers of the health profession culture.

Health Belief Systems

Generally, theories of health and disease (or illness) causation are based on a group's prevailing worldview. Worldview includes a group's health-related values, beliefs, and practices, sometimes referred to as its *health belief system*. Each system has its own corresponding aggregate health beliefs. People embrace three major **health belief systems** or worldviews:

1. *Magico-religious*
2. *Scientific/biomedical*
3. *Holistic*

In the magico-religious and holistic systems, disease is perceived as an entity separate from the *self*, caused by an agent external to the body but capable of "getting in" and causing damage. The causative agent becomes attributed to a variety of natural and supernatural phenomena. Frequently, people may adhere to or believe in aspects of two or all three of the systems at any given time. For example, a person who is ill may understand the illness has an identified causative agent but at the same time may pray to recover quickly as well as embark on a sacred journey to visit a vortex specialist to realign body, mind, and spirit.

Magico-Religious Health Paradigm

In the **magico-religious paradigm**, the world is an arena controlled by supernatural forces. The fate of the world and those in it, including humans, depends on the actions of God, the gods, or other supernatural forces of good versus evil. In some cases, the human individual is at the mercy of such forces regardless of behavior. In other cases, the gods punish humans for their transgressions. Many Latino, African/African American, native or aboriginal, and Middle Eastern cultures are grounded in the magico-religious paradigm (Quiroz & van Andel, 2018). *Magic* involves the calling forth and control of supernatural forces for and against others. Some African and Caribbean cultures have aspects of magic in their belief system, such as voodoo. In some Western (North American, Central American, South American, and European) cultures, metaphysical reality intersects within mainstream society. For example, Christian Scientists believe that physical healing can be effected through prayer alone.

Writing about the history of medicine, Ackernecht (1946) stated that "...magic or religion seems to satisfy better than any other device a certain eternal psychic or 'metaphysical' need of mankind, sick and healthy, for integration and harmony." Magic and religion are logical in their own way but are not based on empiric premises; they defy the reality of the physical or scientific world known from the use of human senses, particularly observation. In the magico-religious paradigm, disease is viewed as the action and result of supernatural forces that cause intrusion of a disease-producing foreign body or health-damaging spirit.

Throughout the world in the magico-religious paradigm, five categories of events are believed to be responsible for illness: *sorcery, breach of taboo, intrusion of a disease object, intrusion of a disease-causing spirit,* and *loss of soul* (Clements, 1932). One or any combination of these belief categories may be offered to explain the origin of disease. Alaska Natives refer to *soul loss* and *breach of taboo* (i.e., breaking a social norm, such as committing adultery). West Indians and some Africans and African Americans believe that the malevolence of sorcerers is the cause of many conditions. Belief in *mal de ojo* (or the *evil eye*), common in Hispanic and other cultures, is viewed as the projected intrusion of a disease-causing spirit by one person onto another, particularly vulnerable persons such as children (Sanchez, 2018).

In the magico-religious paradigm, illness is initiated by a supernatural agent with or without justification, or by another person who practices sorcery or engages the services of sorcerers. The cause-and-effect relationship is not organic; rather, the cause of health or illness is mystical. Health is bestowed as a perceived reward signifying blessing and goodwill by the deity of belief. Illness may be seen as a sign of possession or punishment; alternatively, it may signify special favor permitting the affected person an opportunity to accept the deity's plan (e.g., "*God's will*"). Hence, in many Christian religions, the faithful communally gather to pray for God to heal the ill or to practice healing rituals such as *laying on of hands* or *anointing the sick* with oil. Furthermore, health and illness are commonly viewed as belonging first to the community and then to the individual. Thus, one person's actions may directly or indirectly influence the health or illness of another person or the entire community.

Scientific/Biomedical Health Paradigm

In the scientific/biomedical paradigm, life is controlled by a series of physical and biochemical processes that humans can study and manipulate. Several specific forms of symbolic thought processes characterize the **scientific paradigm**. The first is *determinism*, which states that a cause-and-effect relationship exists for all natural phenomena. The second, *mechanism*, assumes that it is possible to control life processes through mechanical, genetic, and other engineered interventions. The third form is *reductionism*, in which all life can be reduced or divided into smaller parts; studying the unique characteristics of these isolated parts is thought to reveal aspects or properties of the whole (i.e., the human genome and its component parts). The final thought process is *objective materialism*, wherein reality is only what can be observed and measured. Further distinctions between *subjective* and *objective* realities are made within this paradigm.

When the scientific paradigm is applied to matters of health, it is often referred to as the *biomedical model*. The scientific/biomedical paradigm considers only forces that can be observed and measured. Dominant Western cultural groups in the United States, Canada, Europe, Australia, and New Zealand espouse this paradigm. In the biomedical model (generally practiced as either **allopathic** or **osteopathic medicine**), all aspects of human health are viewed through the natural sciences (biology, chemistry, physics, and mathematics). This mindset also fosters the belief that psychological and emotional processes can be reduced to the study of biochemical exchanges. Effective treatments consist of physical and chemical interventions, often with lesser or no regard for human values, beliefs, or relationships.

In this model, disease is viewed metaphorically as the breakdown of the human machine due to wear and tear (stress), external trauma (injury, accident), external invasion (pathogens), or internal damages (fluid and chemical imbalances, genetic, immunologic, or other structural changes). Disease causes illness, generally has a specific cause, follows a predictable time course, and requires a specified set of treatments. The scientific/biomedical paradigm parallels the magico-religious belief in external agents but replaces *supernatural forces* with *infectious and genetic agents*.

With the metaphor of the machine, the computer is analogous for the brain. Biomedicine specialists take care of the "parts" and "fixing" a part restores the machine's function ability; engineering becomes a task for biomedical practitioners. The discovery of DNA and development of the human genome have led to the research field of *genetic engineering*, another eloquent biomedical metaphor. The symbols used to discuss health and disease reflect the U.S. cultural values of *dominance* and *mastery*. Thus, when microorganisms attack the body, war is waged against the invaders, money is donated for the campaign against cancer, and illness is a struggle in which the patient must put up a good defense. The biomedical model defines *health as the absence of disease or the signs and symptoms of disease*. To be healthy, one must be free of all disease. In comparison, the World Health Organization (WHO) defined health more holistically as "...a state of complete physical, mental, and social well-being and not merely the absence of disease or infirmity" (WHO, 1948, p. 100). This oft-cited definition has remained unaltered since 1948, although the topical foci have changed across time (WHO, 2023).

Holistic Health Paradigm

In the **holistic paradigm**, the *forces of nature* must be kept in *natural* balance or *harmony*. Human life is but one aspect of nature and the general order of the cosmos. Everything in the universe has its place with a role to perform according to the natural laws maintaining order. Disturbing these laws creates imbalance, chaos, and disease. The holistic paradigm has existed for centuries in many parts of the world, particularly in Native American and Asian cultures. It has gained wider acceptance in the United States and Canada because it complements the increased sense that the biomedical model fails to account fully for naturally occurring causations and other factors such as cultural values, psychological effects, and social determinants of health (SDOH).

The holistic paradigm seeks to maintain a sense of balance between humans and the larger universe. Explanations for health and disease are based on imbalance or disharmony among the human, geophysical, and metaphysical forces of the universe. For example, in the biomedical model, the cause of tuberculosis is clearly identified as an invasion of mycobacterium. In the holistic paradigm, whereby disease is the result of multiple environment–host interactions, tuberculosis is caused by the interrelationship of poverty, malnutrition, overcrowding, poor sanitation/ventilation/hygiene, and mycobacterium.

The term *holistic*, coined by Smuts (1926), described an attitude or mode of perception wherein the whole person was viewed in the context of the total environment. Its Indo-European root word, *kailo*, means "whole, intact, or uninjured," and from this root have come the words *hale, hail, hallow, holy, whole, heal*, and *health*. Thus, the essence of health and healing became the quality of *wholeness* humans associate with healthy functioning and well-being. In this paradigm, health is viewed as a positive process encompassing more than absent signs and symptoms of disease. Health is not restricted to biologic or somatic wellness but rather involves broader environmental, sociocultural, and behavioral determinants. In this model, diseases of civilization such as unemployment, racism, poverty, urban decay, and pollution are just as much illnesses as are biomedical diseases such as obesity, asthma/allergies, depression, and suicide. This holistic view of health parallels the growing and more prevalent biomedical/Western medicine embrace for SDOH as significant factors influencing health and wellbeing.

The belief system of Florence Nightingale, who emphasized nursing's control of the environment so that patients could heal naturally, was holistic. Transcultural nursing, founded by Madeleine Leininger, and the Theory of Culture Care Diversity and Universality are also holistic paradigms (McFarland & Wehbe-Alamah, 2018, 2019).

Illness is believed to be the outward expression of *disharmony*. This disharmony may result from seasonal changes, emotional imbalances, a disrupted pattern, or other chain of events. Illness is not caused by an intruding agent but is perceived as a natural part of life's rhythmic course. Transitioning in and out of balance is accepted as a natural process that happens continually throughout the life span. Health and illness are dimensions of the same process, in which the individual organism responds to the changing environment. In the holistic paradigm, illness is inevitable and thus perfect health is not the goal. Rather, achieving an optimal adaptation to the environment by living according to society's rules and caring appropriately for one's body is the desired outcome. The holistic paradigm places a greater emphasis on preventive care and maintenance measures than typically occurs in biomedicine.

Metaphors used in this paradigm including the *healing power of nature, health foods, mindfulness*, and *Mother Earth* reflect the human connection with the cosmos and nature. A strong metaphor in the holistic paradigm is exemplified by the Chinese concept of yin and yang, in which the forces of nature are balanced to produce harmony (Xiang et al., 2017). The *yin* force in the universe represents the female aspect of nature. It is characterized as the negative pole, encompassing darkness, cold, and emptiness. The *yang* or male force, characterized by fullness, light, and warmth, represents the positive pole. An imbalance of these forces creates illness.

Another common metaphor for health and illness in the holistic paradigm is the hot/cold theory of disease, founded on the ancient Greek concept of the four body humors: yellow bile, black bile, phlegm, and blood. *Humors* are vital components of the blood found in varying amounts throughout the human body. The four humors work together to ensure the optimum nutrition, growth, and metabolism. When the humors are balanced in a healthy individual, the state of *ecrasia* exists. When the humors are in a state of imbalance, this is referred to as *dyscrasia* (Osborn, 2021). The treatment of disease becomes a process of restoring the body's humoral balance through the addition or subtraction of substances that affect each of these four humors. Foods, beverages, herbs, and drugs are all classified as *hot* or *cold* depending on their effect, not their actual physical state. Disease conditions are also classified as either hot or cold. Imbalance or disharmony is believed to cause internal damage and altered physiologic functions. Medicine is directed at correcting this imbalance as well as restoring body functions. Although the concept of hot and cold is found in Asian, Latino, Black, Arab, Muslim, and Caribbean societies, each cultural group defines what it believes to be hot and cold entities, and little agreement about them exists across cultures.

Health and Illness Behaviors

The series of behaviors typifying the health-seeking process have been labeled *health and illness behaviors.* These behaviors are expressed in the roles people assume after identifying a symptom. Related to these behaviors are the roles individuals assign to others and the status given to the role-players. People assume various types of behaviors once they have recognized a symptom. **Health behavior** is any activity undertaken by a person who believes themself to be healthy to prevent or detect disease at an asymptomatic stage. **Illness behavior** is any activity undertaken by a person who feels ill to define the state of their own health and discover a suitable remedy. **Sick role behavior** is any activity undertaken by a person who considers themself ill to get well or to deal with the illness.

Three sets of factors influence the course of behaviors and practices carried out to maintain health and prevent disease: (1) one's beliefs about health and illness; (2) personal factors such as age, education, knowledge, or experience with a given disease condition; and (3) cues to action, such as advertisements in the media, the illness of a relative, or the advice of friends. Mechanic (1978) outlined the determinants of **illness behavior** model with 10 facets of illness behavior important to understanding the help-seeking process (see Table 4-1). Awareness of these motivational factors (including

cultural influences) provides insights enabling nurses to offer more appropriate assistance to clients traversing the illness process.

Types of Healing Systems

The term *healing system* refers to the accumulated sciences, arts, and techniques of restoring and preserving health that are used by any cultural group. In complex societies in which several cultural traditions flourish, healers tend to compete with one another and/or to view their scopes of practice as separate from one another. In some instances, however, practitioners may make referrals to different healing systems. For example, a nurse may contact a rabbi to assist a Jewish patient with spiritual needs, or a *curandero* may advise a Mexican American patient to visit a professional healthcare provider for an antibiotic when traditional practices do not heal a wound.

Self-Care

For common minor illnesses and injuries, most people initially try **self-care** with over-the-counter medicines, topical agents, megavitamins, herbs, exercise, and/or foods that they believe have healing powers. Many self-care practices have been handed down from generation to generation, frequently by oral tradition. Self-care is the largest component of the U.S. healthcare system with **dietary supplements** accounting for approximately $35 billion annually (Haspel, 2020). The use of over-the-counter medications, or nonprescription medications, is the most common form of self-care among U.S. adults, higher among females than males (Mishra et al., 2023). Dietary supplements such as herbs, vitamins, minerals, oils, topical agents, and other substances are used extensively across all cultures and social strata in the United States. Box 4-1 provides tips for making informed decisions and evaluating information about dietary supplements that may also be a useful guide for health professionals during client interactions. When

Table 4-1 | Mechanic's Determinants of Illness Behavior

Determinant	Description
Quality of symptom	The more frightening or visible the symptom, the greater the likelihood that the individual will intervene.
Seriousness of symptom	The perceived threat of the symptom must be serious for action to be taken. Often, others will step in if the person's behavior is considered dangerous (e.g., suicidal behavior) but will be unaware of potential problems if the person's behavior seems natural ("he always acts that way").
Disruption of daily activities	Behaviors that are very disruptive in work or other social situations are likely to be labeled as illness much sooner than the same behaviors in a family setting. An individual whose activities are disrupted by a symptom is likely to take that symptom seriously (e.g., acne just before a date) even if at another routine time the person would consider the same symptom as less important.
Rate and persistence of symptom	The frequency of a symptom is directly related to its importance; a symptom that persists is also likely to be taken seriously.
Tolerance of symptom	The extent to which others, especially family, tolerate the symptom before reacting varies; individuals also have different tolerance thresholds.
Sociocognitive status	A person's information about the symptom, knowledge base, and cultural values all influence that person's perception of illness.
Denial of symptom	Often, the individual or family members need to deny a symptom for personal or social reasons. The amount of fear and anxiety present can interfere with perception of a symptom.
Motivation	Competing needs may motivate a person to delay or enhance symptoms. A person who has no time or money to be sick will often not acknowledge the seriousness of symptoms.
Assigning of meaning	Once perceived, the symptom must be interpreted. Often, people explain symptoms within normal parameters ("I'm just tired").
Treatment accessibility	The greater the barriers to treatment—whether psychological, economic, physical, or social—the greater the likelihood that the symptom will not be interpreted as serious or that the person will seek an alternative form of care.

Adapted from Mechanic, D. (1978). *Medical sociology* (2nd ed.). The Free Press. Copyright © 1978 by David Mechanic, with permission.

BOX 4-1   Tips for Making Informed Decisions and Evaluating Information About Dietary Supplements

Basic Points to Consider

1. **Q. How do I know if I need a dietary supplement?**
   - **A.** Many products are marketed as dietary supplements, and it is important to remember that supplements include not only vitamins and minerals but also herbs and other botanicals, probiotics, fish oil, and other substances.

- Some supplements may help ensure that you get adequate amounts of essential nutrients or help promote optimal health and performance if you do not consume a variety of foods, as recommended by MyPlate and the *Dietary Guidelines for Americans*.
- However, dietary supplements are not intended to treat, diagnose, mitigate, prevent, or cure disease. In some cases, dietary supplements may have unwanted effects,

(continued)

especially if taken before surgery or with other dietary supplements or medicines, or if you have certain health conditions.

- Do not self-diagnose any health condition. Work with your healthcare provider to determine how best to achieve optimal health. Also check with your healthcare provider before taking a supplement, especially if you take any medicines or other dietary supplements or if you have any health conditions.

2. **Q. How can I get more information about a particular dietary supplement such as whether it is safe and effective?**
   - **A.** Scientific evidence supporting the benefits of some dietary supplements (for example, vitamins and minerals) is well established for certain health conditions, but others need further study.
   - Research studies in people to prove that a dietary supplement is safe are not required before the supplement is marketed, unlike for drugs. This is due to the way dietary supplements are regulated by the U.S. Food and Drug Administration (FDA). It is the responsibility of dietary supplement manufacturers/distributors to ensure that their products are safe and that their label claims are truthful and not misleading. If the FDA finds a supplement to be unsafe once it is on the market, only then can it take action against the manufacturer and/or distributor, such as by issuing a warning or requiring the product to be removed from the marketplace.
   - The manufacturer does not have to prove that the supplement is effective, unlike for pharmaceutical medications. The manufacturer can say that the product addresses a nutrient deficiency, supports health, or reduces the risk of developing a health problem, if that is true. If the manufacturer does make a claim, it must be followed by the statement "This statement

has not been evaluated by the Food and Drug Administration. This product is not intended to diagnose, treat, cure, or prevent any disease."

- Dietary supplements are not intended to treat, diagnose, mitigate, prevent, or cure disease. In some cases, dietary supplements may have unwanted effects, especially if taken before surgery or with other dietary supplements or medicines, or if you have certain health conditions. Supplements should not replace prescribed medications or the variety of foods important to a healthful diet.
   o Some supplements may interact with prescription and over-the-counter medicines.
   o Some supplements can have unwanted effects with surgery.
   o Adverse effects from the use of dietary supplements should be reported to the FDA at https://www.fda.gov/safety/report-problem-fda or by contacting their state or regional consumer complaint coordinator identifiable at https://www.fda.gov/Safety/ReportaProblem/ConsumerComplaintCoordinators/default.htm.

3. **Q. How can I evaluate product websites and labels safely and accurately?**
   - **A.** By federal law, manufacturers of dietary supplements are responsible for ensuring their products are safe before being marketed:
   o What expert or organization sponsors or validates the website?
   o What is the purpose of the website?
   o Is the source of the information identified, and does the site contain accessible references?
   o Does the information appear current and accurate?
   o Are the claims significantly different than found elsewhere (i.e., too good to be true)?

| **BOX 4-1** | **Tips for Making Informed Decisions and Evaluating Information About Dietary Supplements (continued)** |

- Think twice about believing what you read. Here are some assumptions that raise safety concerns:

  "Even if a product may not help me, it at least will not hurt me."

  "When I see the term 'natural,' it means that a product is healthful and safe."

  "A product is safe when there is no cautionary information on the product label."

  "A recall of a harmful product guarantees that all such harmful products will be immediately and completely removed from the marketplace."

- Contact the manufacturer for specific product information before purchasing.
- In addition to talking with your healthcare provider about dietary supplements, you can search online for information about a particular supplement. It is important to ensure that you obtain information from reliable sources such as:
  o ODS dietary supplement fact sheets
  o Nutrient Recommendations: Dietary Reference Intakes (DRI) and Recommended Dietary Allowances (RDA)
  o Dietary supplement warnings and safety information from the U.S. Food and Drug Administration
  o Consumer information from the Federal Trade Commission
- For tips on evaluating sources of healthcare information on the internet, please see the following document: *How to Evaluate Health Information on the Internet: Questions and Answers* at https://ods.od.nih.gov/HealthInformation/How_To_Evaluate_Health_Information_on_the_Internet_Questions_and_Answers.aspx

Sources: U.S. Department of Health and Human Services, Food and Drug Administration, Center for Food Safety and Applied Nutrition. (2020, August 6). *Report a problem to the FDA.* https://www.fda.gov/safety/report-problem-fda; U.S. Department of Health and Human Services, National Institutes of Health, Office of Dietary Supplements. (2021, March 23). *Frequently asked questions.* https://ods.od.nih.gov/HealthInformation/ODS_Frequently_Asked_Questions.aspx

self-care becomes ineffective, people are more likely to seek care from *professional* and/or *folk* (indigenous, generic, traditional, lay) healing systems (see Evidence-Based Practice 4-1).

Professional Care Systems

According to Leininger (1997) and McFarland and Wehbe-Alamah (2015, 2018), **professional care** (also referred to as scientific/biomedical care) is formally taught, learned, and transmitted knowledge and practice skills and approaches for treating acute and chronic illness that involves maintaining health and wellness in professional institutions and healthcare systems with multidisciplinary clinicians and staff. Professional care is characterized by specialized education and knowledge, wherein practitioners take primary responsibility for care provision and outcomes with an expectation of remuneration for services rendered. Nurses, physicians, physical therapists, and other licensed healthcare clinicians constitute the professional care providers in most health systems in the United States, Canada, Europe, Australia, New Zealand, and Japan, other parts of the world.

Folk Healing System

A folk healing system is a set of beliefs that has a shared social dimension and reflects what people typically do when they are ill versus what society says they should do according to a set of social standards (Sandberg et al., 2018). According to McFarland and Wehbe-Alamah (2015, 2018), all cultures of the world have a lay healthcare system, which is sometimes referred to as indigenous, folk, lay, or generic. The key consideration that

Health Literacy as a Social Determinant of Health

Health literacy as a social determinant of health has widespread public health implications. It is essential for optimal self-care and is not directly related to intelligence or level of education. Many researchers have defined health literacy as the wide range of skills and competencies that people develop to seek out, comprehend, evaluate, and use health information and concepts to make informed choices, reduce health risks, and improve quality of life. However, Fleary and Ettienne (2019) determined that "Income (~30%) and education (~37%) were the highest contributors to overall disparities in health literacy" (p. e49).

Health literacy is an independent and mediating determinant of health (Fleary & Ettienne, 2019; Nutbeam & Lloyd, 2021). Individual health literacy becomes compromised under situations of duress such as illness, pain, stress, high emotion, altered cognitive states, and with aging (Prins & Monnat, 2015). As explained by Nutbeam and Lloyd (2021):

> Literacy is not a fixed asset. It can be improved through education and is specific to both content and context. Individuals vary in their ability to learn and will respond in diverse ways to different forms of communication and media. Although the possession of generic literacy skills in reading, writing, and understanding text improves an individual's ability to access, understand, and act on new information, these skills do not guarantee that a person can consistently apply them in situations requiring specific content knowledge or in unfamiliar settings. In different settings, more specialized knowledge and skills may be required. This understanding of the dynamic nature of literacy has led to the recognition of different specialist literacies, such as financial, science, or digital literacy. This distinction reflects the fact that individuals have varying capacity to apply their general literacy skills in different contexts. From this perspective, health literacy may be considered one of many domains of literacy. (p. 161)

The facilitators for safe and effective disease self-management included speaking and listening skills that promote better clinician–patient communication; math (numeracy) skills, such as sliding scales for insulin dosage based on blood glucose levels; reading skills to comprehend educational materials about disease processes and treatment; social support from family members, such as spouse and adult children; and social support from neighbors and friends who have higher levels of literacy than does the patient and, in some instances, more financial resources.

Clinical Implications

- Nurses and other members of the healthcare team should recognize that patients' cultural health belief systems and explanatory models are interrelated with their health and linguistic literacy, educational background, and socioeconomic status.
- Cultural health beliefs exert important influences on the self-management of chronic diseases such as diabetes and hypertension.
- Cultural health beliefs are part of internally consistent explanatory models constructed by the patient in an effort to make sense of their diagnosis and the clinical manifestations of the underlying cause(s) of illness.
- If the patient's cultural health beliefs are not aligned with a biomedical explanation, the patient may decide to adhere to their own beliefs and refrain from following the provided biomedical advice and recommendations by nurses, physicians, and other health professionals.

References: Fleary, S. A., & Ettienne, R. (2019). Social disparities in health literacy in the United States. *Health Literacy Research and Practice*, 3(1), e47–e52; Nutbeam, D., & Lloyd, J. E. (2020). Understanding and responding to health literacy as a social determinant of health. *Annual Review of Public Health*, 42(2021), 159–173; Prins, E., & Monnat, S. (2015). Examining associations between self-rated health and proficiency in literacy and numeracy among immigrants and U.S.-born adults: Evidence from the Program for the International Assessment of Adult Competencies (PIACC). *PLoS ONE*, 10(7), e1–e25. https://doi.org/10.1371/journal.pone.0130257

defines folk systems is their history of tradition: many **folk healing systems** have endured over time through oral transmission of beliefs and practices from one generation to the next. A folk healing system uses healing practices that are often divided into *secular* and *sacred* components.

Most cultures have **folk healers** (sometimes referred to as traditional, lay, indigenous, or generic healers) who may make house calls, usually speak the native tongue of the client, and often charge significantly less than professional/ nontraditional healthcare providers (Leininger, 1997; McFarland & Wehbe-Alamah, 2015, 2018). In addition, many cultures (and some healthcare systems) have lay midwives (e.g., *parteras* for Hispanic women), *doulas* (support women for new mothers and babies), or other healthcare providers available for meeting the needs of clients. Table 4-2 identifies indigenous or folk healers for selected groups.

Table 4-2 Healers and Their Scope of Practice		
Cultural/Folk Practitioner	**Preparation**	**Scope of Practice**
African American/Black		
"Old lady"	Usually, an older woman who has successfully raised her own family; knowledgeable in child care and folk remedies	Consulted about common ailments and for advice on child care; found in rural and urban communities
Spiritualist	Called by God to help others; no formal training; usually associated with a fundamentalist Christian church	Assists with problems that are financial, personal, spiritual, or physical; predominantly found in urban communities
Voodoo priest and priestess or *Houngan* and *Mambo*	May be trained by other priests/ priestesses In the United States, the eldest son of a priest becomes a priest; the daughter of a priest(ess) becomes a priestess if she is born with a veil (amniotic sac) over her face	Knowledgeable about properties of herbs; interpretation of signs and omens; able to cure illness caused by voodoo; uses communication techniques to establish a therapeutic milieu like a psychiatrist; treats African American/Black American, Mexican American, and Native American clients
Amish		
Braucher or *baruch-doktor*	Apprenticeship	Amish persons who use a combination of modalities including physical manipulation, massage, herbs, teas, reflexology, and *brauche*, a folk healing art with origins in the 18th- and 19th-century Europe; especially effective in the treatment of bed-wetting, nervousness, and women's health problems; may be generalist or specialist in practice; some set up treatment rooms; some see non-Amish as well as Amish patients
Lay midwives	Apprenticeship	Care for pregnant persons before, during, and after childbirth
Appalachia		
Granny woman, herb doctor	Lay practitioner familiar with Appalachian culture	Healer usually accessible, familiar with the culture, provides accepted cultural remedies and well known to the family
Chinese		
Herbalist	Knowledgeable in diagnosis of illness and herbal remedies	Both diagnostic and therapeutic; diagnostic techniques include interviewing, inspection, auscultation, and assessment of pulses

(continued)

Table 4-2 | Healers and Their Scope of Practice (continued)

Cultural/Folk Practitioner	Preparation	Scope of Practice
Acupuncturist	3½–4½ years (1,500–1,800 hours) of courses on acupuncture, Western anatomy and physiology, Chinese herbs; usually requires a period of apprenticeship, learning from someone else who is licensed or certified. Licensure required in the United States	Diagnosis and treatment of yin/yang disorders by inserting needles into *meridians*, pathways through which life energy flows; when heat is applied to the acupuncture needle, the term *moxibustion* is used. May combine acupuncture with herbal remedies and/or dietary recommendations. Acupuncture is sometimes used as a surgical anesthetic
Greek		
Magissa "magician"	Apprenticeship	Woman who cures *matiasma* or evil eye; may be referred to as doctor
Bonesetter	Apprenticeship	Specialize in treating uncomplicated fractures
Priest (Orthodox)	Ordained clergy. Formal theological study	May be called on for advice, blessings, exorcisms, or direct healing
Hispanic		
Family member	Possesses knowledge of folk medicine	Common illnesses of a mild nature that may or may not be recognized by modern medicine
Curandero	May receive training in an apprenticeship; may receive a "gift from God" that enables the healer to cure; knowledgeable in use of herbs, diet, massage, and rituals	Treats most of the traditional illnesses; some may not treat illness caused by witchcraft for fear of being accused of possessing evil powers; usually admired by members of the community
Espiritualista or spiritualist	Born with the special gifts of being able to analyze dreams and foretell future events; may serve apprenticeship with an older practitioner	Emphasis on prevention of illness or bewitchment through the use of medals, prayers, amulets; may also be sought for cure of existing illness
Yerbero	No formal training; knowledgeable in growing and prescribing herbs	Consulted for preventive and curative use of herbs for both traditional (folk, lay, cultural) and Western illnesses
Sobador	Knowledgeable in massage and manipulation of bones and muscles	Treats many traditional illnesses, particularly those affecting the musculoskeletal system; may also treat nontraditional illnesses
Native American Native Alaskan Native Hawaiian		
Shaman Medicine Man *Learned One*	Spiritually chosen. Apprenticeship	Uses incantations, divination practices, prayers, and herbs to cure a wide range of physical, psychological, and spiritual illnesses
Crystal gazer, hand trembler (Navajo)	Spiritually chosen. Apprenticeship	Diviner diagnostician who can identify the cause of a problem, either by using crystals or by placing hand over the sick person; does not implement treatment

Adapted from Hautman, M. A. (1979). Folk health and illness beliefs. *The Nurse Practitioner*, 4(4), 23–31; Small, C. C. (2020). Appalachians. In J. N. Giger & L. G. Haddad (Eds.), *Transcultural nursing: Assessment and intervention* (8th ed., pp. 262–279). Elsevier; Specter, R. E. (2017). Health and illness in the American Indian and Alaska Native population. In R. E. Spector (Ed.), *Cultural diversity in health and illness* (9th ed., pp. 150–166). Pearson, with permission.

When clients use folk healers, these practitioners should be an integral part of the healthcare team and participate in as many aspects of the client's care as possible. For example, a nurse might include the folk healer in obtaining a health history and in determining what treatments already have been used toward bringing about healing. In discussing traditional remedies, it is important to be respectful and to listen attentively to healers who combine spiritual and herbal remedies for a wide variety of illnesses, both physical and psychological in origin. Chapter 12 provides detailed information about the religious beliefs and spiritual healers in major religious groups.

Complementary, Integrative, and Alternative Health System

Complementary, integrative, and alternative health is an umbrella term for hundreds of therapies used by individuals and cultures worldwide. Some of these therapies have ancient origins in Egyptian, Chinese, Greek, Indian, and American aboriginal (Mayan, Aztecan, Native American, and First Nations) cultures. Other practices such as chiropractic medicine (Rhee et al., 2018) and **naturopathy** have gained increased mainstream acceptance. Allopathic or biomedicine and osteopathic medicine remain the reference points by which all other therapies are considered *complementary* (in addition to), *integrative* (combined selected magico-religious or holistic therapies with scientifically documented efficacy), or *alternative* (instead of).

Integrative healthcare was defined by Leininger (2002) as "...the safe, congruent, and creative ways of blending together holistic, generic, and professional care practices" for beneficial client outcomes to improve health and wellbeing. McFarland and Wehbe-Alamah (2019) asserted that integrative holism encompasses nursing and extended multidisciplinary and interdisciplinary professional healthcare practices that "blend with client-specific cultural and generic care values, beliefs and preferences for promoting healing and wellness" (p. 542). The use of an integrative

approach to health and wellness across the United States has grown within care settings including primary and specialty care practices, hospitals, hospices, and military health facilities.

Consider a client who has been diagnosed with breast cancer. Worldwide, increasing numbers of individuals use complementary or integrative therapies to manage symptoms, prevent toxicities, and improve quality of life during chronic illness (Bolton et al., 2020; Chatterjee, 2021; Latte-Naor & Mao, 2019). An estimated 80% of North American persons with or surviving cancer self-report using complementary and integrative therapies following diagnosis (American Society of Clinical Oncology, Inc. [ASCO], 2021; Foley et al., 2021). In clinical practice guidelines regarding the supportive care of patients treated for breast cancer, oncology-recommended complementary or integrative therapies include acupuncture/acupressure, massage therapy, meditation, reflexology, hypnosis, music therapy, yoga, tai chi, biofeedback, and selected approved supplements for the management of disease-related pain and chemotherapy-associated nausea and other adverse side effects (Luo et al., 2020; Lyman et al., 2018; Xiang et al., 2017). In addition, complementary or integrative therapies provide therapeutic supportive care for stress, fatigue, and other disease and treatment symptoms or effects, thereby improving quality of life, a belief held by approximately two-thirds of oncology patients and clinicians (ASCO, 2021). Using a special diet in lieu of undergoing specialist-recommended or oncologic treatment is an example of *nonrecommended* alternative solo therapy.

Complementary Health Approaches

Physical activity provides healthful effects for a multitude of physical and mental health issues and is important in health promotion and disease prevention (Abildso et al., 2023). However, in the United States, physical activity rates among adults remains suboptimal, with rural–urban and regional disparities in meeting the combined leisure time physical activity guidelines, with "...no more than 28% of U.S. adults aged 18–64 [having] met combined aerobic and muscle-strengthening guidelines activities in 2018 during leisure-time physical activity" (Abildso et al., 2023). Persons in Eastern or rural regions had significantly lower use compared with residents in Western or metropolitan locations. Other mind–body techniques considered complementary and integrative include meditation, tai chi, prayer, mental healing, aromatherapy, and creative outlet therapies such as art, music, or dance. Box 4-2 identifies and describes some of the complementary and alternative therapies most commonly used by people in the United States and Canada to promote health and prevent and treat disease.

Johns Hopkins Medicine (2023) categorizes complementary and integrative health approaches as follows:

1. *Traditional alternative medicine* beliefs are built on complete systems of theory and practice and have evolved earlier and apart from other conventional medical approaches used in the United States or Canada. Traditional healthcare systems include acupuncture, **Traditional Chinese Medicine**, **Ayurvedic medicine**, homeopathy, and naturopathy.
2. *Body touch* practices include a diverse group of techniques administered by a trained practitioner or teacher that are designed to enhance the mind's capacity to affect bodily functions and symptoms. The most commonly used body touch practices include chiropractic or osteopathic manipulation, acupuncture, massage, and body movement therapies such as tai chi and yoga. Meditation can be a component.
3. *Diet and herbs* include botanicals or herbal medicine, dietary supplements, and nutrition. In their study, Mishra et al. (2023) found 58.5% of adult participants reported using dietary supplements, most commonly multivitamins (31.5%) and Vitamin D (18.5%).
4. *Mind or mind–body* connection practices include deep breathing, meditation, progressive relaxation, and hypnosis.

Mindfulness and/or spirituality are often integrated components (Strehli et al., 2021). Adult use of meditation in the United States increased from 4.1% in 2012 to 14.2% in 2017 (Clarke et al., 2018).

5. *Senses* are believed to affect overall health. Practices include guided imagery, visualization, aromatherapy, and art, dance, or music therapy.
6. *External energy therapies* involve the use of energy fields in two ways:
   - *Biofield therapies* are intended to affect energy fields that surround and penetrate the human body. (The existence of such fields has not yet been scientifically proven.) Some forms of energy therapy manipulate biofields by applying pressure and/or manipulating the body by placing the hands in or through these fields. Examples include qigong (tai chi), Reiki, and therapeutic touch.
   - *Bioelectromagnetic-based therapies* involve the unconventional use of electromagnetic fields, such as pulsed fields, magnetic fields, or alternating-current or direct-current fields.

Efficacy of Complementary Health Approaches

Through rigorous scientific investigation, the National Center for Complementary and Integrative Health works to discover the usefulness and safety of complementary and integrative health approaches and their roles in improving health and healthcare (USDHHS, 2023a). These approaches are classified by their primary therapeutic input or delivery: Nutritional; psychological; physical; or combination (psychological/physical or psychological/nutritional) (USDHHS, 2023b). The Center's current research foci include health restoration, resilience, disease prevention and health promotion across the lifespan; implementation science for complementary and integrative health, including management of pain including military personnel and veterans; integrative approaches for symptom management

BOX 4-2   Selected Complementary and Alternative Therapies

Acupuncture refers to a family of procedures involving stimulation of anatomic points on the body by a variety of techniques. The acupuncture technique that has been most studied scientifically involves penetrating the skin with thin, solid, metallic needles that are manipulated by the hands or by electrical stimulation. When heat is applied to the needles, it is referred to as moxibustion.

Aromatherapy involves the use of essential oils (extracts or essences) from flowers, herbs, and trees to promote health and well-being.

Ayurvedic medicine includes diet and herbal remedies and emphasizes the use of body, mind, and spirit in disease prevention and treatment.

Chiropractic is a noninvasive system of therapy focused on the relationship between bodily structure (primarily that of the spine) and function and how that relationship affects the preservation and restoration of health. Although chiropractors use a variety of treatment approaches, they primarily perform adjustments (manipulations) to the spine or other parts of the body with the goal of correcting alignment problems, alleviating pain, improving function, and supporting the body's natural ability to heal itself.

Dietary supplements are products (other than tobacco) taken by mouth that contain a *dietary ingredient* intended to supplement the diet. *Dietary ingredients* may include vitamins, minerals, herbs or other botanicals, amino acids, and substances such as enzymes, organ tissues, and metabolites. *Dietary supplements* come in many forms including extracts, concentrates, tablets, capsules, gelcaps, liquids, and powders. The United States and Canada have special requirements for labeling and in both countries these products are regulated as *foods* not drugs.

Guided imagery refers to a wide variety of techniques, including simple visualization and direct suggestion using imagery, metaphor and storytelling, fantasy exploration and game playing, dream interpretation, drawing, and active imagination where elements of the unconscious are invited to appear as images that can communicate with the conscious mind (Academy for Guided Imagery, 2022).

Homeopathic medicine is an alternative medical system. In homeopathic medicine, there is a belief that "like cures like," meaning that small, highly diluted quantities of medicinal substances are given to cure symptoms, even though the same substances given at higher or more concentrated doses would actually cause those symptoms.

Massage therapists manipulate muscle and connective tissue to enhance function of those tissues and promote relaxation and well-being.

Naturopathy is an alternative medical system based on the premise that there is a healing power in the body that establishes, maintains, and restores health. Practitioners work with the patient with a goal of supporting this power through treatments such as nutrition and lifestyle counseling, dietary supplements, medicinal plants, exercise, homeopathy, and traditional Chinese medicine.

Osteopathic medicine is a form of conventional medicine that, in part, emphasizes diseases arising in the musculoskeletal system. There is an underlying belief that all of the body's systems work together, and disturbances in one system may affect function elsewhere in the body. Some osteopathic physicians practice osteopathic manipulation, a full-body system of hands-on techniques to alleviate pain, restore function, and promote health and wellbeing.

Qigong ("chee-GUNG") or **tai chi** ("tie-CHEE") is a component of Traditional Chinese Medicine that combines movement, meditation, and regulation of breathing to enhance the flow of qi (pronounced "chee" and meaning *vital energy*) in the body, improve blood circulation, and enhance immune function (Hung et al., 2018).

(continued)

BOX 4-2 | **Selected Complementary and Alternative Therapies (continued)**

Reiki ("RAY-kee") is a Japanese word representing *universal life energy*. Reiki is based on the belief that when spiritual energy is channeled through a Reiki practitioner, the patient's spirit is healed, which in turn heals the physical body.

Therapeutic touch is based on the premise that the healing force of the therapist affects the patient's recovery; healing is promoted when the body's energies are in balance. By passing their hands over the patient, healers can identify energy imbalances.

Traditional Chinese Medicine (TCM) is the current name for an ancient system of healthcare from China. TCM is based on a concept of balanced *qi*, or *vital energy*, which is believed to flow throughout the body. Qi regulates a person's spiritual, emotional, mental, and physical balance and is influenced by the opposing forces of yin (negative energy) and yang (positive energy). Disease is proposed to result from the flow of qi being disrupted and yin and yang becoming imbalanced. Among the components of TCM are herbal and nutritional therapy, restorative physical exercises, meditation, acupuncture, and remedial massage.

Yoga is a term derived from a Sanskrit word meaning *yoke* or *union*. Yoga involves a combination of breathing exercises, meditation, and physical postures that are used to achieve a state of relaxation and balance of mind, body, and spirit.

Sources: Academy for Guided Imagery. (2022). *What is guided imagery?* http://acadgi.com/about_sitemap/power_of_guided_imagery/; Hung, H-M., Yeh, S-H., & Chen, C-H. (2018). Effects of Qigong exercise on biomarkers and mental and physical health in adults with at least one risk factor for coronary artery disease. *Biological Research for Nursing, 18*(3), 264–273; Peregoy, J. A., Clarke, T. C., Jones, L. I., Stussman, B. J., & Nahin, R. L. (2014, April 16). *Regional variation in use of complementary health approaches by U.S. adults. NCHS Data Brief No. 146*, 1-8. U.S. Department of Health and Human Services, Centers for Disease Control and Prevention, National Center for Health Statistics; U.S. Department of Health and Human Services, National Institutes of Health, National Center for Complementary and Alternative Medicine. (2018, October 30). *Use of complementary health approaches in the U.S.* https://nccih.nih.gov/research/statistics/NHIS/2012

for persons with or surviving cancer; complex interactions involving nutritional interactions; mechanisms and biomarkers of body and mind approaches; whole person health and wellbeing; interoception; and quality of life (USDHHS, 2023c). The Center also works on supporting clinical trials of complementary and integrative health approaches, strives to build the complementary/integrative health research workforce, and enhances communication strategies and tools to improve scientific literacy and understanding of clinical research (USDHHS, 2023a).

Research on complementary health approaches has focused on medicinal plants; chiropractic care for low back pain; acupuncture, yoga, tai chi for pain management and/or wellbeing; cell processes and diseases (e.g., cancer, asthma, hypertension, cardiovascular disease, obesity);

role of nutrition; the oxidative degradation of lipids; and diabetes and insulin. For further evidence-based information related to the efficacy of specific health approaches and the reliability and validity of the studies conducted, visit the Cochrane Library (https://www.cochranelibrary.com/); it serves as the repository for the Cochrane Collaboration, a worldwide organization that prepares systematic reviews of healthcare research.

Summary

Cultural belief systems develop from the shared experiences by members of a social group and are expressed symbolically. The use of symbols to define, describe, and relate to the world around us is one of the basic characteristics of being human. The major cultural belief systems embraced by people worldwide are *magico-religious, scientific/biomedical,* and *holistic health paradigms or worldviews*. In the magico-religious cultural belief system, a supernatural agent or agents are believed to bestow health and illness: health may be perceived as a reward given as a sign of blessing and goodwill, while illness may be viewed as a sign of punishment. Most physicians and nurses are formally educated in the scientific or biomedical belief system wherein life is controlled by a series of physical and biochemical processes that can be studied and manipulated by humans through allopathic/osteopathic medicine and other professional care professionals and systems. In holistic cultural belief systems, the forces of nature must be kept in natural balance or harmony. Human life is only one aspect of nature and a part of the general order of the cosmos. Disturbing the laws of nature creates imbalance, chaos, and disease. Order is maintained through balance according to holistic yin/yang and hot/cold theories of health and illnesses.

REVIEW QUESTIONS

1. Describe in your own words the meaning for each of the following terms: (a) cultural belief system, (b) worldview, and (c) paradigm.
2. What are the primary characteristics for each of the three major health belief systems: magico-religious, scientific/biomedical, and holistic paradigms?
3. What are the main differences between professional care and folk care systems?
4. What is allopathic medicine?
5. What is the primary mission of the U.S. National Center for Complementary and Integrative Health (NCCIH)?
6. Describe the six major categories of complementary or integrative approaches.

CRITICAL THINKING ACTIVITIES

1. Select a complementary health approach that you would like to know more about (such as acupuncture, Ayurveda, chiropractic, yoga, tai chi, or naturopathy). Search the internet for information about this practice, then use a library to locate current research literature. After you have learned more about the practice, contact a healer who uses that health approach and ask the following questions:
   a. How did you prepare to be a practitioner of _____?
   b. What do you believe are the major benefits of _____ to clients or patients?
   c. What health-related conditions do you believe respond best to _____?
   d. Are there any risks to clients resulting from the use of _____?
2. The World Health Organization (2013) estimated that 80% of people worldwide access complementary or integrative healthcare for acute and chronic illnesses and to maintain health and wellness (pp. 26–28). Select a common illness (such as upper respiratory infection, arthritis, gastrointestinal upset, or a similar condition), then identify the various complementary and integrative approaches to allopathic medicine that clients might use. What is the efficacy of each modality that you have identified? How effective do you think the complementary and alternative practices are compared with those of allopathic medicine? Compare the cost of each practice as well as its efficacy. What are the risks compared to benefits?
3. View the video "Scientific Results of Yoga for Health and Well-being" that can be found via the NCCIH website or at https://www.youtube.com/watch?v=uOB7pHRBXAY&t=7 as part of their Online Continuing Education Series (USDHHS, 2020, October 6). The presentation will help you to learn more about the

use of yoga and tai chi to improve balance and prevent falls, especially among older adults. After viewing the video, identify the areas for which you are convinced adequate evidence exists to support integrating yoga as a complementary health approach into your nursing practice.

4. The herb *Echinacea* is frequently used for the prevention and treatment of the common cold. If a patient asked your opinion about the use of *Echinacea*, how would you reply? Would you recommend use of this herb to treat a cold? Explain why or why not.

5. Select a disease for which you think a complementary or alternative intervention might be helpful (such as breast cancer, hypertension, osteoarthritis, or other chronic condition). Seek a reputable professional website with current, directly relevant information and resources. Critically appraise the potential benefits and adverse effects of a chosen intervention for clients with this disease. Indicate whether you believe sufficient evidence exists to support recommending the intervention to a client.

REFERENCES

Abildso, C. G., Daily, S. M., Meyer, M. R. U., Perry, C. K., & Eyler, A. (2023). Prevalence of meeting aerobic, muscle-strengthening, and combined physical activity guidelines during leisure time among adults, by rural-urban classification and region—United States, 2020. *U. S. Department of Health and Human Services, Centers for Disease Control and Prevention, Morbidity and Mortality Weekly Report 2023, 72*(4), 85–89.

Academy for Guided Imagery. (2022). *What is guided imagery?* http://acadgi.com/about_sitemap/power_of_guided_imagery/

Ackernecht, E. H. (1946). Natural diseases and rational treatment in primitive medicine. *Bulletin of the history of medicine, XIX*, 467–497. Reprint: (1971). Naturalistic and supernaturalistic diagnosis and treatments. In *Medicine and ethnology: Selected essays* (pp. 135–161). Johns Hopkins Press.

American Society of Clinical Oncology, Inc. (2021, June 15). *Use of integrative medicine by patients with breast cancer* [Blog]. https://ascopost.com/news/june-2021/use-of-integrative-medicine-by-patients-with-breast-cancer/

Bolton, R. E., Fix, G. M., Lukas, C. V.-D., Elwy, A. R., & Bokhour, B. G. (2020). Biopsychosocial benefits of movement-based complementary and integrative health therapies for patients with chronic conditions. *Chronic Illness, 16*(1), 41–54.

Chatterjee, A. (2021). Why do chronic illness patients decide to use complementary and alternative medicine? A qualitative study. *Complementary Therapies in Clinical Practice, 43*(2021), 101363.

Clarke, T. C., Barnes, P. M., Black, L. I., Stussman, B. J., & Nahin, R. L. (2018). *Use of yoga, meditation, and chiropractors among U.S. adults aged 18 and over. NCHS Data Brief, No. 325*. U.S. Department of Health and Human Services, Centers for Disease Control and Prevention, National Center for Health Statistics.

Clements, F. E. (1932). Primitive concepts of disease. *American Archaeology and Ethnology, 32*(2), 185–252.

Fleary, S. A., & Ettienne, R. (2019). Social disparities in health literacy in the United States. *Health Literacy Research and Practice, 3*(1), e47–e52.

Foley, H., Steel, A., McIntyre, E., Harnett, J., Sibbritt, D., & Adams, J. (2021). Disclosure of conventional and complementary medicine use to medical doctors and complementary medicine practitioners: A survey of rates and reasons amongst those with chronic conditions. *PloS one, 16*(11), e0258901. https://doi.org/10.1371/journal.pone.0258901

Haspel, T. (2020, January 27). Most dietary supplements don't do anything. Why do we spend $35 billion a year on them? *Washington Post* https://www.washingtonpost.com/lifestyle/food/most-dietary-supplements-dont-do-anything-why-do-we-spend-35-billion-a-year-on-them/2020/01/24/947d2970-3d62-11ea-baca-eb7ace0a3455_story.html

Hautman, M. A. (1979). Folk health and illness beliefs. *The Nurse Practitioner, 4*(4), 23–31.

Hung, H.-M., Yeh, S.-H., & Chen, C.-H. (2018). Effects of Qigong exercise on biomarkers and mental and physical health in adults with at least one risk factor for coronary artery disease. *Biological Research for Nursing, 18*(3), 264–273.

Johns Hopkins Medicine. (2023). *Types of complementary and alternative medicine.* https://www.hopkinsmedicine.org/health/wellness-and-prevention/types-of-complementary-and-alternative-medicine

Latte-Naor, S., & Mao, J. J. (2019). Putting integrative oncology into practice: Concepts and approaches. *Journal of Oncology Practice, 15*(1), 7–15.

Leininger, M. M. (1997). Founder's focus alternative to what? Generic vs. professional caring, treatments and healing modes. *Journal of Transcultural Nursing, 91*(1), 37.

Leininger, M. M. (2002). Transcultural nursing administration and consultation. In M. M. Leininger & M. R. McFarland

(Eds.), *Transcultural nursing: Concepts, theories, research, and practice* (3rd ed., pp. 563–573). McGraw-Hill.

Luo, X.-C., Liu, J., Fu, J., Yin, H.-Y., Shen, L., Liu, M.-L., Lan, L., Ying, J., Qiao, X.-L., Tang, C.-Z., & Tang, Y. (2020). Effect of Tai Chi Chuan in breast cancer survivors: A systematic review and meta-analysis. *Frontiers in Oncology, 10*(607), 1–15.

Lyman, G. H., Greenlee, H., Bohlke, K., Bao, T., DeMichele, A. M., Deng, G. E., Fouladbakhsh, J. M., Gil, B., Hershman, D. L., Mansfield, S., Mussallem, D. M., Mustian, K. M., Price, E., Rafte, S., & Cohen, L. (2018). Integrative therapies during and after breast cancer treatment: ASCO endorsement of the SIO clinical practice guideline. *Journal of Clinical Oncology, 36*(25), 2647–2657.

McFarland, M. R., & Wehbe-Alamah, H. B. (2015). *Leininger's culture care diversity and universality: A worldwide nursing theory* (3rd ed.). Jones & Bartlett Learning.

McFarland, M. R., & Wehbe-Alamah, H. B. (2018). *Transcultural nursing: Concepts, theories, research, and practices* (4th ed.). McGraw-Hill.

McFarland, M. R., & Wehbe-Alamah, H. B. (2019). Leininger's theory of culture care diversity and universality: An overview with an historical perspective and a view toward the future. *Journal of Transcultural Nursing, 30*(6), 540–557.

Mechanic, D. (1978). *Medical sociology* (2nd ed.). Free Press.

Mishra, S., Gahche, J. J., Ogden, C. L., Dimeler, M., & Potischman, N. (2023, April 18). *Dietary supplement use in the United States: National Health and Nutrition Examination Survey, 2017-March 2020* (pp. 1–14). U.S. Department of Health and Human Services, Centers for Disease Control and Prevention, National Center for Health Statistics, National Center for Health Statistics, NCHS Data Brief No.183.

Nutbeam, D., & Lloyd, J. E. (2021). Understanding and responding to health literacy as a social determinant of health. *Annual Review of Public Health, 42*(2021), 159–173.

Osborn, D. K. (2021). *Greek medicine: The four humors.* http://www.greekmedicine.net/b_p/Four_Humors.html

Peregoy, J. A., Clarke, T. C., Jones, L. I., Stussman, B. J., & Nahin, R. L. (2014, April 16). *Regional variation in use of complementary health approaches by U.S. adults* (pp. 1–8). U.S. Department of Health and Human Services, Centers for Disease Control and Prevention, National Center for Health Statistics, National Center for Health Statistics, NCHS Data Brief No. 146.

Prins, E., & Monnat, S. (2015). Examining associations between self-rated health and proficiency in literacy and numeracy among immigrants and U.S.-born adults: Evidence from the Program for the International Assessment of Adult Competencies (PIACC). *PLoS ONE, 10*(7), e1–e25. https://doi.org/10.1371/journal.pone.0130257

Quiroz, D., & van Andel, T. (2018). The cultural importance of plants in Western African religions. *Economic Botany, 72*(3), 251–262.

Rhee, T. G., Marottoli, R. A., VanNess, P. H., & Tinetti, M. E. (2018). Patterns and perceived benefits of utilizing seven major complementary health approaches in U.S. older adults. *Journals of Gerontology: Medical Sciences, 73*(8), 1119–11124.

Sanchez, A. A. (2018). An examination of the folk healing practice of *curanderismo* in the Hispanic community. *Journal of Community Health Nursing, 35*(3), 148–161.

Sandberg, J. C., Quandt, S. A., Graham, A., Stub, T., Mora, D. C., & Arcury, T. A. (2018). Medical Pluralism in the Use of Sobadores among Mexican Immigrants to North Carolina. *Journal of immigrant and minority health, 20*(5), 1197–1205. https://doi.org/10.1007/s10903-017-0660-y

Small, C. C. (2020). Appalachians. In J. N. Giger & L. G. Haddad (Eds.), *Transcultural nursing: Assessment and intervention* (8th ed., pp. 262–279). Elsevier.

Smuts, J. C. (1926). *Holism and evolution.* MacMillan.

Specter, R. E. (2017). Health and illness in the American Indian and Alaska Native population. In R. E. Spector (Ed.), *Cultural diversity in health and illness* (9th ed., pp. 150–166). Pearson.

Strehli, I., Burns, R. D., Bai, Y., Ziegenfuss, D. H., Block, M. E., & Brusseau, T. A. (2021). Mind-body physical activity interventions and stress-related physiological markers in educational settings: A systematic review and meta-analysis. *International Journal of Environmental Research and Public Health, 18*(1), 224.

U.S. Department of Health and Human Services, Food and Drug Administration, Center for Food Safety and Applied Nutrition. (2020, August 6). *Report a problem to the FDA.* https://www.fda.gov/safety/report-problem-fda

U.S. Department of Health and Human Services, National Institutes of Health, National Center for Complementary and Alternative Medicine. (2018, October 30). *Use of complementary health approaches in the U.S.* https://nccih.nih.gov/research/statistics/NHIS/2012

U.S. Department of Health and Human Services, National Institutes of Health, National Center for Complementary and Alternative Medicine. (2020, October 6). *National #YogaMonth livestream recording: The science and practice of yoga.* https://www.youtube.com/watch?v=uOB7pHRBXAY&t=7s

U.S. Department of Health and Human Services, National Institutes of Health, National Center for Complementary and Alternative Medicine. (2023a, June). *About NCCIH.* https://www.nccih.nih.gov/about#:~:text=The%20mission%20of%20NCCIH%20is,improving%20health%20and%20health%20care

U.S. Department of Health and Human Services, National Institutes of Health, National Center for Complementary and Alternative Medicine. (2023b, June 17). *Be an informed consumer.* https://www.nccih.nih.gov/health/be-an-informed-consumer

U.S. Department of Health and Human Services, National Institutes of Health, National Center for Complementary and Alternative Medicine. (2023c, June 17). *Research funding priorities.* https://www.nccih.nih.gov/grants/research-funding-priorities

U.S. Department of Health and Human Services, National Institutes of Health, Office of Dietary Supplements. (2021, March 23). *Frequently asked questions*. https://ods.od.nih.gov/HealthInformation/ODS_Frequently_Asked_Questions.aspx

World Health Organization. (1948). *Preamble to the Constitution of the World Health Organization* as adopted by the International Health Conference, New York, NY, June 19–22, 1946.

World Health Organization. (2013). *WHO traditional medicine strategy 2014–2023*.

World Health Organization. (2023). *Health and wellbeing*. https://www.who.int/data/gho/data/major-themes/health-and-well-being

Xiang, Y., Lu, L., Chen, X., & Wen, Z. (2017). Does Tai Chi relieve fatigue? A systematic review and meta-analysis of randomized control trials. *PLoS ONE, 12*(4), e1–e22. https://doi.org/10.1371/journal.pone.0174872

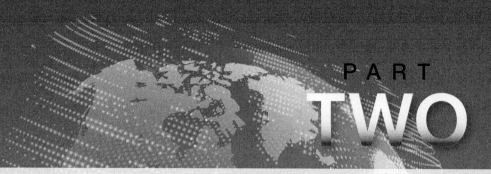

Lifespan

Transcultural Perspectives in Childbearing

• Melva Craft-Blacksheare

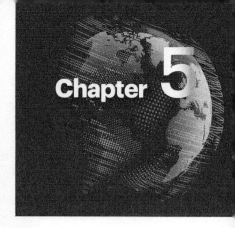

Chapter 5

Key Terms

Birth control–related mistrust
Birthing plan
Childbearing
Emergency contraception
Female genital mutilation/cutting

Intimate partner violence
Maternal morbidity
Maternal mortality
Multicultural families
Participatory women group
Pica

Postpartum depression
Pregnancy
Stereotyping
Taboos
Unintended pregnancy

Learning Objectives

1. Analyze how culture influences the beliefs and behaviors of the childbearing family during pregnancy.
2. Recognize the childbearing beliefs and practices of diverse cultures.
3. Examine the needs of women, birthing persons, and childbearing families, as well as how LGBTQ+ family structures influence childbirth and childrearing.
4. Explore how cultural ideologies of childbearing populations can affect pregnancy outcomes.

Introduction

This chapter discusses how culture, family, and social factors influence childbearing. The experiences of women and other birthing persons and their support systems during **pregnancy**, birth, and the postpartum period are examined. Nursing practice recommendations are offered to facilitate the provision of culture-specific care to childbearing people and their families.

Overview of Cultural Belief Systems and Practices Related to Childbearing

Over the past three decades, there has been a dramatic change in contemporary pregnancy and childbirth practices in U.S. society. Today's global population is increasingly mobile, resulting in new cultural approaches to health and childbirth including a blending of cultural expectations and practices within U.S. culture. Often, parents from two cultures join together to raise a family, with each parent's cultural norms merging to define the family norms (known as **multicultural families**; see Figs. 5-1 to 5-3). Due to global population shifts, cultural beliefs regarding childbearing must be examined to allow nurses to provide culturally congruent care throughout each patient's pregnancy, birth, and postpartum periods. Clearly, offering only mainstream U.S. maternity care will not necessarily align with the nursing needs of today's multicultural patients.

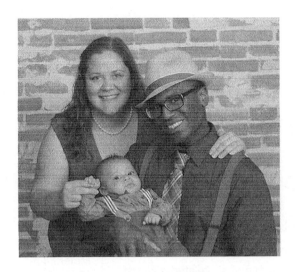

Figure 5-2. African European American family.

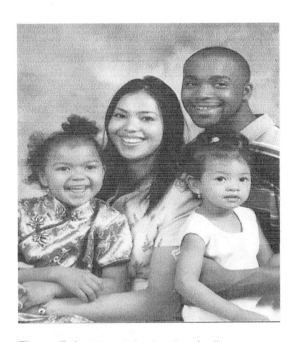

Figure 5-1. African Asian American family.

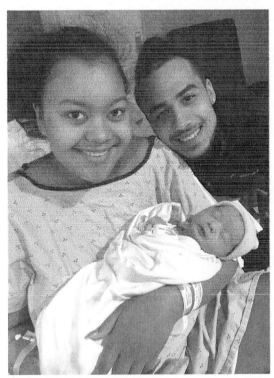

Figure 5-3. African, Asian, Latinx, Middle Eastern, and American family.

Pregnancy and Childbirth Practices in the United States

In their systematic, qualitative review of 35 studies from 19 countries, Downe et al. (2018) explored what mattered to women during childbirth. The authors concluded that women most valued having a positive birth experience that fulfilled or exceeded their personal and sociocultural beliefs and expectations.

Childbearing is a universal phenomenon that crosses all cultures, ethnicities, and socioeconomic levels. Childbirth is often a time of celebration. Indeed, in many cultures, a newborn is not just a new member of the family but also a gift to society. Childbirth is a time of transition and changing needs that are determined by the cultural norms, values, and socioeconomic influences that surround the childbearing person, their family, and community. Therefore, nurses must know how to assess childbearing patients' cultural needs in order to provide appropriate care.

Historically and in many cultures, birth is considered a wellness event—a time of health and celebration. However, in modern times, it is often considered a hospital event, especially in the United States where more than 98% of infants are born in hospitals (George et al., 2022). Hospital deliveries are routinely followed by trained obstetrical nurses, obstetricians, perinatologists, and pediatricians. In most U.S. hospitals, postpartum stays are 36 hours for a typical vaginal delivery and 72 hours for an uncomplicated cesarean delivery. Induction of labor in the United States has more than tripled since it first began to be recorded from live birth certificates in 1989; from 9% of births in 1989 to 31.37% of births in 2020 (Simpson, 2020).

Additionally, 85% of all deliveries in the United States involve continuous electronic fetal monitoring that monitors the baby for the entire labor (Horsager-Boehrer, 2020). Other routine hospital care includes epidurals for vaginal births and anesthesia for cesarean sections. Hospitals generally have a particular culture of rules and regulations related to OB patient care. However, when a laboring patient presents to the hospital with a **birthing plan** (an individualized list of preferred actions to facilitate a desired childbirth), the optimal outcome will include finding common ground between birthing expectations and the hospital's rules and culture. According to MacDorman and Declercq (2016), out-of-hospital births (births at home or in birthing centers) in the United States increased from 0.87% in 2004 to 1.50% in 2014. Twenty-nine percent of the out-of-hospital births occurred in the alternative, freestanding birthing centers where certified nurse-midwives (CNMs), certified midwives (CMs), and obstetricians who promote family-centered care emphasize pregnancy as a normal process requiring minimal technological intervention. During the same period, the remaining percentage of out-of-hospital births took place at home and were attended by lay, professional, or certified midwives (MacDorman & Declercq, 2016).

According to MacDorman et al. (2022), out-of-hospital births in the United States have increased even more in recent years, increasing by 20% from 2019 to 2020 (see Evidence-Based Practice 5-1). For birthing families, the COVID-19 pandemic brought an impetus of fear entering hospitals and restrictions on family and support participants for patients giving birth. During this time, birth center births increased by 13.2%, home births by 22.9%, and planned home births by 23.3%. Hospital births decreased by 3.6% from 2019 to 2020.

Compared to other countries, the United States spends more on healthcare and maternal health than any other type of hospital care (Parente, 2018; Shaw et al., 2016). Despite these expenditures, pregnant people in the United States have a higher risk of pregnancy-related complications compared to pregnant people in 40 other countries. **Maternal morbidity** and **maternal mortality** are byproducts of U.S. health disparities due to the unequal availability of social, economic, and educational opportunities (see Evidence-Based Practice 5-2).

U.S. Community Births Increased by 20% From 2019 to 2020

The COVID-19 pandemic exacerbated stories of the fear of entering a hospital with an abundance of COVID-19 patients and fear of being ignored or mistreated by overworked healthcare workers, so instead, more birthing families than in recent years chose to give birth in the community. The term "community birth" identifies planned home and birth center births.

The authors reviewed birth data from the National Center for Health Statistics to determine variables such as presence of birth attendant, race, Hispanic origin, obstetric estimate gestation, and location of birth.

Two categories of midwife data were collected on the birth certificate: certified nurse-midwife (CNM)/certified midwife (CM) and non-CNM/CM midwife. Non-CNM/CM midwife includes any other type of midwife besides CNM/CM, which is typically a certified professional midwife but could also be a licensed midwife or direct-entry midwife.

In 2020, there were 71,870 community births in the United States, including 45,646 home births and 21,884 birth center births. During this time, planned home births increased by 23.3% and birth center births increased by 13.2%. The increases occurred in every U.S. state, for all racial groups:

- Non-Hispanic Black women—29.9% increase
- Native American women—29.6%
- Latinx women—23.5%
- Non-Hispanic White women—17.6%

Demographic and medical characteristics of 2020 home birth participants were as follows:

- Compared to 33.4% of hospital births, 36.5% of birth center births were to mothers with a bachelor's degree or higher.
- Compared to 32% of birth centers and 38.5% of hospital births, 17.8% of planned home births were to mothers having first live birth.

- Very few planned home (0.8%) or birth center (1.0%) births were to women who smoked during pregnancy, compared to 5.6% of women with hospital birth.
- Women with planned home (2.0%) or birth center (1.7%) births were preterm, compared to 12.1% of hospital births.
- Compared to 8.3% of hospital births, 1.3% of planned home births and 1.0% of birth center births were low birth weight.
- Greater than ½ (52.5%) of planned home births were attended by non-CNM/CM midwives, and another ⅓ (31.1%) by CNM/CM midwives, 6% were delivered by physicians, and in 15.9% of these births, the attendant was marked as "other" (which may include a family member, emergency medical technician, etc.).
- Thirty-eight percent of birth center births were delivered by non-CNM/CM midwives, 52.8% by CNM/CM midwives, and 3.6% by physicians.
- In contrast, 89.5% of hospital births were delivered by physicians and 9.9% by CNM/CM midwives.

The authors noted that the percentage of community births almost doubled between 2004 and 2019, before the pandemic. This growth, along with the increasing numbers of trained midwives and the increase in the number of birth centers, created the foundation for an increase in the assurance of community birthing. They noted, "Many respondents had a preexisting interest in community birth and the pandemic reinforced their choice."

The pandemic created a less supportive environment for hospital birth as many hospitals established policies that limited support persons, including partners and doulas.

References: MacDorman, M. F., Barnard-Mayers, R., Declercq, E. (2022). United States births increased by 20% from 2019 to 220. *Birth*, *49*, 559-568. https://doi.org/10.1111/birt.12627

Health Disparities Among the African American Population

Maternal–Fetal Medicine Facts

- From 2006 to 2010, African American women in the United States were three times more likely to suffer a pregnancy-related death than were White and Hispanic women. African American women accounted for 14.6% of live births but 35.5% of pregnancy-related deaths.
- Between 2011 and 2016, there were 42.4 deaths per 100,000 live births for Black non-Hispanic women in comparison to 13 deaths per 100,000 live births for White non-Hispanic women. Black non-Hispanic women are 3.3 times more likely to die from pregnancy-related causes.
- Compared to White women, African American women are more likely to experience preventable maternal death.
- African American women experience physical *weathering*, meaning their bodies age faster than do White women's due to exposure to chronic stress linked to socioeconomic disadvantages and discrimination. This weathering makes pregnancy riskier for African American women than White women and at an earlier age.
- The social and economic consequences of racism in everyday life experiences, social structures, and healthcare institutions have been linked to poor maternal and infant outcomes.
- African American infants die at twice the rate of White infants. Infant mortality is 5.0 deaths per 1,000 live births for White infants and 11.2 per 1,000 live births for African American infants.
- Preterm births occurred at a rate of 9.1% for White women compared to 14% for African American women.
- African American women are significantly less likely than women of other races to express an understanding that genetic testing is optional, not required.
- African American women are less likely than women of other races to receive recommended influenza vaccinations during pregnancy.
- African American women have 30% higher odds of having an early cesarean section compared to White women.

- While low educational attainment can have a negative effect on birth outcomes, for African American women, higher educational attainment does not improve infant survival rates. In other words, African American women with doctorates and professional degrees still have higher infant mortality rates than do White women who never finished high school.
- The maternal health crisis cannot adequately be addressed without taking into account how racism and bias manifest in the healthcare system and in turn contribute to the high rates of maternal mortality and morbidity among Black women.
- A recent analysis of California women enrolled in Medicaid showed that African American women were less likely than White or Latina women to receive postpartum contraception, and when they did receive it, they were less likely to receive a highly effective method.

Clinical Implications

- Social determinants of health must be addressed through policies that raise incomes and provide access to educational attainment; healthcare; safe, affordable housing; and safe environments.
- It is crucial that nurses assess patients for culture-specific needs and desires and provide culturally sensitive and supportive healthcare.
- The number of minority healthcare professionals should be increased to equate with growing ethnic/racial populations.
- Cultural competence education should be required in all professional health curriculums.

References: Eichelberger, K., Doll, K., Edpo, G. E., & Zerden, M. (2016). Black lives matter: Claiming a space for evidence-based outrage in obstetrics and gynecology. *American Journal of Public Health, 106*(10), 1771–1772. https://doi.org/10.2105/AJPH.2016.303313; National Partnership for Women & Families. (2018). *Black women's maternal health: A multifaceted approach to addressing persistent and dire health disparities, Issues brief.* http://www.nationalpartnership.org/research-library/maternal-health/black-womens-maternal-health-issue-brief.pdf; Smith, I., Bentley-Edwards, K. L., El-Amin, S., & Darity, W. (2018). *Fighting*

(continued)

Health Disparities Among the African American Population (continued)

at birth: Eradicating the Black-White infant mortality gap. https://socialequity.duke.edu/sites/socialequity.duke.edu/files/site-images/EradicatingBlackInfantMortality-March2018%20FINAL.pdf; Taylor, K. (2020) Structural racism and maternal health among Black women. *The Journal of Law, Medicine & Ethics, 48*(3): 506-517 https://doi.org/10.1177/1073110520958875; Oribhabor, G., Nelson, M., Buchanan-Pearl, K., & Cancarevic, I. (2020). A mother's cry: A race to eliminate the influence of racial disparities on maternal morbidity and mortality rates among Black women in America. *Cureus, 12*(7), e9207. https://doi.org/10.7759/cureus.9207; Craft-Blacksheare, M., & Kahn, P. (2023). Midwives' and other perinatal health workers' perceptions of the Black maternal mortality crisis in the United States. *Journal of Midwifery & Women's Health, 68*(1), 62-70. https://doi.org/10.1111/jmwh.13433

Globalization results in the spread of varied cultural beliefs and practices. Gender roles and the roles of social support groups often vary from culture to culture. Many groups have distinct cultural practices including African Americans, Native Americans, Latinos/Hispanic Americans, Middle Eastern Americans, Asian Americans, and Orthodox Jewish Americans. Additionally, subcultures exist related to religious background, regional variations (i.e., urban or rural backgrounds), and sexual orientation. It is paramount that those providing care do not assume that a person from a particular racial/ethnic group will act in a certain way. This assumption is the basis for stereotyping that likely will be viewed in a negative way by the client. Healthcare facilities should have cultural information available regarding the clients they serve. Nurses should inquire about patients' cultural practices and preferences and incorporate these in the patient's care plans.

In addition to cultural variations, patients' particular rituals and support systems also may differ. Unfortunately, nurses and healthcare professionals often expect all clients to act according to the dominant culture. As part of health assessments, nurses should inquire about support systems, cultural practices, taboos, and rituals that are important to patients during childbearing.

Although the U.S. population includes variations in ethnic origin, social class, family structure, and social support, many healthcare providers erroneously assume that pregnancy and childbirth are experienced the same way by all people. Additionally, nurses may believe that some traditional and cultural maternity practices are old-fashioned and therefore do not have a place in modern medicine. It is important to realize that many people strive to maintain their cultural childbearing and child-rearing customs. For example, birthing at home with a community midwife may seem unsafe to nurses working in the obstetrical unit of a U.S. hospital. However, home births are a safe, viable option that allows pregnant people to give birth in a familiar, comfortable environment. Figure 5-4 depicts a low-risk mother in her living room with her midwife. For home births, all prenatal appointments and labor support take place in the birthing parent's home, where delivery is anticipated with a birthing pool setup in the living room space (see Fig. 5-5) or use of existing bath (Fig. 5-6). Nonbirthing parents or support people are encouraged to be extremely involved with the birthing process, as you see in Figure 5-7.

Fertility Control and Culture

A pregnancy-capable person's fertility—their ability to conceive a biologic child—depends on several factors: nutrition, sexual behavior, endocrinology, timing, emotions, and culture. The significance of culture is paramount because sex and reproduction are often related to the surrounding cultural system. Certainly, cultural practices can influence fertility decisions. Fertility-related cultural practices include the desire to extend the family lineage, early

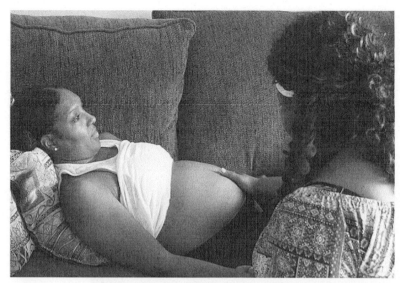

Figure 5-4. Client with home birth midwife.

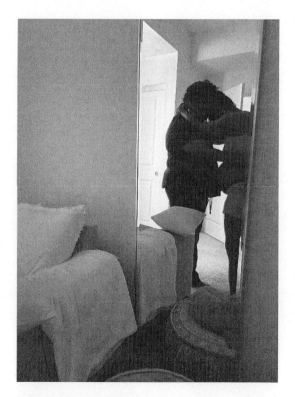

Figure 5-5. Labor support at home birth.

marriages, a preference for producing children of a certain sex, polygamy, and sexual rituals. Practices related to gender roles that affect fertility include subordination of women, economic dependence, and multiple home roles. According to Arousell and Carlbom (2016), an increasing number of contemporary research publications acknowledge religion and culture's influence on sexual and reproductive behavior including healthcare utilization. Gender-sensitive and culturally sensitive family planning services could provide fertility support, birth interval planning, sexually transmitted infection (STI) prevention, and population control maintenance. The following section focuses on the societal elements that influence these factors.

Unintended Pregnancy

The Institute of Medicine defines **unintended pregnancy** as any pregnancy that is mistimed, unplanned, or unwanted at the time of conception (Brown & Eisenberg, 1995).

Finer and colleagues' (2018) research used a new measuring tool, the unintended pregnancy

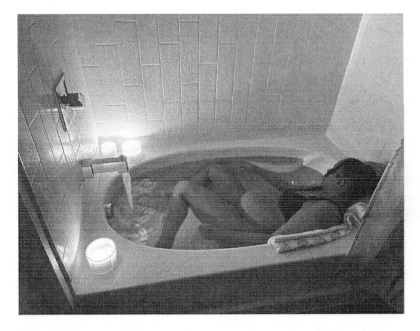

Figure 5-6. Home birth in existing bathtub.

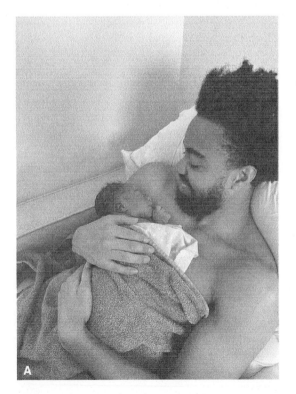

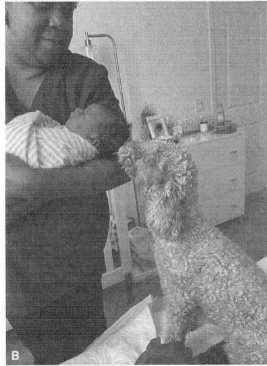

Figure 5-7. **A.** A father enjoying skin-to-skin contact during a home birth. **B.** Home birth: a family affair.

risk index (UPRI), which is based on attitudinal and behavioral measures of women's prospective pregnancy desire, and compared it to the unintended pregnancy rate, which is typically calculated retrospectively. The study design compared three rounds of the National Survey of Family Growth to calculate trends in the UPRI and compare them to the retrospective rate. Based on a women's perspective of pregnancy desire as well as fecundity, sexual activity, and contraceptive use patterns, the UPRI estimates the annual risk of becoming unintentionally pregnant on a scale from 0 to 100. Among all women aged 15 to 34, the UPRI ranged from 7.4 in 2002 to 5.7 in 2013. Even though this rate decreased, large disparities by income and race/ethnicity remain. Therefore, reducing the unintended pregnancy rate remains a national public health goal.

After analyzing data from two survey studies, Rosenthal and Lobel (2018) found that, compared to White women, African American and Latina women reported a greater frequency of and concern over stereotype-related gender racism (ongoing discrimination based on historically rooted stereotypes about their sexuality and motherhood) and **birth control–related mistrust** due to historical abuses. The first study's results ($n = 135$) showed stereotype-related gender racism and birth control–related mistrust among African American and Latina women and none among White women. In addition, the results of the second study ($n = 343$) showed that in general, everyday discrimination and stereotype-related gender racism correlated positively with pregnancy-specific stress for African American and Latina women (Rosenthal & Lobel, 2018). The clinical implications of these findings include the need to educate women's health practitioners about stereotype-related gender racism and birth control–related mistrust to improve the care they provide to these populations. In addition, it would be beneficial to train health practitioners to prevent stereotypes from influencing their perceptions of these women and screen them for gendered racism experiences.

Interventions aimed at reducing the aforementioned disparities in unintended pregnancies should target at-risk groups of people. It is possible that the observed racial and ethnic disparities resulted from psychosocial and economic determinants that must be addressed to improve health outcomes among these groups.

According to the Guttmacher Institute (Frost et al., 2019) in 2010, U.S. public investment in family planning services resulted in $13.6 billion in net savings, helping women avoid unintended pregnancies and a range of other negative reproductive health outcomes, such as STIs, cervical cancer, infertility, and HIV. An economic model developed by Filonenka et al. (2019) estimated the direct annual medical costs of unintended pregnancy for all women of reproductive age (15 to 44). Their results illustrated a conservative annual direct medical cost estimated to be at least $5.5 billion with 54.2% of cost ($3.0 billion) occurring in young women aged 20 to 29. Despite the declines in unintended pregnancy rates, the annual cost of unintended pregnancy in the United States increased from a cost of $4.6 billion in 2011 to $5.5 billion in 2018.

Continuation of Unintended Pregnancy

According to Cutler et al. (2018), ambivalence about an unintended pregnancy has been defined as "contradictory or unresolved feelings about whether or not to continue the pregnancy" (p. 75). Pregnancy ambivalence is a risk factor for high-risk sexual behavior and is associated with poor pregnancy outcomes. Those with unintended pregnancies report increased levels of anxiety, stress, and depression along with receiving late prenatal care (Cutler et al., 2018). Herd et al. (2016) examined women's long-term well-being after continuation of an unintended pregnancy by obtaining data from a 60-year longitudinal study of Wisconsin high school graduates from the class of 1957. The aim of the study was to assess later-life depressive symptoms and episodes among women who reported unintended pregnancies before Roe v. Wade. In this cohort of mostly married White women, continuation of unintended pregnancies was strongly associated with poorer mental health outcomes in later life (Herd et al., 2016).

The *Turnaway Study* (Foster, 2020) researched the consequences of having or being denied an abortion by following 1,000 women over a 10-year period. Every outcome of women who received an abortion was the same or, more frequently, better off than the women who were denied an abortion. Women who received an abortion had better physical and mental health, aspirational plans for the coming year, and a better financial situation. Compared to planned births, births from unintended pregnancies were associated with adverse maternal, infant, and child health outcomes such as delayed prenatal care and premature birth. Births from unintended pregnancies also increased the mothers' risk for smoking cigarettes and using alcohol (Guttmacher Institute, 2016).

Contraceptive Methods

Troutman, Rafique and Plowden (2020) discussed a study that identified women aged 18 to 24 with the highest risk of unintended pregnancy. Additionally, using cost models, it was further estimated that if 10% of women aged 20 to 29 using oral contraception changed to long-acting reversible contraception (LARC), the total costs associated with unintended pregnancy would decrease by $288 million per year.

While they are sexually active and do not want to become pregnant, many do not use a contraceptive method correctly and consistently to prevent pregnancy.

Sixty-seven percent of contraceptive users use nonpermanent methods, primarily hormonal methods (the pill, patch, implant, injectable, and vaginal ring) as well as intrauterine devices (IUDs) and condoms. The remainder rely on female (25%) or male (8%) sterilization.

Women most likely to use the pill are White, in their teens and 20s, college graduates, cohabiting, childless, and never married.

In their demographic research to understand the trends and differentials on U.S. female sterilization research, Johnsen and Sweeney (2022) note that Black, Hispanic, and less-educated women are more likely than White or college-educated women to undergo sterilization. Notably, these differentials unveil a long history of coercive sterilization aimed in particular at low-income women and women of color in the United States. Additionally, estimates suggest that women sterilized at age 30 or younger are twice as likely to desire for sterilization reversal.

According to the Guttmacher Institute (2018), 68% of Catholics, 73% of Protestants, and 74% of Evangelicals who are at risk for an unintended pregnancy use a highly effective method (e.g., sterilization, IUD, or the pill or other hormonal methods). Even though Catholicism encourages natural family planning, only about 2% of at-risk Catholics rely on this method, the same percentage as those who attend church once a month or more.

Emergency contraception (EC), available in the United States, is used to prevent pregnancy after unprotected intercourse or contraceptive failure. To be effective, it must be used within 24 and up to 120 hours after unprotected intercourse. This method is available as a single-dose regimen (1.5 mg levonorgestrel taken once) or a two-dose regimen (two tablets of 0.75 mg levonorgestrel taken 12 hours apart). The single-dose regimen was first made available over the counter in 2013. In addition to hormonal EC, inserting a copper IUD up to 120 hours after unprotected intercourse can be used as an EC method (Holland et al., 2018).

Global Contraception Concerns

The Global Strategy for Women's Children's and Adolescents' Health (2016–2030) initiative promotes ending preventable child and maternal deaths. In their commentary, Fikree et al. (2017) addressed the Global Consensus Statement (*Expanding Contraceptive Choice for Adolescents and Youth to Include Long Acting and Reversible Contraception* [LARC]) by providing evidence on the safety and effectiveness of LARCs for young people. The authors estimated that more than 12 million married and unmarried adolescents (aged 15 to 19) would give birth in 2016 and that pregnancy and childbirth complications are the second leading cause of death in this age group. Evidence supports the fact that early childbearing significantly hinders social and economic prospects for young women. Facilitating the ability of sexually active young people to choose an effective and satisfying contraceptive method will ensure they can exercise their right to prevent, delay, or space pregnancy (Fikree et al., 2017).

Refugees and Reproductive Health

According to World Vision Today in 2023, the Syrian war in 2011 has created the largest refugee and displacement crisis of our time. More than half of the country's population is displaced. Syrian refugees have sought asylum in more than 130 countries; however, most live in regional countries, such as Turkey, Jordan, Lebanon, Iraq, and Egypt.

Women and girls are especially vulnerable, with lack of access to services and collapse of social structures leading to poor sexual and reproductive health (SRH) outcomes. Pregnant women have a greater risk of premature labor, antenatal complications, and infections. In Lebanon, studies have shown that Syrian refugee women are at increased risk of sexual and gender-based violence, reproductive tract infections, and pregnancy.

Syrian children are also vulnerable to sexual abuse and exploitation living in unfamiliar and overcrowded conditions in refugee camps and informal tent settlements. Unfortunately, some families desperate for income are prone to arrange marriages for their young daughters in exchange for dowries.

Prior to the creation of the Women's Refugee Commission and the Inter-agency Working Group on Reproductive Health in Crisis (IAWG), women living in refugee situations received little assistance when encountering the many barriers to reproductive care. To address this issue, the IAWG has taken a leadership role in research, technical guidance, and guideline development. Because of this work, the IAWG published the *Inter-agency Field Manual on Reproductive Health in Humanitarian Settings*, which was updated in 2018 (see Box 5-1). This manual provides information to help humanitarian staff provide reproductive health interventions during humanitarian emergencies. The IAWG also created the *Minimum Initial Service Package* (MISP), a list of priority activities to be implemented at the onset of every humanitarian emergency.

See Evidence-Based Practice 5-3 for a discussion of reproductive care issues faced by refugee women.

BOX 5-1   **IAWG Inter-Agency Field Manual on Reproductive Health in Humanitarian Settings, 2018**

- **Ensure** the health sector/cluster identifies an organization to lead the implementation of the MISP.
- **Prevent** sexual violence and **respond** to the needs of survivors.
- **Prevent** the transmission of and **reduce** morbidity and mortality due to HIV.
- **Prevent** excess maternal and newborn morbidity and mortality.
- **Prevent** unintended pregnancies.

- **Plan** for comprehensive SRH services integrated into primary healthcare as soon as possible.
- **Work** with the health sector/cluster partners to address the six health system building blocks, including service delivery, health workforce, health information system, medical commodities, financing and governance, and leadership.

Source: Inter-Agency Working Group (IAWG) on Reproductive Health in Crisis. (2018). *Inter-agency field manual on reproductive health in humanitarian settings.* https://iawg.wpengine.com/wp-content/uploads/2019/07/IAFM-English.pdf

Refugee Women's Experiences With Contraceptive Care After Resettlement in High-Income Countries: A Critical Interpretive Synthesis

A small fraction of the almost 80 million people displaced in 2019 included 26 million refugees. Refugee women who resettled in high-income countries often share histories of economic hardship, forced displacement, gender-based violence, and common barriers to reproductive healthcare. In a critical interpretative synthesis, the authors compiled and analyzed studies on refugee women's contraceptive preferences and their experiences of contraceptive care conducted in all high-income countries of resettlement.

Critical interpretive synthesis is a review methodology that offers a systematic, empirical method for combining qualitative and quantitative forms of research involving an "ongoing critical orientation" to the studies reviewed and contexts in which they were conducted.

Sixty-two studies conducted in high-income countries contained data related to contraception for resettled refugee women. Twenty-five studies were conducted in Australia, 15 in the United States, 9 in Canada, 1 in Israel, and 16 in European countries. Most studies acknowledged a lack of generalizability as a potential limitation, emphasizing that refugees are not a homogenous population and that research conducted with one population in one setting does not necessarily apply to all refugees.

Quantitative studies demonstrated attention to potential sources of bias arising from the method of data collection employed. In contrast, not all qualitative studies considered the methods and environment in which data were collected, whereas some women may fear repercussions that disclosed information would be reported to immigration services or the government.

Study's Findings

- Many refugee women come from cultures that value large families and high fertility—these women cited several reasons such as pressure to conform to social norms, economic benefits, and security a family provides.
- Refugee women had lower rates of biomedical contraceptive use than the general population;

this was associated with a higher rate of unintended pregnancies and abortions.
- Side effects of hormonal contraceptives, which include weight gain, irregular or heavy bleeding menstrual suppression, and impact on fertility after discontinuation, were also a concern.
- Religious beliefs did not impact contraceptive use in a homogenous way.
- Several studies strongly emphasized male partners' roles in contraceptive use and some focused on their potential to inhibit women's reproductive agency.
- Barriers to contraceptive care included structural factors that prevent patients from reaching healthcare facilities (access care).
- The highly regimented, strict schedule of healthcare provision in high-income countries is more anomalous than the "polychromic" orientation to time that is found in most societies worldwide. Many respondents felt providers were rushed and did not listen to them during the appointment.
- Communication difficulties were found to be one of the most significant barriers for refugee women seeking reproductive healthcare. Women did not often understand providers, explanations, or written instructions; therefore, they were not provided with sufficient information to make an informed choice.
- Refugee women reported experiences of racism and discrimination in reproductive health settings. Many felt stigmatized by being pregnant and having high parity.
- Islamophobia and assumptions about Muslim women's lack of agency influenced some clinical interactions.

Clinical Implications

- Contraceptive care for resettled refugees remains limited by the lack of epidemiologic data available on the unique needs of this population.
- Studies attempt to acknowledge potential biases; however, there remains significant room for improvement.

Refugee Women's Experiences With Contraceptive Care After Resettlement in High-Income Countries: A Critical Interpretive Synthesis (continued)

- Refugee health research includes cultural and religious differences of ethnicities from around the globe, and the challenge of appreciating nuance and variability within the different groups rather than homogenizing each population.

Reference: Chalmiers, M., Karaki, F., Muriki, M., Mody, S. K., Chen, A., & de Bocanegra, H. T. (2022). Refugee women's experiences with contraceptive care after resettlement in high-income countries: A critical interpretive synthesis. *Contraception*, 108, 7–18. https://doi.org/10.1016/j.contraception.2021.11.004

Religion and Fertility Control

Most major religions offer members guidance in SRH matters. Scholars have studied the meaning of sexuality and family planning strategies among the major religious traditions of Judaism, Christianity, Islam, Hinduism, Sikhism, and Buddhism. Each religion offers a distinct belief system. Depending upon their personal interpretations of their faith, religious followers can be considered devout, conservative, or liberal followers of their religion.

Regarding birth control, the Catholic Church endorses only natural family planning methods (i.e., the rhythm method and cycle beads). Such methods require partner agreement and support to refrain from intercourse during the fertile period. Additionally, the user must understand and become familiar with their menstrual cycle in order to avoid or plan a pregnancy.

Arousell and Carlbom (2016) reported on Moreau and colleagues' findings that regular religious practice among Muslims was associated with a later sexual debut among young people. However, the same study found that sexually active adolescents who regularly practiced their religion were less likely to use contraception. In these situations, controls executed by family and social and religious groups may act as barrier that prevents sexually active adolescents from adopting preventative behaviors. The Muslim value system discourages young followers from deviating from sexual norms or gender roles or becoming sexually active before marriage, believing that this shows dishonor to their family (Arousell & Carlbom, 2016).

Westoff and Bietsch (2015) analyzed religion influences on reproductive behavior in 29 sub-Saharan African countries. The health surveys conducted over 10 years (2004–2014) categorized the religions as either Muslim or non-Muslim. Results indicated that Muslim fertility rates were higher than were non-Muslim rates. The fertility rate of married Muslim women was higher for those who married at a younger age (17.7 vs. 19.0 years). Polygyny is more common among Muslim women (35%) compared to non-Muslim women (22%). While Islamic law allows a man to have more than one wife, this practice is illegal in Turkey and Tunisia. Higher education levels and urban or rural residence both are associated with marriage and fertility. The percentage of Muslim women with no schooling is higher than for non-Muslim women. The average number of children desired by young Muslim women is 5.1 compared to 4.4 desired by non-Muslim teenagers. Education is inversely related to the number of children desired. Additionally, in most of the 17 countries, the percentage of married Muslim women currently using a contraceptive method is lower than that of non-Muslim women. Finally, in most countries, Muslim women have shorter birth intervals than do non-Muslim women (Westoff & Bietsch, 2015).

Cultural Influences on Fertility Control

Unfortunately, it is common for health professionals to have misconceptions about pregnancy prevention and contraception in cultures different from their own. To ensure that all persons receive optimal care, nurses are challenged to eradicate stigmas, language barriers, stereotyping, discrimination, and patients' lack of information about the health system from care settings (Cesario, 2017).

Salari's (2018) research examined how cultural attitudes affected the fertility decisions of second-generation immigrant women who were born in the United States but kept their heritage language. The results indicated that their original culture had a direct impact on their fertility decisions, with their total fertility rates reflecting the values of the original culture, not their new culture. Additionally, cultural transmission is found to be statically significant among women whose social network is comprised of people of the same culture (Salari, 2018).

The socialization hypothesis relies on the assumption that the values, norms, and family behaviors of migrants reflect those dominant in their childhood. According to Wilson and Kuha (2017), this hypothesis explains the fertility of "foreign-born persons" who arrive under the age of 16, demonstrating fertility patterns of their country of origin more than those in the country of destination. However, in the study of migrants' Fertility in Italy, Impicciatore et al. (2020) suggest that the disruption hypothesis indicates migration is stressful for a person due to a drastic change in daily life conditions, interruption of social networks, and temporary separation from spouse. In this situation, migrants tend to have particularly low levels of fertility due to the disruptive factors and difficulties of migration itself and a new environment.

Therefore, a client in the family planning office who has lived in the United States for 10 years may embrace their heritage cultures' value system as it relates to fertility and childbearing rather than the dominant culture of the Western culture where they now reside. Health providers must be aware of cultural groups existing in the community, not assume but appropriately assess the individuals, and have the ability to ask appropriately about their family planning preferences in alignment with their cultural needs.

Between 2008 and 2016, Mutumba et al. (2018) examined how communities influenced the fertility decisions of 15- to 24-year-old women from 52 countries: 32 in Africa, 6 in Southeast Asia, 5 from the Eastern Mediterranean region, 20 from the Western Pacific region, 5 from the European region, and 8 from the Americas. These researchers concluded that prenatal attitudes—which act as social scripts that people who can get pregnant are expected to follow—may discourage contraceptives by increasing pressure for young people assigned female at birth to prove their fertility or promote prevailing fears and misconceptions that modern contraceptive methods may reduce fertility. These results also indicated that young women who live in communities with families who have more children than they consider ideal were less likely to report using modern contraceptive methods. However, young women with the following characteristics were more likely to use modern contraceptive measures: having received higher education, residing in a wealthier household, living in urban areas with greater mass media exposure, and having a higher number of living children (Mutumba et al., 2018).

Nurses providing family planning services should strive to be culturally sensitive to help their patients feel comfortable examining their own attitudes, beliefs, and sense of gynecologic well-being regarding fertility control. Nurses should acquire patients' history of previous contraceptive use including identifying their satisfaction or problems with the methods they used. Providing an explanation of contraceptive benefits, side effects, and risks is crucial. If necessary, an interpreter should be used to address language barriers.

Pregnancy and Culture

All cultures recognize **pregnancy** as a special transition period in a person's life. Most societies have customs and beliefs that dictate a person's behavior, activities, and lifestyle during the childbearing period. Due to the U.S. population's varied cultural and ethnic backgrounds, childbirth customs not only reflect the dominant society but also allow for the accommodation and blending of other cultural practices to satisfy maternal and family wishes. The following section describes some of the biologic and cultural variations that could influence nursing care during pregnancy.

Biologic Variations

Nurses who provide care to pregnant women need to learn about biologic variations resulting from genetic and environmental backgrounds. In the United States, pregnant African American patients are screened for sickle cell disease (SCD), a serious, chronic hemolytic anemia resulting from homozygosity for the mutant allele of the hemoglobin S gene. While SCD prevalence is approximately 1 in 400 African American women, the carrier frequency of the heterozygote sickle cell trait (SST) is 1 in 10. Because pregnant people with SST are at an increased risk for asymptomatic bacterial urinary tract infections, pyelonephritis, and preterm labor, frequent urine cultures are obtained during their antenatal care. If a pregnant patient has an SST, a paternal blood test is taken and genetic counseling offered. If the father is heterozygous for the gene, there is a one in four chance that the infant will be born with the disease. Even though sickle cell disease (SSD) and SST predominately occur among people of African descent, SSD is also found among people from the Mediterranean region, South America, and India. A cultural immigration history may be beneficial to determine the necessity of testing for SST (see Evidence-Based Practice 5-4).

Diabetes is another biologic variation related to pregnancy. While diabetes has serious implications for the pregnant person and fetus, survival rates have improved over the last few decades.

Diabetes is a national public health problem where American Indian/Alaskan natives (AI/AN) are disproportionately affected.

According to the CDC's National Diabetes statistic report (2020) among U.S. adults aged 18 years or older, the prevalence of diagnosed diabetes for 2007–2018 was highest among AI/AN at 14.7%. The prevalence for people of Hispanic origin was 12.5%, non-Hispanic Blacks 11.7%, non-Hispanic Asians 9.2%, and non-Hispanic Whites 7.5%.

According to Terry et al. (2020), all gestational diabetes mellitus (GDM) is the most common complication of pregnancy, affecting up to 18% of all pregnancies in the United States. AI/AN women have twice the rate of GDM versus non-Hispanic White women.

Pregnant people with any form of diabetes are at risk for fetal and neonatal complications. Those with pregestational type 1 diabetes are at an increased risk for preeclampsia and adverse neonatal outcomes. Because there is an increased risk of urinary tract infections with every type of diabetes, asymptomatic bacteriuria screening should be performed to help reduce the impact of this problem. In addition, hydramnios (increased amniotic fluid) and fetal macrosomia (baby ≥4,000 g) are more common among pregnant people with diabetes.

Carson et al. (2015) conducted a qualitative research study in which 97 participants from two Oklahoma tribes were interviewed to obtain information about variables that could negatively affect diabetes prevention or control. Data analysis revealed the following themes: diabetes self-care adherence as well as fear of neonatal complications, injections, amputation, blindness, and death. Many participants repeated stories about the disease they heard from friends and family members. The researchers concluded that patients might have explanatory models, influenced by their social network members that differ from the practice-based explanatory models health practitioners use. Additionally, effective communication and culturally sensitive care help promote patient adherence to recommended treatments (Carson et al., 2015).

Sickle Cell Disease and Pregnancy Outcomes: A Study of the Community-Based Hospital in a Tribal Block of Gujarat, India

Sickle cell disease (SCD), a hereditary blood disorder, is a serious public health concern that presents mainly in tropical countries, primarily Africa. SCD is also prevalent in Central America, Saudi Arabia, India, and Mediterranean countries. The purpose of this study was to report on the analysis of tribal maternal admissions in the community-based hospital of SEWA Rural (Kasturba Maternity Hospital) in Jhagadia Block, Gujarat, India. Data were collected from March 2011 to September 2015, during which there were 14,640 total tribal maternal admissions and 10,519 deliveries. Overall, 12% (131 out of 10,519) of tribal deliveries were sickle cell admissions and 0.6% (1,645 out of 10,519) of tribal delivery admissions had the sickle cell trait. The percentage of stillborns among SCD deliveries was 9.2%, compared to 4.2% of non–sickle cell patients. Additionally, almost half of sickle cell deliveries required a blood transfusion. Forty-five percent of sickle cell deliveries were preterm births compared to only 17.3% of non-SCD patients. The odds of severe anemia, stillbirth, blood transfusion, cesarean section, and low birth weight were significantly higher for sickle cell admissions compared to non–sickle cell admissions. These findings indicated that there is a high risk of adverse pregnancy outcomes for pregnant people with SCD. Identification of tribal women with SCD and SCT is crucial for decreasing morbidity/mortality.

Clinical Implications

- This study highlights the need for sickle cell screening and care for people in remote and tribal rural areas in India.
- Pregnant people with SCD need regular third-trimester fetal growth screening.
- Providing blood transfusions for people with SCD (as needed) may help reduce adverse maternal outcomes.
- Health professionals must assess a client's country of ancestral origin to determine if sickle cell blood testing is warranted.

Reference: Desai, G., Anand, A., Shah, P., Shah, S., Dave, K., Bhatt, H., Desai, S., & Modi, D. (2017). Sickle cell disease and pregnancy outcomes: A study of the community-based hospital in a tribal block of Gujarat, India. Journal of Health, Population and Nutrition, 36(1), 3. https://doi.org/10.1186/s41043-017-0079-z

Cultural Variations Influencing Pregnancy

This section discusses Western cultural practices and variations that can influence pregnancy outcomes: alternative family structures, maternal role attainment, nontraditional support systems, cultural beliefs about parental activity during pregnancy, and food taboos and cravings. Nurses must be able to assess a client's cultural practices related to childbearing to determine if they are harmful or benign. Nurses also must never assume that clients "don't look like" they engage in practices outside those of the mainstream population or "don't look like" they are from a particular ethnic group or culture (**stereotyping**). It is important to incorporate questions about cultural practices related to pregnancy, childbirth, and newborn care in the initial assessment and throughout the prenatal period.

Female genital mutilation/cutting (FGM/C) is a dangerous ancient cultural practice that can affect pregnancy. FGM/C, also known as female excision, is a violation of human rights.

According to a recent UNICEF publication (2022), one in three girls aged 15 to 19 living in 31 countries have undergone FGM. This deeply entrenched social norm is rooted in gender inequality. The international community has codified its commitment to eliminate the practice by 2030 under Target 5.3 of the sustainable development goals (SDGs). The number of girls and women alive today who have undergone this practice is estimated at 200 million. Over the past decade, the FGM practice has been estimated to decrease from 41% to 34%.

Even though there has been an overall decline in FGM/C over the last three decades, not all countries have made significant progress and the pace of the decline has been uneven. UNICEF's data illustrate that the progress is insufficient to keep up with increasing population growth. Community members practicing this custom believe that FGM/C will ensure a girl's proper upbringing, future marriage, and honor to the family. Others associate this ritual with religious beliefs, although no religious scriptures require it. The fact that parents allow their daughters to undergo this procedure despite being aware of the harm it causes illustrates the power of this cultural practice. Many are afraid that refraining from the practice will risk their daughter's marriage prospects as well as their family status (see Evidence-Based Practice 5-5).

LGBTQ+ Family Structures

Family composition or family structure refers to how family members are related to each other and society. Structure can refer to the form (e.g., single- or two-parent families), partners (e.g., cohabitation or marriage), or composition (traditional nuclear, extended, or communal family). Regardless of the nurse's perception of what constitutes a family, they must accept whomever clients define as their family members and their relationships with them. In North American culture, the concept of what constitutes a "traditional" family has changed drastically over the last 30 years. Although the dominant cultural expectations for North Americans are for marriage and childbearing to take place within a nuclear family, cultural changes have made it more acceptable to delay childbearing in lieu of a college education and a formal career. This cultural change has encouraged many couples to have smaller families, people who can get pregnant to freeze their embryos (to prevent problems with infertility due to later childbearing), and single people to use donor sperm or surrogacy and raise children as single parents.

A review of the literature indicates there is a growing number of families that include members of sexual and/or gender minority (SGM) groups. According to Griggs et al. (2021), approximately 19% of adults who are members of SGM groups are presently raising 3 million children, hoping to become pregnant, foster, use surrogacy, or adopt in the future.

The American Congress of Obstetricians and Gynecologists (ACOG) (2018) reaffirmed its support for marriage equality for all adults and its intent to "understand, recognize, and address the challenges the (LGBTQ+) community experiences in accessing reproductive healthcare, including family building."

In 2015, the U.S. Supreme Court established the right to same-sex marriage in all states (Obergefell v. Hodges). More than 280,000 same-sex married tax filers in the United States were present after the Windsor and Obergefell Supreme Court case, but little is known about how they build families.

Downing (2019) estimated the prevalence of fertility treatments for lesbian couples and heterosexual (cisgender) couples from 2012 to 2016 using Massachusetts data for live births. The use of fertility services and technologies was identified via hospital data and birth certificate worksheets completed by parents. Pregnancies were identified as resulting from one of the following: reproductive technology, intrauterine insemination, intracervical insemination, and anonymous donor sperm.

The results compared pregnancies of heterosexual (cisgender) sex couples ($n = 233,158$) and pregnancies of lesbian couples ($n = 1,439$), which were 112 times higher for the use of any type of fertility treatments, 9 times higher for fertility-enhancing drugs and assisted reproductive technology (in vitro fertilization), 33 times higher for intrauterine insemination, and 44 times higher for intracervical insemination. Additionally, when comparing pregnancies with anonymous donor sperm, four in five were to lesbian couples (854 to 1,081).

Female Genital Mutilation and Cutting: A Systematic Literature Review of Health Professionals' Knowledge, Attitudes, and Clinical Practice

Due to increased immigration, health professions in high-income countries including the United Kingdom, Europe, North America, and Australia care for patients with female genital mutilation/cutting (FGM/C). This study reviewed health providers' knowledge, clinical practice, and attitudes regarding FGM/C. Most health professionals were aware of the practice of FGM/C, but few correctly identified the four FGM/C categories defined by WHO. Knowledge about FGM/C legislation varied: 25% of professionals in a Sudanese study, 45% of Belgian labor ward staff, and 94% of health professions from the United Kingdom knew that FGM/C was illegal in their country.

Clinical Implications

Female genital mutilation is classified into four major types:

- **Type 1:** Often referred to as clitoridectomy, this is the partial or total removal of the clitoris (a small, sensitive, and erectile part of the female genitals) and, in very rare cases, only the prepuce (the fold of skin surrounding the clitoris).
- **Type 2:** Often referred to as excision, this is the partial or total removal of the clitoris and the labia minora (the inner folds of the vulva), with or without excision of the labia majora (the outer folds of skin of the vulva).
- **Type 3:** Often referred to as infibulation, this is the narrowing of the vaginal opening through the creation of a covering seal. The seal is formed by cutting and repositioning the labia minora, or labia majora, sometimes through stitching, with or without clitoris removal.
- **Type 4:** This includes all other harmful procedures to the female genitalia for nonmedical purposes, for example, pricking, piercing, incising, scraping, and cauterizing the genital area.

Immediate Complications

- Severe pain
- Excessive bleeding

Cultural and Social Factors for Performing FGM

The reasons for performing FGM/C vary from one region to another, as well as over time, and include a mix of sociocultural factors within families and communities. The following are some of the most commonly cited reasons for this practice:

- Where FGM is a social norm, strong motivations to perpetuate the practice include social pressure to conform to what others do and have been doing, the need to be accepted socially, and the fear of community rejection. In some communities, FGM is unquestioned and performed almost universally.
- FGM is often considered a necessary part of raising a girl and a way to prepare her for adulthood and marriage.
- FGM is often motivated by beliefs about what is considered an acceptable sexual behavior. It aims to ensure premarital virginity and marital fidelity. In many communities, FGM is believed to reduce a woman's libido and therefore believed to help her resist extramarital sexual acts. When a vaginal opening is covered or narrowed (type 3), women's fears that opening it will be painful and that doing so will be discovered are expected to discourage extramarital sexual intercourse.
- FGM is more likely to be carried out in communities where it is believed that being cut increases marriageability.
- FGM is associated with cultural ideals of femininity and modesty, which include the notion that girls are "clean" and "beautiful" after the removal of body parts considered unclean, unfeminine, or male.
- Though no religious scripts prescribe the practice, practitioners often believe the practice has religious support.
- Religious leaders take varying positions on FGM: some promote it, some consider it irrelevant to religion, and others contribute to its elimination.

Female Genital Mutilation and Cutting: A Systematic Literature Review of Health Professionals' Knowledge, Attitudes, and Clinical Practice (continued)

- Local power and authority structures—such as community leaders, religious leaders, circumcisers, and even some medical personnel—can contribute to upholding the practice.
- In most societies where FGM is practiced, it is considered a cultural tradition, which often is used as an argument for its continuation.
- In some societies, recent adoption of the practice is linked to copying the traditions of neighboring groups. Sometimes, it has started as part of a wider religious or traditional revival movement.

Key Facts About Female Genital Mutilation

- FGM includes procedures that intentionally alter or cause injury to the female genital organs for nonmedical reasons.
- The procedure has no health benefits.
- The procedures can cause severe bleeding and problems urinating and later cysts, infections, as well as childbirth complications and increased risk of newborn deaths.
- More than 200 million girls and women alive today have been cut in 30 countries where FGM is concentrated (Africa, the Middle East, and Asia).

- FGM is mostly carried out between infancy and age 15.
- FGM is a violation of human rights.

FGM in Humanitarian Settings

- Studies demonstrate that drivers of FGM may precede humanitarian crises such as patriarchy and gender inequality, reduced education and employment opportunities for girls, marriageability, esthetics, and lack of laws banning the practice.
- Many migrants stop performing FGM type III but continue to perform FGM types I, II, and IV. One explanation is that milder forms like type IV will be undetectable and unpunishable by law in high-income countries where FGM is illegal.

References: Elnakib, S., & Metzler, J. (2022). A scoping review of FGM in humanitarian settings; an overlooked phenomenon with lifelong consequence. *Conflict and Health, 16*(1), 49. https://doi.org/10.1186/s13031-022-00479-5; World Health Organization (WHO). (2018b). *Female genital mutilation.* http://www.who.int/news-room/fact-sheets/detail/female-genital-mutilation; Zurynski, Y., Sureshkumar, P., Phu, A., & Elliot, E. (2015). Female genital mutilation and cutting: A systematic literature review of health professionals' knowledge, attitudes, and clinical practice. *BMC International Health and Human Rights, 15*, 32. https://doi.org/10.1186/s12914-015-0070-y

This higher rate of in vitro fertilization and fertility drugs among lesbian couples may be cost-prohibitive and emotionally taxing, which could lead to complications, and increase the risk of multiple births and preterm delivery.

Lesbian, bisexual women, and transgender (LBT) couples have the ability to negotiate who gives birth in a relationship. Malmquist and Nieminen (2021) explored how (LBT) couples negotiate the question of who gives birth, in couples with two potential birth parents, and where one or both partners have a pronounced fear of childbirth (FOC). They interviewed 17 self-identified LBT people about their expectancies and experiences of pregnancy and childbirth. FOC was negotiated as one of many aspects that contributed to the decision of who would be the birth-giving partner. Several participants decided to become pregnant despite their fears, due to the desire to be the genetic parent. Others negotiated with their partner about who was least vulnerable, while others decided to refrain from pregnancy, due to FOC, and were delighted that their partner would give birth. The partner's experience was in some cases not addressed in postnatal care. However, it is important that healthcare staff address both partners' prenatal expectancies and postnatal experiences.

Reproductive Health of Transgender Men

Transgender men are individuals who were assigned female at birth and self-identify along the male spectrum. Transgender men may choose to affirm their gender socially, physically, and/or legally as they align their internal and external experiences of gender; however, they may also choose to retain the reproductive organs they were born with.

LGBTQ+ community members have historically avoided healthcare services due to social and clinical discrimination. For example, Gatos (2018) found that transgender men who retain their cervixes are less likely to receive cervical cancer screening than cisgender women.

Rebecca and MacLean in 2021 conducted a literature review to explore the reproductive health needs of transgender men related to reproductive desires, contraception, family planning, fertility preservation, pregnancy, birth, and lactation. Thirty-six articles were identified and 27 were included in the review. Four common themes emerged: *Existing Barriers to Care, Unique Considerations to Guide Optimal Care, Gestational and Postpartum Challenges for Transgender Men, and Research Gaps on the Reproductive Health Needs of Transgender Men.*

Existing Barriers to Care

It was identified that barriers may lead to disempowerment, avoidance of care, and poor health outcomes (Brandt et al., 2019). Additionally, a lack of safe and inclusive healthcare environments, social stigma, discrimination, providers inexperienced in transgender health, a lack of financial and insurance coverage for gender-affirming treatments, and misgendering (the improper use of chosen names, pronouns, or gender identity descriptors) were also identified as essential issues (Charter et al., 2018; Francis et al., 2018; MacDonald, 2019).

A review of the literature suggests that pregnancy-capable transgender men in the United States accessed midwifery care more than did the cisgender population (Richardson et al., 2019). The unique finding of this group gravitating toward midwifery care should be examined by other providers to further understand how the midwifery model of care understands and supports their needs in order to incorporate this finding into all practices.

Unique Considerations to Guide Optimal Care

Personalized healthcare is desired by all patients; however, transgender men require individualized care related to gender transitioning, contraception, pregnancy birth, and chest feeding, which refers to feeding an infant at the chest (Francis et al., 2018; Richardson et al., 2019).

Gestational and Postpartum Challenges for Transgender Men

Transgender individuals commonly experience discrimination in highly gendered clinical environments; for example, the maternity unit (which is female-oriented) can pose an even greater risk of experiencing oppressive care (Richardson et al., 2019) versus an all-inclusive gender orientation) the "birthing unit." Additionally, pregnancy-capable transgender men have reported being misgendered in clinical environments, which caused them to hide their identity out of fear of discrimination (Richardson et al., 2019).

Research Gaps on the Reproductive Health Needs of Transgender Men

Charter and colleagues (2018) explored the feelings of discrimination, isolation, and invisibility pregnant and birthing transgender men face. They emphasize the failure of the healthcare system, which lacks specific guidelines, best practices, and support for this population. These results emphasize the vulnerability of transgender men in cisgender-normative perinatal environments.

Nurses and other healthcare providers must provide the same prenatal, labor, and postpartum support to transgender pregnant and birthing men as cisgender women. This population may feel more comfortable accessing preconception and perinatal care if health environments and provider care is gender-affirming.

It is important not to make assumptions about an individual's gender identity, chosen names, pronouns, sexual orientation, or sex assignment at birth nor to assume that an individual will openly disclose this information. A significant finding highlights that healthcare providers may already be caring for transgender men and not be aware (MacDonald, 2019). Krempasky and colleagues (2020) propose that health histories for all patients should use a gender-inclusive approach, not only for those identifying as transgender. Providers need to ask and document the individual's gender identity, sexual orientation, chosen names, and pronouns (see Evidence-Based Practice 5-6).

Evidence-Based Practice 5-6

Caring for Transgender Men and Other Individuals Who Identify as LGBTQ+

Background

- People who are LGBTQ+ come from all walks of life, which includes all ages, races, ethnicities, and socioeconomic statuses, and live in various parts of the United States.
- Their health needs are unique and as a group, they tend to disproportionately suffer from social inequality and poorer health outcomes and are at risk for illnesses and disease when compared with those who are not members of an SGM group in part due to structural inequities, stigma, and discriminations.
- Individuals report a lack of cultural competence from nurses and other providers including images and language inclusive of only cisgender and heterosexual couples or families as well as a lack of information and availability of research on SGM perinatal health.

Pregnancy Care

- Support an all-encompassing approach to couples who identify as LGBTQ+ from a place of respect, trust, and open communication to promote an environment of inclusivity.
- Inquire about pronouns and words they use to identify their body parts and make sure to use them (chest feeding [breast-feeding], front pelvic opening [vagina]).
- Understanding that the transgender population is more at risk for depression and suicidal ideation places an emphasis on the heightened vulnerability of pregnant transgender men.

Clinical Implications

- Take an active role by prioritizing education to understand and support transgender bodies, identities, and individuals' reproductive needs.
- Creating a culture of holistic and nonbiased care for SGM populations should be incorporated into the curriculum throughout nursing school.
- Registered nurses, advanced practice nurses, nurse-midwives, and other healthcare providers should be provided with accurate information and ample trans sensitivity training opportunities to be proficient and supportive of LGBTQ+ individuals.
- Health profession schools curriculums and the health service industry should provide education available in various forms, such as simulation scenarios, case studies, self-reflection opportunities, formal training sessions, and online learning.
- Nurses can act as change champions to advocate for gender-affirming perinatal assessments and the inclusion of transgender men in perinatal care models.

References: Griggs, K., Waddill, C., Bice, A., & Ward, N. (2021). Care during pregnancy, childbirth, postpartum, and human milk feeding for individuals who identify as LGBTQ+. *MCN. The American Journal of Maternal Child Nursing, 46*(1), 43–53; Center for Disease Control and Prevention. (2018). Lesbian, gay, bisexual, and transgender health. https://www.cdc.gov/lgbthealth/; Farrow, A. (2015). Lactation support and the LGBTQI community. *Journal of Human Lactation, 31*(1), 26–28. https://doi.org//10.1177/0890334414554928

Maternal Role Attainment

Based on cross-cultural observations and psychological research, John Bowlby (1999) formulated the theory of attachment as a relationship between a young child and a caregiver that is necessary for strong social and emotional development. Klaus and Kennell (1982) further described the importance of maternal and infant interactions, known as bonding behaviors, directly after birth in forming this attachment. Recognizing the importance of maternal–infant bonding for child development, the American Academy of Family Physicians (AAFP) promotes family-centered care, which most hospitals practice today. In the 1980s, bonding rooms—where parents moved to a private room after delivery to hold and marvel at their newborn prior to standard separation—became the norm. Bonding rooms preceded LDRP/LDR (labor, delivery, recovery, postpartum) rooms where bonding takes place today. Not separating the newborn from the family is common practice in many U.S. hospitals. Obstetrical nurses in LDR settings facilitate maternal role attainment by encouraging evidence-based procedures such as allowing the newborn to rest skin-to-skin on the mother after delivery, breast-feeding in the first hour, and deferring newborn weighing and other procedures that used to be performed immediately after birth.

An example of successful maternal role attainment is seen in a study conducted with mothers who conceived via IVF. Research indicates that women with infertility issues often experience high levels of stress and anxiety, as well as low self-esteem. Abadi et al. (2018) divided a sample of 60 women who had IVF into control and intervention groups. Each group completed the *Maternal Self-Report Inventory* (MSRI). The intervention group then participated in a four-session maternal preparation program designed to enhance maternal self-esteem. The premise of the program was that higher self-esteem facilitates maternal role fulfillment that promotes mother–infant attachment that, in turn, facilitates positive fetal development. Immediately and 1 month after program completion, both groups took the MSRI again. The intervention group's scores were higher than the control group, indicating program's effectiveness in promoting the maternal role fulfillment. The study findings showed that the program improved the self-esteem of mothers undergoing IVF. The study's clinical implications suggest that nurses working with women conceiving via IVF can help enhance maternal self-esteem and motherhood facilitation by implementing maternal preparation programs as part of their care (Abadi et al., 2018).

Nontraditional Support Systems

In the United States, most pregnant people seek prenatal care from a physician and plan a hospital delivery. According to data collected by the American College of Nurse-Midwives (ACNM), in 2017, CNMs and CMs attended 351,968 births—a slight increase compared to 2016. Additionally, CNMs/CMs attended 85% of all midwife-attended births and 9.1% of total U.S. births. The numbers are relatively small compared to the rest of the industrialized world in which more than 70% of pregnant women are cared for by midwives who achieve better birth outcomes compared to the United States (Lake & Epstein, 2008). Because of mainstream U.S. medicine's historically curative focus, many U.S. medical care providers view pregnancy as a physiologic state that can become pathologic at any movement. With medicine's shift toward disease prevention and health promotion, many nurse practitioners and midwives who view pregnancy as a normal physiologic process do not see pregnant people as sick patients in need of physician-provided curative services unless a medical condition arises. Many cultural groups also perceive pregnancy as a normal physiologic process. Some pregnant people avoid prenatal care classes at medical centers due to their fear of receiving unnecessary medical interventions.

Since the introduction of Lamaze childbirth education classes in the 1970s, pregnant people and their partners or support people have placed an increasing emphasis on the quality of prenatal care and the childbirth experience. While middle-class White women initiated this trend, many traditional cultural groups have continued their indigenous and cultural practices including African American, Hispanic, Filipino, Asian American, and Native American groups.

It is essential that nurses conduct a thorough cultural assessment to identify whether the pregnant person plans to use nontraditional support systems, mainstream U.S. healthcare, or a blend of both during their pregnancy. Since childbearing is viewed as "women's work" among some cultures, male partners of pregnant women are often not expected to attend prenatal appointments. In contrast, in other cultures, male partners not only attend prenatal appointments but also expect all pregnancy-related questions to be directed to them. Nurses unfamiliar with this custom need to adjust their approach to provide culturally congruent care. Additionally, nurses should discuss patients' use of any herbs or folk medicines. Finally, helping pregnant patients develop a prenatal care plan can allow nurses to gain an understanding of the cultural traditions that are important to the patient during this period.

A pregnant person's choice about the type of support they want during labor is often culturally significant and must be explored during the antenatal period. Pregnant people should be encouraged to discuss their needs with the provider and formulate a written birth plan. Research demonstrates that laboring people greatly value and benefit from the presence of someone they trust to provide emotional, psychological, and practical support and advice (Kabakian-Khasholian et al., 2017). Having continuous labor support also has several clinical benefits: shorter labor, increased rates of spontaneous vaginal birth, decreased use of intrapartum analgesia, fewer cesarean sections, and increased patient satisfaction with the childbirth experience. The World Health Organization's (WHO, 2018a) recommendations encourage all laboring people to have their companion of choice present during labor and childbirth to improve the quality of their care.

Cultural Beliefs Related to Antenatal Care

First-trimester care is encouraged in traditional U.S. antenatal (also known as prenatal) care. According to *National Vital Statistics Reports,*

77% of women began prenatal care in the first trimester and 4.6% in the third trimester, and 1.6% received no prenatal care (Osterman & Martin, 2018). The WHO implemented new guidelines and recommendations when they introduced the 2014 WHO Antenatal Care Model (ANC). The four-visit focused ANC (FANC) model recommended that pregnant people have at least four visits with a healthcare provider. However, this model was replaced in 2016 due to evidence supporting the efficacy of having eight contacts with a healthcare provider during pregnancy to include screening for anemia, gestational diabetes, and UTIs (WHO, 2016). Box 5-2 compares the WHO's two ANC schedules.

Another way for pregnant people to receive care and support is through **participatory women groups** (PWGs). PWGs, defined by Gram et al. (2018), employ trained facilitators to hold scheduled community meetings where groups of local women are led through a cycle of problem identification, action planning, strategy implementation, and outcome evaluation. Qualitative evidence from providers in high-income countries suggests that such group sessions are enjoyable and informative for clients and efficient use of provider time (Downe et al., 2018). Pilot studies of PWG have occurred in Ghana, Malawi, and Tanzania. Trials of participatory learning and action groups were also conducted in Bangladesh, India, Malawi, and Nepal. Trained individuals whose aim was to identify, prioritize, and address concerns women faced about pregnancy, childbirth, and postpartum care facilitated these groups. Community women shared information on a monthly basis, and groups participated in activities related to the specific health topic covered that month (WHO, 2016). Centering Pregnancy is a popular PWG model used in the United States. Due to the evidence that PWGs can help reduce maternal and perinatal mortality, the WHO supports this prenatal care approach (WHO, 2016).

Nursing personnel are in an excellent position to teach patients and promote positive prenatal

BOX 5-2	Comparing World Health Organization Antenatal Care Schedules

WHO FANC Model	2016 WHO ANC Model
First trimester	
Visit 1: 8–12 weeks	Contact 1: up to 12 weeks
Second trimester	
Visit 2: 24–26 weeks	Contact 2: 20 weeks
	Contact 3: 26 weeks
Third trimester	
Visit 3: 32 weeks	Contact 4: 30 weeks
Visit 4: 36–38 weeks	Contact 5: 34 weeks
	Contact 6: 36 weeks
	Contact 7: 38 weeks
	Contact 8: 40 weeks
Return for delivery at 41 weeks if not given birth	

Source: World Health Organization (WHO). (2016). *WHO recommendations on antenatal care for a positive pregnancy experience.* http://www.who.int/reproductivehealth/publications/maternal_perinatal_health/anc-positive-pregnancy-experience/en/

care outcomes. Initially, nurses working in a prenatal setting should examine their own cultural beliefs and practices about pregnancy in order to compare them to and understand other culture's practices. The most important part of reviewing cultural practices is determining if they are safe. Pregnant people who are ingesting culturally accepted foods should be informed if such substances could be harmful to a developing fetus. Immigrants' countries of origin also should be documented, as well as the country of origin of pregnant people who are the second generation in the primary country. Such information is important in discovering potentially harmful cultural and indigenous practices that are uncommon in U.S. society. For example, performing a lead-exposure assessment is imperative for patients who have emigrated from a country where lead-based cosmetics, pottery, spices, or gas are used (see Box 5-3).

In the U.S. healthcare system, antenatal blood tests, ultrasounds, and pelvic exams are common components of routine care. However, nurses should not expect these practices to be common in other cultures. For example, a nurse should help ease the anxiety of a patient receiving a Pap t test for the first time at age 30 by explaining the procedure and showing the instruments to be used. If while doing so the client indicates not wanting to know more but just wanting "to get it over with," these feelings should be honored and accepted.

Myunghee et al. (2018) conducted a qualitative study to understand the prenatal genetic testing decision-making processes among pregnant Korean American women in the United States. Ten Korean American women whose provider recommended they undergo amniocentesis during pregnancy participated in the study. All participants were born in Korea and immigrated to the United States. Four themes emerged from the data analysis: facing the challenges of decision-making, seeking support, determining one's preferred role in the decision-making process, and feeling uncomfortable with the patient's degree of autonomy in the U.S. healthcare system. Most participants felt it would have been easier to make a decision if they were guided by trustworthy

BOX 5-3	Risk Factors for Lead Exposure in Pregnant and Lactating People

- Recent emigration from or residency in areas where ambient lead contamination is high; people from countries where leaded gasoline is still being used (or was recently phased out) or where industrial emissions are not well controlled
- Living near a point source of lead including lead mines, smelters, or battery recycling plants (even if the establishment is closed)
- Working with lead or living with someone who does; people who work in or who have family members who work in an industry that uses lead (e.g., lead production, battery manufacturing, paint manufacturing, shipbuilding, ammunition production, or plastic manufacturing)
- Using lead-glazed ceramic pottery; people who cook, store, or serve food in lead-glazed ceramic pottery made in a traditional process (usually imported by individuals outside the normal commercial channels)
- Eating nonfood substances (pica); people who eat or mouth nonfood items that may be contaminated with lead, such as soil or lead-glazed ceramic pottery
- Using alternative or complementary substances, herbs, or therapies; people that use imported home remedies or certain therapeutic herbs traditionally used by East Indian, Indian, Middle Eastern, West Asian, and Hispanic cultures that may be contaminated with lead
- Using imported cosmetics or certain food products; people who use imported cosmetics, such as kohl or surma or certain imported foods or spices that may be contaminated with lead
- Engaging in certain high-risk hobbies or recreational activities; people who engage in high-risk activities (e.g., stained glass production or pottery making with certain leaded glazes and paints) or have family members who do
- Renovating or remodeling older homes without lead-hazard controls in place; people who have been disturbing lead paint, have been creating lead dust, or have been spending time in such a home environment
- Consumption of lead-contaminated drinking water; people whose homes have leaded pipes or source lines with lead
- Having a history of previous lead exposure or evidence of elevated body burden of lead; people who may have high body burdens of lead from past exposure, particularly those who have deficiencies in certain key nutrients (calcium or iron)
- Living with someone identified with an elevated lead level; people who may have exposure in common with a child, close friend, or other relatives living in the same environment

Source: Centers for Disease Control and Prevention (CDC). (2010). *Guidelines for the identification and management of lead exposure in pregnant and lactating women*. U.S. Department of Health and Human Services. https://www.cdc.gov/nceh/lead/publications/leadandpregnancy2010.pdf

people (e.g., mother, sister, God, or fate), while others were unsure if they could make the decision and were uncertain whether it was even theirs to make. Some participants indicated it was scary that the obstetrician left the decision-making power in their hands. One participant explained that, in Korea, the provider would make the decision and she would honor it. Communication

barriers were evident. Nine of the college-educated participants had trouble understanding the genetic counselor and obstetrician even with a translator: "All I could do was listen to [the translator] talk over my head." If the providers involved in this study were more sensitive to Korean culture, they could have allowed more time for test clarification and explained the shared decision-making in the U.S. system. This study supports the practice of healthcare professionals providing trusting, cultural-sensitive healthcare that allows pregnant patients to ask questions and feel comfortable making autonomous decisions.

Food Taboos and Food Cravings

Due to the body's increasing demand for energy and nutrients during pregnancy, it is important that pregnant people have a nutritious dietary intake. Many cultures have food **taboos** that expand during pregnancy and the postpartum period (Withers et al., 2018). One cultural practice is that a pregnant person should eat what they crave because "the baby must need this." Unfortunately, food taboos can contribute to unhealthy nutritional practices in pregnancy. For example, in Africa, the giant African snail and grass cutter or cane rat are inexpensive, rich sources of animal protein that can serve as vital nutrition in a balanced diet. However, due to cultural beliefs, they are not readily consumed even though they are available (Ekwochi et al., 2016). **Pica**—eating nonnutritious substances such as clay, red dirt, and starch—is often seen in the Southern United States and among African American populations. Pica has been described for centuries (Hippocrates, 1849) and is found in most cultures. While there can be a relationship between pica and low hemoglobin levels, this is not the case for everyone. Latina American women have been known to have cravings for rocks, sand, ice, chalk, and charcoal during pregnancy (Roy et al., 2018). It is extremely important that nurses assess for food taboos and pica during the initial visit as part of the pregnant patient's dietary intake. The nurse should discuss the importance of the nutrients essential to maintaining a healthy pregnancy and the growing fetus' development. In their study of pregnancy-related food taboos in rural and urban areas of Tamil Nadu, Banu et al. (2016) found that younger women (less than 30) were more likely to eat a balanced diet, take prenatal vitamins with folic acid, take iron

and calcium tablets, and attend antenatal care and health education classes. The older women in the study tended to incorporate customary practices and give less credence to eating a balanced diet and receiving antenatal care (Banu et al., 2016). Some food items avoided during pregnancy and the related beliefs seen in this study are listed in Box 5-4.

It is imperative that nursing professionals determine who the dominant person is in the client's home. In modern U.S. culture, women often plan and address their own prenatal health needs. In other cultures, however, the pregnant woman's husband/male partner, mother-in-law, mother, or grandmother may handle these issues. If the client lives in a community without blood relatives, her support person could be a community woman elder who attends all her prenatal visits. It is vital that the support person is recognized in accordance with HIPAA laws. While today's nurses are comfortable with the culture of the U.S. healthcare system, it can be overwhelming to an immigrant from a low- or middle-income country. Nurses should help pregnant patients feel comfortable when introducing them to the U.S. healthcare system. A pregnant client may express a concern about a taboo and its consequences, such as "If you breast-feed the baby before the breast milk is in (colostrum), the baby will become sick." In this case, the nurse—recognizing that the client is referring to the vitamin- and nutrient-rich colostrum—can explain the scientific evidence about the benefits of this fluid and encourage the client to breast-feed. However, the nurse must realize that breast-feeding is the client's decision, regardless of scientific evidence.

Substance Use

In the United States, a patient's social history is taken as part of prenatal care. This assessment includes asking the patient about cigarette smoking, alcohol consumption, and illicit drug use. In order to complete a thorough assessment, particularly for a client with ties to another culture,

BOX 5-4   Food Taboos During Pregnancy

Food Taboos During Pregnancy: Rural and Urban Tamil Nadu

Food	Beliefs
Ripe papaya	Causes loose stool, abdominal pain
Raw papaya	Causes abortion
Pineapple	Causes cough
Grapes, banana, and custard apple	Causes cold
Grapes (black)	Causes child to be born with a dark complexion
Curd, buttermilk	Causes cough and cold
Maize/corn	Abdominal pain
Yam	Allergy to the child
Hot beverages (especially coffee)	Causes child to be born with a dark complexion
Chicken	Causes loose stools, uterine contractions

Source: Ekwochi, U., Osuroah, C. D. I., Ndu, I. K., Ifediora, C., Asinobi, I. N., & Eke, C. B. (2016). Food taboos and myths in South Eastern Nigeria: The belief and practice of mothers in the region. *Journal of Ethnobiology and Ethnomedicine*, *12*, 7. https://doi.org/10.1186/s13002-016-0079-x

Food Taboos and Myths for Pregnant Women and Children in Nigeria and Ghana

Food	Beliefs
Snail	Makes baby sluggish in life and spit too much saliva Ghana: do not eat snails out of respect for ancestors
Bush meat like glasscutter (*Thryonomys swinderianus*)	Causes labor to be difficult and prolonged delivery
Starch foods like *garri* (cassava flakes)	Baby will have excess weight making delivery difficult except by surgery
Do not give eggs to children under age 2	It will cause them to start stealing because it is very sweet
Avoid sweet in small children	Children will get worms
Don't allow children to drink garri	Causes eye problems

Source: Banu, K. K., Prathipa, A., Anandarajan, B., Ismail Sheriff, A. M., Muthukumar, S., & Selvakumar, J. (2016). Food taboos during antenatal and postpartum period among the women of rural and urban areas of Tamilnadu. *International Journal of Biomedical and Advance Research*, *7*(8), 393–396. https://doi.org/10.7439/ijbar.v7i8.3539

nurses must be familiar with substances commonly used by that group. For example, khat (*Catha edulis*) is a natural stimulant that is widely cultivated and used in East Africa and the Middle East. The most common way to use khat is chewing the raw leaves. Khat enhances mood and alertness as it is consumed but can contribute to depression, anxiety, and insomnia with longer-term usage. In the areas where khat use is common, its use is widely accepted among pregnant people (Nakajima et al., 2017).

According to Sharma et al. (2016), alcohol and pregnancy are culturally linked. In Africa, rum can be given to Akan (a people group in Southern Ghana and adjacent parts of the Ivory Coast) and Igbo (a people group in Southeastern Nigeria) children. Additionally, in Ghana, births are often celebrated with alcohol at naming ceremonies.

Greek physicians and Gurung (a people group in Nepal) women may use alcohol to help children go to sleep. Finally, Malaysians may bathe their children in stout (beer) in the belief that it protects babies and cures newborn jaundice.

Cultural Preparation for Childbirth

In the media-filled society, there is plethora of information and education available to support a healthy pregnancy. In the United States as well as many industrialized countries, childbearing people attend childbirth education classes with their birth partner or support person.

Patients from culturally diverse backgrounds often want to incorporate culture-specific activities into their care. The fact that pregnancy is viewed in many cultures as a normal event not requiring medical intervention likely contributes to patients opting to receive antenatal care and give birth at home using traditional and indigenous birth attendants. Health professionals must obtain a thorough cultural assessment to determine a pregnant patient's intention to use nontraditional cultural practices during antenatal care and to assess the patient's birth expectations. A birth plan can incorporate cultural desires along with the beneficial aspects of U.S. hospital culture to ensure a safe, satisfying childbirth. Accommodations should be made to support the childbearing families' cultural desires whenever possible.

Nurses who work in communities that cater to specific cultural groups might consider developing childbirth classes that incorporate specific cultural practices. Facilitating open communication between a hospital's healthcare providers and cultural group leaders when developing such programs would be beneficial for the hospital and the cultural groups it serves.

Birth and Culture

Childbirth can happen in one of two ways: vaginal delivery or cesarean section. Culture, religion, family traditions, and values influence birthing plans. A pregnant person's religion could determine what type of provider they use for childbirth. For example, a Muslim woman may request having only female providers for her delivery. Some cultures believe supernatural forces, either benevolent or malevolent, can affect pregnancy and childbirth. In Bangladesh, some people believe in a *jinn* or *bhut* (an evil spirit) that can give the evil eye, a curse, or harm a pregnant woman (Raman et al., 2016). In U.S. culture, birthing often is a family affair that includes the baby's nonbirthing parent, grandparents, siblings, and other family members. The family also plays an active role in the type of birth experience desired. In cultures where birthing is considered "women's work," only the mother-in-law and traditional midwife accompany the laboring woman to the healthcare clinic or special birthing shed. Cultural practices can dictate the birthplace, position, and members present. Boxes 5-5 and 5-6 describe various cultural practices for birth.

The most common healthcare providers for a childbearing person throughout the world are midwives, except in the United States where obstetricians and hospitals dominate childbirth. More than 90% of births are under the care of obstetricians in the United States, compared to Europe where midwives are the main providers for 75% of births (Guerra-Reyes & Hamilton, 2017). However, it was not always like this in the United States. During the 1900s, midwives attended 50% of all U.S. births. This number decreased to 12.5% by 1935 despite half of all African American births being attended by midwives. The Sheppard–Towner Act of 1921 resulted in the widespread regulation of African American "granny" midwives. This act was followed by the 1948 push to standardize medicine and eliminate lay healers, which gained a momentum around the time the American Medical Association was formed. As a result, by 1972, midwives attended only 1% of all U.S. births. Today, the trend toward midwife-attended births is highest among non-Hispanic White women (11%) and African American women (8%) (Yoder & Hardy, 2018).

BOX 5-5	Cultural Influences on Antenatal, Intrapartum, and Postpartum Care in Asian Countries

Country	Belief or Practice
Antenatal	
Pakistani	Avoid hot foods during pregnancy (sugar, nuts, beans, and maize [hot]) as they are abortifacients. Avoid cold foods (buttermilk, oranges, and curd) because they harm the fetus. Prenatal massages are a common practice to promote maternal and infant health. Use amulets and holy water to solve problems instead of seek help from a healthcare provider. Pregnant people from designated lower castes should give birth in a cowshed or specially constructed place.
Indonesia	Eating fish makes breast milk tastes and smells bad. Avoid prenatal vitamins, as they cause excess fetal growth and discourage an easy delivery.
Chinese	Eating shrimp causes the baby to have skin allergies. Eating rabbit meat leads to cleft palate development. Eating meat harms fetal health. Use traditional herbs used for bathing, enemas, ointments, treating nausea and vomiting, and labor stimulation. Use of traditional practitioners, spiritual healers, and religious leaders as to protect a pregnancy. Eating more than half of a banana may cause birth obstruction.
Papua New Guinea	It is the birthing person's responsibility to dispose of the placenta, as pregnancy and birth is "polluting."
Thailand	Eating shellfish and Northern Thai relishes prevents the perineum from drying out after birth. Thai eggplant will cause anal pain after giving birth.
Labor	
India	Feed pregnant people clarified butter, ginger, lentils, milk, or tea to facilitate labor by promoting warmth.
Laotian	Drink holy water and coconut milk. Place holy water or eggs on the abdomen to ease birth.
Nepal	Drink cumin seed soup and glucose water to gain strength for birth.
Birthing	
Bangladeshi	Having a hospital delivery is stigmatizing. Pregnancy is normal, so your baby should be delivered at home. "They don't let you bury placenta in hospital." Hospitals and health centers are a place for treating someone with health problems and disease. Giving birth at a hospital lying on one's back is not preferred. Sitting, squatting, or kneeling during delivery is desired. "If you go to a hospital, you are forced to have surgery."
Nepal, Bangladesh, India, Papua New guinea	Purifications and rituals protect pregnant person from evil spirits and malevolent spirits could cause continuous, forceful bleeding, and blood clots. Pregnant should seek help from traditional healers. Use mustard oil or turmeric for childbirth; rub it on the newborn and the umbilical cord stump (Nepal).

(continued)

BOX 5-5	Cultural Influences on Antenatal, Intrapartum, and Postpartum Care in Asian Countries (continued)

Country	Belief or Practice
Postpartum	
China, Cambodia, Laos, Nepal, Thailand, Myanmar, Singapore, Vietnam	Restrict postpartum person's movement to help with rest and rebuilding of strength, as postpartum people are weak, fragile, and vulnerable to illness. Practice sexual abstinence for 30–40 days, and don't bathe, wash hair, or practice dental hygiene (China, "doing the month"). Refrain from reading, eating, or drinking while standing, moving around excessively, experiencing strong emotions, and doing housework. Consume hot foods and avoid cold foods but during the 1st month postpartum. Avoid cold vegetables (e.g., water spinach, spinach, and pumpkins). Hot foods (e.g., beef, mutton, rice with black pepper, anchovies, salted fish, coffee, and milk) are suitable for postpartum mothers.
Cambodia	Spirits (*priey krawlah pleung*) can attack someone left exposed after birth causing seizures, fainting, and altered consciousness.
Bangladesh, China, Nepal	People should seek help from trained birthing assistants for any postpartum issues.
China	Cold foods create an imbalance of *qi*, which leads to poor circulation, a weak bladder and uterus, and sore back muscles. Cold foods are fruit and raw or cooked vegetables such as cabbage, bamboo shoots, and turnips. Eating spicy, hot food can cause a baby to be born hairless. Drinking coffee and tea decreases infant intelligence.
Myanmar	Burmese women shave the newborns head at 2 months to remove infants "dirtiness" from coming through the birth canal. Breast-feeding to age 2 is culturally indicated.

Source: Withers, M., Kharazmi, N., & Lim, E. (2018). Traditional beliefs and practices in pregnancy, childbirth and postpartum: A review of the evidence from Asian countries. *Midwifery*, *56*, 158–170. https://doi.org/10.1016/j.midw.2017.10.019

BOX 5-6	Childbirth and Postnatal Cultural Practices in Selected Countries

Cord Cutting Rituals

- Cord is cut with a sickle and then antiseptic, cooking oil, ghee (butter), toothpaste, or ash is applied to the umbilical stump (Nepali).
- Cord is cut with a scythe and stump is cleaned with water (Tamang).
- Placenta is buried at the foot of a tree (Gurung).
- Placenta is buried at a junction or under the road (Newari, Tamang).
- Placenta is buried at a junction in Mexico (old Jewish texts tell pregnant woman not to stand alone at the crossroads, as "they may see the fetus taken away by evil powers").
- Placenta is a dirty object and therefore must be buried and fire burned over it to prevent evil spirits and animals from

| **BOX 5-6** | **Childbirth and Postnatal Cultural Practices in Selected Countries** (continued) |

reaching it. If any part of the woman touches the placenta, the lochia might dry up causing harm to her baby and possibly neonatal death (Lao).

- The placenta must "roast" to provide heat to stimulate the mother's healing (Burmese and Lao).
- Cord cut after the placenta is delivered; the cord cutter remains unholy and cannot go for prayer for 40 days (Bangladesh).
- The child's future health is linked to the placenta.

Rest and Seclusion

- The postnatal mother is not allowed to go into the kitchen until the 9th day; then she is sent to another person's home for about 10 to 15 days and can stay as long as she wishes up to a month (Tamang).
- Mother and new baby are massaged with mustard oil to relax the mother's muscles and help the child grow.
- In the maternal home, the new mother is cared for and fed a diet of lentils and spices (such as cumin) to stimulate breast milk production.
- Women are isolated in the stable or shed during menstruation and pregnancy (Tamang and Newari).

Purification, Naming, and Weaning Ceremonies

- The birth of a baby is believed to be unclean.
- A day is set aside to clean the home and bathe the mother and baby.
- At the ceremony, a Nwaran name is given to the baby based on the astrological sign.
- The ceremony takes place between the 3rd and 12th day after birth.
- The ritual is celebrated on the 9th day for girl and on the 11th day for boy.
- The new mother cannot go out before the ceremony, she can't go to temple, and no one will touch her or take the child directly from her, as she is considered dirty; fire is used to burn the woven mat women lie on during and after childbirth (Bahun).

- After the ceremony, the mother returns to household activities.
- The sleeping child is placed in sari, as the cloth is believed to offer protection from the evil eye.
- The ceremony timing varies by ethnic groups: Nwaran is on the 3rd day for Tamangs, 7th day among Bahun and Chhetri, and on the 9th or 12th day for Newar communities. The higher the caste of the family, the later the ceremony is held.
- In Greece, birth customs include women and babies resting and being isolated for 40 days after birth (during the "lochia period").
- Women in Zaire and India are secluded in a hut.
- For Muslims, the postnatal seclusion period traditionally lasts 40 days.
- In Burma and Turkey, women are more vulnerable to evil spirits during the postnatal period: "the grave of a woman who have just gave birth is open for 40 days."
- In Bangladesh, purdah (female seclusion) lasts 5 to 9 days, and dietary restrictions can last up to 6 months.
- For the Negev Bedouin in Israel, the 40-day postnatal period includes seclusion (homestay) followed by congratulatory visits and food.
- Among Mayans, the period lasts 20 days.
- Among Japanese people, mothers remain in a birth chamber for 3 weeks.
- The Chinese postnatal period ("sitting month" or "doing the month") lasts 30 or 40 days. Traditional Chinese medicine is given to women who are believed to be in a weak state during the postpartum period.
- In Nepal, new mothers stay with their babies continuously for 6 days ("the up sitting") after which bed linens would be changed on the 10th day and the mother would be allowed to perform housekeeping duties.

(continued)

BOX 5-6 | Childbirth and Postnatal Cultural Practices in Selected Countries (continued)

- Burmese women rest for a 40-day period ("the quarantine" time) for purification and rest.
- In many cultures, postnatal women are believed to be "dirty" and "weak" (Japan, China, Canadian Intuits, Turkey, and Bangladesh).
- In England, the postnatal time is called the "lying-in period."
- In Germany, the period is called the wochenbett or "child bed."
- U.S. customs are guided by self-help books that indicate it takes 6 weeks for the uterus to return to a nonpregnant size and bleeding to abate; similar guidelines are used for UK parents.
- Nepali and Mayan women get postpartum massages.
- China found that the 40-day seclusion period can adversely affect woman's mental health (postpartum depression).
- The Church of England has a thanksgiving and cleansing ritual to welcome new mothers back to church.
- In the Scottish highlands, churches hold a cleansing ritual ("kirking") to allow women "polluted" by childbirth to come back to church.
- The Greek orthodox Archdiocese in the United States states, "woman may stay home for 6 weeks after birth according to Leviticus XII: ...."
- Jewish women are allowed back into temple 33 days after the birth of son and 66 days after the birth of daughter.
- Laotian women believe that advance preparation of baby clothes would lead to the newborn's death.

Nutrition and Breast-Feeding

- Special foods may be given during the postnatal period: kwati (beans and meat), dahi-chura (curd and beaten rice with curry meat), and gudpak (a sweet cake, rich in calories made with flour, clarified butter, cashews, and coconut).
- Newborns are given hamma ghuti, balmrita (Ayurvedic medicine herbs), and Jaiphal (nutmeg).
- Women who adhere to traditional foods in Burma and Turkey are not given any water to drink for 2 to 3 days after birth.
- For Cantonese Chinese people, the pregnant mother is considered cold and the fetus hot. In Vietnam, both mother and fetus change from cold in the first trimester to hot in the last. The concept of hot and cold also exists in Laos.
- In Nepal, India, and other places in South Asia, colostrum is not given to an infant until the priest approves it, as it is considered pus.
- In Bangladesh, colostrum is not given, as it is considered "dirty milk." In the first 40 days, breast milk is given along with sweet water (misi pani); wealthier houses give babies goat or cow milk after 40 days.
- In Cairo, Egypt, breast-feeding lasts 40 days.
- In one study, most participants discarded their colostrum, which they felt was inadequate in nutritional value.
- In contrast, the WHO recommends breast-feeding in the 1st hour after birth.

Alcohol Plays an Important Role in the Birth and Postpartum Periods in Nepal

- Alcohol and pregnancy are linked culturally; some women are allowed to sip it during labor.
- Alcohol is given to Akan and Igbo children.
- It is used for celebration at the naming ceremony; it is also thought to confer protection on children.
- Mayans bathe babies in stout (beer) to protect them from jaundice.

Source: Sharma, S., van Teijlingen, E., Hundley, V., Angell, C., & Simkhada, P. (2016). Dirty and 40 days in the wilderness: Eliciting childbirth and postnatal cultural practices and beliefs in Nepal. BMC Pregnancy and Childbirth, 16(1), 147. https://doi.org/10.1186/s12884-016-0938-4

Trends in birth facilities demonstrate that after a gradual decline from 1990 to 2004, the number of out-of-hospital births increased from 35,578 in 2004 to 62,228 in 2017. In 2017, 1 of every 62 births in the United States was an out-of-hospital birth (1.61%). Home births increased by 77% from 2004 to 2017, while birth center births more than doubled (MacDorman & Declercq, 2019).

Prior to labor, nurses should discuss with clients any specific things they would like to do during their labor and birth to determine what, if any, accommodations need to be made (see Box 5-7).

BOX 5-7	World Health Organizations Recommendations: Intrapartum Care for a Positive Childbirth Experience

The WHO's intrapartum care recommendations are encouraged globally, regardless of the setting or the birthing environment's level of healthcare. The recommendations are neither country nor region specific but designed for use with all birthing people. The 56 guidelines are geared toward patient-centered care to optimize the labor and childbirth experience for birthing parents and their babies through a holistic, human rights–based approach. Listed below are a few of the recommendations.

Care Option	Recommendation	Category of Recommendation
Care throughout labor and birth		
Respectful maternity care	Respectful care—which refers to care organized for and provided to all birthing people in a manner that maintains their dignity, privacy, and confidentiality—ensures freedom from harm and mistreatment and enables informed choice and continuous support during labor and childbirth are recommended	Recommended
Effective communication	Effective communication between maternity care providers and people in labor, using simple and culturally acceptable methods, is recommended	Recommended
First stage of labor		
Oral fluid and food	For pregnant people at low risk, oral fluid, and food intake during labor is recommended	Recommended
Second stage of labor		
Method of pushing	Patients in the expulsive phase of the second stage of labor should be encouraged and supported to follow their own urge to push	Recommended
Third stage of labor		
Delayed umbilical cord clamping	Delayed umbilical cord clamping (not earlier than 1 minute after birth) is recommended for improved maternal and infant health and nutrition outcomes	Recommended
Controlled cord traction (CCT)	In settings where skilled birth attendants are available, CCT is recommended for vaginal births if the care provider and the parturient person regard a small reduction in blood loss and a small reduction in the duration of the third stage of labor as important	Recommended

(continued)

BOX 5-7	World Health Organizations Recommendations: Intrapartum Care for a Positive Childbirth Experience (continued)	

Care Option	Recommendation	Category of Recommendation
Uterine massage	Sustained uterine massage is not recommended as an intervention to prevent postpartum hemorrhage (PPH) in women who have received prophylactic oxytocin	Not recommended
Newborn care		
Routine nasal or oral suction	In neonates born through clear amniotic fluid who start breathing on their own after birth, suctioning of the mouth, and nose should not be performed	Not recommended
Skin-to-skin contact	Newborns without complications should be kept in skin-to-skin contact with their mothers during the first hour after birth to prevent hypothermia and promote breast-feeding	Recommended
Breast-feeding	All newborns, including low birth weight babies who are able to breast-feed, should be put to the breast as soon as possible after birth when they are clinically stable and the mother and baby are ready	Recommended

Reference: World Health Organization (WHO). (2018a). *WHO recommendations: Intrapartum care for positive childbirth experience.* http://www.who.int/reproductivehealth/publications/intrapartum-care-guidelines/en/

Cultural Expression of Labor

Culture and religious beliefs can include taboos that can affect how a pregnant person responds to labor. It is important to assess clients' comfort/pain level to determine if they need comfort interventions. Some patients who believe it is a taboo to scream during labor may appear stoic with the pain of contractions. Ghanaian cultural beliefs are that crying out might delay the birth and taking pain medication may not be beneficial. Some cultures believe that shouting and crying with pain is a sign of weakness (Raman et al., 2016). Other cultures view childbirth pain as natural, and therefore the stronger the pain, the better. Because stoicism is often culturally expected, it is important to assess the birthing person's needs throughout the course of labor.

Birth Positions

In the United States, patients birthing in hospitals with obstetricians typically deliver in the lithotomy position. In contrast, people receiving midwifery care in the United States deliver in a variety of positions: lithotomy, side lying, squatting, and hands and knees. Birth positions influenced by culture include sitting, squatting, or kneeling. Bangladeshi people favor all three positions, Mexican American people tend to favor birthing chairs, and Laotian Hmong people generally prefer a squatting position. Refer back to Boxes 5-5 and 5-6 for information on specific birthing positions related to different cultures. During prenatal care, preparation for birth should include conversation about the pregnant person's birthing expectations, including the desired birthing position. Do not assume that a client delivering in a hospital expects to deliver in a lithotomy position. It is important that the nursing staff and delivery provider offer culturally sensitive care during the birthing process.

Cultural Meaning Attached to Infant Sex

Infant sex preferences vary from culture to culture. Historically in U.S. culture, families preferred males as the first born to solidify male inheritance of the family finances and property, carry on the family name, and assume the head-of-household role if the needs arise. With females legally able to inherit family property and having the ability and desire to take responsibility for caring for aging family members, modern society reports family preferences for a mix of sexes among children.

According to Dubuc and Devinderjit (2017), son preference and prenatal sex selection against females have resulted in a significant imbalance in birth–sex ratio in several Asian countries, including India and China. The development of prenatal sex determination techniques by ultrasound screening has made sex-selective abortion possible. In addition, IVF combined with prefertilization selection of male spermatozoa (sperm sorting) allows sex selection of offspring.

Male child preference is still common in South Asia, Africa, the Middle East, China, and Turkey. Rouhi et al. (2017) hypothesized that maternal perception of a family's male child preference was a risk factor for antenatal depression. Their study included a sample of 780 pregnant Iranian women and used the Iranian version of the Edinburgh Postnatal Depression Scale. Maternal perception of male child preference was common and associated with an antenatal depression value of 20.1%. Women who had a daughter from previous pregnancy were more likely to experience depression during the present pregnancy. Even when women and their families preferred female children but were content with having a boy, they feared being criticized by their husbands and his family if they had a female child.

To address these concerns, nurses should consider a patient's cultural background when discussing fetal/newborn sex. Additionally, establishing a trusting relationship with the patient may allow them to verbalize feelings related to the selected sex. Assessment of antenatal or postpartum anxiety and depression related to sex preference should also be evaluated during the antenatal and postpartum periods.

Culture and the Postpartum Period

Most people who deliver in a U.S. hospital are discharged 48 hours after a vaginal birth and 72 hours after a cesarean section. Nurses provide a great deal of teaching during this period, including providing information about breast-feeding and newborn care. With help from the nursing staff, the birthing person should be able to rest, take care of their newborn, and reflect on their birthing experience. It is important for nurses to observe a new parent's interaction with the newborn. A nurse who is unfamiliar with the practice of the mother-in-law acting as the dominant caregiver might think that the mother is not interested in the child. However, it is important to assess and be aware of cultural practices in which it may be taboo for the mother to handle the child and instead one of the baby's grandmothers assumes this role.

In some Muslim cultures, the postnatal seclusion period traditionally lasts 40 days. Performance of religious rituals on the 40th day may include shaving of the newborns hair, due to what is considered to be the unclean passage of the infant through the vagina (Sharma et al., 2016). The Punjabi cultural tradition of *Sawa Mahina* is their period requiring 40 days of complete rest—however, by their choice, mothers can take part in a few domestic chores after several weeks (Qamar, 2017). Japanese women may return to their mother's home during the birth period to receive care from their mother. This tradition is known as *gae ri bunben* (home to the village to give birth). In China, the women "do the month," a resting period expected to restore balance (Withers et al., 2018).

Filipino and Hispanic cultural belief systems include the practice of *balancing opposites*—that there are natural, external factors that must be kept in balance to maintain health. In other words, to restore a disrupted balance, you must apply the opposite. For example, to treat a "hot" condition such as a fever, the person eats cold food (fresh vegetables, meats, and dairy products). Conversely, hot foods (chocolate, aromatic beverages, cheese, and eggs) are consumed to treat a "cold" condition such as a headache (Withers et al., 2018).

Adams and Smith (2018) conducted an integrative review of 13 studies that identified factors affecting postpartum care in the developing countries of Nigeria, Uganda, the Philippines, Jordan, Pakistan, Nepal, Cameroon, South Africa, Egypt, Indonesia, and Bangladesh. Some cultures that regard childbirth as a natural process do not view postpartum care as a standard practice. In Ugandan culture, normalization of the birth process prevented clients from participating in postpartum visits. In Bangladesh, a woman must stay in a private room for 7 to 10 days after birth and therefore cannot leave for care. However, according to Adams et al. (2017), 34% to 50% of rural Malawi women receive a postpartum assessment (including having their blood pressure and temperature measured and their abdomen, vagina, and breasts examined) before discharge from a healthcare facility. Adams and Smith's (2018) review also found that women exposed to mass media were more likely to attend postpartum care appointments. In addition, adults with higher educational and income levels who were not farm workers were more likely to seek postpartum care. The WHO (2015) noted that 99% of global maternal mortality occurs in developing countries, with more than half in sub-Saharan Africa. Nurses are in the best position to inform women about the importance of postpartum care and assess the family's understanding of its importance. Refer back to Boxes 5-5 and 5-6 to review cultural practices and rituals for the postpartum period.

Postpartum Depression

Postpartum depression (PPD) is associated with adverse infant and maternal outcomes such as less breast-feeding and poor maternal–infant bonding (Centers for Disease Control and Prevention [CDC], 2017; Wouk et al., 2016). According to Alexander et al. (2017), PPD is commonly seen in those with a history of depression, relationship issues, a lack of social support, and negative life experiences. According to Ko et al. (2017), PPD affects about one of every nine women in the United States. Greenberg et al. (2015) estimated that the economic burden of depression in the United States is $210.5 billion and can be attributed to workplace-, healthcare-, and suicide-related costs. Clearly, the prevalence of PPD means that it contributes to these costs.

The American College of Obstetricians and Gynecologists (ACOG, 2018) recommends that obstetricians–gynecologists and other obstetric care providers screen patients at least once during the perinatal period for depression using a standardized validated tool.

Park and Kim (2023) compared the predictive validity of the Edinburgh Postnatal Depression Scale (EPDS) and other tools for screening depression in pregnant and postpartum women through systematic review and meta-analysis. They concluded the EPDS showed excellent performance can be used in preference to other tools to screen depression in perinatal women at a primary care setting or a midwifery center.

Nurses should include information about PPD in their discharge teaching and have family members present to inform them of the condition. The birthing person's support system needs to be identified and documented in the care plan. Additionally, birthing parents who experience signs or symptoms of PPD must be given follow-up information.

Treatment for PPD must be individualized, taking into account each patient's unique preferences and cultural needs. Nguyen (2017) conducted a literature review of alternative PPD therapies. In the review of 27 randomized control trials (RCTs), 15 showed significant improvement in the intervention group over the control group, and 10 behavior therapies were found to be effective. Several studies demonstrated the efficacy of Internet- or telephone-delivered interventions, indicating that these modes of delivering education and counseling can be valid solutions that also increase healthcare access (Nguyen, 2017).

Nurses must be cognizant of the signs and symptoms of PPD. Inquiring about a patient's history of PPD, depression, anxiety, and any other mental health issues is an important part of perinatal and postpartum care. For minority groups that are part of a subculture, such as immigrants, nurses should assess the support offered by their community groups to ensure they are not isolated when they return home.

In U.S. healthcare, PPD treatment typically involves prescribing pharmaceuticals. This approach may not be culturally appropriate for all groups. The healthcare team must find culturally acceptable treatments that will support the patient while addressing the problem's underlying cause.

Postpartum Dietary Prescriptions and Activity Levels

Despite being in a hospital setting, patients often follow cultural practices related to the postpartum period. For example, people from some Hispanic cultures see pregnancy and childbearing as a hot state that requires the ingestion of cold foods during the postpartum period. In contrast, people in some Asian cultures will not drink cold water, instead consuming only hot drinks during this period. In many Asian cultures, the person who has given birth does not leave the house for 28 to 40 days, during which time the mother-in-law is responsible for food preparation and infant care. African Americans may have an older female family member in charge of the room environment, monitor visitors, and care for the baby and new mother. It is common to have multiple visitors who bring food to the hospital for the new mother.

Nurses need to observe and inquire what foods are desired and taboo during this period to ensure the patient is receiving sufficient nutrition and fluid intake. The importance of continuing prenatal vitamins should be discussed. If certain foods are not customarily eaten due to cultural beliefs or likes and dislikes, the nurse should formulate a dietary guide of acceptable foods in order to support a healthy postpartum diet. Refer again to Box 5-4 for pregnancy and postpartum food taboos.

Postpartum Rituals

Placental burial rituals are part of postpartum traditions in several sub-Saharan African countries. The ritual is also found in certain Asian cultures and among some members of the African American community. Postpartum clients may request a container to use for the ritual burial of their placenta. It would be helpful if this request is incorporated in their care plan and supported by the facility. If placental burial is a cultural practice, healthcare facilities need to have guidelines about how to store placentas until patient discharge. Nurses working in postpartum areas should be aware of the cultural rituals of their surrounding community. Even though placental burial may seem out of the ordinary to those in mainstream U.S. culture, supporting cultural differences remains important. Review Boxes 5-5 and 5-6 for a list of postpartum rituals.

Cultural Influences on Breast-Feeding and Weaning

Several organizations recommend exclusive breast-feeding for the first 6 months of a baby's life (AAFP, 2014; Association of Women's Health, Obstetric and Neonatal Nurses [AWHONN], 2015; Committee on Health Care for Underserved Women & ACOG, 2007). Research documents the advantages of breast milk for infants (development and immune support) and birthing parents (decreased risk of breast and ovarian cancers) (Victoria et al., 2016). Even when exclusive breast-feeding is not possible, even a small amount of breast milk consumed in the first few days of life is beneficial.

According to the CDC (2023), fewer non-Hispanic Black infants (74.1%) are ever breast-fed compared with Asian infants (90.8%), non-Hispanic White infants (85.3%), and Hispanic infants (83.0%). See Evidence-Based Practice 5-7 for a review of a study that examined factors that influence African American infant-feeding practices.

Alghamdi et al. (2017) conducted an RCT with 540 low-income mothers of non-Hispanic White, African American, and Hispanic ethnicity to examine the racial and ethnic differences in their maternal knowledge, self-efficacy, and propensity to breast-feed. Data analysis showed that White mothers had the highest mean knowledge scores followed by African American and then Hispanic mothers. The results also indicated that Hispanic mothers had significantly lower self-efficacy in infant feeding than did Whites and African Americans, while White and African American mother's scores were similar in this category. After adjusting for mother's age and education, marital, and working status, the odds of breast-feeding were significantly higher among Hispanic mothers than among White and African American mothers. The authors attributed the Hispanic mothers' higher odds of breast-feeding despite having the lowest infant feeding knowledge and self-efficacy scores to their social and cultural breast-feeding expectations (Hohl et al., 2016).

Shin et al. (2018) conducted an RCT of 150 pregnant women of Mexican descent to examine the influence of acculturation and cultural values on their breast-feeding practices. The results showed that a higher score on the Anglo orientation subscale of the Acculturation Rating Scale for Mexican Americans instrument was associated with less breast-feeding at 1-month postpartum and less exclusive breast-feeding. The researchers concluded that if an Anglo orientation is present among mothers of Mexican descent, the nurse can emphasize the fact that breast-feeding is experiencing increasing acceptance in mainstream society and is congruent with Anglo norms.

Pérez-Escamilla et al. (2016) conducted a narrative, systematic review to examine the impact of the Baby-Friendly Hospital Initiative (BFHI) on breast-feeding and child health outcomes in 19 different countries located in South America, North America, Western Europe, Eastern Europe, South Asia, Eurasia, and sub-Saharan Africa. The BFHI is a key component of the WHO/United Nations Children's Fund's Global Strategy for Infant and Young Child Feeding, whose aim is to improve short-, medium-, and long-term breast-feeding outcomes. Community support was found to be a key factor for long-term breast-feeding sustainability.

The World Health Organization (2021) and UNICEF recommend breast-feeding within 1 hour of birth, exclusive breast-feeding for the first 6 months of life, and introduction of nutritionally adequate and safe complementary (solid) foods at 6 months together with continued breast-feeding up to 2 years of age or beyond.

Nurses must remember to be culturally sensitive by not judging women breast-feeding a toddler, instead supporting their right to breast-feed.

Cultural Issues Related to Intimate Partner Violence

The World Health Organization (2012) defines **intimate partner violence** (IPV) as "any behavior within an intimate relationship that causes physical, psychological, or sexual harm to those in the relationship." IPV against women is a global public health problem with many short-term and long-term effects on the physical and mental health of women and their children. Section 5.2 Goal 5 of The SDGs (2015) calls for its elimination by the year 2030. Based on data from the WHO Global Database of Prevalence of Violence against Women, Sardinha et al. (2022) used a Bayesian multilevel model to develop global, regional, and country estimates of partner violence by age, year, and country to jointly estimate lifetime IPV. Studies from 2000 through 2018 were reviewed, which included women aged 15 years or older, measuring physical, sexual, or both, IPV. Studies were representative of 90% of the world's population of ever-partnered women and girls aged 15 years and older. Their findings derived from the WHO Global

A Qualitative Study of Social, Cultural, and Historical Influences on African American Women's Infant-Feeding Practices

DeVane-Johnson et al. (2018) described the cultural factors influencing African American mothers' perceptions about infant feeding. The participants were a purposive sample of 39 African American woman of diverse ages (26 to 45 years), educational backgrounds, and socioeconomic status. Six focus groups were conducted with a non–breast-feeding group (NBFG) and a breast-feeding group (BFG), resulting in the following themes listed below with participant comments.

Theme 1: It Takes a Village

- "I grew up thinking breast-feeding was a White thing, I never saw a Black woman breast-feed." "Everyone in my family bottle feeds, it's just been generationally. That's the way Grandma did it and continued." "But it's just like my aunts are old-fashioned. They're like, no, we're not allowed to do in front of family members." (NBFG)

Theme 2: Real-World Issues

- Work—"I think I feel more working moms, a lot of us really couldn't breast-feed. But I think by us being working, we didn't really have a choice to breast-feed." Other women described the inability to advance in the workplace while pumping and having no place to store milk. (NBFG)
- Pain—"I guess my boobs were really sore, so when my baby started to suck on them, they were really tender, so I stopped, I didn't want him to be on me."

Theme 3: Personal Realities

- "I wanted to make sure someone else could help." "I wanted a little bit of freedom, the bottle was easier." Artificial supplementation gave a sense of "empowerment." Formula feeding was described on social messaging as normal, convenient, and natural. (NBFG)
- "It's enough that you already have the spotlight because you are Black. If you are Black and you nurse, it's an additional, 'Oh my gosh, look at that person with that baby.'" "There's newer

formulas that can replicate what's coming out of me, I have a choice today…"
- "Breast milk adjusts based on the needs of the baby, I want to be as natural as possible. I do not know what's in formula." (BFG)

Theme 4: Historical Stigma

- "The stealing of breast milk from the slaves. They put them down on their stomach and they will squeeze their breast into the jugs until they were empty."
- "Breast-feeding was what they had to do because the economy at that time for Blacks it was not that good. So mother, she breast-feed because she had to."
- "This day and time Black women have a better choice. So that is why I chose to bottle-feed, because I did have a better choice."
- "Some just associate breast-feeding with slavery, wet-nursing, and the lack of choice. So they feel like a formula will be a step up."

Theme 5: Negative Body Image (Breast-Related Self-Esteem and Body Image Issues Affect Infant-Feeding Decisions)

- "I was not happy with my breasts. I got boobs early and I would hunch to try and hide them." One-group member shared her satisfaction with her breasts because they were large yet reported disappointment that they did not produce milk, "I prayed to God every night for big breasts. I really do love my breasts, I just wish they would have done right for my babies." (NBFG)

Theme 6: Breast-Feeding Described as "Nasty" (This Description Was Shared by Both Groups)

- "I chose to bottle-feed because I thought breast-feeding was nasty." "I thought it was nasty like 'Ooh, she got the baby sucking her breast!'" (NBFG)
- One woman said she received a message from her family that breast-feeding was "nasty":

(continued)

A Qualitative Study of Social, Cultural, and Historical Influences on African American Women's Infant-Feeding Practices (continued)

"Breast-feeding is like taboo. I have a sister that's older than me and when she found out that I was breast-feeding, I wasn't allowed to do it at her house because she said it was nasty." (BFG)

Clinical Implications

- Nurses and healthcare professionals working with African American patients must be made aware of the underlying historical stigma that can be related to breast-feeding by some members of this community (e.g., referencing slavery and wet nurses) compared to other racial/ethnic clients.

- Nurses should begin discussing the benefits of breast-feeding early during prenatal care.
- Nurses can promote breast-feeding demonstrations with the use of a shawl or blanket to decrease breast exposure and protect modesty.
- Healthcare professionals should prioritize culturally sensitive care while avoiding cultural or racial stereotypes that limit their ability to provide the highest quality of services.

Reference: DeVane-Johnson, S., Giscombe, C. W., Williams, R., Fogel, C., & Thoyre, S. (2018). A qualitative study of social, cultural, and historical influences on Africa American women's infant-feeding practices. *Journal of Perinatal Education*, 27(2), 71–85. https://doi.org/10.1891/1058-1243.27.2.71

Database comprised 366 eligible studies, capturing responses from 2 million women. Data were obtained from 161 countries, covering 90% of the global population of women and girls (15 years or older). Globally, 27% of ever-partnered women aged 15 to 49 are estimated to have experienced physical or sexual, or both, IPV in their lifetime, with 13% (10% to 16%) experiencing it in the past year before they were surveyed. It was proposed that violence starts affecting adolescent girls and young women early, with 24% of women aged 15 to 18 and 26% aged 19 to 24 having already experienced violence at least once since the age of 15 years. Regional variations exist, with low-income countries reporting higher lifetime, and more pronouncedly, higher past-year prevalence compared with high-income countries.

Maheu-Giroux et al. (2022) indicate that in the last decade, there has been a substantial increase in the number of nationally representative population-based surveys collecting data on IPV. However, the measurement of IPV across surveys and the types of measures used make comparability across studies and countries challenging. Bacchus et al. (2018) find that IPV and

mental health effects, including injuries, depression, anxiety, unwanted pregnancies, and STIs, can also lead to death.

IPV and Pregnancy

Drexler et al. (2022) assert that the etiology of IPV is complex and often centers around power and control. Causes are multifactorial, including individual, relationship, community, and social factors, and often the perpetrator's own experience of violence within their family, community, and society. Exposure to IPV during the perinatal period is associated with increased pregnancy complications, including miscarriage, placental abruption, preterm labor or birth, and low birth weight. Pregnant patients exposed to IPV in pregnancy were three times more likely to experience perinatal death.

Screening for IPV is recommended by the U.S. Preventative Services Task Force (2018) and multiple other organizations and should be universal to all patients during pregnancy. The American College of Obstetricians and Gynecologists (ACOG) along with the American College of Nurse-Midwives (ACNM) and the Association of

Women's Health, Obstetric and Neonatal Nurses (AWHONN) recommends screening at the first prenatal visit, during each trimester and postpartum (Halpern-Meekin et al., 2019).

Wallar et al. (2022) obtained data from the National Center for Health Statistics 2018 and 2019 mortality files to identify all female decedents aged 10 to 44 in the United States. They used data to estimate 2-year pregnancy-associated homicide mortality ratios (deaths/100,000 live births) for comparison with homicide mortality among nonpregnant, nonpostpartum females (deaths/100,000 population) and to mortality ratios for direct maternal causes of death. There were 3.62 homicides per 100,000 live births among females who were pregnant or within 1 year postpartum, 16% higher than homicide prevalence among nonpregnant and nonpostpartum females of reproductive age. Homicide during pregnancy or within 42 days of the end of pregnancy exceeded all the leading causes of maternal mortality by more than twofold. Pregnancy was associated with a significantly elevated homicide risk in the Black population and among girls and younger women (age 10 to 24) across racial and ethnic subgroups.

For their hospital quality improvement project, Bermele et al. (2018) implemented an IPV protocol for screening and case management in a Midwestern hospital's intrapartum unit. All unit nurses were trained about IPV and abuse during pregnancy, and RNs completed learning modules and participated in role-play scenarios. Women who needed support were referred to the unit's social worker. The scores indicated a significant increase in nurses' knowledge from the pretest (75%) to the posttest mean score (94%). Of the patient respondents, 64% reported experiencing abuse ($n = 25$) and were referred to a social worker (Bermele et al., 2018). Healthcare workers caring for childbearing patients should screen them for IPV in a private place, using culturally sensitive questions tailored to the community's population.

Nurses who work in the prenatal setting have an opportunity to initiate a caring, trusting relationship with the pregnant person while gathering information.

Nurse-provided education must stress the detrimental effects abuse can have on the pregnant patient and the unborn child's health. Even if they see their partner as a "victim," they need to learn that this is not a valid reason for accepting abuse. The client should be given information about community support systems and shelters and offered a referral to a social worker. Additionally, if applicable, the nurse should encourage them to speak with a trusted family who can help improve interactions between the partners. Moreover, the nurse should help the individual develop an escape plan should they feel unsafe and need to leave. This plan should indicate where to go, what they should take, and whom they should call. Finally, nurses should ask follow-up questions and offer support at each visit.

IPV Among Marginalized Groups

Hulley et al. (2023) explored barriers experienced among Black, Asian, and Minority Ethnic (BAME) and Immigrant IPV female victims seeking help. 921 women were included in the sample, of whom 630 were immigrants. Forty-seven studies met the selection criteria; United States (34 papers), United Kingdom (4), Hong Kong (3) Australia (2), Norway, Canada, Taiwan, and Sweden (1 each) were selected for inclusion in the review take. The most commonly identified were Latina (Hispanic) (12 papers), African American (9 papers), South Asian (7 papers), and Asian (5 papers). Other identified groups included Vietnamese, African immigrant, and Muslim (3 papers each); Mexican, West African, and Multiracial (2 papers each); and Cambodian, Chinese, Pacific Islander, African Caribbean, Irish, Jewish, Nigerian, and Ethiopian (1 paper each). A wide age range was represented, from early to late adulthood. The synthesis found that these women faced additional barriers as a result of institutional racism, immigration laws, culture and religion, issues related to cultural competence, and lack of diversity within the frontline services. Such barriers, from a range of formal and informal resources, services, and other mechanisms of support, served to exacerbate feelings of fear, threat, isolation, and powerlessness.

Even though the women in the study represented different countries and were heterogeneous in nature, all cultures nonetheless contained their own patriarchal norms, which related to ideas that women were responsible for "keeping the family together" and that women's roles were primarily domestic and "private" in contrast to the "public." Additionally, some acceptance of gendered violence was apparent, together with the importance placed upon maintaining an intact marriage, both in cultural and religious terms (Hulley et al., 2023).

Lee and Lee (2018) conducted a cross-sectional study of 250 pregnant South Korean married women to identify factors predictive of IPV. In South Korea, about 12% of married women report having an IPV experience during their lifetime. The results indicated that 34% of the pregnant women had experienced some form of IPV including psychological, physical, or sexual violence (SV) in the previous 12 months. Non-IPV group participants had a higher rate of employment and intended pregnancy compared to the IPV group. In addition, the non-IPV group had a significantly higher social support score than did the IPV group. IPV was more common among women with a graduate school education than among high school graduates. Unemployment was also significantly associated with IPV. The authors indicated that no investigation of IPV among pregnant women was previously conducted in South Korea. South Korean cultural norms dictate that women avoid exposing IPV. The authors suggested the need to screen and report violence toward pregnant women by their partners and provide social support during prenatal examinations. They also advocated for the legal system to mandate reporting of IPV cases in prenatal care settings (Lee & Lee, 2018).

Male dominance and female submission were significant themes among Chinese respondents surveyed about IPV. One of these respondents recalled her husband's announcement that "the woman whom I marry should be as docile as a sheep, and should never talk back" (Chiu, 2017, p. 1301). According to Jordan and Bhandari (2016), South Asian cultural values also prize masculinity, believed to derive from virility and the ability to control women.

Within Latin American culture, "machismo" sets the expectation for men to be dominant, the decision-maker, and the provider, whereas "marianismo" refers to women's responsibility for maintaining relations and peace (Hulley et al., 2023). The following survivor quote highlights ways these concepts work toward keeping women in abusive relationships:

> If your husband says something that you do not like, your obligation is to shut up and put up with it, because he is your husband, I mean you already got married, you are there and you put up with it. (Silva-Martinez, 2016, p. 531)

Some cultural norms included male violence toward women, which often prevented women from recognizing abuse. South Asian respondents noted that culturally, partner abuse is a private family issue, largely overlooking it, thus considering the behavior normal (Sabri et al., 2018).

"Familismo" in Latin American culture, remaining loyal to family, serves as a powerful barrier to exiting an abusive relationship. Hulley et al. (2023) assert that women within strong cultural and religious communities often feared the consequences of leaving their abusive relationship, concerned about the shame and humiliation this would bring to themselves and their families. A respondent from Sabri et al. (2018, p. 247) noted:

> As the cultural Indian girl, I'm not allowed to leave him, because I can change the man by changing my tactics. It will be a disgrace to the family. The children will have a black spot on their name, and no one will marry them when they grow older.

Shame is described as a powerful agent of social control in South Asian culture and a key deterrent to the disclosure of mistreatment. The family often reinforced the necessity of preserving family honor through the use of threats (Hulley et al., 2023): My father said, "If you divorce, you are dead to me, do not come back home" (Tonsing & Barn, 2017, p. 633).

Hulley et al.'s (2023) synthesis of two papers on religion/spirituality focused on samples of

Muslim women's experiences on how religion was often useful in assisting women to cope with the abuse. Acts and suggestions of visiting a place of worship also provided some women with feelings of peace and reduced isolation. Religion and spirituality often provided sources of empowerment and strength to remain in the relationship rather than the strength to leave.

Hulley et al. (2023) found that African women, even after being divorced by an abusive first husband, often remarried quickly due to fear of negative stereotypes and community ostracization as single women.

Due to cultural influence, the impact of racism, and the internalization of stereotypes, African American women commonly keep family/personal issues to themselves. They are also aware of the impact that racism has on their friends and family members and do not wish to subject them to further oppression by other actors, such as the police (Monterrosa, 2019, p. 16). The "Strong Black Woman" stereotype of tough, domineering, and insensitive women who are hard to handle and who necessitate the use of physical control by men impeded Black Women's help-seeking, through fear of being disbelieved, being perceived as vulnerable/weak and unworthy of care and concern (Monterrosa, 2019).

Discrimination is also experienced by immigrants to the United States, as South Asian women claimed that being an immigrant, not having a job, and being a single mother, they struggled to rent an apartment due to discriminatory landlords (Kiamanesh & Hauge, 2019). Additionally, it is well-known that perpetrators use a range of threats to deter their victims from leaving violent relationships. The threat of deportation was sometimes explicitly used against immigrant women so violent partners and families could control their victims (Hulley, 2023).

IPV and American Indian women

The National Institute of Justice in 2016 looked at how prevalent psychological aggression and physical violence by intimate partners, stalking, and SV were among American Indian and Alaska Native (AI/AN) women. It examined the perpetrators' race and the impact of violence. Using a national representative sample from the National Intimate Partner and Sexual Violence Survey, a total of 2,473 adult women identified themselves as AI/AN, either alone or in combination with another racial group. 83% of the women were affiliated or enrolled with a tribe or village. Fifty-four percent had lived within reservation boundaries or in an Alaska Native village in the past year.

Results show that more than four in five AI/NA women (84.3%) have experienced violence in their lifetime. This includes 56.1% who experienced SV, 55% who have experienced physical violence by an intimate partner, 48.8% who have experienced stalking, and 66.4% who have experienced psychological aggression by an intimate partner. Overall, more than 1.5 million AI/NA women have experienced violence in their lifetime (Rosay, 2016).

President Biden's Executive Order on Improving Public Safety and Criminal Justice for Native Americans and Addressing the Crisis of Mission or Murdered Indigenous People, published Nov. 15, 2021, acknowledges that "Native Americans face unacceptably high levels of violence, and are victims of violent crime at a rate much higher than the national average." The president specifically highlights that Native American women are disproportionately the victims of sexual and gender violence, including intimate partner homicide, and that approximately half of Native American women have experienced physical violence by an intimate partner.

Luebke et al. (2023) conducted an ethnography research study to address a gap in the literature surrounding the phenomenon of IPV against AI women living in urban and metropolitan Wisconsin. This study aims to understand the needs and barriers of help-seeking AI women. Help-seeking is defined as the process that a survivor utilizes to disclose, garner support, and/or secure formal services for partner abuse (Goodson & Hayes, 2018; Stork, 2008).

Semistructured interviews with 34 AI IPV survivors living in Wisconsin urban areas were conducted. Findings highlight context-specific structural barriers to help-seeking after experiences of IPV heightened by the COVID-19 pandemic (Luebke et al., 2023).

The Wisconsin urban metropolitan area was experiencing an uptick in homicides before the pandemic, with twice as many homicides seen in 2020 incomparable to the previous year. Two of every five of homicides were related to domestic violence (Lutheran, 2020). Consistent with global trends, IPV and sexual assault advocates in Wisconsin began to report an increase in self and police referrals to their agencies by women experiencing IPV after the pandemic began (Lutheran, 2020). Women who are victims of IPV are at a particularly increased risk for harm due to the "stay at home" measures put in place to combat COVID-19, because home is not necessarily the safest place for them. This message may traumatize the victim, due to being trapped at home with their abuser, and increased isolation which also minimizes the women's ability to seek help. Fear of seeking shelter or services may also be exacerbated by fear of contracting and becoming ill with COVID-19 (Lutheran, 2020). Ethnic and minority populations were at a higher risk of contracting COVID-19 or experiencing severe COVID-19–related illnesses (CDC, 2020). This is due specifically to the health inequities formed at the intersections of structural racism and poverty, which for AIs are also rooted in ongoing colonization (CDC, 2021).

Financial-related barriers and barriers to accessing existing resources were the most prominent themes describing barriers to help-seeking across all interviews. Subthemes that fell under the main theme of financial-related barriers include feelings that "I didn't have anywhere to go and no way to get help, I don't have any insurance," barriers to accessing existing resources, distrust, and discrimination, lack of culturally relevant care, and personal barriers such as fear of retaliation or fear of increased violence (Luebke et al., 2023).

Highlights of the study indicated that many urban-based AI survivors who desire to leave a violent situation have limited access to culturally specific IPV-related services. Several survivors in the study reiterated that they refused help after experiencing violence due to previous negative interactions with healthcare, allied, or law enforcement professionals (Luebke et al., 2023).

According to the CDC/tribes organizations (2022), there are 574 federally recognized American Indian and Alaska Native (AI/AN) tribes spread across the United States. The tribes represent diverse groups of people with unique cultures, languages, histories, and practices (see Fig. 5-8). AI/AN people have many differences; however, they also often share similar experiences with and approaches to maintaining the health and wellness of their communities.

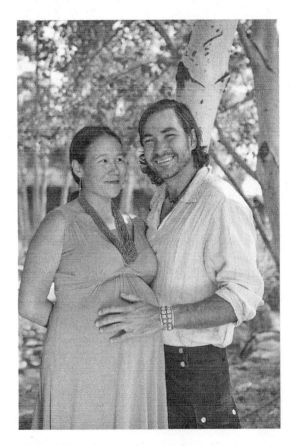

Figure 5-8. Native American pregnant couple. (Mona Makela/https://www.shutterstock.com)

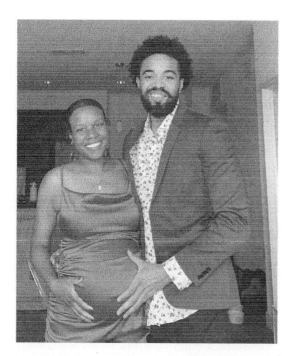

Figure 5-9. African American pregnant couple.

In their qualitative research study, Giacci et al. (2022) conducted narrative interviews with AI/AN women from four tribal reservation communities. The purpose of the interviews was to explore connections among SRH, IPV, SV, reproductive coercion (RC), and historical trauma. Fifty-six women were interviewed (aged 17 to 55; 77% were aged 40 years and younger), and all described multiple exposures to violence and highlighted a lack of disclosure related to sexuality, childhood abuse, SV, and historical trauma. Almost half reported experiencing RC in their lifetime. The use of substances occurred in both the context of SV and for surviving after exposure to violence. The women underscored the extent to which IPV, SV, and RC are embedded in histories of colonization, racism, and ongoing oppression.

IPV and African American Women

Many African Americans participate in a culture that focuses on the importance of family

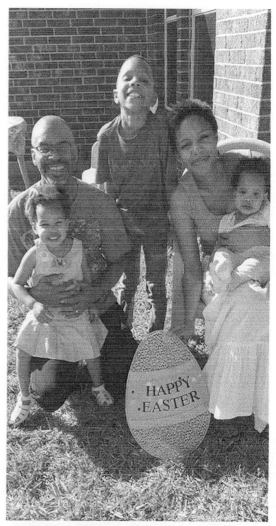

Figure 5-10. African American family.

and church. Family includes not only mother, father, sister, and brother but also the extended kinship of grandparents, aunts, uncles, cousins, and close individuals who, while not "blood" related, play an important role in the family system. The church has traditionally been a sanctuary for members of the African American community, offering spiritual worship, fellowship, education, guidance, and counseling (see Figs. 5-9 and 5-10).

African American women are more likely than women of other racial and ethnic groups in the United States to be murdered by their intimate partner (Violence Policy Center, 2020). Further, African American women experience IPV-related homicide at younger ages. The average age that an African American woman is murdered by her intimate partner is 36 years old, which is 5 years younger than the national average (Violence Policy Center, 2020). However, they are more likely to remain with their abusive partner rather than seek help from service providers, due in part to the racism and racial discrimination they experience during help-seeking (Bent-Goodley, 2013; Petrosky et al., 2017). Waller et al. (2022) performed a systematic review to provide a critical examination of the literature to understand the intersections of IPV and help-seeking behavior among African American women. A total of 85 empirical studies were identified and 21 were included in the systematic review. The review illuminated both formal and semiformal help-seeking pathways.

Literature notes that survivors typically secure assistance from formal providers within the criminal justice, shelter, and healthcare systems. However, African American survivors additionally heavily rely upon the Black church for guidance and support (Lacey et al., 2020). According to Cox and Diamant (2018), African American women are the most religious population in the United States and more readily rely upon prayer for strength while secretly suffering from abuse, garner inner spiritual strength, and rely upon Biblical readings, prayers, and spirituality for private support rather than accepting public assistance from the community or clergy (Waller et al., 2022).

A review of the 21 studies found that African American women generally forgo police intervention because they believe they can handle the situation better than officers, and more than half of women avoided police intervention due to fear officers would mishandle the situation (Waller et al., 2022). Deutsch and colleagues (2017) conducted a series of focus groups and found that

African American women tend to be uncooperative with the legal process because they feel like they will neither be believed nor fully supported. Survivors further expected that their cases would not be adequately adjudicated and they feared they would be abused by the legal system (Deutsch et al., 2017). In their review, Waller et al. (2022) reported African American women's experiences of a range of racial microaggressions, particularly at issue since White workers in IPV shelters are known to systematically overlook African American women's needs and relegate them to residing in subpar temporary shelters that are located in unsafe neighborhoods where crime and poverty rates are high and where White women are never referred. Additionally, African American survivors said that they overwhelmingly felt like the White shelter workers perceived them as less than deserving of any of the emergency benefits that are provided to them (Nnawulezi & Sullivan, 2014). Waller et al. (2022) conclude that intersectionality is a useful framework to illuminate barriers to this population's help seeking because it provides a lens whereby their overlapping vulnerabilities may be elucidated and how these vulnerabilities impact their ability to secure urgent aid. Race, class, and gender oppression are experienced simultaneously and are inextricably linked.

Despite its prevalence, IPV is not considered an acceptable action in African American culture. As with other marginalized minority groups, African Americans may feel disengaged from the dominant society due to systemic racism, which intensifies the likelihood of poor educational attainment, low incomes, job stress, or unemployment. In addition, drug and alcohol use is also common among abusers (Waller et al., 2022).

IPV and Latina Women

As an ethnic group, Hispanics share a heritage that includes strong family and religious elements. As with any cultural group, differences exist, with subgroups maintaining distinct

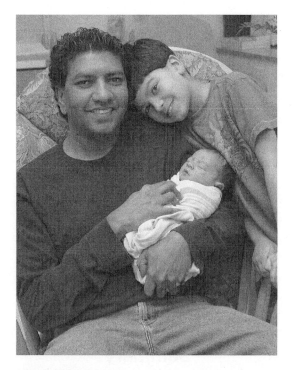

Figure 5-11. Hispanic dad, brother, and newborn. (7Glenda/https://www.shutterstock.com)

cultural beliefs and customs. For Hispanics, relatives and older family members are respected and often consulted on decisions involving health and illness (see Fig. 5-11).

Compared with non-Latina Whites, Latinas are more likely to experience severe negative consequences of IPV, such as increased risk for transmission of HIV or other STI infections (CDC, 2018), depression, and posttraumatic stress disorder. They are also less likely than non-Latina Whites to have access to, seek, and receive adequate mental healthcare to treat the psychological effects of IPV. However, having higher levels of education and being employed are associated with greater reporting of IPV. Da Silva et al. (2021) identify the traditional Latino patriarchal social systems and societal values, which emphasized men's dominance and women's submission may lead some to perceive violence as normative. Marianismo beliefs

prescribe various dimensions of Latina femininity and depict Latina women as nurturing, self-sacrificing, virginal, and emotionally stronger than men. Additionally, subordinate to others and silencing self to maintain harmony beliefs are hypothesized to contribute to IPV among Latinas by encouraging submissiveness, self-silencing, and preservation of the family unit, often at the expense of individual well-being (Rountree et al., 2016).

Da Silva et al.'s (2021) study examined whether endorsement of marianismo beliefs mitigated or exacerbated psychological distress after experiences of IPV among Latina women. The sample consisted of 205 Miami-Dade County, Florida, Latina women involved in a romantic relationship since their arrival to the United States, who were asked about potential IPV experiences. The average participant had resided in the United States for approximately 16 months, with an age range of 18 to 23 years. The majority completed a high school diploma (57%) or received a bachelor's or trade school degree (30%). Slightly less than two-thirds of the sample reported being unemployed (61%), and among those who worked, hours per week varied greatly. Overall, 77% of the sample were unmarried, and 23% were married. The ethnic classification of participants is as follows: Cuban 42%, Columbian 11.2%, Nicaraguan 6.8%, Honduran 6.3%, Venezuelan 6.35, Peruvian 5.9% Ecuadorian 3.4% Mexican 2.9%, and Panamanian, Dominican, and Chilean 2.4% each. Approximately 87% were document immigrants, and 13% were undocumented.

Da Silva et al.'s (2021) study findings suggest that the construct of marianismo is relevant for young adult recent Latina immigrants to the United States. Although egalitarian gender role beliefs are associated with acculturation to U.S. society, it is important to note that acculturation and enculturation are distinct processes and not poles on a continuum. Recently immigrated Latinas may acculturate to U.S. society to a degree while remaining encultured to their heritage culture, which may diminish or reinforce traditional gender role beliefs. Mental health practitioners should attend to relevant cultural beliefs to facilitate services access and utilization for this vulnerable population.

Intimate Partner Violence Among the LGBTQ+ Community

Lifetime prevalence of IPV in lesbian, gay, and bisexual (LGB) couples appeared to be similar to or higher than in heterosexual ones: 61.1% of bisexual women, 43.8% of lesbian women, 37.3% of bisexual men, and 26.0% of gay men experienced IPV during their life, while 35.0% of heterosexual women and 29.0% of heterosexual men experienced IPV. When episodes of severe violence were considered, the prevalence was similar or higher for LGB adults (bisexual women: 49.3%; lesbian women: 29.4%; gay men: 16.4% compared to heterosexual adults [heterosexual women: 23.6%, heterosexual men: 13.9%] [Rolle et al., 2019]).

Individuals classified as being sexual minority (SM) and gender minority (GM) are conceptualized as individuals whose sexual and gender identity, orientation, or behavior do not conform with the practices of the majority group in U.S. society (Anderson et al., 2023). A recent study by Steele et al. (2020) found that race/ethnicity was a significant predictor of IPV victimization among Black and Latina SM women, even when controlling for socioeconomic status and childhood sexual abuse (which is not true for non-SM women). GM women of color also report encountering stigma, dating violence (psychological, physical, and sexual), and reliance on survival strategies (Gamarel et al., 2022; King et al., 2021). A study on Sexual Gender Minority college students found that race predicted exposure to emotional, physical, and sexual IPV (with Black and "other race" students reporting the highest prevalence of victimization for each form of IPV); Black transgender students had more than six times the risk of emotional and physical IPV versus White cisgender students, and Asian transgender students had more than seven times the risk of sexual IPV versus White cisgender students (Whitfield et al., 2021).

In the context of increasing IPV, stress, and mental health issues during the COVID-19 pandemic, violence against SGM populations is on the rise in the United States (Adamson et al., 2022; Madrigal-Borloz, 2020; Peitzmeir et al., 2022). Policy changes must include improved training and supervision of victim service providers from social workers to healthcare providers, assessment of the inclusivity and safety of language and literature, and quality assurance procedures that protect this population's access to IPV prevention services. Anderson et al.'s (2023) study findings concluded that immediate improvement to existing services, such as the elimination of hetero-presumptive language about partner perpetrators, or the enforcement of policies that allow equitable access to services regardless of perceived gender, is necessary to support this clientele.

Summary

As the United States moves toward a heterogeneous society, health professionals who work with childbearing people must incorporate cultural practices into their care plans. Healthcare providers should perform honest self-evaluations to assess their personal cultural beliefs and biases. All patients deserve compassion, support, and the best healthcare possible, regardless of their race, ethnicity, socioeconomic, gender, or sexual preference/status. As nurses and healthcare providers, we are taught to be nonjudgmental when caring for our patients. Providing culturally competent nonbiased care is crucial for our patient's well-being.

REVIEW QUESTIONS

1. Describe the special needs of an African American childbearing family due to the health disparities of infant mortality and maternal morbidity.

2. A pregnant woman arrives at your clinic for prenatal care. She does not speak English; however, she has her 12-year-old son with her for interpretation of her native language of Spanish. How would you assess the obstetrical history and cultural needs of this patient?

3. How do you assist your community healthcare center to be more involved in providing culturally centered care for the Native American pregnant patients who fear coming for care due to the community's perception of unnecessary labor interventions?

4. You are a postpartum nurse with a Latinx transgender male patient who delivered a 7-pound 3-ounce baby 1 hour ago. Your patient is requesting assistance with chest feeding. How do you provide culturally supportive care?

5. What nursing intervention would you use for a pregnant Asian woman (who speaks some English) who presents to the prenatal clinic with bruising on her left arm and abdomen (found on the initial physical exam)? When you inquire about the bruising, she begins to cry and tells you that she is alone in this country and her family is in Thailand. How do you provide culturally supportive care?

CRITICAL THINKING ACTIVITIES

1. Critically analyze and describe the culturally competent nursing intervention for an African American postpartum woman who desires to breast-feed but is concerned that her sisters and aunt think it is a bad choice. How would you support her decision?

2. Discuss the responses a postpartum nurse would make when she notices an Asian woman refuses to shower and is not eating her breakfast of cereal and orange juice or drinking cool water from the pitcher.

3. You are the labor nurse with a Ghanaian patient who refuses pain medication in labor. She is having strong palpable contractions every 2 minutes and tears are running down her face. What can you do to ensure her comfort?

4. Describe and analyze how the nurse might alter her care approach for a patient whose culture requires the father of the newborn to whisper a prayer in the infant's ear as the first sound they hear initially after birth?

REFERENCES

Abadi, A. S., Zandi, M., Shiva, M., Pourshirvani, A., & Kazemnejad, A. (2018). Effect of preparation for maternal role program on self-esteem of women undergoing in-vitro fertilization. *Evidence Based Care Journal, 7*(4), 63–72.

ACOG (2018). ACOG Committee Opinion No. 757: Screening for perinatal depression. *Obstetrics & Gynecology, 132*(5), e208–e212. https://doi.org/10.1097/AOG.0000000000002927

Adams, Y. J., & Smith, B. A. (2018). Integrative review of factors that affect the use of postpartum care services in developing countries. *Journal of Obstetric, Gynecologic, & Neonatal Nursing, 47*(3), 371–384. https://doi.org/10.1016/j.jogn.2018.02.006

Adams, Y. J., Stommel, M., Ayoola, A., Horodynski, M., Malata, A., & Smith, B. (2017). Use and evaluation of postpartum care services in rural Malawi. *Journal of Nursing Scholarship, 49*(1), 87–95. https://doi.org/10.1111/jnu.12257

Adamson, T., Lett, E., Glick, J., Garrison-Desany, H. M., & Restar, A. (2022). Experiences of violence and discrimination among LGBTQ+ individuals during the COVID-19 pandemic: A global cross-sectional analysis. *BMJ Global Health, 7*(9), e009400.

Administration for Children & Families. (2022). *PSAs highlight domestic violence awareness among Native Americans.* Retrieved October 23, 2022, from https://www.acf.hhs. gov/media/press/2022/psas-highlight-domestic-violence-awareness-among-native-americans

Alexander, L. L., LaRosa, J. H., Bader, H., Garfield, S., & Alexander, W. J. (2017). *New dimensions in women's health* (7th ed.). Jones & Bartlett Learning.

Alghamdi, S., Horodynski, M., & Stommel, M. (2017). Racial and ethnic differences in breastfeeding, maternal knowledge, and self-efficacy among low-income mothers. *Applied Nursing Research, 37*, 24–27. https://doi.org/10.1016/j.apnr.2017.07.009

American Academy of Family Physicians. (2014). *Breastfeeding, family physicians supporting [Position paper].* http://www.aafp.org/about/policies/all/breastfeeding-support.html

American College of Obstetricians and Gynecologists. (2018). ACOG Committee Opinion No. 757: Screening for perinatal depression. *Obstetrics & Gynecology, 132*(5), e208–e212. https://doi.org/10.1097/AOG.0000000000002927

Anderson, E. J., Marlow, H., & Izugbara, C. (2023). Epidemiological profile of intimate partner homicides of sexual and gender minority women in the United States, 2003 to 2017. *Journal of Interpersonal Violence, 38*(11–12), 7143–7169.

Arousell, J., & Carlbom, A. (2016). Culture and religious beliefs in relation to reproductive health. *Best Practice & Research Clinical Obstetrics & Gynaecology, 32,* 77–87. https://doi.org/10.1016/j.bpobgyn.2015.08.011

Association of Women's Health, Obstetric and Neonatal Nurses (AWHONN). (2015). AWHONN position statement. Intimate partner violence. *Journal of Obstetric, Gynecologic, and Neonatal Nursing, 44*(3), 405–408. https://doi.org/10.1111/1552-6909.12567

Bacchus, L. J., Ranganathan, M., Watts, C., & Devries, K. (2018). Recent intimate partner violence against women and health: A systematic review and meta-analysis of cohort studies. *BMJ Open, 8,* e019995. https://doi.org/10.1136/bmjopen-2017-019995

Banu, K. K., Prathipa, A., Anandarajan, B., Ismail Sheriff, A. M., Muthukumar, S., & Selvakumar, J. (2016). Food taboos during antenatal and postpartum period among the women of rural and urban areas of Tamilnadu. *International Journal of Biomedical and Advance Research, 7*(8), 393–396. https://doi.org/10.7439/ijbar.v7i8.3539

Bermele, C., Andresen, P. A., & Urbanski, S. (2018). Educating nurses to screen and intervene for intimate partner violence during pregnancy. *Nursing for Women's Health, 22*(1), 79–86. https://doi.org/10.1016/j.nwh.2017.12.006

Bowlby, J. (1999). *Attachment and loss* (Vol. 1, 2nd ed.). Basic Books.

Brandt, J. S., Patel, A. J., Marshall, I., & Bachmann, G. A. (2019). Transgender men, pregnancy, and the "new" advanced paternal age: a review of the literature. *Maturitas, 128,* 17–21.

Brown, S. S., & Eisenberg, L. (1995). *The best intentions: Unintended pregnancy and the welling of children and families.* National Academies Press.

Carson, L. D., Henderson, J. N., King, K., Klesz, K., Thompson, D., & Mayer, P. (2015). American Indian diabetes beliefs and practices: Anxiety, fear, and dread in pregnant women with diabetes. *Diabetes Spectrum, 28*(4), 258–263. https://doi.org/10.2337/diaspect.28.4258

Centers for Disease Control and Prevention. (2018). *Lesbian, gay, bisexual, and transgender health.* https://www.cdc.gov/lgbthealth/

Centers for Disease Control and Prevention (2020). *National Diabetes Statistics Report, 2020.* Centers for Disease Control and Prevention, U.S. Dept of Health and Human Services.

Centers for Disease Control and Prevention (CDC). (2010). *Guidelines for the identification and management of lead exposure in pregnant and lactating women.* U.S. Department of Health and Human Services. https://www.cdc.gov/nceh/lead/publications/leadandpregnancy2010.pdf

Centers for Disease Control and Prevention (CDC). (2020). *Report: COVID-19 in racial and ethnic minority groups.* https://www.cdc.gov/coronavirus/2019-ncov/need-extra-precautions/racial-ethnic-minorities.html

Centers for Disease Control and Prevention (CDC). (2021). COVID-19 health equity data. *COVID data tracker.* Retrieved December 16, 2021, from https://covid.cdc.gov/covid-data-tracker/#health-equity-data

Centers for Disease Control and Prevention. (2023). *Breastfeeding disparities exist.* https://www.cdc.gov/breastfeeding/data/facts.html#print

Cesario, S. K. (2017). Immigration basics for nurses. *Nursing for Women's Health, 21*(6), 499–505. https://doi.org/10.1016/j.nwh.2017.10.004

Chalmiers, M., Karaki, F., Muriki, M., Mody, S. K., Chen, A., & de Bocanegra, H. T (2022). Refugee women's experiences with contraceptive care after resettlement in high-income countries: A critical interpretive synthesis. *Contraception, 108,* 8–18. https://doi.org/10.1016/j.contraception.2021.11.004

Charter, R., Ussher, J. M., Perz, J., & Robinson, K. (2018). The transgender parent: Experiences and constructions of pregnancy and parenthood for transgender men in Australia. *International Journal of Transgenderism, 9*(1), 64–77. https://doi.org/10.1080/ 15532739.2017.1399496

Chiu, T. Y. (2017). Marriage migration as a multifaceted system: The intersectionality of intimate partner violence in cross-border marriages. *Violence against Women, 23*(11), 1293–1313. https://doi.org/10.1177/1077801216659940

Committee on Health Care for Underserved Women, American College of Obstetricians and Gynecologists (ACOG). (2007). ACOG Committee Opinion No. 361: Breastfeeding: maternal and infant aspects. *Obstetrics and Gynecology, 109*(2 Pt 1), 479–480.

Cox, K., & Diamant, J. (2018, September 26). Black men are less religious than black women, but more religious than white women and men. *Fact Tank.* News in the Numbers. www.pewresearch.org

Craft-Blacksheare, M., & Kahn, P. (2023). Midwives' and Other Perinatal health workers' perceptions of the Black maternal mortality crisis in the United States. *Journal of Midwifery & Women's Health, 68*(1), 62–70. https://doi.org/10.1111/jmwh.13433

Cutler, A., McNamara, B., Qasba, N., Kennedy, H. P., Lundsberg, L., & Gariepy, A. (2018). "I just don't know": An exploration of women's ambivalence about a new pregnancy. *Women's Health Issues, 28*(1), 75–81. https://doi.org/10.1016/j.whi.2017.09.009

Da Silva, N., Verdejo, T. R., Dillon, F. R., Ertl, M. M., & De La Rosa, M. (2021). Marianismo beliefs, intimate partner violence, and psychological distress among recently immigrated, young adult Latinas. *Journal of interpersonal violence*, *36*(7–8), 3755–3777.

Desai, G., Anand, A., Shah, P., Shah, S., Dave, K., Bhatt, H., Desai, S., & Modi, D. (2017). Sickle cell disease and pregnancy outcomes: A study of the community-based hospital in a tribal block of Gujarat, India. *Journal of Health, Population and Nutrition*, *36*(1), 3. https://doi.org/10.1186/s41043-017-0079-z

Deutsch, L. S., Resch, K., Barber, T., Zuckerman, Y., Stone, J. T., & Cerulli, C. (2017). Bruise documentation, race and barriers to seeking legal relief for intimate partner violence survivors: A retrospective qualitative study. *Journal of Family Violence*, *32*, 767–773.

DeVane-Johnson, S., Giscombe, C. W., Williams, R., Fogel, C., & Thoyre, S. (2018). A qualitative study of social, cultural, and historical influences on Africa American women's infant-feeding practices. *Journal of Perinatal Education*, *27*(2), 71–85. https://doi.org/10.1891/1058-1243.27.2.71

Downe, S., Finlayson, K., Oladapo, O., Bonet, M., & Gulmezoglu, A. M. (2018). What matters to women during childbirth: A systematic qualitative review. *PLoS One*, *13*(4), e0194906. https://doi.org/10.1371/journal.pone.0194906

Downing, J. M. (2019). Pathways to pregnancy for sexual minority women in same-sex marriages. *American Journal of Obstetrics & Gynecology*, *221*(3), 281–282.

Drexler, K. A., Quist-Nelson, J., & Weil, A. B. (2022). Intimate partner violence and trauma-informed care in pregnancy. *American Journal of Obstetrics & Gynecology MFM*, *4*(2), 100542.

Dubuc, S., & Devinderjit, S. S. (2017). Gender preferences and fertility effects on sex-composition. Linking behavior and macro-level effects. Paper presented at the Annual Meeting of the Population Association of America, April 27–29, 2017, Chicago, IL.

Eichelberger, K., Doll, K., Edpo, G. E., & Zerden, M. (2016). Black lives matter: Claiming a space for evidence-based outrage in obstetrics and gynecology. *American Journal of Public Health*, *106*(10), 1771–1772. https://doi.org/10.2105/AJPH.2016.303313

Ekwochi, U., Osuroah, C. D. I., Ndu, I. K., Ifediora, C., Asinobi, I. N., & Eke, C. B. (2016). Food taboos and myths in South Eastern Nigeria: The belief and practice of mothers in the region. *Journal of Ethnobiology and Ethnomedicine*, *12*, 7. https://doi.org/10.1186/s13002-016-0079-x

Elnakib, S., & Metzler, J. (2022). A scoping review of FGM in humanitarian settings; an overlooked phenomenon with lifelong consequence. *Conflict and Health* https://doi.org/10.1186/s13031-022-00479-5

Farrow, A. (2015). Lactation support and the LGBTQI community. *Journal of Human Lactation*, *31*(1), 26–28. https://doi.org//10.1177/0890334414554928

Fikree, F. F., Lane, C., Simon, C., Hainsworth, G., & MacDonald, P. (2017). Making good on a call to expand method choice for young people—Turning rhetoric into reality for addressing sustainable development goal three. *Reproductive Health*, *14*(1), 53. https://doi.org/10.1186/s12978-017-0313-6

Filonenko, A., Law, A., Purser, M., Mader, G., & Graham, J. (2019). PIH36 economic burden of unintended pregnancy in the United States. *Value in Health*, *22*, S188–S189.

Finer, L. B., Lindberg, L. D., & Desai, S. (2018). A prospective measure of unintended pregnancy in the United States. *Contraception*, *98*(6), 522–527.

Foster, D. G. (2020). *The turnaway study: Ten years, a thousand women, and the consequences of having—or being denied—an abortion*. Scribner.

Francis, A., Jasani, S., & Bachmann, G. (2018). Contraceptive challenges and the transgender individual. *Women's Midlife Health*, *4*, Article 12. https://doi.org/10.1186/s40695-018-0042-1

Frost, J. J., Zolna, M. R., Frohwirth, L. F., Douglas-Hall, A., Blades, N., Mueller, J., Pleasure, Z. H., & Shivani Kochhar, S. (2019). *Publicly supported family planning services in the United States: Likely need, availability and impact, 2016*. Guttmacher Institute. https://www.guttmacher.org/report/publiclysupported-FP-services-us-2016

Gamarel, K. E., Jadwin-Cakmak, L., King, W. M., Lacombe-Duncan, A., Trammell, R., Reyes, L. A., Burks, C., Rivera, B., Arnold, E., & Harper, G. W. (2022). Stigma experienced by transgender women of color in their dating and romantic relationships: Implications for gender-based violence prevention programs. *Journal of Interpersonal Violence*, *37*(9–10), NP8161–NP8189.

Gatos, K. C. (2018). A literature review of cervical cancer screening in transgender men. *Nursing for women's health*, *22*(1), 52–62.

George, E. K., Shorten, A., Lyons, K. S., & Edmonds, J. K. (2022). Factors influencing birth setting decision making in the United States: An integrative review. *Birth: Issues in Perinatal Care*, *49*(3), 403–409. https://doi.org/10.1111/birt.12640

Giacci, E., Straits, K. J., Gelman, A., Miller-Walfish, S., Iwuanyanwu, R., & Miller, E. (2022). Intimate partner and sexual violence, reproductive coercion, and reproductive health among American Indian and Alaska native women: a narrative interview study. *Journal of Women's Health*, *31*(1), 13–22.

Goodson, A., & Hayes, B. E. (2018). Help-seeking behaviors of intimate partner violence victims: A cross-national analysis in developing nations. *Journal of Interpersonal Violence*, 1–23. https://doi.org/10.1177/0886260518794508.

Gram, L., Skordis-Worrell, J., Manandhar, D., Strachan, D., Morrison, J., Saville, N, Osrin, D., Tumbahangphe, K. M., Costello, A., & Heys, M. (2018). The long-term impact of community mobilization through participatory women's groups on women's agency I the household: A follow-up study to the Makwanpur trial. *PLoS One, 13*(5), e0197426. https://doi.org/10.1371/journal.pone.0197

Greenberg, P. E., Fournier, A., Sisisky, T., Pike, C. I., & Kessler, R. C. (2015). The economic burden of adults with major depression disorder in the United States (2005 and 2010). *Journal of Clinical Psychiatry, 76*(2), 155–162. https://doi.org/10.4088/JCP.14m09298

Griggs, K., Waddill, C., Bice, A., & Ward, N. (2021). Care during pregnancy, childbirth, postpartum, and human milk feeding for individuals who identify as LGBTQ+. *MCN. The American Journal of Maternal Child Nursing, 46*(1), 43–53.

Guerra-Reyes, L., & Hamilton, L. J. (2017). Racial disparities in birth care: Exploring the perceived role of African-American women providing midwifery care and birth support in the United States. *Women and Birth, 30*(1), e9–e16. https://doi.org/10.1016/j.wombi.2016.06.004

Guttmacher Institute. (2016). *Unintended pregnancy in the United States*. https://www.guttmacher.org/fact-sheet/unintended-pregnancy-united-states

Guttmacher Institute. (2018). *Contraceptive use in the United States*. https://www.guttmacher.org/fact-sheet/contraceptive-use-united-states

Halpern-Meekin, S., Costanzo, M., Ehrenthal, D., & Rhoades, G. (2019). Intimate partner violence screening in the prenatal period: Variation by state, insurance, and patient characteristics. *Maternal and Child Health Journal, 23*, 756–767. https://doi.org/10.1007/s10995-018-2692-x

Herd, P., Higgins, J., Sicinski, K., & Merkurieva, I. (2016). The implications of unintended pregnancies for mental health in later life. *American Journal of Health Perspectives, 106*(3), 421–429. https://doi.org/10.2105/AJPH.2015.302973

Hippocrates (1849). *The genuine works of Hippocrates*. Sydenham Society.

Hohl, S., Thompson, B., Escareño, M., & Duggan, C. (2016). Cultural norms in conflict: Breastfeeding among Hispanic immigrants in rural Washington state. *Maternal and Child Health Journal, 20*(7), 1549–1557. https://doi.org/10.1007/s10995-016-1954-8

Holland, A. C., Strachan, A. T., Pair, L., Stallworth, K., & Hodges, A. (2018). Highlights from the U.S. selected practice recommendations for contraceptive use. *Nursing for Women's Health, 22*(2), 181–190. https://doi.org/10.1016/j.nwh.2018.02.006

Horsager-Boehrer, R. (2020). *Is electronic fetal monitoring worthwhile?* Medical Blog–UT Southwestern Medical Center.

Hulley, J., Bailey, L., Kirkman, G., Gibbs, G. R., Gomersall, T., Latif, A., & Jones, A. (2023). Intimate partner violence and barriers to help-seeking among Black, Asian, minority ethnic and immigrant women: A qualitative meta-synthe-sis of global research. *Trauma, Violence, & Abuse, 24*(2), 1001–1015.

Impicciatore, R., Gabrielli, G., & Paterno, A. (2020). Migrants' fertility in Italy: A comparison between origin and destination. *European Journal of Population, 36*(4), 799–825.

Johnsen, S., & Sweeney, M. (2022). Female sterilization in the course: Understanding trends and differentials in early sterilization. *Demographic Research, 47*, 529–544. https://www.demographic-research.org/Volumes/Vol47/18/DOI:10.4054/DemRes.2022.47.18

Jordan, A., & Bhandari, S. (2016). Lived experiences of South Asian women facing domestic violence in the United States. *Journal of Ethnic & Cultural Diversity in Social Work, 25*(3), 227–246. https://doi.org/10.1080/15313204.2015.1134374

Kabakian-Khasholian, T., Bashour, H., El-Nemer, A., Kharouf, M., Sheikha, S., El Lakany, N., Barakat, R., Elsheikh, O., Nameh, N., Chahine, R., & Portela, A. (2017). Women's satisfaction and perception of control in childbirth in three Arab countries. *Reproductive Health Matters, 25*(Suppl. 1), 16–26. https://doi.org/10.1080/09688080.2017.1381533

Kiamanesh, P., & Hauge, M. I. (2019). "We are not weak, we just experience domestic violence"-immigrant women's experiences of encounters with service providers as a result of domestic violence. *Child & Family Social Work, 24*(2), 301–308. https://doi.org/10.1111/cfs.12615

King, W. M., Restar, A., & Operario, D. (2021). Exploring multiple forms of intimate partner violence in a gender and racially/ethnically diverse sample of transgender adults. *Journal of Interpersonal Violence, 36*(19–20), NP10477–NP10498.

Klaus, M., & Kennell, J. (1982). *Parent-infant bonding* (2nd ed.). Mosby.

Ko, J. Y., Rockhill, K. M., Tong, Y. T., Morrow, B., & Farr, S. L. (2017). Trends in postpartum depressive symptoms— 27 states, 2004, 2008, and 2012. *Morbidity and Mortality Weekly Report, 66*(6), 153–158. http://dx.doi.org/10.15585/mmwr.mm6606a1

Krempasky, C., Harris, M., Abern, L., & Grimstad, F. (2020). Contraception across the transmasculine spectrum. *American Journal of Obstetrics and Gynecology, 222*(2), 134–143. https://doi.org/10.1016/ j.ajog.2019.07.043

Lacey, K. K., Jiwatram-Negron, T., & Sears, K. P. (2020). Help-seeking behaviors and barriers among Black women exposed to severe intimate partner violence: Findings from a nationally representative sample. *Violence against women, 27*(6–7), 952–972.

Lake, R. (Executive Producer), & Epstein, A. (Director). (2008). *The business of being born* [Indie Film/Documentary]. http://www.thebusinessofbeingborn.com/the-business-of-being-born/

Lee, S., & Lee, E. (2018). Predictors of intimate partner violence among pregnant women. *International Journal of Gynecology & Obstetrics, 140*(2), 159–163. https://doi.org/10.1002/ijgo.12365

Luebke, J., Kako, P., Lopez, A., Schmitt, M., Dressel, A., Klein, K., & Mkandawire-Vahlmu, L. (2023). Barriers faced by American Indian women in urban Wisconsin in seeking help following an experience of intimate partner violence. *Violence against women, 29*(11), 2080–2103.

Lutheran, A. (2020). "Home isn't always a safe place for everyone": Domestic violence shelters, hotlines, stay open during coronavirus outbreak. *Milwaukee Journal Sentinel.* https://www.jsonline.com/story/news/local/milwaukee/2020/03/22/milwaukee-domestic-violence-shelters-hotlines-open-during-coronavirus-abuse-help-covid-19/2886783001/

MacDonald, T. K. (2019). Lactation care for transgender and non-binary patients: Empowering clients and avoiding aversives. *Journal of Human Lactation, 35*(2), 223–226. https://doi.org/10.1177/ 0890334419830989

MacDorman, M. F., Barnard-Mayers, R., & Declercq, E. (2022). United States births increased by 20% from 2019 to 220. *Birth, 49,* 559–568. https://doi.org/10.1111/birt.12627

MacDorman, M. F., & Declercq, E. (2016). Trends and characteristics of United States out-of-hospital births 2004–2014: New information on risk status and access to care. *Birth, 43*(2), 116–124. https://doi.org/10.1111/birt.12228

MacDorman, M. F., & Declercq, E. (2019). Trends and state variations in out-of-hospital births in the United States, 2004-2017. *Birth, 46*(2), 279–288.

MacLean, L. R. D. (2021). Preconception, pregnancy, birthing, and lactation needs of transgender men. *Nursing for Women's Health, 25*(2), 129–138.

Madrigal-Borloz, V. (2020). *Protection against violence and discrimination based on sexual orientation and gender identity.* United Nations General Assembly [UNGA].

Maheu-Giroux, M., Sardinha, L., Stöckl, H., Meyer, S. R., Godin, A., Alexander, M., & García-Moreno, C. (2022). A framework to model global, regional, and national estimates of intimate partner violence. *BMC Medical Research Methodology, 22*(1), 1–17.

Malmquist, A., & Nieminen, K. (2021). Negotiating who gives birth and the influence of fear of childbirth: Lesbians, bisexual women and transgender people in parenting relationships. *Women and Birth, 34*(3), e271–e278.

Monterrosa, A. E. (2019). How race and gender stereotypes influence help-seeking for intimate partner violence. *Journal of Interpersonal Violence, 36*(17–18), 1–22. https://doi.org/10.1177/ 0886260519853403

Mutumba, M., Wekesa, E., & Stephenson, R. (2018). Community influences on modern contraceptive use among young women in low and middle-income countries: A cross-sectional multi-country analysis. *BMC Public Health, 18*(1), 430. https://doi.org/10.1186/s12889-018-5331-y

Myunghee, J., Thongpriwan, V., Choi, J., Choi, K. S., & Anderson, G. (2018). Decision-making about prenatal genetic testing among pregnant Korean-American women. *Midwifery, 56,* 128–134. https://doi.org/10.1016/j.midw.2017.10.003

Nakajima, M., Jebena, M. G., Taha, M., Tesfaye, M., Gudina, E., Lemieux, A., Hoffman, R., & al'Absi, M. (2017). Correlates of khat use during pregnancy: A cross-sectional study. *Addictive Behaviors, 73,* 178–184. https://doi.org/10.1016/j.addbeh.2017.05.008

National Partnership for Women & Families. (2018). *Black women's maternal health: A multifaceted approach to addressing persistent and dire health disparities, Issues brief.* http://www.nationalpartnership.org/research-library/maternal-health/black-womens-maternal-health-issue-brief.pdf

Nguyen, J. (2017). A literature review of alternative therapies for postpartum depression. *Nursing for Women's Health, 21*(5), 348–359. https://doi.org/10.1016/j.nwh.2017.07.003

Nnawulezi, N. A., & Sullivan, C. M. (2014). Oppression within safe spaces: Exploring racial microaggressions within domestic violence shelters. *Journal of Black Psychology, 40*(6), 563–591.

Oribhabor, G., Nelson, M., Buchanan-Pearl, K., & Cancarevic, I. (2020). A mother's Cry: A race to eliminate the influence of racial disparities on maternal morbidity and mortality rates among Black women in America. *Cureus, 12*(7), e9207. https://doi.org/10.7759/cureus.9207

Osterman, M. J. K., & Martin, J. A. (2018). Timing and adequacy of prenatal care in the United States, 2016. *National Vital Statistics Reports, 67*(3) https://www.cdc.gov/nchs/data/nvsr/nvsr67/nvsr67_03.pdf

Parente, S. (2018). Factors contribution to higher health care spending in the United States compared with other high-income countries. *JAMA, 319*(10), 988–990. https://doi.org/10.001/jama.2018.1149

Park, S. H., & Kim, J. I. (2023). Predictive validity of the Edinburgh postnatal depression scale and other tools for screening depression in pregnant and postpartum women: A systematic review and meta-analysis. *Archives of Gynecology and Obstetrics, 307,* 1331–1345. https://doi.org/10.1007/s00404-022-06525-0

Peitzmeier, S. M., Fedina, L., Ashwell, L., Herrenkohl, T. I., & Tolman, R. (2022). Increases in intimate partner violence during COVID-19: prevalence and correlates. *Journal of Interpersonal Violence, 37*(21–22), NP20482–NP20512.

Pérez-Escamilla, R., Martinez, J. L., & Segura-Pérez, S. (2016). Impact of the Baby-friendly Hospital Initiative on breastfeeding and child health outcomes: A systematic review. *Maternal & Child Nutrition, 12*(3), 402–417. https://doi.org/10.1111/mcn.12294

Petrosky, E., Blair, J. M., Betz, C. J., Fowler, K. A., Jack, S. P., & Lyons, B. H. (2017). Racial and ethnic differences in homicides of adult women and the role of intimate partner violence—United States, 2003–2014. *Morbidity and Mortality Weekly Report, 66*(28), 41–746. http://dx.doi.org/10.15585/mmwr.mm6628a1

Qamar, A. (2017). The postpartum tradition of Sawn Mahina in rural Punjab, Pakistan. *Journal of Ethnology and Folkloristics, 11*(1), 127–150. https://doi.org/10.1515/jef-2017-0008

Raman, S., Nicholls, R., Ritchie, J., Razee, H., & Shafiee, S. (2016). How natural is the supernatural? Synthesis of the qualitative literature from low and middle income countries on cultural practices and traditional beliefs influencing the perinatal period. *Midwifery, 39*, 87–97. https://doi.org/10.1016/j.midw.2016.05.005

Richardson, B., Price, S., & Campbell-Yeo, M. (2019). Redefining perinatal experience: A philosophical exploration of a hypothetical case of gender diversity in labour and birth. *Journal of Clinical Nursing, 28*(3–4), 703–710. https://doi.org/10.1111/jocn.14521

Rosay, A. B. (2016). Violence against American Indian and Alaska native women and men. *NIJ Journal, 277*, 38–45. http://nij.gov/journals/277/Pages/violence-against-american-indians-alaska-natives.aspx

Rosenthal, L., & Lobel, M. (2018). Gendered racism and the sexual and reproductive health of Black and Latina women. *Ethnicity & Health, 25*(1), 1–26. https://doi.org/10.1080/13557858.2018.1439896

Rountree, M. A., Granillo, T., & Bagwell-Gray, M. (2016). Promotion of Latina health: Intersectionality of IPV and risk for HIV/AIDS. *Violence Against Women, 22*, 545–564.

Rouhi, M., Rouhi, N., Vizheh, M., & Salehi, K. (2017). Male child preference: Is it a risk factor for antenatal depression among Iranian women? *British Journal of Midwifery, 9*(25), 572–578. https://doi.org/10.12968/bjom.2017.25.9.572

Roy, A., Furentes-Afflick, E., Fernald, L., & Young, S. (2018). Pica is prevalent and strongly associated with iron deficiency among Hispanic pregnant women living in the United States. *Appetite, 120*, 163–170. https://doi.org/10.1016/j.appet.2017.08.033

Sabri, B., Simonet, M., & Campbell, J. C. (2018). Risk and protective factors of intimate partner violence among South Asian immigrant women and perceived need for services. *Cultural Diversity and Ethnic Minority Psychology, 24*(3), 442–452. https:// doi.org/10.1037/cdp0000189

Salari, M. (2018). The impact of intergenerational cultural transmission on fertility decisions. *Economic Analysis and Policy, 58*, 88–99. https://doi.org/10.1016/j.eap.2018.01.003

Sardinha, L., Maheu-Giroux, M., Stöckl, H., Meyer, S. R., & García-Moreno, C. (2022). Global, regional, and national prevalence estimates of physical or sexual, or both, intimate partner violence against women in 2018. *The Lancet, 399*(10327), 803–813.

Sharma, S., van Teijlingen, E., Hundley, V., Angell, C., & Simkhada, P. (2016). Dirty and 40 days in the wilderness: Eliciting childbirth and postnatal cultural practices and beliefs in Nepal. *BMC Pregnancy and Childbirth, 16*(1), 147. https://doi.org/10.1186/s12884-016-0938-4

Shaw, D., Guise, J., Shah, N., Gemzell-Danielsson, K., Joseph, K. S., Levy, B., Wong, F., Woodd, S., & Main, E. (2016). Drivers of maternity care in high-income countries: Can health systems support women-centered care? *Lancet, 388*(10057), 2282–2295. http://dx.doi.org/10.1016/S0140-6736(16)31527-6

Shin, C.-N., Reifsnider, E., McClain, D., Jeong, M., McCormick, D. P., & Moramarco, M. (2018). Acculturation, cultural values, and breastfeeding in overweight or obese, low-income, Hispanic women at 1 month postpartum. *Journal of Human Lactation, 34*(2), 358–364. https://doi.org/10.1177/0890334417753942

Silva-Mart´inez, E. (2016). El silencio. *Violence against Women, 22*(5), 523–544. https://doi.org/10.1177/1077801215607357

Simpson, K. R. (2020). Cervical ripening and labor induction and augmentation. *Nursing for Women's Health, 24*(4), S1–S41. https://doi.org/10.1016/j.nwh.2020.04.005

Smith, I., Bentley-Edwards, K. L., El-Amin, S., & Darity, W. (2018). *Fighting at birth: Eradicating the Black-White infant mortality gap.* https://socialequity.duke.edu/sites/socialequity.duke.edu/files/site-images/EradicatingBlackInfantMortality-March2018%20FINAL.pdf

Steele, S. M., Everett, B. G., & Hughes, T. L. (2020). Influence of perceived femininity, masculinity, race/ethnicity, and socioeconomic status on intimate partner violence among sexual-minority women. *Journal of Interpersonal Violence, 35*(1–2), 453–475.

Stork, E. (2008). Understanding high-stakes decision making: Constructing a model of the decision to seek shelter from intimate partner violence. *Journal of Feminist Family Therapy, 20*(4), 299–327.

Taylor, K. (2020). Structural racism and maternal health among Black women. *The Journal of Law, Medicine & Ethics, 48*(3), 506–517. https://doi.org/10.1177/1073110520958875

Terry, M. A., Stotz, S. A., Charron-Prochownik, D., Beirne, S., Gonzales, K., & Marshall, G.; Stopping GDM Study Group (2020). Recommendations from an expert panel of health professionals regarding a gestational diabetes risk reduction intervention for American Indian/Alaska Native teens. *Pediatric Diabetes, 21*(3), 415–421.

Tonsing, J., & Barn, R. (2017). Intimate partner violence in South Asian communities: Exploring the notion of 'shame' to promote understandings of migrant women's experiences. *International Social Work, 60*(3), 628–639. https://doi.org/10.1177/0020872816655868

Troutman, M., Rafique, S., & Plowden, T. C. (2020). Are higher unintended pregnancy rates among minorities a result of disparate access to contraception? *Contraception and Reproductive Medicine, 5*. https://doi.org/10.1186/s40834-020-00118-5

UNICEF. (2022). *Female genital mutilation and the humanitarian development nexus: Practical ways to support programme-level implementation.*

United Nations Sustainable Development Group. *Transforming our world: The 2030 agenda for sustainable development A/Res/70/1.* https://sustainable development.un.org

U.S. Preventive Services Task Force. (2018). *Intimate partner violence, elder abuse, and abuse of vulnerable adults: Screening.* https://www.uspreventiveservicestaskforce.org/uspstf/recommendation/intimate-partner-violence-and-abuse-of-elderly-and-vulnerable-adults-screening

Victoria, C. G., Bahl, R., Barros, A. J. D., Franca, G. V. A., Horton, S., Krasevec, J., Murch, S., Sankar, M. J., Walker, N., & Rollins, N. C.; Lancet Breastfeeding Series Group. (2016). Breastfeeding in the 21st century: Epidemiology, mechanisms, and lifelong effect. *Lancet, 387*(10017), 475–490. https://doi.org/10.1016/S0140-6736(15)01024-7

Violence Policy Center. (2020, September). *When men murder women: An analysis of 2018 homicide data.* Violence Policy Center.

Waller, B., Harris, J., & Quinn, C. (2022). Caught in the crossroad: An intersectional Examination of African American Women intimate partner violence survivors' help seeking, trauma. *Violence & Abuse, 23*(4), 1235–1248. https://doi.org/10.1177/152483838021991303

Westoff, C., & Bietsch, K. (2015). Religion and reproductive behavior in Sub-Saharan Africa. *DHS Analytical Studies 48.* ICF International. https://dhsprogram.com/pubs/pdf/AS48/AS48.pdf

Whitfield, D. L., Coulter, R. W., Langenderfer-Magruder, L., & Jacobson, D. (2021). Experiences of intimate partner violence among lesbian, gay, bisexual, and transgender college students: The intersection of gender, race, and sexual orientation. *Journal of Interpersonal Violence, 36*(11–12), NP6040–NP6064.

Wilson, B., & Kuha, J. (2017). Residential segregation and the fertility of immigrants and their descendants. *Population, Space and Place, 24*(3), e2098. https://doi.org/10.1002/psp.2098

Withers, M., Kharazmi, N., & Lim, E. (2018). Traditional beliefs and practices in pregnancy, childbirth and postpartum: A review of the evidence from Asian countries. *Midwifery, 56,* 158–170. https://doi.org/10.1016/j.midw.2017.10.019

World Health Organization (2012). *Understanding and addressing violence against women: Intimate partner violence* (Vol. No. WHO/RHR/12.36). World Health Organization.

World Health Organization (WHO). (2015). *Maternal mortality.* http://www.who.int/news-room/fact-sheets/detail/maternal-mortality

World Health Organization (WHO). (2016). *WHO recommendations on antenatal care for a positive pregnancy experience.* http://www.who.int/reproductivehealth/publications/maternal_perinatal_health/anc-positive-pregnancy-experience/en/

World Health Organization (WHO). (2018a). *WHO recommendations: Intrapartum care for positive childbirth experience.* http://www.who.int/reproductivehealth/publications/intrapartum-care-guidelines/en/

World Health Organization (WHO). (2018b). *Female genital mutilation.* http://www.who.int/news-room/fact-sheets/detail/female-genital-mutilation

World Health Organization (WHO). (2021). *Infant and young child feeding.* https://www.who.int/news-room/fact-sheets/detail/infant-and-young-child-feeding#:~:text=WHO%20and%20UNICEF%20recommend%3A,years%20of%20age%20or%20beyond

Wouk, K., Stuebe, A. M., & Meltzer-Brody, S. (2016). Postpartum mental health and breastfeeding practices: An analysis using the 2010–2011 pregnancy risk assessment monitoring system. *Maternal and Child Health Journal, 21*(3), 636–647. https://doi.org/10.1007/s10995-016-2150-6

Yoder, H., & Hardy, L. (2018). Midwifery and antenatal care for Black women: A narrative review. *SAGE Open, 8*(1) https://doi.org/10.1177/2158244017752220

Zurynski, Y., Sureshkumar, P., Phu, A., & Elliot, E. (2015). Female genital mutilation and cutting: A systematic literature review of health professionals' knowledge, attitudes and clinical practice. *BMC International Health and Human Rights, 15,* 32. https://doi.org/10.1186/s12914-015-0070-y

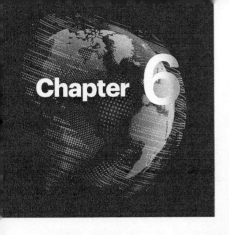

Chapter 6

Transcultural Perspectives in the Nursing Care of Children

• Heather M. Bowers

Key Terms

Adverse childhood
    experiences
Discipline

Extended family
Family
Multicultural
Multiracial

Parental attachment
Play
Poverty
Refugees

Learning Objectives

1. Explain family and community influences on children's cultural development.
2. Identify factors leading to an increase in multicultural children and families.
3. Describe family structures and role expectations.
4. Understand the influence of parenting style and culture on implemented methods of discipline.
5. Analyze the nurse's role in promoting optimal child health while integrating family and community cultural influences.

Introduction

Culture influences children's growth, development, and identities. Family and community influences guide a child's cultural development. Travel, technology, immigration, and adoption are examples of international integration that have led to increased blending of cultural beliefs and practices. The child's culture is formed through the interaction of these influences (see Fig. 6-1). Healthcare providers including nurses are responsible for assessing and providing

education about health and development topics at every encounter with children and families. The unique cultural and community context of families and children must be applied to enhance the effectiveness of these encounters.

Family

One of the main influences in a child's cultural development is the **family**. In Madeleine Leininger's Sunrise Enabler, kinship and social factors are identified as key factors that influence

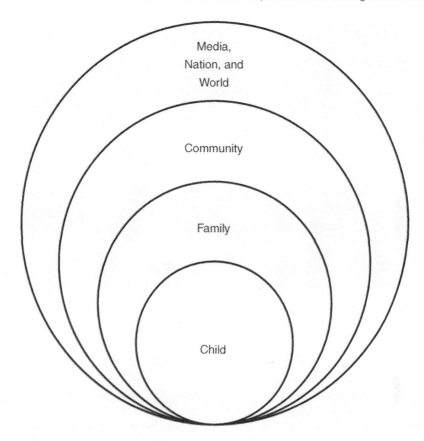

Figure 6-1. The layers of influence on a child's cultural development.

a person's beliefs and expressions of culture (McFarland & Wehbe-Alamah, 2015). This shows the importance of gaining an understanding of the important people influencing a child and family's cultural and healthcare decisions. Family can be defined in many ways based on genetic relationships, roles, functions, households, or community interactions (Giger & Haddad, 2021; Kyle & Carman, 2021). Due to this variety of definitions, when considering a child's family, the nurse should address biologic, legal, and social definitions in addition to the child's perspective.

Family Structures

Prior definitions of family focused on a nuclear family as a man and woman of similar ethnic and generational cultures who married and had children (Giger & Haddad, 2021). However, half of families today do not meet the definition of a nuclear family (American Academy of Pediatrics, 2022). The family arrangements that exist today are not all named or defined. Parents may represent differing cultures or generations (see Fig. 6-2). A married couple may not have children due to either choice or medical reasons (Giger & Haddad, 2021). Parents may become divorced, leading to potential fear and confusion in children based on role changes or household events prior to the divorce (Kyle & Carman, 2021). Single-parent families involve a parent raising children alone for reasons such as choice, divorce, death, or other circumstances (Giger & Haddad, 2021). Blended families also occur as one or two single parents marry and "blend" the family structure, possibly birthing children together. Additional

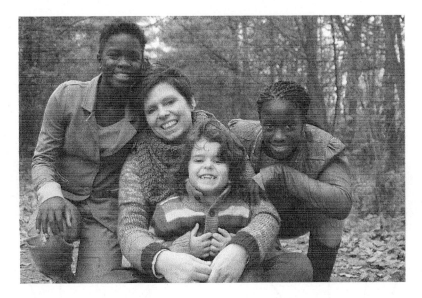

Figure 6-2. A single-parent multicultural family. (From DNF Style/Shutterstock.com)

variations of families include same gender parents, unmarried parents, foster or adoptive parents, siblings parenting their younger siblings, or communal living of people who may or may not be related (AAP, 2022; Giger & Haddad, 2021; Kyle & Carman, 2021).

A family may choose to live with or have close interactions with **extended family** such as grandparents, aunts, uncles, and cousins, either out of necessity or to reinforce the family and cultural identity (Dockery, 2020). There has been an increase in families where grandparents are raising their grandchildren (Giger & Haddad, 2021). The biologic parent may or may not be involved with the grandparent caregiver (Freeman et al., 2019). This family situation can lead to role confusion and complicated family dynamics for all involved. Children raised by grandparents can experience stress related to the situation, especially when the biologic parent is not involved. However, when the biologic parent cannot fulfill their role, children have enhanced outcomes and family connections when raised by extended family members like grandparents compared with other foster care experiences.

Children are also highly influenced by other people in the community (Kearney & Haskins, 2020). Children may see teachers, school staff, and neighborhood role models as supportive figures. Youth may even admire celebrities and other adults they see in the media. Nurses should inquire about sources of support, mentorship, and role models for children. Children are also highly influenced by their peers (Lofton et al., 2019). This peer influence may lead children to make choices in attempts to fit in. Children may act as bullies or strive to avoid being bullied (AAP, 2021). Teens are especially susceptible to engaging in risky behaviors as part of exploring identity development and peer influences (Alderman & Breuner, 2019). Youth who identify as LGBTQ+ can experience additional stigma and bullying from peers and parents, leading to poorer physical and mental health outcomes. Trusted peers and community members are important influences for development, especially during adolescence, so nurses should assess for these roles in a teen's life. Evidence-Based Practice 6-1 describes one evidence-based approach to improve healthcare for youth of varied sexual orientations and gender identities.

Promoting Access to Culturally Competent Healthcare for LGBTQ+ Youth

Many adolescents identify themselves according to their sexuality and gender including lesbian, gay, bisexual, transgender, or queer (LGBTQ+) (Hermosillo et al., 2022). Youth representing this group are susceptible to health disparities due to systemic barriers or personal avoidance in seeking care. Barriers include limitations in insurance coverage, financial resources, and availability of culturally competent care. Avoidance may occur out of fear of discrimination, previous unsupportive experiences with health professionals, or lower health literacy. These systemic and individual factors lead to inconsistent primary healthcare experiences and poorer sexual and mental health outcomes in LGBTQ+ youth.

Development of an Evidence-Based Program

Despite identification of the need for health professionals to display competence in caring for LGBTQ+ clients, many nurses lack training, confidence, and experience in providing care to this population (Hermosillo et al., 2022). Evidence-based recommendations to increase the comfort of LGBTQ+ youth clients include asking questions about sexual and gender identity, designing a welcoming space through selection of inclusive signs and restrooms, and promoting media to increase health education and awareness of access to supportive care environments.

In response to the identified need to increase access to healthcare for LGBTQ+ youth, a clinic on the West Side of Chicago implemented a multifaceted project (Hermosillo et al., 2022). One area of focus was a continuing education plan for staff. The continuing education included best practices for assessment and documentation of information related to sexual and gender identity, awareness of implicit bias, and the importance of apologizing when needed. The second focus involved redesigning the clinic to be more inclusive including art selections, available magazines, revision of documents including consent forms, and clearly displaying the nondiscrimination policy. The third focus was on community outreach including electronic marketing that highlighted that the clinic's care was targeted for those identifying as LGBTQ+. This marketing was shared with the local school system and the relevant student organization.

Program Evaluation and Implications

A review of charts indicated that the percentage of LGBTQ+ adolescent clients increased from 7% to 10% (Hermosillo et al., 2022). Staff demonstrated increased knowledge of documentation of sexuality and gender identity through an increase in mean pretest and posttest scores, though mean scores for three questions relating to terminology and documentation decreased from the pretest to posttest. This shows the need for ongoing education including terminology and best practices for documentation. Inconsistent documentation of sexuality and gender identity assessment led to identification of the need for updated templates in the electronic health record and continued staff education. Long-term evaluation including the effectiveness of the clinic redesign and electronic marketing materials is needed. Identified limitations to the project include the impact of the pandemic and the lack of LGBTQ+ stakeholders involved in designing the project. Nursing students and practicing nurses should seek education on culturally competent care for this population.

Reference: Hermosillo, D., Cygan, H. R., Lemke, S., McIntosh, E., & Vail, M. (2022). Achieving health equity for LGBTQ+ adolescents. *Journal of Continuing Education in Nursing, 53*(8), 348–354. https://doi.org/10.3928/00220124-20220706-05

Family Interactions

Families have varying expectations for interaction, communication, and play. These expectations may be rooted in broader cultures or related to community and employment situations (Kearney & Haskins, 2020; Lansford, 2022). Limitations in resources can lead to parental stress and lesser attachment to children, especially if parents spend more time working than with children. Employment policies such as parental leave time at birth or throughout the child's life can impact **parental attachment** (Lansford, 2022).

Expectations for physical contact vary across cultures (Lansford, 2022). Some cultures emphasize prompt response to infant cries and increased skin-to-skin time including co-sleeping (Lansford, 2022; Mandlik & Kamat, 2020). This includes cultures where harvesting and similar physical labor are important tasks for parents who may carry infants in slings while working. Families from other cultures may prioritize separation through the use of strollers, infant seats, and separate sleeping rooms (Lansford, 2022). These parents may also emphasize the development of self-soothing practices by infants and young children (Mandlik & Kamat, 2020).

Child role expectations and developmental timelines also vary across cultures. In cultures with a greater focus on manual tasks, children may be expected to help with chores such as carrying water from an early age (Lansford, 2022). Parents in these cultures often prioritize work over education, especially in response to financial demands. In other cultures with conveniences like piped water, parental expectations for their children prioritize education and cognitive development. These cultures may also prioritize school attendance and career development.

Communication with children, including during **play**, is important for the development of language skills and understanding of societal expectations (Rochanavibhata & Marian, 2022). Cultures vary in the style and length of conversations between parents and children. In cultures with a focus on cognitive development, parents are more likely to engage in singing, talking, reading, and playing (Lansford, 2022). Through play, some families demonstrate a cultural emphasis on independence, assertiveness, and more distant personal relationships, with children in these cultures more likely to give commands and display disagreement (Rochanavibhata & Marian, 2022). Other families demonstrate an emphasis on interdependence and closer interpersonal relationships, with children voicing polite requests and displaying agreement with others. Another variation of communication during play is seen in the focus of the terminology that is used. Parents in some cultures emphasize language about what the child is doing while other cultures emphasize language identifying objects and building vocabulary. However, in another cultural variation, some parents minimize speaking to children related to a belief that infants are possessed by evil spirits through being spoken to by adults (Lansford, 2022).

Interaction styles vary across cultures, influencing the roles and communication styles that children adopt. Some cultures place an emphasis on collaboration while others emphasize hierarchy and independent roles (Dayton et al., 2022). Families may demonstrate positive coping strategies such as problem solving and social support or negative coping strategies such as avoidance, ignorance, or emotional outbursts (Mayo et al., 2022). In cultures that prioritize independence, families promote children's pursuits of personal ambitions and dreams (Motti-Stefanidi, 2018). In cultures with a collectivist approach, families are more likely to dictate the life plans of children to align with family expectations for priorities, obedience, respect, and dignity.

Families have varying expectations for communication and education of children related to their health education and physical development. Sexuality and puberty are topics that some cultures consider taboo or private (Gozansky, 2018). Previously, these topics were left for families to choose to avoid or to educate children about. In some countries, schools are allowed to include fact-based educational approaches on sexuality and puberty. Children often receive education on sexuality and puberty through media, which can be related to a cultural expectation or the curiosity of children who consider fact-based school approaches as inadequate. Nurses should assess the accuracy of information that children are receiving and promote open communication and accurate information from parents.

Family Discipline

Cultural perspectives influence parenting styles and methods of **discipline** (Sahithya et al., 2019). Authoritarian styles have a greater focus on strict obedience, respect, and discipline. Democratic parenting styles focus on the development of open relationships that allow independence and expression. Parenting styles may include a combination of these approaches.

Parenting styles also align with expectations for communication and authority. Some cultures expect autonomy, responsibility, and self-reliance for youth while other cultures expect full obedience to authority even into early adulthood (Durà-Vilà & Hodes, 2017). Cultural influences also guide when adolescents are expected to independently make decisions, including life choices for education, career, finances, family, and religious practices. Families enforcing strict adherence to religious practice may experience tension as adolescents desire to explore their own beliefs and make their own life decisions.

Parents utilize a variety of methods of discipline (Lansford, 2022). The selection of a discipline method is often rooted in the parent's perspective on parental authority and beliefs about necessary or effective means of discipline. These disciplinary measures range from nonviolent discipline through socialization and building respect to corporal punishment. While corporal punishment is illegal in many countries, some parents still believe that it is the only effective means of discipline. While 60% of children around the world have reported receiving some form of physical punishment, the highest incidences of physical punishment and corporal punishment are concentrated in countries where this discipline remains legal (World Health Organization, 2021). In some cultures, physical discipline can be performed by parents and by those in the community such as school staff. Nurses and healthcare providers are in a key position to explore parents' choices for discipline and share recommendations for appropriate discipline measures.

Immigrants and Refugees

In 2020, an estimated 36 million children were identified as international migrants (UNICEF, 2021b). This number included millions of children, some without their families, who were seeking refuge or asylum after being displaced from their home countries (**refugees**) (UNICEF, 2021b). While some of these children have been forced to leave their home countries due to situations like war, terrorism, and famine, other children and families have chosen to migrate in pursuit of a better life (Motti-Stefanidi, 2018).

When reaching a host country, families are often limited to working jobs with lesser pay (Motti-Stefanidi, 2018). This can lead to children working to support the family or older children taking on a greater role in managing the household including caring for siblings while the parent is at work (Yakhnich & Michael, 2022). Migrant youth may take on additional burdens including serving as a language translator for parents and helping the family to navigate the complex educational and healthcare systems of the destination (Nguyen-Truong et al., 2019; Yakhnich & Michael, 2022). Differences between the expectations and beliefs of the home country and destination country can lead to tension (Lansford, 2022). Family tensions may increase as children distance themselves from their parents while assimilating into the culture of the destination country (Yakhnich & Michael, 2022). Cultural differences can also lead to tension with healthcare professionals who may not understand cultural health practices of their patients' home countries (Lansford, 2022).

Cultural Identity

Children form cultural identities as part of their development. Children are first introduced to culture through family experiences (Atkin & Yoo, 2019). Families can share their culture with children through cooking traditional foods, attending cultural events, participating in religious practices, or traveling to other countries. Families may also select media including books, toys, music, and other art forms to teach children about various cultures.

The number of children whose parents represent multiple racial groups is increasing, leading to an increase in children who identify as bicultural, multicultural, or multiracial (Atkin & Yoo, 2019; Giger & Haddad, 2021). This can lead to confusion in the development of the child or family's cultural identity. The child may feel confused and a sense of not fitting with any racial group, leading to further confusion about one's role in society (Atkin & Yoo, 2019). Families are left to make decisions about how to support the child's cultural identity by emphasizing one or multiple familial cultural influences. Tension may be enhanced as the child grows and desires to develop a culture different from what the family established. Parents of **multiracial** children also face a tension between preparing the child for discrimination versus avoiding such topics despite child inquiries. Despite the hesitation, open communication within families is important.

Many children are adopted by families that represent other cultures from the same or other countries (Benoit et al., 2018). This can also introduce complexity, as the family must decide whether to focus on the child's birth culture or to raise the child in the culture of the adoptive family. The adoptive family may lack an understanding of the child's birth culture. The development of a bicultural or **multicultural** identity allows the child to develop a connection through knowledge and skills for both cultures. Case Study 6-1 describes the nurse's role in fostering open conversation between Jamal and his parents who represent another culture.

Parents use cultural health practices to display care for their children, but health professionals who don't understand may see the practices as abuse or neglect (Lansford, 2022). Many of these practices are related to beliefs that illnesses come from sources such as air, emotion, temperature, diet, or spiritual forces (Fowler et al., 2022). Nurses may not be familiar with practices such as cupping and coining that families may implement to promote healing (Lansford, 2022). Other cultural remedies include teas, oils, and massages (Fowler et al., 2022). Cultural beliefs may also influence family perspectives on health topics including fevers, vaccines, and sleep practices (Mandlik & Kamat, 2020). Parents often wish to discuss their cultural health practices and beliefs with their health providers, but often do not out of fear that the provider will not understand or agree with the practice (Fowler et al., 2022). Nurses should welcome discussions with families about cultural health practices and beliefs, promoting the family's trust in the healthcare system (Mandlik & Kamat, 2020). Even when nurses do not understand the cultural practices and beliefs of a family, nurses must recognize that the parents are acting out of a desire to care for their child and integrate cultural health practices in plans of care (Oliveira & da Rocha, 2019). Evidence-Based Practice 6-2 provides insight for communicating with Spanish-speaking mothers of hospitalized children when the nurse has a different language and culture.

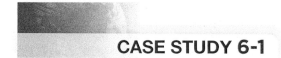

CASE STUDY 6-1

The Talk

The nurse is providing care for 11-year-old Jamal. Jamal, who is Black, was adopted as an infant by a White family. During the initial screening, the nurse notices that Jamal seems hesitant to talk about school, friends, or even family. Upon further questioning, he comments "I just feel like I don't fit in. On social media I see all of these scary things happening to Black people. Then when I was walking home from the park last week the police stopped me and asked a bunch of questions about what I was doing there. I have tried to talk to my parents, but they don't understand. They say it's all in my head or that only people who do bad things get stopped by the police."

The nurse feels uncertain about how to respond. She knows that the parents should be involved in a conversation like this, but because she does not know how to proceed, she approaches her charge nurse. The charge nurse replies, "I have seen many Black children impacted by the events in the media and by their own experiences. We can come up with some points to discuss with his parents."

When the nurse returns to Jamal's room, his parents are present. The nurse asks the parents if they've talked to Jamal about his experiences. They reply "Did he tell you about that race stuff again? He makes this stuff up. Color is not as big of a deal as he makes it out to be."

The nurse reassures Jamal's parents that his experiences and feelings are real, and their response is also normal. The nurse replies that parents should have age-appropriate conversations about race with their children. Infants as young as 6 months can recognize differences including features attributed to race with beliefs about race and culture adopted by the age of 12 (Anderson & Dougé, 2019). Youth have experienced increased media exposure to race-based bias and violence including attacks by law enforcement officials on unarmed Black persons (Anderson et al., 2022). In addition, many Black people have lived experiences of discrimination in their communities or

from law enforcement in addition to experiencing persistent inequities rooted in systemic racism (Anderson et al., 2022; Sullivan et al., 2021). Studies have found that in many cities in America, Black and Latino youth are more likely to experience force and to be arrested by law enforcement officers (Maroney & Zuckerman, 2018). Based on this, Black parents often have conversations with their children about race to build ethnic pride while also focusing on safety and survival (Anderson et al., 2022). White parents are less likely to discuss race with their children, promoting a stance of color blindness that denies different experiences rooted in race (Sullivan et al., 2021). In comparison with White parents, Black parents are more concerned that their children will experience bias and are more likely to discuss racism and race-based inequalities with their children, with public awareness of this difference heightened after George Floyd's death (Sullivan et al., 2021).

The mother acknowledges that Jamal's experiences and feelings might be different from her own and asks, "How do I talk to Jamal about this? Where do I even start?"

The nurse has identified some evidence-based recommendations for race discussions with children. Parents should first identify their own racial biases and then can talk to their children about racial differences, bias, confronting racism, and showing kindness to diverse people (Anderson & Dougé, 2019). Age-appropriate strategies can include identifying differences in a positive way, having open conversations with children, and creating an atmosphere where children feel comfortable talking about their experiences and asking questions (Anderson & Dougé, 2019).

The nurse has also reviewed the evidence and identified some of the key points related to "The Talk" that Black parents regularly have with their children. This conversation often focuses on racial differences, racial profiling, bias, and strategies for diffusing tense encounters with the goal of safety (Anderson et al., 2022). Parents should create space for open conversations and use questions to get information about the child's experiences, including in school or with law enforcement (Anderson et al., 2022; Saleem, 2019). During an experience of discrimination or when approached by law enforcement, the primary goal is maintaining safety through keeping hands visible, remaining calm, cooperating, answering questions, and not running no matter how the child feels (Anderson et al., 2022; Maroney & Zuckerman, 2018). Once the experience is over and the child is safe, a parent or another trusted adult should be notified (Anderson et al., 2022; Maroney & Zuckerman, 2018). Whether or not the child or parent has experienced these situations, parents should acknowledge that the encounters portrayed in media and told by those in the community are real (Anderson et al., 2022). Children can be taught about their rights and informed about ways to take action to promote accountability and awareness (Anderson et al., 2022). However, parents should also promote balance by sharing positive experiences with people of other races and with law enforcement (Anderson et al., 2022). Parents can even collaborate with other parents or teachers at the child's school to have conversations about race, concerns of racism, and ways to incorporate diversity in the classroom and the school environment (Saleem, 2019).

Outcome: Jamal's parents thank the nurse for taking the time to share this information. They also apologize to Jamal for not believing his experiences or acknowledging his feelings.

Jamal's family have begun to have open conversations about his feelings and experiences.

The nurse has recognized the importance of addressing topics like diversity, racism, and bias. After seeing how Jamal was impacted by his experiences, the nurse recommends to the charge nurse that questions about racism and race-related stress are added to the nursing admission screening. As she was reviewing evidence, she found that recent publications to guide nursing practice include a focus on diversity, equity, inclusion, and preparing nurses to act as change agents who advocate and promote health policy that addresses health inequalities, discrimination, systemic injustices, and disparities in social determinants of health (American Association of Colleges of Nursing, 2021; National Association of Sciences, Engineering, and Medicine, 2021). She requests the establishment of a committee that will develop staff education to increase awareness of these topics and share ideas for advocacy.

References: American Association of Colleges of Nursing. (2021). *The essentials: Core competencies for professional nursing practice.* https://www.aacnnursing.org/AACN-Essentials; Anderson, A., & Dougé, J. (2019). *Talking to children about racial bias.* American Academy of Pediatrics. https://www.healthychildren.org/English/healthy-living/emotional-wellness/Building-Resilience/Pages/Talking-to-Children-About-Racial-Bias.aspx; Anderson, L. A., O'Brien Caughy, M., & Owen, M. T. (2022). "The talk" and parenting while Black in America: Centering race, resistance, and refuge. *Journal of Black Psychology*, *48*(3-4), 475–506. https://doi.org/10.1177/00957984211034294; Maroney, T., & Zuckerman, B. (2018). "The Talk," Physician version: Special considerations for African American, male adolescents. *Pediatrics*, *141*(2), 1–3. https://doi.org/10.1542/peds.2017-1462; National Academies of Sciences, Engineering, and Medicine. (2021). *The future of nursing 2020-2030: Charting a path to achieve health equity.* The National Academies Press. https://doi.org/10.17226/25982; Saleem, F. (2019, September 17). *Is your teen racially and culturally comfortable at school?* Successful Black Parenting. https://successfulblackparenting.com/2019/09/17/is-your-teen-racially-and-culturally-comfortable-at-school/; Sullivan, J. N., Eberhardt, J. L., & Roberts, S. O. (2021). Conversations about race in Black and White US families: Before and after George Floyd's death. *Proceedings of the National Academy of Sciences*, *118*(38), 1. https://doi.org/10.1073/pnas.2106366118

Supporting the Needs of Spanish-Speaking Parents of Hospitalized Children

Communication between pediatric nurses and the parents of hospitalized children is important for providing optimal care. However, language can be a barrier that hinders the communication between the nurse and the parents even in parents who can speak some English (Stephen et al., 2023). To learn more about the impact of language barriers and cultural needs of Spanish speaking parents with limited English proficiency, one study interviewed parents who were from Mexico, lived in the United States, and had children who were hospitalized.

Three themes were identified from the interview responses (Stephen et al., 2023). One was the important role of the mother to manage the child's care and the family at home. As the mother prioritized staying with the hospitalized child, other family members had to care for any other children at home. This separation from other family members was a source of concern for the mother. However, mothers prioritized their role of caring for their child through feeding, diapering, monitoring the child for pain or fear, and notifying the nurse when assistance was needed. The mothers also shared a desire to consistently be updated on the child's status and included in the child's plan of care and interventions, but this did not happen often due to the language barrier. Another theme was negative emotions including fear and worry related to the unknown. Even though some nurses spoke Spanish or used an interpreter, there were still information gaps and a desire to learn how to care for the child's needs. The third theme was the importance of compassionate, attentive care.

Mothers prioritized affect above clinical skills when determining how caring a nurse was. The mothers identified caring nurses as those who included mothers in decision making and communicated with mothers and children.

Clinical Implications

Nurses should seek to build relationships with patients and their parents even in the presence of a language barrier (Stephen et al., 2023). Nurses can display a caring, attentive demeanor even without words. Interpreters should be used to keep the mother updated on the patient's status, provide education on caring for the child, and address the mother's questions or concerns. Nurses must always keep in mind the CLAS standards (Office of Minority Health, 2018) that require organizations to offer language assistance to individuals with limited English proficiency and use competent individuals to provide language assistance rather than untrained individuals. In addition, nurses should address the concerns of the mother regarding her children and other family members who are at home.

References: Office of Minority Health. (2018). *The national CLAS standards*. https://www.minorityhealth.hhs.gov/omh/browse.aspx?lvl=2&lvlid=53; Stephen, J. M., Zoucha, R., Cazzell, M., & Devido, J. (2023). Cultural care needs of Spanish speaking parents with limited English proficiency whose children are hospitalized: An ethnonursing study. *Journal of Pediatric Nursing*, 69, 62–70. https://doi.org/10.1016/j.pedn.2022.12.019

Children With Disabilities

Estimates are that more than 240 million children around the world experience some form of disability or impairment (UNICEF, 2021a). These disabilities may be present from birth or develop during childhood. Disabilities can lead to impairments in function, activity, or participation. Despite the 2030 Agenda for Sustainable Development's emphasis on not leaving people behind, children in many societies are left behind due to barriers to support, education, nutrition, play, and social protection. The varied needs of these children, combined with environmental barriers and lower socioeconomic status, lead to an increased risk of infection and poorer physical outcomes. Children from minority ethnicity and low socioeconomic backgrounds are more susceptible to health disparities and inequitable access to care (Morone et al., 2022). Families caring for children with complex medical needs may feel a sense of burden that is enhanced when encountering barriers or limited resources (Im & Kim, 2021). These children and their families need a supportive community (Morone et al., 2022). Nurses are in a key role to advocate for supportive policies, cultural practices, educational opportunities, and environments for equitable opportunities for these children (UNICEF, 2021a).

Food and Nutrition

Nutrition is important for healthy growth and development of children, and food selection can be an important part of a family's culture. Some families prioritize traditional foods and cooking methods as part of maintaining culture or as a form of cultural healing remedy (Chatham & Mixer, 2021). Many children voice a preference for foods representative of the family's culture (Lofton et al., 2019). Children's food preferences are also influenced by the broader culture, as media portrays celebrities or other youth eating or cooking different foods. While social media can be a tool to learn about new foods or increase the social aspects of food for youth, inaccurate information may be presented. Food can also be used to build community or show hospitality (Opalinski et al., 2017). One way that food can be used in these community settings is to recruit youth participation in community events, but the foods selected for this purpose are often high in fat and carbohydrates. Nurses should provide education about nutritional options while integrating a family's beliefs and a child's preferences. Nurses can also advocate for healthy food options at community events.

Childhood obesity is increasing in many countries, which is concerning due to correlations with decreased physical and mental health outcomes (Cunningham et al., 2022). Childhood experiences with lower socioeconomic status and increased food insecurity correlate with increased rates of childhood obesity (Cunningham et al., 2022; Gross & Mendelsohn, 2019). In the United States, the highest increase in childhood obesity rates has been in children from ethnic minorities including non-Hispanic Black children (Chatham & Mixer, 2021; Cunningham et al., 2022). In the United States, these ethnic minority groups are often disproportionately impacted by social, neighborhood, and economic barriers to healthy foods (Chatham & Mixer, 2021). Some neighborhood and socioeconomic barriers that impact child obesity include a lack of transportation or other resources for after-school sports, lack of access to safe parks for outdoor play, or selection of low-cost but energy-dense foods instead of produce and other healthy foods, which may be related to cost or limited availability (Chatham & Mixer, 2021; Morone et al., 2022). Nurses can advocate for equitable access to safe activity and affordable healthy foods.

Community and Life Experiences

The environment and community can be sources of **adverse childhood experiences** (National Center for Injury Prevention and Control, 2021). These can include family situations including violence or suicide, family exposure to mental illness or incarceration, and community impacts such as homelessness, discrimination, food insecurity, and systemic racism that can lead to generational poverty. These experiences can lead to lifelong negative impacts due to toxic stress and competing focuses. Children from minority Black, Hispanic, or lower socioeconomic backgrounds experience a higher incidence of adverse childhood experiences (Goldstein et al., 2021). In the absence of supportive adults, these children also suffer more significant impacts from these experiences. Nurses should inquire about the adverse experiences children are exposed to, assess sources of support, and advocate for community policies and resources to address these experiences.

Poverty

Poverty is a significant barrier to healthy growth and development. Children are disproportionately impacted by poverty, with poverty rates exacerbated through disasters including the recent COVID-19 pandemic (Schmidt et al., 2021). When comparing the cognitive development of children across socioeconomic statuses, disparities are evident even prior to 2 years of age (Wodtke et al., 2022). Children from countries with higher poverty rates and lower education rates have increased morbidity and mortality (Poulain et al., 2020). Experiencing poverty as children can lead to stress experiences with long-term outcomes including poorer mental health, physical health, financial, and educational outcomes with increased vulnerability

to infections (Mayo et al., 2022; Schmidt et al., 2021). Parents may experience depression, arguments, or substance use disorders while responding to the stresses of poverty, increasing the stressful experiences for the children in these families (Mayo et al., 2022). Families may live in communities with additional stressors including crowding, noise pollution, or violence. Children living in communities with low socioeconomic status are faced with increased poverty levels, violence, health hazards including unsafe drinking water and older buildings that may contain lead, and environmental barriers such as pollution or inadequate parks (see Fig. 6-3) (Poulain et al., 2020; Wodtke et al., 2022). In addition, children from communities with socioeconomic disadvantage have significantly lower school readiness scores and reduced vocabularies (Lipscomb et al., 2019; Wodtke et al., 2022). Poverty also exacerbates inequalities in power and resources, leading to greater community disparities (Schmidt et al., 2021).

Children may experience homelessness. These children may be staying in cars, abandoned

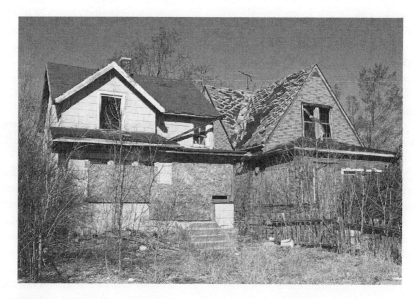

Figure 6-3. Abandoned buildings that may be present in a low-income neighborhood, leading to potential safety hazards for children. (From Henryk Stadura/Shutterstock.com)

buildings, homeless shelters, transitional housing, shared housing, or temporary lodging such as motels (Gultekin et al., 2020). In the United States, during the 2020–2021 school year over one million children were identified as homeless (NCHE, 2022). Children who have experienced homelessness have increased rates of asthma, obesity, abnormal blood lead levels, infectious diseases, malnutrition, behavioral health challenges, delays in development and social skills, and toxic stress responses (Gultekin et al., 2020). Nurses should assess children's living arrangements and advocate for availability of safe and affordable housing.

Violence

Around the world, children are exposed to violence in many forms including wars, school shootings, domestic violence, and community violence. Thousands of American children are injured or killed through firearm violence every year (Rajan et al., 2019). Beyond the physical injuries to these children, additional impacts include the effects of hearing gunshots and experiencing the loss of a loved one. Minority youth, especially those identified as Black, and youth from low socioeconomic status backgrounds have reported higher rates of exposure to homicide (Turner et al., 2021). Exposure to violence can be an adverse childhood experience leading to a posttraumatic stress response (Rajan et al., 2019). A significant correlation exists between a child experiencing homicide of a family or friend and displaying symptoms of trauma (Turner et al., 2021). Indirect exposure to community violence has correlated with negative health effects, decreased memory, increased aggression and hyperactivity, and impairments in learning and self-regulation (Bergen-Cico et al., 2018). Even the perception of living in unsafe neighborhoods has correlated with decreased standardized exam performance (Bergen-Cico et al., 2018). Nurses should gather information about the communities where their patients live and be advocates for resources to promote community safety and support.

Summary

Nurses care for patients and families from a variety of cultural backgrounds. Families and communities are influential in child growth and development through roles and organization, communication styles, expectations for play and work, health practices, and access to resources. Travel, technology, immigration, and adoption are some factors that lead to integrated cultural practices and beliefs. Nurses can provide culturally sensitive care to children by integrating cultural healing methods and providing education that is culturally sensitive. Nurses should also assess the communities that children come from and advocate for increased safety and access to resources.

REVIEW QUESTIONS

1. Compare and contrast the nuclear family with three other family structures.
2. Identify parental approaches to communication, interaction, and play. Describe how these approaches relate to the child's social development and parental choice of discipline.
3. Evaluate the influence of community factors in children's cultural development. Explain the impact of chronic illness, poverty, and violence on the children's physical and cultural development.

CRITICAL THINKING ACTIVITIES

1. Have a conversation with a peer from a different cultural background from your own. Discuss your peer's family structure, parenting style, family interactions, choices of discipline, and health practices. Compare and contrast your peer's experience with your own family experience.

2. Refugee families may encounter many barriers when settling in a destination country. What resources are available in your local

community to support refugee families? Are these resources easy to navigate, especially for those who do not speak the dominant language? Consider access to food, housing, employment, healthcare, childcare, and education.

3. When caring for a child with a chronic illness or disability, ask the parents about access to care and support. What are the family's greatest strengths? What are the family's greatest needs? What are the family's beliefs for the long-term outcomes of the child? Does your community have the resources this family needs?

4. A child's cultural identity is influenced by many family, peer, and community factors. Reflect on your own cultural practices and beliefs including expectations for childhood roles, communication, and responses to health and illness. How did your practices and beliefs develop? How do they compare with the family and community you grew up with? Have they changed over time?

5. Children may encounter many adverse childhood experiences in their home and larger community including exposure to poverty and violence. Explore ways that nurses can be involved with individual patients and the larger community to minimize community exposure to adverse childhood experiences and mitigate the long-term negative effects of these experiences.

REFERENCES

Alderman, E. M., & Breuner, C. C. (2019). Unique needs of the adolescent. *Pediatrics*, *144*(6), 1–12. https://doi.org/10.1542/peds.2019-3150

American Academy of Pediatrics (AAP). (2021, October 4). *Bullying: It's not ok.* https://www.healthychildren.org/English/safety-prevention/at-play/Pages/Bullying-Its-Not-Ok.aspx

American Academy of Pediatrics (AAP). (2022). *Types of families.* https://www.healthychildren.org/English/family-life/family-dynamics/types-of-families/Pages/default.aspx

Atkin, A. L., & Yoo, H. C. (2019). Familial racial-ethnic socialization of multiracial American youth: A systematic review of the literature with MultiCrit. *Developmental Review*, *53*, 100869. https://doi.org/10.1016/j.dr.2019.100869

Benoit, L., Harf, A., Sarmiento, L., Skandrani, S., & Rose Moro, M. (2018). Shifting views and building bonds: Narratives of internationally adopted children about their dual culture. *Transcultural Psychiatry*, *55*(3), 405–427. https://doi.org/10.1177/1363461518764250

Bergen-Cico, D., Lane, S. D., Keefe, R. H., Larsen, D. A., Panasci, A., Salaam, N., Jennings-Bey, T., & Rubinstein, R. A. (2018). Community gun violence as a social determinant of elementary school achievement. *Social Work in Public Health*, *33*(7–8), 439–448. https://doi-org.ezproxy.liberty.edu/10.1080/19371918.2018.1543627

Chatham, R. E., & Mixer, S. J. (2021). Methods, ethics, and cross-language considerations in research with ethnic minority children. *Nursing Research*, *70*(5), 383–390. https://doi.org/10.1097/NNR.0000000000000537

Cunningham, S. A., Hardy, S. T., Jones, R., Ng, C., Kramer, M. R., & Venkat Narayan, K. M. (2022). Changes in the incidence of childhood obesity. *Pediatrics*, *150*(2), e2021053708. https://doi.org/10.1542/peds.2021-053708

Dayton, A., Aceves, A. I., & Rogoff, B. (2022). Collaboration at a microscale: Cultural differences in family interactions. *British Journal of Developmental Psychology*, *40*(2), 189–213. https://doi.org/10.1111/bjdp.12398

Dockery, A. M. (2020). Inter-generational transmission of Indigenous culture and children's wellbeing: Evidence from Australia. *International Journal of Intercultural Relations*, *74*, 80–93. https://doi.org/10.1016/j.ijintrel.2019.11.001

Durà-Vilà, G., & Hodes, M. (2017). Socio-cultural variation in attitudes to adolescents' decision-making. *Mental Health, Religion & Culture*, *20*(10), 954–972. https://doi.org/10.1080/13674676.2017.1402173

Fowler, A. L., Mann, M. E., Martinez, F. J., Yeh, H.-W., & Cowden, J. D. (2022). Cultural health beliefs and practices among Hispanic parents. *Clinical Pediatrics*, *61*(1), 56–65. https://doi.org/10.1177/00099228211059666

Freeman, J. D., Elton, J., & Lambert South, A. (2019). A second-chance at being a parent: Grandparent caregivers' reported communication and parenting practices with co-residential grandchildren. *Journal of Family Communication*, *19*(3), 261–276. https://doi.org/10.1080/15267431.2019.1632864

Giger, J. N. & Haddad, L. G. (2021). *Transcultural nursing: Assessment and intervention* (8th ed.). Elsevier.

Goldstein, E., Topitzes, J., Miller-Cribbs, J., & Brown, R. L. (2021). Influence of race/ethnicity and income on the link between adverse childhood experiences and child flourishing. *Pediatric Research*, *89*(7), 1861–1869. https://doi.org/10.1038/s41390-020-01188-6

Gozansky, Y. (2018). Showing puberty: Overcoming the taboo in children's television. *Sex Education*, *18*(5), 555–570. https://doi.org/10.1080/14681811.2018.1441019

Gross, R. S., & Mendelsohn, A. L. (2019). Food insecurity during early childhood: Marker for disparities in healthy growth and development. *Pediatrics, 144*(4), 1–3. https://doi.org/10.1542/peds.2019-2430

Gultekin, L. E., Brush, B. L., Ginier, E., Cordom, A., & Dowdell, E. B. (2020). Health risks and outcomes of homelessness in school-age children and youth: A scoping review of the literature. *Journal of School Nursing, 36*(1), 10–18. https://doi.org/10.1177/1059840519875182

Hermosillo, D., Cygan, H. R., Lemke, S., McIntosh, E., & Vail, M. (2022). Achieving health equity for LGBTQ+ adolescents. *Journal of Continuing Education in Nursing, 53*(8), 348–354. https://doi.org/10.3928/00220124-20220706-05

Im, Y., & Kim, D. H. (2021). Family management style and psychosocial health of children with chronic conditions. *Journal of Child & Family Studies, 30*(2), 483–492. https://doi.org/10.1007/s10826-020-01870-7

Kearney, M. S., & Haskins, R. (2020). How cultural factors shape children's economic outcomes. *Future of Children*, 1–6. https://doi.org/10.1353/foc.2020.0005

Kyle, T. & Carman, S. (2021). *Essentials of pediatric nursing* (4th ed.). Wolters Kluwer.

Lansford, J. (2022). Annual research review: Cross-cultural similarities and differences in parenting. *Journal of Child Psychology & Psychiatry, 63*(4), 466–479. https://doi.org/10.1111/jcpp.13539

Lipscomb, S. T., Miao, A. J., Finders, J. K., Hatfield, B., Kothari, B. H., & Pears, K. (2019). Community-level social determinants and children's school readiness. *Prevention Science, 20*(4), 468–477. https://doi.org/10.1007/s11121-019-01002-8

Lofton, S., McNaughton, D. B., Julion, W. A., Bergren, M. D., & Norr, K. F. (2019). Using the PEN-3 model to explore cultural factors that influence food choice for African-American youth. *ABNF Journal, 30*(1), 6–11.

Mandlik, N., & Kamat, D. (2020). Medical anthropology in pediatrics: Improving disparities by partnering with families. *Pediatric Annals, 49*(5), e222–e227. https://doi.org/10.3928/19382359-20200421-02

Mayo, C. O., Pham, H., Patallo, B., Joos, C. M., & Wadsworth, M. E. (2022). Coping with poverty-related stress: A narrative review. *Developmental Review, 64*, 101024. https://doi.org/10.1016/j.dr.2022.101024

McFarland, M. R. & Wehbe-Alamah, H. B. (2015). The theory of culture care diversity and universality. In M. R. McFarland & H. B. Wehbe-Alamah (Eds.), *Culture care diversity and universality: A worldwide nursing theory* (3rd ed., p. 1–34). Jones & Bartlett Learning.

Morone, J. F., Cronholm, P. F., Teitelman, A. M., Hawkes, C. P., & Lipman, T. H. (2022). Underrepresented voices: Impacts of social determinants of health on Type 1 Diabetes family management in single-parent. Black families. *Canadian Journal of Diabetes, 46*(6), 602. https://doi.org/10.1016/j.jcjd.2022.05.012

Motti-Stefanidi, F. (2018). Resilience among immigrant youth: The role of culture, development and acculturation. *Developmental Review, 50*, 99–109. https://doi.org/10.1016/j.dr.2018.04.002

National Center for Homeless Education (NCHE). (2022). *Student homelessness in America School Years 2018-19 to 2020-21.* https://nche.ed.gov/data-and-stats/

National Center for Injury Prevention and Control. (2021). *Adverse childhood experiences prevention strategy.* https://www.cdc.gov/injury/pdfs/priority/ACEs-Strategic-Plan_Final_508.pdf

Nguyen-Truong, C. K. Y., Leung, J., & Micky, K. (2019). Cultural narratives of Micronesian islander parent leaders: Maternal and children's health, the school system, and the role of culture. *Asian/Pacific Island Nursing Journal, 4*(4), 173–182. https://doi.org/10.31372//20190404.1078

Oliveira, E. A. R., & da Rocha, S. S. (2019). The parents' cultural care towards promoting child development. *Revista de Pesquisa: Cuidado e Fundamental, 11*(2), 397–403. https://doi.org/10.9789/2175-531.2019.v1112.397-403

Opalinski, A. S., Dyess, S. M., & Gropper, S. S. (2017). Food culture of faith communities and potential impact on childhood obesity. *Public Health Nursing, 34*(5), 437–443. https://doi.org/10.1111/phn.12340

Poulain, T., Vogel, M., & Kiess, W. (2020). Review on the role of socioeconomic status in child health and development. *Current Opinion in Pediatrics, 32*(2), 308–314. https://doi.org/10.1097/MOP.0000000000000876

Rajan, S., Branas, C. C., Myers, D., & Agrawal, N. (2019). Youth exposure to violence involving a gun: Evidence for adverse childhood experience classification. *Journal of Behavioral Medicine, 42*(4), 646–657. https://doi.org/10.1007/s10865-019-00053-0

Rochanavibhata, S., & Marian, V. (2022). Culture at play: A cross-cultural comparison of mother-child communication during toy play. *Language Learning & Development, 18*(3), 294–309. https://doi.org/10.1080/15475441.2021.1954929

Sahithya, B. R., Manohari, S. M., & Vijaya, R. (2019). Parenting styles and its impact on children; a cross cultural review with a focus on India. *Mental Health, Religion & Culture, 22*(4), 357–383. https://doi.org/10.1080/13674676.2019.1594178

Schmidt, K. L., Merrill, S. M., Gill, R., Miller, G. E., Gadermann, A. M., & Kobor, M. S. (2021). Society to cell: How child poverty gets "Under the skin" to influence child development and lifelong health. *Developmental Review, 61*, 100983. https://doi.org/10.1016/j.dr.2021.100983

Turner, H. A., Finkelhor, D., & Henly, M. (2021). Exposure to family and friend homicide in a nationally representative sample of youth. *Journal of Interpersonal Violence, 36*(7-8), NP4413–NP4442. https://doi.org/10.1177/0886260518787200

United Nations Children's Fund (UNICEF). (2021a). *Seen, counted, included: Using data to shed light on the well-being of children with disabilities.* https://data.unicef.org/resources/children-with-disabilities-report-2021/

United Nations Children's Fund (UNICEF). (2021b, April). *Child migration.* https://data.unicef.org/topic/child-migration-and-displacement/migration/

Wodtke, G. T., Ramaj, S., & Schachner, J. (2022). Toxic neighborhoods: The effects of concentrated poverty and environmental lead contamination on early childhood development. *Demography, 59*(4), 1275–1298. https://doi.org/10.1215/00703370-10047481

World Health Organization. (2021, November 23). *Corporal punishment and health.* https://www.who.int/news-room/fact-sheets/detail/corporal-punishment-and-health

Yakhnich, L., & Michael, R. (2022). "I don't want my children to work so hard": Perceptions of parent-child relationships and future parenting among immigrant young adults. *Journal of Cross-Cultural Psychology, 53*(5), 451–470. https://doi.org/10.1177/00220221221093813

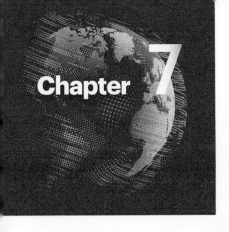

Chapter 7

Transcultural Perspectives in the Nursing Care of Adults

• Joyceen S. Boyle and John W. Collins

Key Terms

Adulthood
Caregiving
Developmental crises
Developmental tasks

Generativity
Health-related situational
   crisis
HIV/AIDS
Middle adulthood
Midlife crisis

Physiologic development
Psychosocial development
Sandwich generation
Social age
Social roles
Young adulthood

Learning Objectives

1. Evaluate how culture influences adult development.
2. Explore how health-related situational crises or transitions might influence adult development.
3. Analyze the influences of culture on caregiving.
4. Evaluate cultural influences in adulthood that assist individuals and families to manage during health-related situational crises or transitions.
5. Explain how gender and specific religious beliefs and practices might influence an adult's health and/or illness during situational crises or transitions.

Introduction

This chapter discusses transcultural perspectives of health and nursing care associated with developmental events in the adult years. The focus is primarily on **young adulthood** and **middle adulthood**. The first section of this chapter presents an overview of cultural influences on **adulthood**, with an emphasis on how health/illness situational crises or transitions might be influenced by cultural variations. The second section provides the context for and gives an example of a health-related situational crisis. The influences of culture on individual and family responses to health problems, caregiving, and health/illness transitions and crises are discussed.

Health/illness transitions have been referred to in the past as developmental tasks, those transitions that occur in a healthy successful adulthood. A health/illness situational crisis refers to changes or turmoil as individuals struggle to cope with a sudden life-threatening illness. Erikson (1963), who studied human development, used the term "**developmental tasks**" or "**developmental crises**" to describe those times in an individual's life when changes occur, such as marriage or the birth of a child. Nursing theorist A. I. Meleis chose the term "transitions," believing that term more adequately describes life changes and is a conceptually more appropriate term for nursing theory (Im, 2021). In this chapter, *transitions* refer to those health or illness events that occur within adulthood and require an individual to make lifestyle modifications. Transitions can occur gradually over a period of time, or they may be preceded by a situational crisis. A situational crisis includes a greater level of turmoil and anxiety and is more threatening to an individual and family. An example of a health/illness situational crisis might be a sudden myocardial infarction experienced by a 48-year-old man. Until his condition is stabilized, both he and his family will be in a crisis situation, worried and very anxious about his life. When his condition stabilizes and is no longer life threatening, both he and his family members will experience a more gradual health/illness transition. This transition will include changes in behavior, such as appropriate exercises, dietary changes that promote weight reduction, and the addition of prescribed medications. Whether the client experiences a crisis or a transition, they will need culturally competent and contextually meaningful nursing care.

Overview of Cultural Influences on Adulthood

Health/illness crises and/or transitions during adulthood are of interest to nursing because they include responses to health and illness. In addition, health/illness transitions influence how individuals respond to health promotion and wellness by shaping individual lifestyles, including eating habits, exercise, work, and leisure activities. Consider, for example, how pregnancy (a transition into parenthood) influences many people to improve their diet, begin moderate exercise, abstain from alcohol, and generally take better care of themselves for the health of the baby.

During the adult years, gradual physical and psychosocial changes occur and reflect the expected processes of aging. These physical changes, or **physiologic development**, are evident in the hormonal changes that take place in adulthood. **Psychosocial development**, or the development of personality, may be more subtle but is equally important. Both physiologic development and psychosocial development are influenced by cultural values and norms, and they occur throughout a lifetime.

Physiologic Development During Adulthood

Individuals who undergo menopause experience one of the more profound physiologic changes, which gradually decreases ovarian function with subsequent depletion of progesterone and estrogen. While these physiologic changes occur over time, the psychosocial concepts of self-image and self-concept may also change. The influence of culture is relevant because people learn to respond to menopause within the context of their families and culture. The *perception* of menopause and *aspects* of the experience of menopausal symptoms appear to vary across cultures. It has sometimes been assumed that people from non-Western cultures do not experience the menopausal problems seen in Western society because their status increases as they age; however, this assumption has been challenged. In mainstream cultures in Canada and the United States, youth and beauty are valued and aging is viewed with trepidation. North American medicine has tended to treat the symptoms of menopause with hormone replacement therapy, surgical interventions, and/or pharmaceutical products. Although there are not many studies on the perimenopausal transition across cultural groups, there seem to be cultural differences in the reporting of symptoms associated with treatments for menopausal symptoms. One recent study has shown that such factors as family income, perceived general health, and perimenopausal status were factors associated with and predictors of depressive symptoms among women of four major ethnic groups. Further, sports and exercise activities were negatively associated with depressive symptoms, while occupational, household, and caregiving physical activity were associated positively with depressive symptoms (Arigo et al., 2020; Im et al., 2015). This reinforces an earlier statement that individuals experiencing menopause and their families respond differently to menopause and aging within the context of their families and culture.

Males also have physical and emotional changes from the decreased levels of hormones. Loss of muscle mass and strength and a possible loss of sexual potency occur slowly. However, developmental differences among different sexes have not been extensively examined cross-culturally, and most existing theoretical and conceptual models of adult health do not provide insight into cultural variations. The cultural belief that aging, however gradual, is a normal process and not a cause for medical and/or surgical intervention may be more apparent in diverse cultural groups.

Psychosocial Development During Adulthood

Adulthood was termed the "empty middle" by Bronfenbrenner (1977), a recognized developmental psychologist. His use of this term was an indication of Western culture's lack of interest in the adult years. Traditionally, these years were viewed as one long plateau that separates childhood from old age. It was assumed that decisions affecting marriage and career were made in the late teens and that drastic changes in developmental processes seldom occurred afterward. For many years, most developmental theorists saw adulthood as a period to adapt to and come to terms with aging and one's mortality. Western thinking has changed considerably since Bronfenbrenner's observations. Psychosocial development in middle age is now viewed as a vigorous and changing stage of life involving many challenges and transformations.

Sociocultural factors in Western society have precipitated tremendous changes, producing crises, changes, and other unanticipated events in adult lives. Divorce, remarriage, career changes, increased mobility, and other societal changes have had a profound impact on the adult years. Further, many middle-aged adults may be caught in the **sandwich generation**, the years where they still have concerns with adult children (and sometimes grandchildren) while also becoming increasingly concerned with the care of aging parents. Middle life can be a time of reassessment, turmoil, and change. Society acknowledges this with common terms such as **midlife crisis** or even *empty nest syndrome*, along with other terms that imply stress, dissatisfaction, and unrest. Adults in midlife may experience anxiety as they realize they have been overly occupied with raising children but no longer have the close relationship with their spouse or partner that originally drew them together. Awareness of cultural values may be heightened as they wrestle with decisions between divorce or staying in the relationship.

However, adulthood is not always a tumultuous, crisis-oriented state; many middle-aged persons welcome the space, time, and independence that middle age often brings. Midlife can be a time of challenge, enjoyment, and satisfaction for many people. According to Meleis, we now tend to view a "midlife crisis" as a time of transition that can be a positive experience, including the mastery of new skills and behaviors that helps an individual change and grow in response to a new environment (Im, 2021).

Chronologic Standards for Appropriate Adult Behavior

Much of the contemporary work on adult development was done in the 1960s and 1970s by developmental psychologists such as Bronfenbrenner (1977), Havighurst (1980), and Neugarten (1968), all of whom proposed different theories about adult development. We still rely on some of this early work as we attempt to understand the complexities of adult development. Neugarten (1968) observed that each culture has specific chronologic standards for appropriate adult behavior. These standards prescribe the ideal ages to leave the protection of one's parents, choose a vocation, marry, have children, and, in general, get on with life. The events associated with these standards do not necessarily precipitate crises, but they do bring about change. What is more important is the timing of these events. As a result of each culture's sense of social time, individuals tend to measure their accomplishments and adjust their behavior according to a kind of social clock. Awareness of the social timetable is frequently reinforced by the judgments and urging of friends and family, who may say, "It's time for you to…" or "You are getting too old to…" or "You should act your age." However, an example of recent societal change is seen as late baby boomers and Generation Xers have touted that "50 is the new 30," emphasizing that the typical roles and responsibilities once thought to be anchored to specific decades of life are subject to change (Mapes, 2016; Owoc, 2023).

Problems often arise when social timetables change for unpredictable reasons. An example is the recent trend of adult children, once married but recently divorced, unemployed, or both, returning to live with their parents, often bringing along their own children. This arrangement is very common in U.S. society with one in three 18- to 34-year-olds living with parents in their parents' home (Vespa, 2017). A recent study among 16- to 35-year-old adult children who initially moved out of their parents' home indicated that 61% subsequently moved back in with parents for a temporary but extended stay (the data exclude adult children who stayed fewer than 3 consecutive months; Gillespie, 2020). Additionally, grandparents caring for grandchildren is now a common phenomenon in Western society (Clark et al., 2022; Vespa, 2017). Also, life events like being widowed in young adulthood or losing one's job in midlife due to an economic downturn are examples of events in adulthood that are likely to cause stress and conflict because they occur outside of the anticipated social timetable.

Culture exerts important influences on human development by providing a means for recognizing stages in the continuum of individual development throughout the lifespan. Culture defines **social age**, or what is considered an appropriate behavior in each stage of the life cycle. In nearly all societies, adult role expectations are placed on young people when they reach a certain age. Several cultures have defined rites of passage that mark the line between youth and adulthood. In the United States, markers of beginning adulthood may include reaching the legal age to obtain a driver's license, to drink alcohol, or to join the military forces, but coming of age is rarely tied to a defined moment or event among many Western populations.

Menarche (first menstruation) is a milestone in physiologic development and a psychologically significant event that provides a dramatic demarcation between childhood and adulthood. However, this is not an event that is celebrated openly in Western culture; most children are too embarrassed to talk openly about it with anyone but their parents who have experienced menstruation or close friends. There are no definitive boundaries that mark adulthood for young people, although legal sanctions confer some rights and responsibilities at the ages of 18 and 21 years. There is no single criterion for determining when Western young adulthood begins, given that different individuals experience and cope with growth and development differently and at different chronologic ages. For example, a young person who joins the military forces at age 18 and serves their country in another part of the world may have a different experience than the 18-year-old who lives with their parents, has a part-time job, and attends a local community college.

Adulthood is usually divided into young adulthood (late teens, 20s, and 30s) and middle adulthood (40s and 50s), but the age lines can be fuzzy. Generally, a young adult in their late teens and early 20s struggles with independence and issues related to intimacy and relationships outside the family. Role changes occur when the young adult is pursuing an education, experiencing marriage, starting a family, and establishing a career. A middle adult most often concentrates on career and family matters. However, as previously mentioned, adulthood is not necessarily an orderly or predictable pattern. Experiences at work have a direct bearing on the middle-aged adult's development through exposure to job-related stress, levels of physical and intellectual activity, and social relationships formed with coworkers. "Re-careering" or changing careers during middle adulthood is becoming more common as certain careers are eliminated due to increasing technology and automation, while new high-demand career fields are popping up overnight. Additionally, recent societal changes being observed are that baby boomers and Generation Xers in middle age are voluntarily changing careers or are retooling their education and pursuing second careers in the fourth and fifth decade of life. The transition from middle age into retirement for many is delayed as boomers and Xers continue in the active workforce beyond traditional retirement age, thereby impacting societal changes, global economic and political issues, and family dynamics (Sullivan & Al Ariss, 2019).

Because of both forced and voluntary career changes, the sometimes-required relocation, educational retooling, and financial impacts can make family life chaotic, with role changes and other developmental transitions occurring with dizzying frequency. Some life changes can lead to developmental crises (McLeod, 2018; Sullivan & Al Ariss, 2019). According to Erikson (1963), developmental crisis occurs when an individual experiences typical and expected challenges that are age appropriate. Examples of adult developmental crises are as follows:

- A young adult may have difficulties separating from their parents and establishing independence. These difficulties usually manifest as "homesickness" and dissipate as the young adult gains the ability to adjust to a new lifestyle such as college, the military, or employment away from home. The major developmental task of young adulthood is the resolution of intimacy versus isolation, with intimacy being the goal of happy relationships and being comfortable with one's commitments.
- Middle adults may experience difficulties in adjusting to career, marriage, and parenthood, but these usually resolve with time and the development of a trusting intimate relationship. A new "normal" of balancing career and family develops as the individual adapts to the middle adult years. The major developmental task of middle adulthood is the resolution of **generativity** versus stagnation. Resolution of the "crises" or conflict between these two conflicting forces results in attainment of generativity, or the feeling of having created things that will outlast one's lifetime through parenting, working in one's career, participating in community activities, or working cooperatively with peers, spouse or partner, family members, and others to reach mutually determined goals.
- Older adults may find the "golden years" difficult as they are faced with the realization that they are getting older and may feel like they have made some wrong choices or have left many things undone. Further, they may find it difficult to experience the

feeling of not being productive and contributing to society via their career. Resolution of the "crises" or conflict between ego integrity versus despair is successfully resolved as the older adult develops satisfaction with the level of accomplishment and life success they have achieved. Mature adults, having resolved this crisis, have a well-developed philosophy of life that serves as a basis for stability in their lives, and the numerous **social roles** they have attained, such as spouse or partner, parent, child of aging parent, worker, friend, organization member, and responsible citizen (McLeod, 2018; Sullivan & Al Ariss, 2019).

A health/illness situational crisis is often focused and specific and can occur at any time during any developmental stage. Sometimes, a situational crisis can be precipitated by an illness, such as a diagnosis of type 2 diabetes, or the death of a family member. A situational health/illness crisis is usually time-limited, although additional transitions may occur. How well individuals cope with and manage the challenges of health/illness crises and transitions in adulthood is influenced by cultural values, traditions, and backgrounds.

Developmental Tasks

Throughout life, each individual is confronted with developmental tasks, those responses to life situations encountered by all persons experiencing physiologic, psychological, spiritual, and sociologic changes (Erikson, 1963). Although the developmental tasks of childhood are widely known and have long been studied, the developmental tasks of adulthood are less familiar to most nurses.

Several theorists have studied and defined the developmental or *midlife* tasks of adulthood. Among others, personality theorists Erikson and Fromm cite maturity as the major criterion or task of adulthood (Erikson, 1963; Fromm, 1969). These various theories have

implications for how we define "development," "maturity," and "wisdom." Each of these social roles involves expected behaviors established by the values and norms of society. Through the process of socialization, the individual is expected to learn the behaviors appropriate to the new role. It is important to note that many developmental theories have connotations of stability and blandness associated with adulthood, although this probably is not the case. The constellation of characteristics enumerated by Erikson and other theorists has been attributed to predominantly White Anglo-Saxon Protestant (WASP) views and behaviors. For many cultural groups in Western society, the mastery of Erikson's developmental tasks is not easily managed and is not always applicable, and in some cases, it may even be undesirable. For some groups, developmental tasks may be accomplished through culturally defined patterns that are different from or outside of the norm of what is expected in the dominant culture (Erikson, 1963).

Childbearing is a special time for most cultures, and there are cultural prescriptions to ensure the well-being of both the mother and the child. Childbearing that occurs in young and middle adulthood is a prime example of the interface between culture, religion, childbearing practices, and transcultural nursing care. Evidence-Based Practice 7-1 discusses how an observant Jewish woman and her family, in labor, delivery, and postpartum, should have nursing care that allows her to abide by Jewish laws, customs, and practices that influence everyday life as well as those that pertain to childbearing.

Studies focusing on the developmental experiences of women have led some authors to suggest that developmental stages and the associated developmental tasks of adulthood often published have been derived primarily from studies of men, suggesting that women experience adult development differently (Belenky, 1997). Women's traditional location of responsibility was in the home, in heterosexual relationships, nurturing children and husbands as well

Jewish Laws, Customs, and Practice in Labor, Delivery, and Postpartum Care

This article provides a comprehensive and thorough guide to specific laws, customs, and practices of traditionally, religious observant Jewish people that assist the transcultural nurse or midwife to provide culturally congruent and sensitive care during labor, delivery, and the postpartum period. Providing culturally congruent care includes cultural knowledge; in this case, the nurse or midwife needs to understand the Jewish laws, customs, and practices that guide everyday life, as well as those that pertain to childbearing. These cultural issues include adherence to the laws that influence intimacy issues between husband and wife in heterosexual marriages, or *niddah*; dietary laws, or *kashrut*; and observance of the Sabbath. Detailed tables are provided that list the following: (1) observant Jewish customs, laws, and practices during labor, delivery, and postpartum; (2) annual Jewish holidays and fast days; and (3) a cultural assessment for Jewish clients in labor, delivery, and postpartum. Case studies are presented that describe cultural competence challenges for nurses who want to learn about the Jewish culture and how to provide culturally competent care to Jewish women during childbirth.

Clinical Implications

- Recognize that observant Jewish couples are committed to maintaining their religious laws, customs, and practices as much as possible throughout the labor, delivery, and postpartum experiences.
- Understand that childbirth is a time that is highly influenced by cultural values and beliefs.
- The religious laws, customs, and practices that will be most apparent during labor, delivery, and postpartum will pertain to prayer, communication between spouses, dietary laws, the Sabbath, modesty issues, and labor and birth customs.
- The culturally competent nurse follows the cues of the religious family, tailoring their health and nursing care in a manner that allows the family to practice their traditions in their specific designed manner while employing professionalism and creativity in providing quality patient care.

Reference: DeVito, J. (2019). Understanding the Orthodox Jewish family during childbirth. *Nursing Forum*, *54*, 220–226. https://doi.org/10.1111/nuf.12320

as parents. Patrick et al. (2020) point out that this view is changing, prompted by societal changes and informed by scholars who are addressing women's psychosocial development in new ways. We also see emerging cultural pressures on women who now are expected to balance nurturing and rearing of children, keeping the home, all while maintaining full-time employment in the workplace (Lamar et al., 2019).

Culture and Adult Transitions

More recent theories on adulthood (Demick & Andreoletti, 2003; Kjellstrom & Stalne, 2017) suggest that development is an evolutionary expanse involving different eras and transitions. Within nursing, Meleis proposed a framework to study life transitions (Im, 2021). The focus is on developmental and situational transitions, including those brought about by an illness.

The next section discusses several important adult life transitions and examines how culture and life events influence adult growth and change during these transitions. Successful progression through developmental tasks and/or life transitions may occur slowly over many years and is important in terms of quality of life and life satisfaction. Culture influences these transitions, and nurses must be able to evaluate their adult clients and help them adjust and change in culturally appropriate ways. These adult life transitions are often based on what we could call "middle-class, White American culture." In their study of cultural influences on life transitions, Baird and Boyle reported that diverse cultures may experience different life transitions or experience life transitions in different ways depending on the cultural group (Baird, 2012; Baird & Boyle, 2012). The following section focuses on various cultural groups and how they might experience adult life transitions. The terms "transitions" and "developmental tasks or goals" are used interchangeably and refer to selected activities at a certain period in life that are directed toward a goal. According to Erikson, unsuccessful achievement of a goal is thought to lead to inability to perform tasks associated with the next period or stage in life (Erikson, 1963); thus, successful development transitions are important.

Developmental Transitions: Achieving Career Success

Many persons in traditional Western culture define career success in financial terms, while others may see it as providing service or making a contribution to the lives of their fellow citizens. Achieving success in one's career, including adequate financial remuneration as well as satisfaction and enjoyment, is considered an important developmental task or goal in adulthood. However, there are many groups who struggle to attain this goal. Immigrants to the United States, Canada, or Europe may find it very difficult to find employment that pays an adequate salary or offers opportunities for advancement or job satisfaction. North America and Europe, as well as other parts of the world, have experienced a tremendous influx of immigrants and refugees from Southeast Asia, Latin America, Eastern Europe, the Middle East, Africa, and other geographical areas over the last 30 years ("U.S. immigration trends," 2017). Although immigrants and refugees may aspire to career success or to earn a higher salary, those may be difficult goals to attain. They may have difficulty with the language, with the skills, and with the educational level required,

as well as other factors necessary for holding a good job in their new country.

Other factors, such as gender roles, also influence the attainment of satisfaction in career choices. More women are working outside of the home, and, for married women, there may be a different division of time and energy for both spouses that pose challenges. Women's presence in the workforce has increased dramatically, from 29.7 million in 1970 to 75.7 million in 2020, and this has had a significant impact on childcare and family finances. Although women have made significant gains in certain occupations, many women continue to be employed in low-paying jobs with little chance for advancement. Many are employed in occupations that have been traditionally oriented toward women (*Women in the labor force: a databook*, 2017; *Women in the labor force: a databook*, 2021), and the salaries are less than what men earn in similar positions. Working in a low-paying job that does not offer opportunities for advancement or intellectual challenges does not lead to career success or recognition from one's peers.

Many immigrant and refugee families experience role conflict and stress as gender roles begin to change during contact with Western culture. For example, sometimes, the male head of household who has immigrated is unable to find employment; if he was a professional in his former country, he may be reluctant to accept the menial jobs that are traditionally filled by immigrants or refugees when they first migrate to another country. Frequently, low-status jobs are more available to immigrant women, yet, for many of these women, their traditional roles are closely tied to the home and family. When an immigrant or refugee woman from a culture with such gender roles begins to work outside of the home, her role changes and those changes alter the traditional power structure and the roles within the family (DeSantis, 1997). The lack of adequate social supports, such as affordable daycare for children and adequate compensation for work, and the additional physical and emotional stress result in an unacknowledged toll on immigrant and refugee families. Box 7-1 lists some characteristics of immigrant and refugee families.

BOX 7-1   Some Characteristics of Immigrant and Refugee Families

1. Traditional family values are evident; for example, roles of men and women are differentiated. Women's role is often in the home with the family. Men are heads of the household and typically the family providers.
2. Families tend to be extended; if members do not actually live in the same household, they visit and contact each other frequently. New immigrants and refugees tend to keep in fairly close contact with family members in the home country.
3. Many immigrants come to the United States because they already have family members here.
4. Many immigrants and refugees are experiencing poverty and struggle to earn an adequate income. Often, men in refugee communities have been professionals in their home country but are unable to be employed in the same capacity in their new host country. Women are often more easily employed outside of

the home, and they often find employment as domestic or service workers. For many refugee or immigrant women, working outside of the home is a new experience for them. To earn a salary and provide for their families can be very empowering for these women.
5. Refugees may be fleeing war and political persecution. Many may experience symptoms of posttraumatic stress syndrome.
6. Traditional health and illness beliefs may influence behavior. Immigrant and refugee families may combine traditional health practices with modern Western healthcare. The use of traditional practices is fairly common in some groups.
7. Language is often a significant barrier for the first few years that immigrants and refugees live in the United States and Canada. Children tend to learn English and become acculturated faster than do their parents.

At present in the United States, members of certain groups, such as people experiencing poverty, ethnic minorities, newly arrived immigrants or refugees, people experiencing homelessness, those with mental illnesses, or people who are unemployed, are not afforded equitable opportunities for satisfying, interesting jobs or the status derived from succeeding in a career. Thus, although the work role is valued in American society, the attainment of a successful career that includes financial success and personal fulfillment may not be realistic for some minority groups, immigrants, or even certain individuals within the majority culture, some of whom are returning to school in the hope of preparing for a second career. A bright spot in career transition of adult learners returning to college classrooms is that the cultural perspectives they add to a once homogenous student body contributes to a microcosm of ages, ethnicities, and life

experiences that enriches cultural understanding among all students in the class (J. Sonnega, PhD, personal communication, September 28, 2012).

Developmental Transitions: Achieving Social and Civic Responsibility

Social and civic responsibilities are in part culturally defined. Generally speaking, American and Canadian cultures value the voluntary contributions of their citizens in various agencies and organizations that serve the community or society in general. For this discussion, achieving social and civic responsibilities can be viewed as participation in those activities in adulthood that contribute to the "good of society." Usually, this means activities and commitments outside of the immediate family. These can vary considerably from serving as a board member for a community agency, such as a homeless shelter, to volunteering to teach in a literacy program or donating blood at the local blood bank. Not all members of Western cultures value achieving an elected office in, for example, the local parent–teacher organization (PTO) or Rotary Club; other cultures may find these goals baffling and, instead, emphasize activities and contributions within the cultural group. For example, in some groups, religious obligations are given priority over civic responsibilities. Some traditional religious groups have not encouraged the emergence of women in leadership roles within the church structure or the wider society, although this is now being accepted within many religious groups.

Sometimes within traditional cultures, women who seek roles outside the family are criticized because recognition and acknowledgment outside the family group may conflict with the traditional role of women. Some religious and ethnic or cultural groups believe that a woman's place is in the home, and women who attempt to succeed in a career or participate in activities outside the home or group are frowned on by other members of the group. Civic responsibilities that relate to children or domestic matters may be viewed as more culturally appropriate for women to assume, whereas other civic activities may be viewed as more within the scope of opportunities and obligations of men. However, some Middle Eastern and Southeast Asian cultures emphasize and value responsibilities and contributions to the extended family or clan rather than to the wider society. Researchers (Banulescu-Bogdan, 2020) have reported that refugee women in the United States continue to socialize almost exclusively with other refugee women, often extended family/clan or tribe members. They are more comfortable with others who not only share their traditional culture and language and life events but are also going through similar situational transitions, sometimes called *the immigrant experience* (Banulescu-Bogdan, 2020).

Many refugee women are single or widowed with children. Married women whose spouses have been killed or have stayed behind to fight in various conflicts are often forced to flee with children and/or older family members. Women refugees carry a substantial burden during the migration process and are essential in helping the family members settle into a new country (Baird, 2012). Coping with life in a new country becomes the focus of their daily lives. Finding a job, getting children into school, learning English, and other resettlement activities become challenging transitions for them. Many refugee women are justifiably very proud of their accomplishments. They learn new job skills, a new language, and how to drive a car, all accomplishments that are not always recognized by members of their new society. For the refugee women and her family, these are significant achievements; however, they can be quite stressful. Often, informal social networks, such as having family members and friends nearby, are very helpful and supportive. The social and civic responsibilities that we have associated with adulthood in Western cultures may not be appropriate for many other cultural groups. Concepts such as social connectedness and integration, resilience, and strength might help us better understand adult development and transitions in refugee and immigrant families (Berry et al., 2022; Garcia & Birman, 2022).

Developmental Transition: Marriage and Raising Children to Adulthood

Marriage and raising children usually take place in early to middle adulthood. The age at which young persons marry and become independent varies by custom or cultural norm, as well as by socioeconomic status. Generally speaking, in Western culture, young adults of lower socioeconomic status leave school, begin work, marry, and become parents and grandparents at earlier ages than do middle-class or upper-class young adults (Landberg et al., 2019). Indeed, many North American families encourage early independence by urging their children to attend college or to find employment away from home. Other cultural groups, such as some from the Middle East and Latin America, place more emphasis on maintaining the extended family. Even after marriage, a newly married couple may choose to live very close to both spouses' families and to visit relatives several times each day. Families from some cultural groups, including some Hispanics, or traditional religious groups, such as the Hutterites or the Amish, may be reluctant to allow their young daughters to leave home until they marry. In many Muslim families, girls do not leave home until they are married.

Increased mobility in American and Canadian societies has impacted family life as many young families now live far away from grandparents, and the traditional influences of grandparents on young grandchildren are decreasing. Sometimes, because of geographical distance, grandparents barely know their grandchildren, although digital photos via internet access, cell phones, video calling, and other technological devices are helping to keep grandparents up to date with the growth and activities of their grandchildren. However, technological advances do little to provide young parents with the assistance from grandparents in the child-rearing responsibilities. Many parents of young children must rely on daycare centers to care for children while both parents work, further impacting cultural norms once held by close-knit families.

Changes in terms of women's participation in the workforce began in the 1960s and 1970s when it became increasingly difficult for a single-income household to support a comfortable, middle-class lifestyle (*Women in the labor force: a databook*, 2021). In addition, many young women attend college or universities and want to become established in their careers before they marry or have children. With both parents working, children are often placed in childcare facilities. These factors have had a tremendous impact on gender roles and responsibilities within the marriage and on how children are raised.

Developmental Transition: Changing Roles and Relationships

Relationships between marriage partners, between and among genders, within social networks of family and friends, between parents and children, and gender roles within these relationships are all influenced by cultural norms and traditions. In Western culture, the relationship between a married couple is often enhanced in middle adulthood, although divorce at this time is not infrequent in the United States. The frequent need for both spouses to work may conflict with traditional roles and cause feelings of guilt on the part of both spouses. In heterosexual partnerships, some women continue to assume all responsibility for domestic chores while working outside the home, and they experience considerable stress and fatigue as a result of multiple role demands. If either or both spouses are working in low-paying jobs and still struggling to make ends meet, or if the jobholder is laid off or loses their job, adulthood may not be a time of enjoyment and leisure activities. Some adults may experience what is known as a "life changing event," a particularly dramatic event such as an accident, illness, divorce, death of a spouse, or other difficult relational or physical life event. The struggle to adjust to such an event and make meaning out of it often inspires profound and lasting personal growth and change. Of course, not everyone experiences transformative growth after a traumatic event; for some individuals, such an event might trigger depression, a sense of despair, and a downward trajectory in terms of quality of life.

The relationship between married adults can vary considerably by culture. For example, not all cultures emphasize an emotionally close interpersonal relationship between spouses. In some Hispanic cultures, in heterosexual relationships, women develop more intense relationships or affective bonds with their children or relatives than with their husbands. Latino men, in turn, may form close bonds with siblings or friends—ties that meet the needs for companionship, emotional support, and caring that in other cultures might be expected from their wives (Zoucha & Zamarripa-Zoucha, 2021).

Gender roles and how men and women go about establishing personal ties with either gender are heavily influenced by culture. Touch between men (walking arm in arm) as well as physical touch between women is acceptable in many societies. In contemporary American society, women are more likely to have intimate, self-disclosing friendships with other women than men have with other men; a man's male friends are likely to be working, drinking, or playing "buddies." In Southern Europe and the Middle East, men are allowed to express their friendship with each other with words and embraces; expressions of affection between men are less common in American culture.

Affiliation and friendship needs in adulthood and the satisfaction of these needs are facilitated or hindered by cultural expectations. Social support, family ties, and friendship needs can be met through the extended family and kinship system or through other culturally prescribed groups such as churches, singles bars, work, and civic associations. Social networking websites are an increasingly popular way to connect with friends and family as well. An individual's health may be affected by these social ties: persons who have a reliable set of close friends and an extensive network of acquaintances are usually healthier emotionally and physically than are persons without supportive networks and close friends. Facebook, LinkedIn, and other social networking sites might meet social needs of younger persons or even older adults (Keles et al., 2020).

Roles and relationships change between adult children and their parents as both become older. Caring for and launching their own children and caring for their own aging parents place some middle-aged adults between the demands of caregiving from parents and those from children. Primarily, caregivers have been women, and the stress resulting from the demands of caregiving places them at increased risk of health problems (*Caregiving in the U.S., 2020*, 2020). In traditional cultures that value and maintain extended family networks, the responsibilities of caring for both children and older parents can be shared with other family members (see Fig. 7-1). This decreases the responsibilities being placed on any one family member.

Adjusting to the aging of parents and the associated responsibilities, as well as finding appropriate solutions to problems created by aging parents, is a challenge created by situational, developmental, and even health–illness transitions. Placing an aged parent in a nursing home or extended care facility may be a decision made with reluctance and only when all other alternatives have been exhausted. Such actions may be totally unacceptable to some members of certain

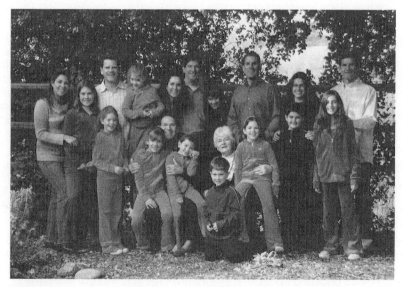

Figure 7-1. The extended family of Teresa and Neil Cooper of Carlsbad, California. This family is multiethnic in each generation, yet maintaining close family ties is a priority that has continued through three generations.

cultural groups, in which family and community networks would facilitate the complex care required by an older relative needing daily assistance. Such cultural norms would exert a great deal of social pressure on an adult child, or especially a daughter (in cultures where gender roles designate this as a woman's responsibility), who was unable to fulfill this obligation.

Cultural values also influence professional healthcare roles and relationships. How individuals are approached and greeted as well as the kind and type of relationship established may be closely tied to cultural expectations and norms.

A casual, first-name basis has become the norm in many healthcare situations, with medical receptionists and often other health professionals calling patients by their first names. While this may be appropriate at the check-in desk because of Health Insurance Portability and Accountability Act (HIPAA) regulations, it can be inappropriate in other instances. Healthcare professionals should always inquire about the appropriate manner to use in approaching clients and their family members. Table 7-1 provides some suggestions and guidelines to use in approaching clients and using their names in professional relationships.

Table 7-1 | Guidelines for Names

Culture	Guidelines
Some Arabic cultures	Both male and female children are given a first name. The father's first name is sometimes used as the middle name; the last name is the family name. Usually, a person is called formally by the first name, such as Mr. Mohammed or Dr. Anwar.
Chinese	The family name is stated or written first followed by the given name (the opposite of European and North American tradition). Only very close friends use the given name. Politeness and formality are stressed; always use the whole name or family name. Use only the family name to address men, for example, if the family name is Chin and the man's given name is Wei-jing, address the man as Chin. Women in China do not use their husband's name after marriage. Many Chinese people take an English name that they use in their North American host country. Use a title (such as Mr., Mrs., Ms., Dr., etc.) preceding the English name; using only the first name is considered rude.
Latin American	The use of surnames may differ by country. Many Latin Americans use two surnames, representing both parents' sides of the family. The name "Maria Cordoba Lopez" indicates that her father's name is Cordoba and her mother's surname is Lopez. When Maria marries, she will retain her father's name and add the last name of her spouse, becoming Maria Cordoba de Recinos. Many Latin American immigrants drop their mother's surnames after they immigrate to the United States because having two last names can be inconvenient. In approaching clients of traditional Latino cultures, it is appropriate to use the Spanish terms *señor* or *señora*, followed by the primary surname (the husband's for clients in heterosexual marriages), if the nurse is comfortable with those terms.
Native North American	Native North American names differ by tribal affiliation. Many tend to follow the dominant cultural norms. In the Navajo culture, a healthcare provider may call an older Navajo client "grandfather" or "grandmother" as a sign of respect. In the past, some tribes have tended to convert traditional names into English surnames, for example, Joe Calf Looking and Phyllis Greywolf.

The above mentioned examples are very general. If in doubt, always ask: it can be embarrassing for both the nurse and the client if the nurse uses a name in an inappropriate manner. Generally speaking, it is *always best and most appropriate* to be formal and to use the surname with the appropriate title such as Mr. or Mrs. (or other culturally appropriate titles) preceding the name, unless the client has indicated that they prefer to be called by their first name.

Adapted from Purnell, L. D. (2013). *Transcultural health care: A culturally competent approach* (4th ed.). F.A. Davis.

Health-Related Situational Crises and Transitions

Situational transitions often occur when a serious illness is diagnosed, or other traumatic events happen to individuals and their families. Some developmental theorists refer to the initial period as a "situational crisis" when a serious illness is diagnosed, or traumatic event occurs. Such a diagnosis or event often leads to fear and anxiety in the client and family members. As clients and family members learn more about the precipitating condition, they realize that many of their fears are unfounded as they gain more confidence in managing the illness condition. The "crisis" dissipates but still the illness remains and must be managed appropriately. The client and family must "transition" to living with a chronic illness. It is not uncommon for a situational transition, precipitated by an illness event, to occur in middle age or late adulthood. The leading causes of death in the United States are heart disease, cancer, COVID-19, accidents, stoke, chronic lower respiratory diseases, Alzheimer disease, and diabetes, most of which are usually diagnosed in adulthood (Murphy et al., 2021). These conditions affect individuals, but they also occur within a family system and affect children, spouses, aging parents, and other close relatives. Because middle-aged adults may be caring for aging parents, adult children, and even grandchildren, the illness of any one individual must be evaluated carefully for the myriad of ways in which it affects all members of the family. Evidence-Based Practice 7-2 describes the experiences of Latina wives as their husbands recovered from radical prostatectomy. The shock of the cancer diagnosis and the long-term effects of the surgery precipitated a situational transition that affected both husbands and wives.

Evidence-Based Practice 7-2

Purposeful Normalization When Caring for Husbands Recovering From Prostate Surgery

This study describes the experiences of Latina women as their husbands recovered from radical prostatectomies. Purposeful normalization can be viewed as a situational transition. The women's lives changed dramatically when their husbands were diagnosed with cancer. Cultural beliefs related to gender roles and sexual functioning are some of the strongest values and traditions within a cultural system. The husbands' depression, irritability, and erectile dysfunction posed special challenges to the Latina women in this study. Prostate cancer is the most frequently diagnosed noncutaneous cancer in men in the United States.

Despite high incidence rates, overall survival rates are very high and increasing all of the time. Issues such as postsurgical incontinence and erectile dysfunction, along with the fact that many prostrate survivors are married men, have prompted many to describe prostate cancer as a *couple's disease.* Partnered men have significantly better mental health, lower symptom distress, and fewer urinary problems than do unpartnered men. Still, many wives experience significant distress when faced with their partner's diagnosis and treatment. This study interviewed 28 partners of *Latino* men who had a radical prostatectomy. The primary aim was to describe the experiences of low-income Latina women as their husbands recovered from radical prostatectomies. The overarching process was identified as normalization with some themes working against normality while others worked toward it.

(continued)

Purposeful Normalization When Caring for Husbands Recovering From Prostate Surgery (continued)

Working Against Normality: Threats to normality of the women's lives began immediately when their husbands were diagnosed with cancer. Some concerns diminished with time, such as the initial shock and fear and dealing with the side effects. They feared losing their husband. Dealing with the symptoms and the side effects caused the women to feel anxious and frustrated. The husbands' depression and irritability, as well as erectile dysfunction, posed special challenges.

Working Toward Normality: The Latina women described many themes that kept them feeling a sense of "normal." They worked hard to conceal their own emotions and to show their husbands that they had everything under control. They tried to move forward, putting changes brought about by their husband's illness behind them. They tried to make dietary changes that they believed were helpful—such as eating more vegetables and fruits and cutting down on sugar. Their families were supportive with the grown children visiting and making frequent phone calls. Grandchildren visited and were a source of joy and comfort. Women found great support in their religious faith that helped them make changes in a positive way.

Clinical Implications

- Understand that caregiving can be extremely stressful and that caregivers need support, understanding, and help in this role. Simply acknowledging the emotional impact of both the illness itself and of caring for the patient can be helpful.
- Talk to wives/caregivers about actively shaping the emotional responses they feel and how they can help their husbands deal with the changes they are experiencing.
- Encourage caregivers to contribute to recovery by empowering them to make healthy changes in their lifestyle, such as eating healthy food, getting appropriate amounts of sleep, and perhaps simple exercise such as walking short distances together with their husband.
- Become comfortable when discussing symptoms such as erectile dysfunction and helping clients and their partners consider alternative forms of intimacy.
- Actively encourage family members to visit and to telephone frequently. Help clients plan for grandchildren to spend the night.

References: Williams, K. C., Hicks, E. M., Chang, N., Connor, S. E., & Maliski, S. L. (2014). Purposeful normalization when caring for husbands recovering from prostate surgery cancer. *Qualitative Health Research, 24*(3), 306–316; Green, A., Winter, N., DiGiacomo, M., Oliffe, J. L., Ralph, N., Dunn, J., & Chambers, S. K. (2022). Experiences of female partners of prostate cancer survivors: A systematic review and thematic synthesis. *Health & Social Care in the Community, 30*, 1213–1232. https://doi.org/10.1111/hsc.13644

Cultural beliefs and values influence health promotion, disease prevention, and the treatment of illness. Families influence the health-related behavior of their members because definitions of health and illness, and reactions to them, form during childhood within the family context. When an illness has social and/or cultural connotations, or involves sexual issues, shame, and/or stigma, the response from the client and the family may be more pronounced.

Evidence-Based Practice 7-3 describes how sexual education has sometimes been a "flash point" in numerous communities, and many parents have objected to such programs in the school setting. Shambley-Ebron et al. (2016) conducted a study with preadolescent African American girls that also included the girls' mothers. A targeted 8-week educational program involving both mothers and daughters tapped into the cultural and gender

Cultural Preparation for Womanhood in Urban African American Girls: Growing Strong Women

Poor sexual health is a significant contributor to morbidity in young African American women. Human immunodeficiency virus/acquired immune deficiency syndrome (HIV/AIDS) and other sexually transmitted infections (STIs) are tragic and costly in all populations; however, African Americans bear an excess burden of poor health due to these conditions. Understanding how knowledge about sexual health is transmitted to African American girls is needed to develop effective and culturally relevant preventive interventions.

This study explored the ways that African American mothers transmitted sexual values and information to their daughters. The author interviewed 14 mothers who had young daughters, 8 to 16 years of age. The data were qualitatively analyzed, and three major themes about *Growing Strong Black Women* were identified: truth-telling, building strength through self-esteem, and spirituality as helper.

Helping their daughters grow into strong, successful, and healthy women was viewed by the mothers as a task that was primarily their responsibility. This responsibility was enacted through an ongoing process of providing truthful answers and open communication, helping their daughters develop a healthy self-esteem that would promote independence, and providing a foundation of spirituality and religious beliefs to enable their daughters to deal with the societal issues that face young African American girls and women. Mothers were honest with their daughters with regard to sexuality, their changing bodies, and relationships with men. Sometimes, mothers told their daughters painful stories of their own experiences. Other times, they sought out literature to explain how their bodies worked or how STIs occurred. Mothers reinforced their daughters' self-esteem and helped them develop confidence in their own abilities to

be successful in life. They encouraged them to become active in church and school activities, to develop a faith and belief in God, and to participate in religious practices such as prayer and attendance at religious services.

Clinical Implications

- Supportive networks for young African American girls can be broadened and strengthened by involving teachers, nurses, and women from their church groups as support persons to help them achieve their goals relative to age-appropriate relationships and sexual behaviors.
- African American mothers (indeed, all mothers) of teenage girls need accurate information about sexual health and STIs. Nurses can work with churches and various community groups to provide information and support to parents.
- Culture and gender are unique and distinct aspects of the lives of young African American girls and must be taken into account when planning preventive interventions for health and well-being.
- Nursing interventions that focus on building self-esteem and supporting the future aspirations of young African American girls can be useful to reinforce parental teachings and help young girls move into adulthood successfully.
- The use of spirituality and religiosity appears consistently in the literature as ways to help young African American girls deal appropriately with life experiences.

Reference: Shambley-Ebron, D., Dole, D., & Karikari, A. (2016). Cultural preparation for womanhood in urban African American girls: Growing strong women. *Journal of Transcultural Nursing, 27,* 25–32. https://doi.org/10:1177/1043659614531792

beliefs and practices to educate girls about **HIV/AIDS** prevention. Input for educational intervention was solicited from women in the community, including the mothers of the young girls. The findings from these studies indicate that culture

and gender influences play a critical role in how young African American girls develop culturally appropriate strategies to deal with sexuality and healthy womanhood. Further, these studies are an example of how education about sensitive topics such as HIV/AIDS prevention can be conducted (Crooks et al., 2020).

The content in this section provides the context for and gives an example of a **health-related situational crisis**. The influences of culture on individual and family responses to health problems, caregiving, and health/illness transitions and crises are discussed.

Caregiving

Caregiving occurs when a (typically) unpaid person, usually a family member, helps another family member who has a chronic illness or disease. Many caregivers are women who are caring for their aged and ill parents or husbands. Caregiving, as used in this chapter, implies the provision of long-term help to an impaired family member or close friend. Caregiving is usually labor intensive, time-consuming, and stressful; the exact effects on the physical and emotional health of caregivers are still being documented. Although positive outcomes, such as feelings of reward and satisfaction, do occur for caregivers, caregivers still experience negative psychological, emotional, social, and physical outcomes (*Caregiving in the U.S., 2020*, 2020). When caregiving for other family members takes place during middle adulthood, the roles for both the caregiver and the recipient may change as new challenges emerge. The caregiver may be forced to quit their job as caregiving responsibilities increase when the person being cared for becomes more infirm or ill and the need for assistance in tasks of daily living increases.

Culture fundamentally shapes how individuals make meaning out of illness, suffering, and dying. Cultural beliefs about illness and aging influence the interpretation and management of caring for people who are ill and older adults, as well as the management of the trajectory of caregiving. Family members provide care for the vast majority of those in need of assistance. The demands of caregiving can result in negative emotional and physical consequences for caregivers. How they cope with stress, social isolation, anxiety, feelings of burden, and the challenges of caregiving will all be influenced by cultural values and traditions.

Shambley-Ebron et al. (2016) have documented that these general problems and characteristics of caregivers are compounded for African American women by the special circumstances of their lives and the lives of the people for whom they care (Crooks et al., 2020). In the case of African American caregivers, prejudice, discrimination, health disparities, and poverty often all interact to increase stress and pose challenges that frequently result in poor health. Like other caregivers, African American caregivers are mostly female; most recipients of care from African American caregivers are females as well (e.g., mothers, grandmothers, aunts) (*Caregiving in the U.S., 2020*, 2020).

Studies of African American caregivers have found that they tend to use religious beliefs and/or spirituality to help them cope with the stress of caregiving; Collins and Hawkins (2016) found that a major source of support for African American caregivers was their personal relationships with "Jesus," "God," or "the Lord." These authors suggest that spirituality is both personal and empowering for some African Americans and is related to the deepest motivations in life, including seeing God as their healer, provider, and sustainer (Park et al., 2018). Spirituality is often expressed in the context of daily life, not necessarily by formal attendance at religious events. Numerous researchers have noted that the specific nature of the religion–health connection among African Americans is of great interest to health professionals as it holds promise for integrating church-based health interventions.

Culture and ethnicity can influence beliefs, attitudes, and perceptions related to caregiving, including how often individuals engage in self-care versus seeking formal health services, how many medications they take, how often they rest and exercise, and what types of foods they consume when ill. Ethnic and/or cultural differences have rarely been analyzed in caregiver research; only recently have nurse researchers and others focused on specific cultural groups to study caregiving (*Caregiving in the U.S., 2020*, 2020) and the ethnocultural factors that are so important in planning support for caregivers (Crist et al., 2018).

REVIEW QUESTIONS

1. Describe examples of health transitions in your family members and friends. Which types of transitions can you identify in your clients/patients? Do you think it is helpful to think of "transitions" as opposed to "developmental tasks or stages"? Why?

2. How does culture influence transitions of adulthood? For example, explain what might be learned when completing a cultural assessment of a woman from a traditional culture such as those in the Middle East, who may experience adulthood differently than adult women in Western cultures.

3. Discuss how gender might influence adult development in a White, middle-class family.

4. Describe how social factors such as mobility, increased education, and changes in the economy have influenced adult development in American and Canadian cultures.

5. How might caregiving for a family member bring about a situational transition for a middle-aged adult? Would this differ in cultural groups such as Chinese Americans or Mexican Americans? How?

6. Describe how culture influences the role of the caregiver in some African American cultures. What can you find in the literature about caregiving in other cultural groups?

CRITICAL THINKING ACTIVITIES

1. Interview a middle-aged colleague, a client, or a person from another cultural group. Ask about adult roles within the family and how they are depicted. How are these role descriptions typical of traditional roles that are described in the literature? If not, how are they different? What are some of the reasons why they have changed?

2. Interview a middle-aged client from another cultural group. Ask about the client's experiences within the healthcare system. What were the differences the client noted in health beliefs and practices? Ask the client about their health needs during middle age.

3. Using the Andrews/Boyle Transcultural Nursing Guide for Individuals and Families provided in Appendix A, conduct a cultural assessment of a middle-aged client of another cultural group. Critically analyze how the client's culture affects the client's role within the family and the timing of developmental transitions. How might the assessment data differ if the client were older? Younger?

4. Review the literature on Mexican American culture. Describe the traditional Mexican American family. What are the cultural characteristics of Mexican Americans to consider in assessing the developmental transitions of adulthood in this group?

5. You are assigned a new patient, a 24-year-old man, from El Salvador named Jose Calderon. At morning report, you learn that he has been a gang member in El Salvador, and because he wanted to stop all gang-related activities, his life was threatened. He fled to the United States and has been granted political asylum. You are told that he has extensive tattoos on his body. What do you know about gang membership in Central America? In the United States? How does membership in a gang address the needs of adolescents? What are the cultural factors that are important to consider when you are planning nursing care for a patient like Jose? For example, how do you view body tattoos? What are the issues related to political asylum, immigration, and the like? How might you assist Jose to meet his developmental needs? What might be the problems he will encounter in the U.S. society or in our healthcare system?

REFERENCES

Arigo, D., Brown, M. M., Pasko, K., Ainsworth, M. C., Travers, L., Gupta, A., Downs D. S. Smyth, J. M. (2020). Rationale and design of the women's health and daily experiences project: Protocol for an ecological momentary assessment study to identify real-time predictors of midlife women's physical activity. *JMIR Research Protocols, 9*(10), e19044. https://doi.org/10.2196/19044

Baird, M. B. (2012). Well-being in refugee women experiencing cultural transition. *Advances in Nursing Science, 35*(3), 249–263. https://doi.org/10.1097/ANS.0b013e31826260c0

Baird, M. B., & Boyle, J. S. (2012). Well-being in Dinka refugee women of southern Sudan. *Journal of Transcultural Nursing, 23*(1), 14–21. https://doi.org/10.1177/1043659611423833

Banulescu-Bogdan, N. (2020). *Beyond work: Reducing social isolation for refugee women and other marginalized newcomers.* Transatlantic Council on Migration.

Belenky, M. F. (1997). *Women's ways of knowing: The development of self, voice, and mind* (10th anniversary ed.). Basic Books.

Berry, J. W., Lepshokova, Z., & Grigoryev, D.; MIRIPS Collaboration. (2022). How shall we all live together? Meta-analytical review of the mutual intercultural relations in plural societies project. *Applied Psychology, 71*(3), 1014–1041.

Bronfenbrenner, U. (1977). Toward an experimental ecology of human development. *American Psychologist, 32*(7), 513–531. https://doi.org/10.1037/0003-066X.32.7.513

Caregiving in the U.S., 2020. (2020). https://www.caregiving.org/wp-content/uploads/2021/01/full-report-caregiving-in-the-united-states-01-21.pdf

Clark, K. C., Kelley, S. J., Clark, P. C., & Lane, K. (2022). Needs of grandparents raising grandchildren: A qualitative study. *The Journal of School Nursing.* https://doi.org/10.1177/10598405221115700

Collins, W. L., & Hawkins, A. D. (2016). Supporting caregivers who care for African American elders: A pastoral perspective. *Social Work and Christianity, 43*(4), 85–103.

Crist, J. D., Montgomery, M. L., Pasvogel, A., Phillips, L. R., & Ortiz-Dowling, E. M. (2018). The association among knowledge of and confidence in home health care services, acculturation, and family caregivers' relationships to older adults of Mexican descent. *Geriatric Nursing.* https://doi.org/10.1016/j.gerinurse.2018.05.005

Crooks, N., Wise, A., & Frazier, T. (2020). Addressing sexually transmitted infections in the sociocultural context of black heterosexual relationships in the United States. *Social Science and Medicine, 263*, 113303. https://doi.org/10.1016/j.socscimed.2020.113303

Demick, J., & Andreoletti, C. (2003). *Handbook of adult development.* Kluwer Academic/Plenum Publishers.

DeSantis, L. (1997). Building healthy communities with immigrants and refugees. *Journal of Transcultural Nursing, 9*(1), 20–31. https://doi.org/10.1177/104365969700900104

DeVito, J. (2019). Understanding the Orthodox Jewish family during childbirth. *Nursing Forum, 54*, 220–226. https://doi.org/10.1111/nuf.12320

Erikson, E. H. (1963). *Youth: Change and challenge.* Basic Books.

Fromm, E. (1969). *Escape from freedom.* Henry Holt and Company, LLC.

Garcia, M. F., & Birman, D. (2022). Understanding the migration experience of unaccompanied youth: A review of the literature. *American Journal of Orthopsychiatry, 92*(1), 79–102. https://doi.org/10.1037/ort0000588

Gillespie, B. J. (2020). Adolescent intergenerational relationship dynamics and leaving and returning to the parental home. *Journal of Marriage and Family, 82*(3), 997–1014.

Green, A., Winter, N., DiGiacomo, M., Oliffe, J. L., Ralph, N., Dunn, J., & Chambers, S. K. (2022). Experiences of female partners of prostate cancer survivors: A systematic review and thematic synthesis. *Health & Social Care in the Community, 30*, 1213–1232. https://doi.org/10.1111/hsc.13644

Havighurst, R. J. (1980). Life-span developmental psychology and education. *Educational Researcher, 9*(10), 3–8. https://doi.org/10.2307/1174928

Im, E., Ham, O. K., Chee, E., & Chee, W. (2015). Physical activity and depressive symptoms in four ethnic groups of milife women. *Western Journal of Nursing Research, 37*(6), 746–766. https://doi.org/10.1177/0193945914537123

Im, E.-O. (2021). Afaf Ibrahim Meleis: Transitions theory. In M. R. Alligood (Ed.), *Nursing theorists and their work* (p. 306). Elsevier Health Sciences.

Keles, B., McCrae, N., & Grealish, A. (2020). A systematic review: The influence of social media on depression, anxiety and psychological distress in adolescents. *International Journal of Adolescence and Youth, 25*(1), 79–93. https://doi.org/10.1080/02673843.2019.1590851

Kjellstrom, S., & Stalne, K. (2017). Adult development as a lens: Applications of adult development theories in research. *American Psychological Association, 22*(2), 266–278. https://doi.org/10.1037/bdb0000053

Lamar, M. R., Forbes, L. K., & Capasso, L. A. (2019). Helping working mothers face the challenges of an intensive mothering culture. *Journal of Mental Health Counseling, 41*(3), 203–220. https://doi.org/10.17744/mehc.41.3.02

Landberg, M., Lee, B., & Noack, P. (2019). What alters the experience of emerging adulthood? How the experience of emerging adulthood differs according to socioeconomic status and critical life events. *Emerging Adulthood, 7*(3), 208–222. https://doi.org/10.1177/2167696819831793

Mapes, D. (2016, October 14). *America's favorite age? It's 50, new poll says.* https://www.today.com/health/americas-favorite-age-its-50-new-poll-says-8C11144329

McLeod, S. (2018). *Erik Erikson's stages of psychological development.* Simply Psychology. https://www.simplypsychology.org

Murphy, C. P., Kochanek, K. D., Xu, C., & Arias, E. (2021). Mortality in the United States, 2020. *NCHS Data Brief, no 427.* National Center for Health Statistics.

Neugarten, B. L. (1968). Perspectives of the aging process. Developmental perspectives. *Psychiatric Research Reports*, *23*, 42–48.

Owoc, E. (2023). *The New 30 – At 50, Why not Look the Way You Feel?* https://www.agelessmed.com/the-new-30-at-50-why-not-look-the-way-you-feel/

Park, C. L., Holt, C. L., Le, D., Christie, J., & Williams, B. R. (2018). Positive and negative religious coping styles as prospective predictors of well-being in African Americans. *Psychology of Religion and Spirituality*, *10*, 318–326. https://doi.org/10.1037/rel0000124

Patrick, J. H., Hayslip Jr., B., & Hollis-Sawyer, L. (2020). *Adult development and aging: Growth, longevity, and challenges*. SAGE Publications.

Shambley-Ebron, D., Dole, D., & Karikari, A. (2016). Cultural preparation for womanhood in urban African American girls: Growing strong women. *Journal of Transcultural Nursing*, *27*(1), 25–32. https://doi.org/10.1177/1043659614531792

Sullivan, S. E., & Al Ariss, A. (2019). Employment after retirement: A review and framework for future research. *Journal of Management*, *45*(1), 262–284. https://doi.org/10.1177/0149206318810411

U.S. Immigration Trends. (2017). https://www.migrationpolicy.org/about/contact-and-directions

Vespa, J. (2017). *The changing economics and demographics of young adulthood: 1975–2016* (pp. 20–579). U.S. Census Bureau. http://hispanicad.com/sites/default/files/p20-579.pdf

Williams, K. C., Hicks, E. M., Chang, N., Connor, S. E., & Maliski, S. L. (2014). Purposeful normalization when caring for husbands recovering from prostate cancer. *Qualitative Health Research*, *24*(3), 306–316. https://doi.org/10.1177/1049732314523842

U.S. Bureau of Labor Statistics. (2017). Women in the labor force: A databook. *Report no. 1071.* https://www.bls.gov/opub/reports/womens-databook/2017/pdf/home.pdf

U.S. Bureau of Labor Statistics. (2021). Women in the Labor Force: A Databook. *Report no. 1092.* Division of Information and Marketing Services. https://www.bls.gov/opub/reports/womens-databook/2020/home.htm

Zoucha, R., & Zamarripa-Zoucha, A. (2021). People of Mexican heritage. In L. D. Purnell & E. A. Fenkl (Eds.), *Textbook for transcultural health care: A population approach; cultural competence concepts in nursing care* (pp. 613–636). Springer International Publishing.

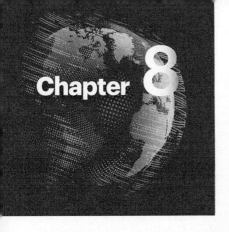

Chapter 8

Transcultural Perspectives in the Nursing Care of Older Adults

• Mary Lou Clark Fornehed, Karina E. Strange, and Sandra J. Mixer

Key Terms

Aging in place
Caring
Chronic illness

Communication
Culturally congruent care
Economic challenges
End-of-life

Palliative care
Social determinants of health
Social support
Spirituality

Learning Objectives

1. Demonstrate knowledge of the sociodemographic shift in the older adult population and how population changes necessitate improved gerontological nursing care.
2. Analyze how socioeconomic, spiritual, technical, kinship, communication factors, and cultural values and beliefs influence older adult health.
3. Describe the needs of diverse older adults on a continuum of care (e.g., health promotion, community, assistive and long-term care, and palliative/hospice care and in various settings).
4. Develop nursing interventions that are based on cultural values and individual preferences throughout older adulthood, dying, and death.

Introduction

This chapter is organized into sections that address the culture care influences on older adult health as depicted in Leininger's Sunrise Enabler in Chapter 1. Older adult culture care influences discussed in this chapter are biologic factors; environmental context; economic factors; language and communication; kinship, social factors, and community; traditional beliefs and practices; spirituality, faith, and religion; construct of care; holistic culturally congruent care; well-being care expressions and practices; disability and illness care expressions and practices; and dying and death care expressions and practices. Case studies provide real-life examples of application for culturally congruent gerontological nursing care.

Culturally diverse individuals, families, and communities have different perceptions of successful aging; these viewpoints are influenced by cultural and social dimensions (McFarland, 2018). Because there is great cultural diversity worldwide, it is beyond the scope of this chapter to address all cultures. Therefore, much of this chapter focuses on U.S. older adults and refers to Western cultures and approaches to gerontological care. Global perspectives are interspersed.

The Older Adult in Contemporary Society: Factors Affecting Healthcare

As the Baby Boomer generation ages (born 1946–1964), the U.S. older adult population is skyrocketing; this population increase has been referred to as the "graying of America" (Vespa, 2019, para. 1). By 2030, the number of older adults is expected to increase by approximately 30% since 2020 (from 56.1 million older adults in 2020 to 73.1 million in 2030) (Vespa et al., 2020). In an unprecedented demographic shift, U.S. older adults will soon outnumber children. Within the next decade, all Baby Boomers will have reached age 65 or older, and approximately 21% of the U.S. population will be composed of older adults (Vespa, 2019). U.S. healthcare infrastructure will be overburdened by the combination of older adult population rise, high percentages of chronic comorbidities, and longer life expectancies (The Stern Center for Evidence-Based Policy, n.d.; Vespa et al., 2020).

The U.S. older adult populating is rapidly aging and becoming more culturally diverse. A Snapshot of U.S. Older Adults Population Projections and Demographics is provided in Table 8-1. Between 2020 and 2060, international migration will overtake natural population increase as the primary driver of U.S. population growth; this shift will lead to significant demographic changes (Vespa et al., 2020). In 2016, there were approximately 44 million foreign-born persons in the United States; by 2060, that number is projected to rise to 69 million.

Table 8-1	Snapshot of U.S. Older Adult (≥65) Population Projections and Demographics

- Constituted 16.8% of the population
- Oldest-old subgroup is the fastest-rising[a]
- 61% of community-dwelling live with a spouse/partner; 27% live alone[a]
- 55% women, 45% men; 16% widows, 5% widowers[a]
- ¼ represent racial/ethnic minority populations[a]
- ⅓ live at or below 200% of the federal poverty level[b]
- 2% live in assisted-living communities[c]
- 20% are caregivers: 13% are 65–74 years; 7% are 75+ years[c]
- 95% have at least one chronic comorbidity; 80% have 2 or more
- ¼ have a behavioral health condition (e.g., anxiety, depression, substance misuse)
- 24% of community-dwelling older adults are socially isolated[d]

[a] Administration for Community Living. (2021). *2020 profile of older Americans*. https://chrome-extension://efaidnbmnnnib-pcajpcglclefindmkaj/https://acl.gov/sites/default/files/aging%20and%20Older%20In%20America/2020Profileolderamericans.final_.pdf
[b] National Council on Aging. (2022b). *Get the facts on older Americans*. https://ncoa.org/article/get-the-facts-on-olderamericans
[c] Samuels, C. (2022, December 13). *Portrait of Americans in assisted living, nursing homes, and skilled nursing facilities*. https://www.aplaceformom.com/caregiver-resources/articles/long-term-care-statistics
[d] National Academies of Sciences, Engineering, and Medicine. (2020). *Social isolation and loneliness in older adults: Opportunities for the health care system*. The National Academies Press. https://doi.org/10.17226/25663

The number of persons who identify as representing two or more races will increase 200% by 2060. Asian and Hispanic populations are also growing at unprecedented rates (Vespa et al., 2020). Such dramatic numerical and cultural demographic changes indicate the pressing need for innovative, cost-effective, and culturally congruent gerontological nursing care (Fulmer et al., 2021). Equipped with the knowledge of evidence-based practices related to trust and rapport with culturally diverse older adult patients, nurses can provide meaningful, safe, and beneficial care in various clinical settings (McFarland, 2018).

Most national and international organizations define the term *older adult* as an individual who is older than 60 or 65 years (American Psychological Association, 2023). However, there is no universal agreement on the age at which a person becomes old. Some researchers subdivide the term *older adults* into "young-old" (65 to 74 years old), "middle-old" (75 to 84 years), and "oldest-old" (≥85 years) (Lee et al., 2018). These subgroups contribute to demographic considerations. Of all adults aged 65 and older, the number of oldest-old individuals is rising most rapidly; an increase of 198.1% is expected by 2060 (Vespa et al., 2020).

The Significance of Terminology/ Syntax Related to Older Adults

Since this chapter focuses on older adults, the authors address the significance of the term "older adult" and other words/phrases that may be used to refer to persons at this age/stage of life. For example, the American Psychological Association (APA) (2020) is very clear that stigmatizing terms such as seniors, elderly, and aged should be avoided when writing research. On the other hand, to provide culturally congruent care, it is important to acknowledge that people are who they say they are (McFarland, 2018).

The term "elder" has been used in many transcultural research studies within diverse cultural groups; for example, Asian (Sudha, 2014), Eastern Band of Cherokee Indians Public Health and Human Services Division (2019), Yu'Pik Eskimo (Embler et al., 2015), American Indian and Alaska Native (AIAN) (Hirchak et al., 2018; Isaacson et al., 2018), indigenous peoples of Latin America (Roche et al., 2018), and others (Kwak et al., 2014). In these and other cultures, the term "elder" is revered and preferred by the people themselves. Throughout this chapter, the term

"older adult(s)" will be used. However, when referencing a cultural group who uses other terms, the authors will honor their words.

Cultural Diversity of the U.S. Older Adult Population

U.S. older adults have diverse life experiences, education levels, employment histories, family support systems, and cultural backgrounds. Furthermore, older adults live in various settings, including independent residences, congregate care facilities, adult family homes, and long-term care institutions (e.g., nursing homes or skilled nursing facilities) (Miller, 2023b). Based on cultural and environmental influences, nurses and other healthcare providers should provide preventive education, **chronic illness** management, care coordination, case management, and hospice care services in culturally meaningful ways.

In all clinical settings, nurses consider how generic (folk) and professional (care–cure) practices influence holistic health, well-being, disability, illness, death, and dying (McFarland, 2018; Wehbe-Alamah, 2018). Older adults' cultural values, beliefs, and lifeways affect interactions with healthcare providers and processes of healthcare decision-making. Holistic nursing care of older adults is enriched by the confluence of physical, mental, psychosocial, and spiritual dimensions (Miller, 2023c; Patrick et al., 2022).

Health disparities influence multiple dimensions of health and healthcare provision; discussion of disparities and social determinants is integrated throughout the text. Health disparities impact older adults for interrelated reasons, including (a) lower income; (b) lack of insurance (including supplemental insurance to Medicare); (c) barriers in access to care; (d) rural residence in medically underserved areas/healthcare provider shortage areas as designated by the Health Resources and Service Administration; and (e) individual decisions to not seek care (Khatana & Groeneveld, 2020; McAfee et al., 2021; Morales et al., 2020; Trinh et al., 2019).

Influences of Biologic Factors

Biologic factors include race/ethnicity, age, sex/gender, genetics, and other physiologic aspects unique to each person. Consideration of biologic factors is especially important since the U.S. older population is predicted to become increasingly diverse (Vespa et al., 2020).

Factors Related to Race and Ethnicity

Race and ethnicity are correlated to multimorbidity, life expectancy, and incidence of health disparities. For example, in a nationally representative sample of Medicare beneficiaries in the United States, chronic conditions associated with hospitalization, admission to skilled nursing facilities, and/or death were cardiovascular diseases in White Americans and chronic kidney disease in Black Americans (Quiñones et al., 2022). There are several reasons for these associations in older adults. The healthcare system in United States has long been fraught with large racial and ethnic disparities associated with access to care, lack of insurance coverage, and costs of healthcare deemed unaffordable (Lopez et al., 2021).

Factors Related to Disability

Disability is another important biologic factor for nurses to consider. Approximately 18.2 million (36%) of U.S. older adults have at least one disability (Mateyka & He, 2022). Nineteen percent have one or more types of impairment in physical functioning (e.g., limited mobility, hearing or vision loss, cognitive decline, and so forth) (ACL, 2021). Older adults greater than 64 years of age reported access to care with health insurance coverage for many disability types and received primary care services (Centers for Disease Control and Prevention [CDC], 2022b). Younger adults were reported to be less likely to have health insurance to cover vision disabilities and were less likely than their older counterparts to see a primary care provider because of high healthcare costs.

Factors Related to Age and Life Expectancy

Age was a critical factor impacting the COVID-19 pandemic. Older adults are at higher risk of severe complications and death related to the COVID-19 virus, especially when compounded with multiple comorbidities. Persons aged 65 and older make up 16.5% of the U.S. population and accounted for 75.8% of COVID deaths in the United States (CDC, 2023). U.S. older adults with comorbidities face a higher risk of severe illness and death from COVID-19 (Dadras et al., 2022).

Life expectancy is influenced by various factors, including race/ethnicity, gender/sex, and geographic location. Overall, the life expectancy in the United States is declining (Hill et al., 2023). For example, compared to White persons, American Indian/Alaska Native (AIAN), and Black individuals have shorter life expectancies and faster declines. AIAN persons have the shortest life expectancy at 65.2 years; the expectancy for Black Americans is 70.8 years; White Americans' life expectancy is 76.4 years; and Hispanic individuals and people of Asian origin have the longest life expectancies at 77.7 and 83.5 years, respectively (Hill et al., 2023). These differences in life expectancies can be explained by the social determinants of health, such as where persons grow up, their poverty level, and where they live and work. These **social determinants of health** predict access to care or lack thereof. Also, while life expectancy is declining in the United States, women will still live longer at 79.1 years compared to the life expectancy of men at 73.2 years (Centers for Disease Control and Prevention, 2022a, 2022b).

From a transcultural nursing perspective, it is important to consider life expectancy in relation to global statistics. Of note are the Longevity Blue Zones, five regions of the world where many older adults live to 100 years or more (Poulain et al., 2021). Currently, the Longevity Blue Zones are Loma Linda, California; Nicoya, Costa Rica; Sardinia, Italy; Ikaria, Greece; and Okinawa, Japan. These areas have high percentages of centenarians. Researchers attribute healthy aging and longevity to lifestyle behaviors such as physical activity, good nutrition (moderate and plant-based intake), stress management, faith community, and sense of purpose contribute to healthy aging in these areas (Buettner & Skemp, 2016; Kreouzi et al., 2022).

Environmental Context Influences

Environmental context critically influences health of older adults and their quality of life (Brossoie et al., 2020). Environmental context includes factors such as access to food, transportation, pharmacies, primary care, dental and vision care, community resources (e.g., senior centers, faith communities, internet access), safety, places for physical activity, geography (e.g., rural/urban, mountains/desert), and living arrangements (McFarland, 2018).

Living Arrangements

Living arrangements impact older adult health and well-being. Independent homes (e.g., house, condo, or apartment), retirement communities, and assisted-living or long-term care facilities are examples of older adult places of residence.

However, older adults often face economic barriers to finding housing that best meets their needs. Findings from the United Health Foundation Senior Report (2022) indicate that 32.7% of U.S. older adults experienced severe housing problems (e.g., small households with an adult $\geq$ 62 years of age). For millions of U.S. older adults, lack of safe and affordable rental housing is a critical problem. Recent research indicates that for over 10 million households with an adult $\geq$ 65 years old, rent payments are greater than 30% of income pay more than one third of income. Half of those households measured spent more than 50% of their monthly

income on housing (Molinsky, 2022). Many older adults choose between paying for housing, food, or medications; financial constraints related to high housing costs hamper the ability to buy medications or healthy food (Molinsky, 2022).

Aging in Place

Aging in place is staying in one's family home and familiar community as long as possible and delaying admission to any kind of institutional care setting (Bigonnesse & Chaudhury, 2019; Cramm et al., 2018). Many older adults have a strong desire to age in place, which has been found to enhance physical, social, and emotional health (National Institute on Aging [NIA], n.d.). Even older adults living with life-limiting illnesses prefer the comfort of home while dying (Fornehed et al., 2020). Reasons for aging in place include (a) remaining in a familiar setting, (b) maintaining independence, (c) managing finances, and (d) its positive impact on older adult health outcomes (National Academies of Sciences, Engineering, and Medicine [NASEM], 2020). In a nationwide random sample of 328 non-Hispanic White older adults, Ahn et al. (2020) found that public/community-based care services could help older adults age in place. Though often a protective factor, aging in place can increase risk of social isolation and loneliness if an older adult does not have transportation, internet access, or social support at home (NASEM, 2020). These factors will be discussed in the section on social support. In addition, aging in place requires careful preparation; for example, decreasing fall risks by removing area rugs and installing grab bars in the bathroom (NIA, n.d.).

Retirement Communities, Assisted Living, and Long-Term Care

Older adults who have good health status, mobility, cognitive functioning, and stable socioeconomic support can more readily remain in their homes or live in continuing care retirement communities (CCRC). These communities provide a continuum of services for the life of an older adult, ranging from independent living to assisted living and to long-term care. CCRCs provide a one-stop option of services and amenities, such as safe outdoor spaces, transportation, social and civic engagement activities, and health services (Ayalon, 2018).

High-functioning older adults may decide to initially live in their own apartments (Carver et al., 2018). At some point when the older adult requires more care, the resident may move to an assisted living unit to receive help with activities of daily living. Assisted-living programs vary by size, structure, sponsorship, amenities, cost, and service availability. When more intensive care is needed or following an acute illness or injury, the resident may transition to a skilled nursing care unit on the CCRC campus: "The transition to a CCRC can be seen as a gain as it provides older adults with opportunities to age in place in an environment that gradually accommodates to their emerging needs" (Ayalon, 2018, p. 269). Considering the rising number of aging persons, long-term care could be reconceptualized as not only a basic safety net for vulnerable older adults but also a way of life where culturally diverse older adults can remain functional and maintain a sense of dignity (World Health Organization [WHO], 2022).

Between 2019 and 2020, there was a significant uptick in low-care nursing home residents: 9.9% to 15.2%, an increase of 54% (United Health Foundation, 2022, p. 23). Low-care nursing home residents are individuals who do not need assistance with certain activities of daily living, including eating, toileting, mobility, and transferring. These older adults benefit from care provided in home, community, or assisted-living settings (United Health Foundation, 2022).

It is estimated that 70% of U.S. older adults will need at least 3 years of care in a long-term care facility. Of those adults, one fifth may need care for 5 or more years (Samuels, 2022). Of note is the number of older adults who are informal caregivers. In the United States, 20% of caregivers are

65 or older. Of those, 13% are 65 to 74 years old and 7% are over the age of 75 years old (Samuels, 2022).

Social Determinants of Health: Components of the Environmental Context

Social determinants of health are the "nonmedical factors" that influence how people live, grow, play, work, and age. Social determinants include (but are not limited to) housing; food insecurity; transportation; income/socioeconomic status; education; and access to healthcare (WHO, 2022; Whitman et al., 2022). Worldwide, social determinants of health as well as social, economic, and political systems significantly impact health and illness throughout the lifespan. In the United States, it is estimated that "clinical care impacts only 20 percent of county-level variation in health outcomes, while social determinants of health (SDOH) affect as much as 50 percent" (Whitman et al., 2022, p. 1). For example, zip code has been associated with life expectancy (Hill-Briggs et al., 2020). Perez et al. (2022) call for an "integrated healthcare plan" that involves screening tools and community care coordination to address social determinants, enhance health of older adults, and minimize the impacts of health disparities (para. 1). The Kaiser Family Foundation found that across multiple measures of social determinants of health, "Black, Hispanic, AIAN, and Native Hawaiian and Other Pacific Islander (NHOPI) people fared worse compared to white people across most examined measures of social determinants of health for which data were available" (Hill et al., 2023).

According to the WHO (2023), there is a worldwide pattern that low socioeconomic status is correlated with poor health outcomes. This prediction could have a huge impact on healthy aging or being well functionally while getting older. By the year 2030, it is estimated that 12% of the world population will be greater than 65 years of age, with a steep increase in the aged trajectory predicted thereafter. With this rapid increase in aging, the disease burden that goes with this could pose a real threat to our health globally (McMaughan et al., 2020).

Food Insecurity

For U.S. older adults, food availability is a major consideration related to environmental context. Good nutrition is an essential method of managing chronic illnesses such as hypertension, high cholesterol, diabetes, and obesity. However, according to the United Health Foundation (2022), 12.6% of U.S. older adults ≥ 60 years old experienced food insecurity, and 9.4% of U.S. older adults ages 65 and older were living in poverty. Food insecurity is associated with chronic comorbidities in a "negative feedback loop" that jeopardizes older adult health and well-being (Pooler et al., 2019, p. 421). People who live in low-income communities and rural areas have limited access to healthy options and tend to buy inexpensive and obesogenic foods (e.g., processed foods) (Centers for Disease Control and Prevention, 2022a, 2022b; Pooler et al., 2019). In 2020, approximately 5.2 million (approximately 6.8%) U.S. older adults were hungry, and older adults of color and those living with disabilities are disproportionately impacted (National Council on Aging [NCA], 2022b).

The Older Americans Act has funded food service programs implemented by the Administration for Community Living's Administration on Aging (n.d.). Food programs such as the Supplemental Nutrition Assistance Program (SNAP) increase many U.S. older adults' access to healthy foods. In a comprehensive evaluation of the Older Americans Act Title III-C Nutrition Services Program, Mabli et al. (2017) found that many older adults would have skipped meals or eaten less if they had not had the Nutrition Services Program. In other studies of the Nutrition Services Program, findings indicated that older adults who received home-delivered meals reported improvements in anxiety and self-rated health, as well as decreased numbers of hospitalizations and falls (Volkert et al., 2022). However, only 48% of U.S. adults ≥ 60 years old who are eligible for this program are enrolled and getting food (NCA, 2022a). Through careful assessment and care coordination, nurses and other healthcare providers can assess for food insecurity and coordinate referrals that may help alleviate an older adult's food insecurity (Pooler et al., 2019). Overall, "...nutrition services help older Americans remain healthy and independent in their communities by providing meals and related services in a variety of community settings and via home-delivery to older adults who are homebound due to illness, disability, or geographic isolation" (Whitman et al., 2022, p. 15).

Transportation

Lack of transportation limits access to community resources, food, medications, and opportunities for socialization (American Association of Retired Persons [AARP], 2020; Pooler et al., 2019). More than 600,000 U.S. older adults use public transportation to go to doctors' appointments (Gimie et al., 2022). Public transportation, rideshares, and/or coordinating rides with loved ones can facilitate an older adult's ability to age in place. Accessible and affordable transportation facilitates healthcare access and promotes socialization. Older adults who do not have good transportation options may need long-term care (National Aging and Disability Transportation Center, 2023). Nurses and other healthcare providers need to consider an older adult patient's means of transportation and whether it is feasible to travel to primary care services, specialists' offices, and pharmacies.

Considerations for Older Adults Who Have Recently Immigrated

Older adult immigrants or refugees may face significant changes when adapting to U.S. cultural norms and healthcare. For example, older adult immigrants may have walked daily in their home countries and eaten diets high in fruits and vegetables. Often, when immigrants move to different settings, they may alter their diets for various reasons, such as financial strain, stress/anxiety eating, and limited access to healthy foods, instead eating prepared and packaged foods (Dao et al., 2022). Older adults who have recently immigrated may distrust or fear the U.S. healthcare system, have limited experience seeking biomedical care, and experience "ongoing post-migration stressors" (Siddiq et al., 2023, p. 147). Interpreter services may be minimal and challenging to use (National Standards for Culturally and Linguistically Appropriate Services [NSCLAS], n.d.; Siddiq et al., 2023, p. 147). Nurses should address the unique culture care needs of recently immigrated older adults by considering (a) length of time spent in a new community and degree of acculturation; (b) proximity to immediate and extended family members; (c) network of friends from country(ies) of origin; and (d) connections with ethnic, social, and health-related institutions (Zhao et al., 2021).

Economic Influences

In the United States, the economics of aging constitute significant challenges for older adults and their families. According to the NCA (2022a), approximately one third of older Americans are considered "economically insecure" and live at or below 200% of the federal poverty level. Of significant concern is that approximately 25% of U.S. older adults have decreased monies for basic needs because their healthcare costs are too high; by extension, they have inadequate funds for food, clothing, and medication (NCA, 2022b). Additionally, stark racial and gender disparities are prevalent within the U.S. older adult population; for example, Black and Hispanic older adults have higher rates of economic insecurity related to the environments in which they work and live. Furthermore, due to unequal pay and time away from the workforce, older women face higher risk of living in poverty (NCA, 2022a).

Many U.S. older adults do not seek preventative healthcare due to exorbitant costs (Jacobsen et al., 2021). One example is dental care, which is generally not covered under Medicare and Medicaid. As of 2021, approximately 16% of U.S. older adults did not have dental care due to cost (Jacobsen et al., 2021). In terms of healthcare expenditures, data indicate that Medicare, Medicaid, and out-of-pocket expenses are growing exponentially and predicted to continue to rise through 2030 (NHE Fact Sheet, 2021). Yearly long-term care costs are estimated at $471.1 billion; only 42% of those expenditures are covered by Medicaid (Samuels, 2022).

These **economic challenges** influence culture care expressions for older adults, including **end-of-life** care. For example, Fornehed et al. (2020) discovered that rural Appalachian care expressions at end-of-life (EOL) were influenced by economic factors. Despite the cultural value and belief about the importance of caring for family members at home, there were times when older adult care would have been best provided in a long-term care facility. However, due to financial constraints, families often felt they had no choice but to bring older adult family members home. In some situations, children had to miss work and stay home to provide care. Unfortunately, this circumstance increases economic burden for the family (Fornehed et al., 2020).

Informal caregivers are individuals who assist older adults with activities of daily living. Generally, informal caregivers are not paid, and it is estimated that 41.8 million Americans provided care for family members, and these services represent approximately $470 billion dollars (Samuels, 2022). These informal caregivers are usually female family members. Informal caregivers face a variety of difficulties caring for their family members. For example, a community assessment of urban African Americans who have dementia found that family caregivers faced multiple challenges. Obstacles included (a) lack of affordable and safe housing, (b) high healthcare costs, (c) inadequate health insurance, (d) insufficient transportation, and (e) feelings of shame and stigma that limited the confidence to access resources and that restricted home care of older family members (Epps et al., 2018).

Formal caregivers provide long-term care and services for a fee. As described above, this type of care includes home healthcare, adult day-care centers, hospice centers, and skilled nursing facilities. Formal services can be billable through Medicare and Medicaid with some out-of-pocket payments required. These services are provided for older adults who meet established eligibility criteria related to morbidity (e.g., need assistance with activities of daily living such as transferring, toileting, eating, dressing, bathing, and taking medications). Such support services can help older adults stay in their preferred community residences (Søvde et al., 2022).

Language and Communication Influences

In their qualitative ethnonursing study, Fornehed et al. (2020) found that **communication** and family decision making at end of life is complex. This complexity stems in part from lack of health literacy. Personal health literacy was redefined for *Healthy People 2030* as the "degree to which individuals have the ability to find, understand, and use information and services to inform health-related decisions and actions for themselves and others" (Office of Disease Prevention and Health Promotion [ODPHP], n.d.). Older adults may struggle with health literacy for several reasons. For example, older adults being treated in healthcare environments get a great deal of information in a short amount of time. Individual factors such as sensory deficits (e.g., hearing or vision impairment) can be significant barriers to gaining and understanding health information. Further, these challenges need to be addressed in a culturally acceptable manner.

Culturally and linguistically appropriate services (CLAS Standards) should be incorporated in care of all people. The CLAS Standards focus on respect and responsiveness to individual cultural similarities and differences (McFarland, 2018; NSCLAS, n.d.). The goal is to improve quality of care and reduce health disparities.

Organizational obstacles include healthcare teams who have little to no education about effectively communicating health information (Riffenburgh & Stableford, 2020; Santana et al., 2021). However, with appropriate training and intentionality, healthcare professionals can ensure that older adult patients understand healthcare decisions, which will significantly affect health and well-being. Clear communication is a crucial first step to facilitate healthcare literacy. Using plain, nonmedical language, speaking slowly, and drawing pictures are strategies that can enhance patient understanding. Often nurses and other healthcare providers use pictures to explain complex health phenomena to patients and families (Riffenburgh & Stableford, 2020; Santana et al., 2021).

Kinship, Social, and Community Influences

Kinship, social, and community connectedness are integral components of an older adult's health and well-being (see Fig. 8-1) (Reich et al., 2020). **Social support** has been defined in three ways: (a) affective support (expressions of respect and love); (b) affirmational support (having endorsement for one's behavior and perceptions); and (c) tangible support (receiving aid or physical assistance, such as accompanying a person to an appointment). Many older adults are deprived of informal social supports due to losses including but not limited to:

- Geographic separation from family members
- Age-related segregation caused by increased nuclear families in neighborhoods
- Loss of spouse or partner due to illness, death, and dying
- Loss of leisure pursuits or entertainment due to illness, loss of income, and/or functional decline

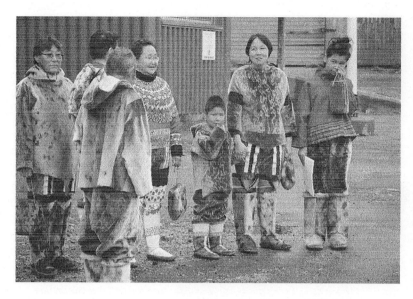

Figure 8-1. Successful aging through social engagements with family. (From TeodorLazarev/ Shutterstock.com)

The Ramifications of Social Isolation and Loneliness on Older Adult Health

When discussing kinship, social, and community influences on older adult health, it is essential to consider the importance of social isolation and loneliness, which have been studied in the United States (National Academies of Sciences, Engineering, and Medicine, 2020) and internationally (Bigonnesse & Chaudhury, 2019; Kemperman et al., 2019; Pinazo-Hernandis et al., 2022). Social isolation is "an objective lack of social contact with others," while loneliness is "the subjective feeling of being isolated," and both are "underappreciated public health risks" (NASEM, 2020, p. xi). Older adults may experience loneliness following events characteristic of late life, for example, death of a spouse, moving to unfamiliar new environments such as long-term care, and functional decline (Miller, 2023c).

The NASEM conducted a comprehensive review of loneliness and social isolation among U.S. older adults ≥ 50 years old. Synthesizing evidence from four decades of research, the NASEM identified significant associations between lack of social connectedness and premature mortality. Interestingly, "there is some evidence that the magnitude of the effect on mortality risk may be comparable to or greater than other well-established risk factors such as smoking, obesity, and physical inactivity" (2020, p. 42). Physical and mental health ramifications of social isolation and loneliness include cardiovascular disease, cognitive decline, depression, anxiety, and diabetes mellitus. Additionally, social isolation and loneliness have been found to impact older adult health behaviors, such as tobacco use, alcohol consumption, poor diet, and lack of exercise (National Academies of Sciences, Engineering, and Medicine, 2020).

Nursing Care to Address Social Isolation and Loneliness of Older Adults

Currently, the NASEM is examining how healthcare providers can care for older adults

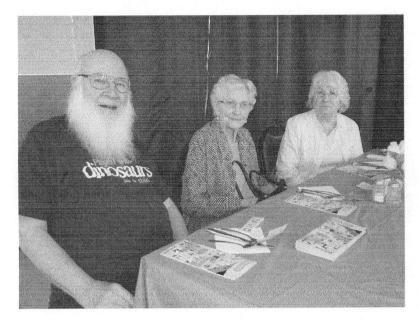

Figure 8-2. Active seniors enjoy a birthday celebration at a community center.

experiencing loneliness and isolation. In particular, the NASEM recommends that nurses follow American Association of Colleges of Nursing guidelines and Essentials (American Association of Colleges of Nursing, 2021), which indicate that nurses should provide culturally congruent holistic care that resonates with an older adult's personal values, beliefs, and lifeways. Furthermore, the NASEM (2020) advises that nurses address biopsychosocial needs of older adults and coordinate care between hospitals and community settings (see Fig. 8-2). When providing culturally congruent gerontological care, nurses and interdisciplinary healthcare team members should address older adult needs for social connectedness and support. Example care actions include (a) helping older adults participate in social/group activities and meals, (b) positioning chairs or wheelchairs so that older adults can interact with one another, and (c) encouraging community-dwelling older adults to participate in support groups about chronic disease management (Miller, 2023c).

Traditional Beliefs and Practices

Older adults may have strong recollections of traditional beliefs and related remedies from childhood. Traditional care practices may be used concurrently with or instead of biomedical approaches by many older adults. An older adult may choose an over-the-counter medication and use other popular remedies before, during, and after prescribed biomedical care practices/approaches. Older individuals may also use folk medicine prepared by "healers" from their cultures. To assess the older client's concurrent use of traditional practices, folk medicine, or popular medicine, nurses can actively listen and ask older adult patients about generic/folk/traditional actions they take to treat their conditions. Case Study 8-1 illustrates that assessing alternative sources of symptom management is useful for codeveloping a culturally congruent care plan with the older adult.

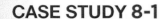

CASE STUDY 8-1

Hospice Care and Metastatic Breast Cancer

Ms. L.V. is an 82-year-old widowed female who has a past medical history (PMH) of breast cancer with right mastectomy and radiation 12 years ago. Other PMH includes hypertension, osteoarthritis, hypothyroidism, and previous left hip arthroplasty. Ms. L.V. has done very well but fell and broke her left femur 1 week ago. After imaging was completed, the healthcare team determined that her fracture was pathologic, and she likely had bone metastasis of her breast cancer. After further workup, she was told that her breast cancer had spread to her bones, lungs, and brain. Ms. L.V. has two daughters who live within 30 minutes of her house. She has been very active in her garden until 3 weeks ago, when she started having low back pain. She is active in her church community and has several good friends that she talks with weekly and who help her in the garden. Ms. L.V. also lives in a very rural area of the United States and drives 2 hours for an oncology appointment. Ms. L.V.'s femur is fixed so she can ambulate; after discharge she travels with her daughters to see the oncologist who initially treated her breast cancer.

Once her metastatic cancer treatment options have been discussed with Ms. L.V. and her daughters, she tells the oncologist that she is considering

hospice care. Her husband passed away from lung cancer and did not have hospice. However, she remembered how much pain he experienced, and she does not want her last days to be like her spouse's. One of the daughters says she had a friend talk with her about hospice care and all agreed they wanted Ms. L.V. to be comfortable. Ms. L.V. is tearful and tells the doctor she has lived a "good and long life" and wants to "die a good death if possible."

Ms. L.V. and her daughters go to the Hospice and Palliative Care Nursing website (https://www.nhpco.org/hospice-care-overview/hospice-facts-figures/) where they read about the goals of hospice care. How can Ms. L.V. obtain a referral for hospice? What services will she receive from hospice? Ms. L.V. is concerned about being in pain, so symptom control is very important to her and her daughters. If you were the hospice nurse, how would you speak to the patient and her family about common symptoms she may have and how to control these as well as pain control?

One of the daughters speaks up and says she knows of a neighbor who received hospice and "they killed him with all the medicine." As the hospice nurse, how would you address this concern with the daughter? Ms. L.V. reports that she has been using "a salve" a neighbor fixed for her, and it has "really worked" for her back pain. How would you address the use of this folk or nontraditional medicine? Lastly, who can ultimately make the decision to accept hospice care? Are the daughters involved in this decision? How would you discuss hospice with the family and assure them their mother will be comfortable?

Spirituality, Faith, and Religion

Multidisciplinary research indicates that spirituality and religion are broad, overlapping constructs (Dunn & Robinson-Lane, 2020; Victor & Treschuk, 2020). Generally, **spirituality** is described as a personal phenomenon; conversely,

religion is associated with sacred doctrine and collective rituals (Jones, 2020). Interestingly, an individual's spirituality may or may not be connected to religion. A growing number of U.S. adults identify as "spiritual but not religious" (Wixwat & Saucier, 2021). For the purposes of this chapter, we use the term *spirituality* for consistency and to reflect the inclusion of

Table 8-2	Culturally Congruent Spiritual Care for Older Adults

- Provide spiritual care in a culturally congruent manner that aligns with an older adult's values, beliefs, and practices (e.g., incorporate generic/folk practices such as involving a chaplain or traditional healer).
- Provide spiritual care throughout each stage of older adulthood to promote health and well-being, manage illness, thrive despite disability, and transition to death and dying.
- Avoid stereotyping individual spiritual values, beliefs, and practices.
- Consider whether/how spiritual care provision extends to family members, friends, faith-community, loved ones, and informal or formal caregivers.
- Facilitate older adult connectedness with faith community by considering transportation to worship services, internet connections, visual and audio resources (e.g., Bible and other faith-based tools).
- Remember that nurses are responsible for using regulatory and professional standards/guidelines (e.g., the Essentials and Joint Commission) to provide spiritual care.

spiritual, faith, and religious beliefs and practices. Depending on individual, familial, and community worldviews, spiritual beliefs and practices are interconnected.

Decades of multidisciplinary research indicate that spirituality intensifies as adults age and face challenges of late life, including bereavement, social isolation, and functional decline (Burkhardt, 1989, 1993; Jernigan, 2001; Koenig, 2015; Miller, 2023a; Moberg, 2005; Patrick et al., 2022; Reed, 1991; Ross, 1997). Spirituality enhances resilience of older adults (Manning et al., 2019) and facilitates coping with challenging health conditions, losses in personal relationships, diminished sense of purpose, and chronic stress. In these ways, spirituality plays an important role in successful/healthy aging (Miller, 2023c). Additionally, cultural worldviews influence older adults' spiritual beliefs and practices (McFarland, 2018). Therefore, there is no universal approach to spiritual nursing care. Interdisciplinary teams can effectively address the unique spiritual needs and preferences of individual patients (Peteet et al., 2019).

Nurses striving to provide culturally congruent care should consider that religious, spiritual, and philosophical factors impact culture care meanings, expressions, patterns, and practices of older adults as they maintain health or cope with illness, disability, death, and dying (McFarland, 2018). Along with physiologic, sociocultural, lifestyle, and economic factors, nurses should assess spiritual beliefs and practices of individuals, families, and communities (American Nurses' Association, n.d.; McFarland, 2018). Providing culturally congruent spiritual care for older adults is outlined in Table 8-2. To enhance spiritual assessment and care, the spiritual dimension should be incorporated in nursing practice, science, and education (American Holistic Nurses Association, 2022; Hawthorne & Gordon, 2020). Spiritual care education enhances spiritual care competence among undergraduate nursing students (Bush et al., 2022), and spiritual care trainings in the workplace have been found to enhance practicing nurses' spiritual care knowledge (American Holistic Nurses Association, 2022; Green et al., 2020; Hawthorne & Gordon, 2020). Additionally, nurse faculty need guidelines about teaching culturally congruent spiritual assessment and care (Bush et al., 2022). See Case Study 8-2.

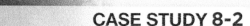

CASE STUDY 8-2

Assessing Spirituality

Mrs. Smith is an 85-year-old woman who was born and raised in Yalobusha County, one of the most religious counties in Mississippi. Like all her older loved ones, Mrs. Smith was raised in an evangelical Baptist church. Throughout her childhood, she learned that faith and prayer are integral components of health; therefore, Mrs. Smith engages her faith beliefs and practices for healthcare decision making. When the COVID-19 pandemic began, Mrs. Smith and her friends prayed daily for God to keep their loved ones safe and healthy. In addition to prayer, Bible studies, and spending time with her church family, Mrs. Smith followed the guidelines for COVID-19 prevention. She wore masks, attended church services online, and communicated through video chat with her children and grandchildren.

In late spring 2021, Mrs. Smith has her 6-month check-up. Her nurse, Tiffany, asks Mrs. Smith whether she has gotten her COVID-19 vaccinations. Mrs. Smith explains that she is hesitant to get the vaccines for several reasons. Primarily, she does not understand how the vaccines work, and she is afraid of terrible side effects. Additionally, Mrs. Smith discusses her belief in God and her daily prayers for good health of herself and loved ones.

Using open-ended questions and active listening, Tiffany understands and acknowledges the importance of faith in Mrs. Smith's life and how prayer has influenced her healthcare decision-making for many years. In response to Mrs. Smith's questions, Tiffany teaches her patient about how vaccination enhances immune responses. Tiffany senses that the decision about vaccination is challenging and that Mrs. Smith could benefit from an interdisciplinary approach. The nurse asks Mrs. Smith's doctor and the clinic chaplain to join the conversation and answer Mrs. Smith's questions. Mrs. Smith learns that her comorbidities of hypertension, diabetes, and lung disease increase her risk for severe illness and death. As the healthcare team listens to and honors Mrs. Smith's priorities and perspectives, they cultivate a trusting relationship with her. Ultimately, Mrs. Smith tells her healthcare team that she will go home, pray about her decision, and notify the team when she is ready. The nurse, doctor, and chaplain ensure that Mrs. Smith has no more questions. She tells her team that she feels equipped with reliable information, and she feels prepared to discuss her decision with God and her loved ones. Her healthcare team demonstrates respect and provides culturally congruent care for Mrs. Smith as she makes this very important decision.

Construct of Care

Care constructs are abstract and concrete phenomena that indicate how older people support one another. **Caring** includes professional and folk ideas that might be used to heal, comfort, and support an older person's well-being. When abstract, caring can be invisible and often difficult for a nurse to identify. Care constructs have now been confirmed in multiple qualitative ethnonursing studies that provide nurses with crucial information as they care for culturally diverse older adults (McFarland & Wehbe-Alamah, 2019). Qualitative research using the ethnonursing method has demonstrated more than 170 care constructs from more than 58 cultures (McFarland, 2018). Fornehed et al. (2020) describes five care constructs related to caring practices of families in rural Appalachia who make decisions for severely ill older adults. These practices were family involvement, communication, comfort, hope, and faith.

Holistic Culturally Congruent Care of Older Adults

Integrating generic and professional care in the aging population can safely and creatively blend holistic care practices that will benefit older adults within the context of their cultural beliefs and lifeways (McFarland & Wehbe-Alamah, 2019). Nurses who deliver transcultural care to this population understand the importance of integrated care and multidisciplinary approaches. For example, nurses can work in interdisciplinary teams with case managers, social workers, pharmacists, registered dieticians, speech pathologists, physical therapists, and respiratory therapists, among others.

Over decades, modern medicine technologies have improved, but nurses know that not all persons have access to these technologies. Many cultures use generic or folk care in the form of herbs, liniments, and practices to heal, cure, or relieve symptoms of various illnesses, and these traditional practices are passed down for generations. Nurses have become increasingly aware of folk medicine and the importance of looking beyond biomedical care to include folk practices that older adults were taught over generations. An important consideration for nurses is that folk care may delay an older adult from seeking care at a health facility; unfortunately, this may result in an individual seeking care late in the illness trajectory (Fornehed et al., 2020).

Well-being Care Expressions and Practices

Many older adults seek health information and make behavioral changes to maintain independence as they age. Older adults who use self-help strategies to stay healthy generally report better psychological well-being and physical functioning than do older adults who do not use these approaches (Taylor et al., 2018).

Nurses can provide helpful information about the benefits of exercise, smoking cessation, and healthy eating habits. Additionally, nurses may also ask older clients about circumstances that inhibit exercise (e.g., fear of walking in unsafe neighborhoods) and then help clients find ways to incorporate exercise into daily life. Furthermore, nurses who are aware of cultural variations can appreciate that older individuals have diverse value orientations underlying their decisions related to healthy behaviors. Older adults may also learn how to cope with chronic illness and assess new illness symptoms.

Community nurses can coordinate with families caring for older adults who need formal support services (e.g., visiting nurse services, chore services, and adult day care) and informal support services (e.g., family members who provide relief care, neighborhood volunteers, and meal delivery) (see Fig. 8-3). Families of older ethnic minority adults have various reactions to and access of formal services owing to their knowledge, potential residential segregation,

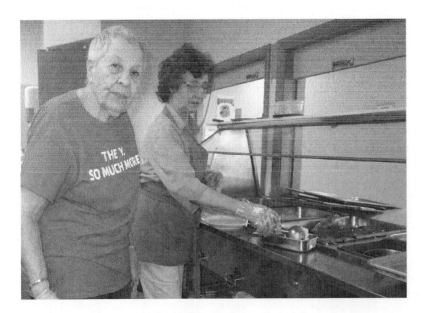

Figure 8-3. Older adults volunteering at a community center.

confidence, inadequate health insurance, and comfort in the use of service providers (Bonds & Lyons, 2018; Crist et al., 2018; Epps et al., 2018). In addition to assessing the well-being of the older adult client, nurses also assess a caregiver's capacities, needs, and resources in planning for extended care of an older adult at home. For example, a nurse may support a caregiver who is a working parent sandwiched between the care of an older relative and also caring for adolescent children. A caregiver could also be a retired worker in their 60s who has a chronic illness.

The developing array of home-based care organizations that offer personal care (e.g., home health aide care) and supportive services (e.g., transportation) present options for the growing population of older adults who want to live in their home communities. The levels and types of services that are available necessitate an expanded role for nurses to work in ambulatory care settings and assist older clients as they determine the best care option/setting. The terms screening, geriatric assessment, and/or health risk appraisal may be used for a systematic process when a nurse identifies the strengths and limitations of an older client's physical, mental, and psychosocial spiritual condition (Simpson & Pedigo, 2018).

Many local and faith-based agencies can train volunteers to care for older adults; these community care approaches may be used in conjunction with formal care services that help older adults with many comorbid problems function at home. For many older adults, the value of independence is so strong that a person would rather live alone, even in poor health, than become a burden to their family. Moreover, some older adults feel stigmatized by residence in a congregate care facility and would prefer to live in an independent location in the community (Søvde et al., 2022). See Case Study 8-3.

CASE STUDY 8-3

The Influence of Mr. Brown's Environment on his Health and Well-Being

Despite his 85 years and multiple chronic conditions, Mr. Brown is highly energetic, independent, and attentive to his health. He diligently records his blood pressure twice daily and takes the blood pressure logs to his cardiologist every 3 months. But at his June visit, Mr. Brown's nurse, Tiffany, notices that he forgot to bring his blood pressure logs, looks disheveled, and has high blood pressure during the clinic visit. Dr. Green, his primary care provider, sends new prescriptions to Mr. Brown's pharmacy and makes an appointment with Mr. Brown in a month.

Mr. Brown misses his appointment, which the healthcare team notes is unusual for him. Mr. Brown does not schedule another appointment for 3 months. When he arrives, Tiffany and Dr. Green sense there is a problem. Mr. Brown reports that he has stopped taking his blood pressure at home, never got the new prescriptions. His clothes are ragged, and he has lost weight. Mr. Brown's face is gaunt, and he is no longer smiling or humorous. Tiffany and Dr. Green sense that Mr. Brown has "given up."

Neither Tiffany nor Dr. Green knows about the recurrent shootings in Mr. Brown's neighborhood, which have increased in frequency and rendered his environment unsafe. This environmental shift has deeply impacted Mr. Brown's daily routines. He used to contribute to managing his blood pressure, cholesterol, and glucose levels by walking around the neighborhood park. Now, he stays at home and watches television for hours each day. He stopped walking to the grocery store and the pharmacy because both are in particularly dangerous areas of the community. Over time, as the neighborhood has become more violent, Mr. Brown only feels safe walking to the corner store, which has no fresh produce. Mr. Brown buys canned soup, white bread, deli meats, and processed sweets. Since his wife died 1 year ago and his son moved away, Mr. Brown's church friends have become his family/primary support system. Mr. Brown has stopped going to church for fear of being exposed to drug deals and violent situations. Additionally, Mr. Brown is living on a fixed income and cannot afford to have the internet at home; he cannot use email or online platforms to connect with people from the safety of his apartment.

During his October visit, Tiffany and Mr. Brown actively listen and ask open-ended questions to determine the root problem of Mr. Brown's declining health. Shyly, Mr. Brown tells them about his current circumstances. Tiffany and Dr. Green coordinate with the social worker and mental health counselor at the clinic. They help Mr. Brown find low-income senior housing in a safer neighborhood. In his new environment, Mr. Brown feels comfortable walking to the grocery store, pharmacy, and local library where he attends church services online and remains connected with his friends.

Following this experience as an interdisciplinary team, the nurse, primary care physician, social worker, and counselor gather to discuss how—even in neighborhoods only 5 miles apart—older adults' cultural perspectives vary widely and should be assessed accordingly. Tiffany decides to hang a map of the city inside the exam room so patients can point to their neighborhoods. Information about an older adult's environmental context is used by nurses to further assess needs, that is, food availability, transportation, pharmacy, and community resources to coordinate patient-centered culturally congruent care.

When older adults choose to relocate to new residences late in life, these decisions can lead to increased unfamiliarity in new neighborhoods. New residents then take the opportunity to interact with peers. For many older adults, participation in community activities, cultural events, or recreational sites is very fulfilling (see Fig. 8-4). Other prospective residents might prefer the stimulation of intergenerational contact outside of an age-restricted residence. As they decide where/how to live and grow old, older adults work through developmental tasks to discover where they feel satisfied and fulfilled (Reich et al., 2020; Søvde et al., 2022).

Intergenerational programs support older adults as they become involved with local communities and educational systems. These programs include the Older American Volunteer Program, the Retired and Senior Volunteer Program, and the Foster Grandparents Program. There are also intergenerational childcare centers that facilitate beneficial relationships among children and older adults in local communities. Evaluations of multigenerational programs found that older volunteers demonstrated high level of life satisfaction, including psychosocial adjustment, positive social exchanges, and self-esteem (Carver et al., 2018).

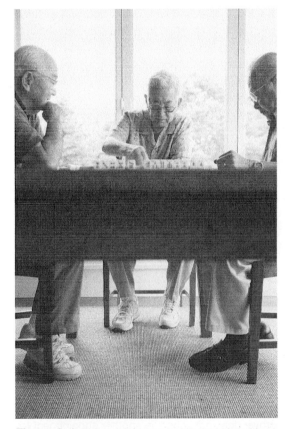

Figure 8-4. Retirees enjoy an activity in their residential community. (From Blend Images/Shutterstock.com.)

Disability and Illness Care Expressions and Practices

Over time, evidence-based clinical guidelines have been developed to enhance care for older adults with acute and chronic conditions who reside in community and institutional settings. Several print and visual media sources can guide the nurse in assessing an older client. For example, print media should be short and precise using everyday language. Serif fonts with "tails" are easier to read for the older client. The use of upper and lowercase letters with lots of white space around the writing is also much easier to read. As they age, many older adults receive three types of care based on changing needs: (1) intensive personal health service; (2) health maintenance and restorative care; and (3) coordinated nursing, social services, and ancillary services that are provided episodically for community-dwelling older adults. Many older adults require care and assistance to manage chronic conditions. A current major public health goal is to encourage adults to adopt and follow health-promoting actions in younger years to minimize the risk for developing chronic conditions.

The roles that family members take in caring for and supporting their elders vary according to cultural, socioeconomic, and demographic characteristics. Nurses and other healthcare professionals can ask families about whether they retain generic/folk/traditional values and/or blend biomedical approaches to care. Nurses working with older adults should be sensitive to the evolving needs of family caregivers.

Dying and Death Care Expressions and Practices

Depending on environment and cultural worldview, older adults with life-limiting or terminal illness have preferences when dying. Nurses provide culturally and spiritually congruent care as diverse older adults face death and dying (Embler et al., 2015; Fornehed et al., 2020; Mixer et al., 2014). For example, Fornehed et al. (2020) found that rural Appalachian persons wanted family to assist with end-of-life decision-making; they sought comfort in their last days by tending gardens, checking livestock, or watching television shows. Some older adults sought comfort in hospice care; however, not all participants felt that hospice was helpful in a family member's last days. The inability to predict the illness trajectory and the fear of losing all assets that had been so hard-earned played a huge role in making decisions at EOL for rural Appalachians.

Lack of palliative and EOL education regarding communication with severely ill older adults can be a significant barrier to culturally appropriate care. Some terminally ill aged adults and their families have reported that it is difficult to obtain the information needed to make well-informed decisions for a care plan that meets the needs of the person who is dying. Poor communication with the family and severely ill individuals could also mean that the older adult and family members rely on "a miracle (p. 192)" and a "sliver of hope (p. 192)" for recovery (Fornehed et al., 2020).

Many nurses view culturally congruent EOL care as complex. Beaver et al. (2021) addressed the importance of accepting ill persons for who they were and where they were at that time in their lives; such acceptance facilitates therapeutic relationships and culturally appropriate care provision. Understanding that terminally ill people and their families move along an illness trajectory at different rates and that generic (folk) care lends the feeling of normalcy, nurses and the interdisciplinary team should respect and accommodate the terminally ill aged adult's faith expressions and practices along with assessing the diverse economics of all terminally ill persons by gaining understanding of family resources (Fornehed et al., 2020). Finally, culturally appropriate **palliative care** and EOL care is needed for interdisciplinary team members in acute and community settings so that families and people with severe illnesses understand their options when making these decisions. Recommendations for providing culturally congruent EOL care for older adults is outlined in Table 8-3.

Table 8-3	Recommendations for Providing Culturally Congruent End-of-Life (EOL) Care for Older Adults

- Understand that EOL care is contextualized within an older adult's values, beliefs, and practices and extends to family members, friends, faith-community, loved ones, and informal or formal caregivers.
- Actively listen and communicate using easily understood terminology, visual aids, and written materials to promote patient and family understanding of life-limiting illness and palliative/hospice services.
- Preserve generic/folk care that helps create a "sense of normalcy" to support and comfort older adults.
- Accommodate faith practices among older adults and loved ones.
- Assess the older adult and family for economic factors that may influence access to EOL care in the desired setting (e.g., home, assisted living, skilled nursing facility, or acute care); then facilitate resources.

Note: Some recommendations have been adapted from earlier studies (Fornehed, M. L. C., Mixer, S. J., & Lindley, L. C. [2020]. Families' decision making at end of life in rural Appalachia. *Journal of Hospice & Palliative Nursing, 22*[3], 188–195; Mixer, S. J., Fornehed, M. L., Varney, J., & Lindley, L. C. [2014]. Culturally congruent end-of-life care for rural Appalachian people and their families. *Journal of Hospice and Palliative Nursing, 16*[8], 536–535. https://doi.org/10.1097/NJH.0000000000000114).

Summary

Taken together, the influences, expressions, and care practices described have a compounding impact on older adult holistic health, well-being, disability, illness, dying, and death. **Culturally congruent care** for older adults reflects that individuals are products of and participants in an encompassing societal framework. Cultural backgrounds of older adults influence variations in their culture care expressions and practices. Culture serves as a guide for the older adult to determine health-related choices and actions that are appropriate and acceptable. Within cultural groups, individual variation is evident in responses to the physiologic signs and the psychosocial demands of increasing age. As part of their assessment, nurses in acute care or community settings often ask several questions related to older adulthood:

1. Is the older adult isolated from or enmeshed in a caring network of relatives and friends?
2. Has a culturally appropriate network replaced family members in performing some tasks for the older adult client?
3. Does the older adult expect family members to provide care, including nurturance and emotional support, which family members are unable to provide?
4. Does language create a barrier in the older client's receipt of services from formal (and informal) resources?

Older adult clients have often developed their own informal support systems (e.g., help from neighbors) for coping with illness and age-related changes/challenges. Formal resources may be used to sustain the informal support systems to promote the lifestyle preferred by the older client. Nurses caring for older adult clients should tend to the client's family and social roles and develop care plans that maintain and restore the individual to their usual roles and patterns of activity. In the future, nurses will assess and support more older clients as they progress along a continuum of services and types of residence.

Clients may be reluctant to use services for various reasons, such as cultural and linguistic differences or previous negative experiences in healthcare settings. To overcome such barriers perceived by older clients, nurses can be advocates and teach clients to be self-advocates for services and eligibility. Nurses may also assume a care coordinator role to link interdisciplinary services such as physical and occupational therapy, nutrition services, or social support services to safely sustain older adults with health needs in community settings (Shaw et al., 2018).

REVIEW QUESTIONS

1. What resources, needs, and limitations should the nurse assess to develop a care plan for a recently discharged 82-year-old chronically ill man with end-stage chronic obstructive lung disease who is returning to low-income housing with hospice?

2. As the nurse who does health assessments for older adults who attend a community comprehensive day program, what information should the nurse assess to identify culturally appropriate care plans or service delivery plans for older rural Appalachian clients?

3. The inpatient intensive care unit where you are the nurse manager serves a multinational group of older clients who are admitted for life-limiting illness. What cultural assessments do you teach the staff to use in identifying the spiritual needs of clients and their families?

CRITICAL THINKING ACTIVITIES

1. If you are a case manager for a managed care organization, you receive many authorization requests for in-home nursing services to assist older adults who have been discharged home following hospitalization for acute illnesses or surgery. List the factors that you will consider and the types of data that you need to make an informed decision about the nursing and health-related services and the duration of services that the older client should receive while at home.

2. In many communities, nurses provide hospice services to residents in long-term care facilities or to older adults living in other settings.

Contact a community-based hospice nurse to request information about how the services meet older adults' needs for caring, hope, and belongingness, as well as reflection and recollection that are expressed late in life.

3. With your awareness that cultural traditions and life experiences influence many older adults who prefer independent living, prepare a letter as a home health nurse to the appropriate official to request government-funded home health services for older adults.

REFERENCES

Administration for Community Living. (2021). *2020 profile of older Americans.* https://chrome-extension://efaid-nbmnnnibpcajpcglclefindmkaj/https://acl.gov/sites/default/files/aging%20and%20Disability%20In%20America/2020Profileolderamericans.final_.pdf

Ahn, M., Kwon, H. J., & Kang, J. (2020). Supporting aging-in-place well: Findings from a cluster analysis of the reasons for aging-in-place and perceptions of well-being. *Journal of Applied Gerontology, 39*(1), 3–15. https://doi.org/10.1177/0733464817748779

American Association of Colleges of Nursing. (2021). *The essentials: Core competencies for professional nursing education.* https://www.aacnnursing.org/AACN-Essentials

American Association of Retired Persons [AARP]. (2020). https://www.aarp.org/home-garden/transportation/info-11-2010/getting_around_guide_public_transit.html

American Holistic Nurses Association. (2022). *What is holistic nursing?* https://www.ahna.org/About-Us/What-is-Holistic-Nursing

American Medical Association Manual of Style Committee (2007). *AMA manual of style: A style guide for authors and editors* (10th ed.). Oxford University Press.

American Nurses Association. (n.d.). *The nursing process.* https://www.nursingworld.org/practice-policy/workforce/what-is-nursing/the-nursing-process/

American Psychological Association. (2020). *Publication Manual of the American Psychological Association* (7th ed.). American Psychological Association.

American Psychological Association. (2023). *A snapshot of today's older adults and facts to help dispel myths about aging. Older adults: Health and age-related changes.* American Psychological Association. https://www.apa.org/pi/aging/resources/guides/older

Ayalon, L. (2018). Transition and adaptation to the continuing care retirement community from a life course perspective: Something old, something new, and something borrowed.

Journal of Applied Gerontology, 37(3), 267–288. https://doi.org/10.1177/0733464816637851

Beaver, C., Bidwill, S., Hallauer, A., Kopp, P., Perkins, D., Rice, C., Weithman, L. & Rebar, C. (2021). Providing culturally congruent care. *Nursing, 51*(12), 58–59. https://doi.org/10.1097/01.NURSE.0000800108.58421.a4

Bigonnesse, C., & Chaudhury, H. (2019). The landscape of "aging in place" in gerontology literature: Emergency, theoretical perspectives, and influencing factors. *Journal of Aging and Environment, 34*(3), 233–251. https://doi.org/10.1080/02763893.2019.1638875

Bonds, K., & Lyons, K. S. (2018). Formal service use by African American individuals with dementia and their caregivers: An integrative review. *Journal of Gerontological Nursing, 44*(6), 33–39.

Brossoie, N., Robnett, R. H., & Chop, W. (2020). Age matters: Profiles of an aging society. In *Gerontology for the health care professional* (4th ed., pp. 1–25). Jones & Bartlett.

Buettner, D., & Skemp, S. (2016). Blue zones: Lessons from the world's longest lived. *American Journal of Lifestyle Medicine, 10*(5), 318–321. https://doi.org/10.1177/1559827616637066

Burkhardt, M. A. (1989). Spirituality: An analysis of the concept. *Holistic Nursing Practice, 3*(3), 69–77.

Burkhardt, M. A. (1993). Characteristics of spirituality in the lives of women in a rural Appalachian community. *Journal of Transcultural Nursing, 4*(2), 12–18.

Bush, R. S., Baliko, B., & Raynor, P. (2022). Building spiritual care competency in undergraduate psychiatric mental health nursing students: A quality improvement project. *Journal of Holistic Nursing, 41*(3), 256–264. https://doi.org/10.1177/08980101221103104

Carver, L. F., Beamish, R., Phillips, S. P., & Villeneuve, M. (2018). A scoping review: Social participation as a cornerstone of successful aging in place among rural older adults. *Geriatrics, 3*(4), Article 4. https://doi.org/10.3390/geriatrics3040075

Centers for Disease Control and Prevention. (2022a). *Life expectancy in the U.S. dropped for the year in a row in 2021*. https://www.cdc.gov/nchs/pressroom/nchs_press_releases/2022/20220831.htm

Centers for Disease Control and Prevention. (2022b, July). *Racial and ethnic approaches to community health (REACH)*. https://www.cdc.gov/nccdphp/dnpao/state-local-programs/reach/

Centers for Disease Control and Prevention. (2023). *Demographic trends of COVID-19 cases and deaths in the US reported to CDC*. https://covid.cdc.gov/covid-data-tracker/#demographics

Cramm, J. M., Van Dijk, H. M., & Nieboer, A. P. (2018). The creation of age-friendly environments are especially important to frail older people. *Aging & Society, 38*(4), 700–720.

Crist, J. D., Montgomery, M. L., Pasvogel, A., Phillips, L. R., & Ortiz-Dowling, E. M. (2018). The association among knowledge of and confidence in home health care services, acculturation, and family caregivers' relationships to older adults of Mexican descent. *Geriatric Nursing, 39*(6), 689–695.

Dadras, O., Ahmad, S., Alinaghi, S., Karimi, A., Shamsabadi, A, Qaderi, K., Ramezani, M., Mirghaderi, S. P., Mahdiabadi, S., Vahedi, F., Saeidi, S., Shojaei, A., Mehrtak, M., Azar, S. A., Mehraeen, E., & Voltarelli, F. A. (2022). COVID-19 mortality and its predictors in the elderly: A systematic review. *Health Science Reports, 5*(4), e723. https://doi.org/10.1002/hsr2.657

Dao, M. C., Yu, Z., Maafs-Rodríguez, A., Moser, B., Cuevas, A. G., Economos, C. D., & Roberts, S. B. (2022). Perceived intrinsic, social, and environmental barriers for weight management in older Hispanic/Latino adults with obesity. *Obesity Science and Practice, 9*, 145–157. https://doi.org/10.1002/osp4.631

Dunn, K. S., & Robinson-Lane, S. G. (2020). A philosophical analysis of spiritual coping. *Advances in Nursing Science, 43*(3), 239–250. https://doi.org/10.1097/ANS.0000000000000323

Eastern Band of Cherokee Indians Public Health & Human Services Division. (2019). *Eastern Band of Cherokee Indians Tribal Health Assessment 2018* (pp. 1–128). https://phhs.ebci-nsn.gov/wp-content/uploads/2021/10/THA-2018-FINAL-060119.pdf

Embler, P., Mixer, S. J., & Gunther, M. (2015). End-of-life culture care practices among Yup'ik Eskimo. *Online Journal of Cultural Competence in Nursing and Healthcare, 5*(1), 36–49. https://doi.org/10.9730/ojccnh.org/v5nIa3

Epps, F., Weeks, G., Graham, E., & Luster, D. (2018). Challenges to aging in place for African American older adults living with dementia and their families. *Geriatric Nursing, 39*(6), 646–652. Retrieved from www.gnjournal.com

Fornehed, M. L. C., Mixer, S. J., & Lindley, L. C. (2020). Families' decision making at end of life in rural Appalachia. *Journal of Hospice & Palliative Nursing, 22*(3), 188–195.

FrameWorks Institute. (2023). https://www.frameworksinstitute.org/publication/gauging-aging-mapping-the-gaps-between-expert-and-public-understandings-of-aging-in-america/

Fulmer, T., Reuben, D. B., Auerbach, J., Fick, D. M., Galambos, C., & Johnson, K. S. (2021, January 21). Actualizing better health and health care for older adults. *Health Affairs, 40*(2), 219–225. https://doi.org/10.1377/hlthaff.2020.01470

Gimie, A. M., Melgar Castillo, A. I., Mullins, C. D., & Falvey, J. R. (2022). Epidemiology of public transportation use among older adults in the United States. *Journal of the American Geriatrics Society, 70*(12), 3549–3559. https://doi.org/10.1111/jgs.18055

Green, A., Kim-Godwin, Y. S., & Jones, C. W. (2020). Perceptions of spiritual care education, competence, and barriers in providing spiritual care among registered nurses. *Journal of Holistic Nursing, 38*(1), 41–51. https://doi.org/10.1177/0898010119885266

Hawthorne, D. M., & Gordon, S. C. (2020). The invisibility of spiritual nursing care in clinical practice. *Journal of Holistic Nursing, 38*(1), 147–155. https://doi.org/10.1177/0898010119889704s

Hill, L., Ndugga, N., & Artiga, S. (2023, March 15). *Key data on health and health care by race and ethnicity.* Kaiser Family Foundation. https://www.kff.org/racial-equity-and-health-policy/report/key-data-on-health-and-health-care-by-race-and-ethnicity/#:~:text=Provisional%20data%20from%202021%20show,77.7%20years%20for%20Hispanic%20people

Hill-Briggs, F., Adler, N. E., Berkowitz, S. A., Chin, M. H., Gary-Webb, T. L., Navas-Acien, A., Thornton, P. L., & Haire-Joshu, D. (2020). Social Determinants of Health and Diabetes: A Scientific Review. *Diabetes care, 44*(1), 258–279. Advance online publication. https://doi.org/10.2337/dci20-0053

Hirchak, K. A., Leickly, E., Herron, J., Shaw, J., Skalisky, J., Dirks, L. G., Avey, J. P., McPherson, S., Nepom, J., Donovan, D., Buchwald, D., & McDonell, M. G.; The HONOR Study Team (2018). Focus groups to increase the cultural acceptability of a contingency management intervention for American Indian and Alaska Native Communities. *Journal of Substance Abuse Treatment, 90,* 57–63. https://doi.org/10.1016/j.jsat.2018.04.014

Home page | ACL Administration for Community Living. (n.d.). http://acl.gov/

Isaacson, M. J., Bott-Knutson, R. C., Fishback, M. B., Varnum, A., & Brandenburger, S. (2018). Native elder and youth perspectives on mental well-being, the value of the horse, and navigating two worlds. *Online Journal of Rural Nursing & Health Care, 18*(2), 265+. https://doi.org/10.14574/ojrnhc.v18i2.542

Jacobsen, G., Cicchiello, A., Shah, A., Doty, M. M., & Williams II, R. D. (2021, October 1). *When costs are a barrier to getting health care: Reports from older adults in the United States and other high-income countries.* The Commonwealth Fund.

Jernigan, H. L. (2001). Spirituality in older adults: A cross-cultural and interfaith perspective. *Pastoral Psychology, 49*(6), 413–437.

Jones, C. L. C. (2020). Spiritual well-being in older adults: A concept analysis. *Journal of Christian Nursing, 37*(4), E31–D38. https://doi.org/10.1097/CNJ.0000000000000770

Kemperman, A., van den Berg, P., Weijs-Perrée, M., & Uijtdewillegen, K. (2019). Loneliness of older adults: Social network and the living environment. *International Journal of Environmental Research and Public Health, 16*(3), 406. https://doi.org/10.3390/ijerph16030406

Khatana, S. A. M., & Groeneveld, P. W. (2020). Health disparities and the coronavirus disease 2019 (COVID-19) pandemic in the USA. *Journal of General Internal Medicine, 35,* 2431–2432.

Koenig, H. G. (2015). Religion, spirituality, and health: A review and update. *Advances in Mind-Body Medicine, 29*(3), 19–26.

Kreouzi, M., Theodorakis, N., & Constantinou, C. (2022). Lessons learned from blue zones, lifestyle medicine pillars and beyond: An update on the contributions of behavior and genetics to wellbeing and longevity. *American Journal of Lifestyle Medicine.* https://doi.org/10.1177/15598276221118494

Kwak, J., Ko, E., & Kramer, B. J. (2014). Facilitating advance care planning with ethnically diverse groups of frail, low-income elders in the USA: Perspectives of care managers on challenges and recommendations. *Health and Social Care in the Community, 22*(2), 169–177. https://doi.org/10.1111/hsc.12073

Lee, S. B., Oh, J. H., Park, J. H., Choi, S. P., & Wee, J. H. (2018). Differences in youngest-old, middle-old, and oldest-old patients who visit the emergency department. *Clinical and Experimental Emergency Medicine, 5*(4), 249–255. https://doi.org/10.15441/ceem.17.261

Lopez, L., Hart, L. H., & Katz, M. H. (2021). Racial and ethnic health disparities related to COVID-19. *Jama, 325*(8), 719–720.

Lundebjerg, N. E., Trucil, D. E., Hammond, E. C., & Applegate, W. B. (2017). When it comes to older adults, language matters: Journal of the American Geriatrics Society adopts modified American medical association style [Editorial]. *Journal of the American Geriatrics Society, 65*(7), 1386–1388. https://doi.org/10.1111/jgs.14941

Mabli, J., Gearan, E., Cohen, R., Niland, K., Redel, N., Panzarella, E., & Carlson, B. (2017, April 21). *Evaluation of the effect of the older Americans act title iii-c nutrition services program on participants' food security, socialization, and diet quality.* https://acl.gov/sites/default/files/programs/2017-07/aoa_outcomesevaluation_final.pdf

Manning, L., Ferris, M., Rosario, C. N., Prues, M., & Bouchard, L. (2019). Spiritual resilience: Understanding the protection and promotion of well-being in the later life. *Journal of Religion, Spirituality, and Aging, 31*(2), 168–186. https://doi.org/10.1080/15528030.2018.1532859

Mateyka, P., & He, W. (2022, October 12). People ages 65 and older with disabilities change residences more often but move shorter distances. United States Census Bureau. https://www.census.gov/library/stories/2022/10/do-disabilities-impact-older-peoples-moves-to-other-locations.html

McAfee, T., Malone, R. E., & Cataldo, J. (2021). Ignoring our elders: Tobacco control's forgotten health equity issue. In *Tobacco control* (Vol. 30, Issue 5, pp. 479–480). BMJ Publishing Group Ltd.

McFarland, M. R. (2018). The theory of culture care diversity and universality. In M. R. McFarland & H. B. Wehbe-Alamah (Eds.), *Leininger's transcultural nursing: Concepts, theories, research & practice* (4th ed., pp. 39–56). McGraw Hill Education.

McFarland, M. R., & Wehbe-Alamah, H. B. (2019). Leininger's theory of culture care diversity and universality: An overview with a historical retrospective and a view toward the future. *Journal of Transcultural Nursing, 30*(6), 540–557. https://doi.org/10.1177/1043659619867134

McMaughan, D. J., Oloruntoba, O., & Smith, M. L. (2020). Socioeconomic status and access to healthcare: Interrelated drivers for healthy aging. *Frontiers in Public Health, 8*, 231. https://doi.org/10.3389/fpubh.2020.00231

Miller, C. A. (2023a). Caring for older adults at the end of life. In C. A. Miller (Ed.), *Nursing for wellness in older adults* (9th ed., pp. 600–614). Wolters Kluwer.

Miller, C. A. (2023b). Health care for older adults in various settings. In C. A. Miller (Ed.), *Nursing for wellness in older adults* (9th ed., pp. 88–101). Wolters Kluwer.

Miller, C. A. (2023c). Psychosocial wellness. In C. A. Miller (Ed.), *Nursing for wellness in older adults* (9th ed., pp. 212–237). Wolters Kluwer.

Mixer, S. J., Fornehed, M. L., Varney, J., & Lindley, L. C. (2014). Culturally congruent end-of-life care for rural Appalachian people and their families. *Journal of Hospice and Palliative Nursing, 16*(8), 536–535. https://doi.org/10.1097/NJH.0000000000000114

Moberg, D. O. (2005). Research in spirituality, religion, and aging. *Journal of Gerontological Social Work, 45*(1–2), 11–40. https://doi.org/10.1300/J083v45n01_02

Molinsky, J. (2022, August 18). *Housing for America's older adults: Four problems we must address.* Joint Studies for Housing Studies of Harvard University. https://www.jchs.harvard.edu/blog/housing-americas-older-adults-four-problems-we-must-address

Morales, D. A., Barksdale, C. L., & Beckel-Mitchener, A. C. (2020). A call to action to address rural mental health disparities. *Journal of Clinical and Translational Science, 4*(5), 463–467.

National Academies of Sciences, Engineering, and Medicine. (2020). *Social isolation and loneliness in older adults: Opportunities for the health care system.* The National Academies Press. https://doi.org/10.17226/25663

National Aging and Disability Transportation Center. (2023). *Unique issues related to older adults and transportation. Older adults & transportation.* https://www.nadtc.org/about/transportation-aging-disability/unique-issues-related-to-older-adults-and-transportation/

National Council on Aging. (2022a). *Economic security for advocates: Get the facts on economic security for seniors.* https://ncoa.org/article/get-the-facts-on-economic-security-for-seniors

National Council on Aging. (2022b). *Get the facts on older Americans.* https://ncoa.org/article/get-the-facts-on-older-americans

National Health Fact Sheet [NHE]. (2021). https://www.cms.gov/research-statistics-data-and-systems/statistics-trends-and-reports/nationalhealthexpenddata/nhe-fact-sheet

National Institute on Aging, Aging in place. National Institute on Aging. Retrieved May 18, 2023, from. https://www.nia.nih.gov/health/topics/aging-place

National Standards for Culturally and Linguistically Appropriate Services [NSCLAS]. (n.d.). https://thinkculturalhealth.hhs.gov/clas

Office of Disease Prevention and Health Promotion. (n.d.). *Health People 2030.* https://health.gov/healthypeople

Patrick, J. H., Carney, A. K., & Ebert, A. R. (2022). Religious and spiritual growth goals: A forgotten outcome. *The International Journal of Aging and Human Development, 94*(1), 41–54. https://doi.org/10.1177/0091415021103485

Perez, F. P., Perez, C. A., & Chumbiauca, N. (2022). Insights into the social determinants of health in older adults. *Journal of Biomedical Sciences and Engineering, 15*(11), 261–268. https://doi.org/10.4236/jbise.2022.1511023

Peteet, J. R., Al Zaben, F., & Koenig, H. G. (2019). Integrating spirituality into the care of older adults. *International Psychogeriatrics, 31*(1), 31–38. https://doi.org/10.1017/S1041610218000716

Pinazo-Hernandis, S., Blanco-Molina, M., & Ortega-Moreno, R. (2022). Aging in place: Connections, relationships, social participation, and social support in the face of crisis situations. *International Journal of Environmental Research and Public Health, 19*(24), 16623. https://doi.org/10.3390/ijerph192416623

Pooler, J. A., Hartline-Grafton, H., DeBor, M., Sudore, R. L., & Seligman, H. K. (2019). Food insecurity: A key social determinant of health for older adults. *Journal of the American Geriatrics Society, 67*(3), 421–424.

Poulain, M., Herm, A., Errigo, A., Chrysohoou, C., Legrand, R., Passarino, G., Stazi, M. A., Voutekatis, K. G., Gonos, E. S., Franceschi, C., & Pes, G. M. (2021). Specific features of the oldest old from the Longevity Blue Zones in Ikaria and Sardinia. *Mechanisms of Ageing and Development, 198*, 111543. https://doi.org/10.1016/j.mad.2021.111543

Quiñones, A. R., McAvay, G. J., Peak, K. D., Vander Wyk, B., & Allore, H. G. (2022). The Contribution of chronic conditions to hospitalization, skilled nursing facility admission, and death: Variation by race. *American Journal of Epidemiology, 191*(12), 2014–2025. https://doi.org/10.1093/aje/kwac143

Reed, P. G. (1991). Spirituality and mental health in older adults: Extant knowledge for nursing. *Family and Community Health, 14*(2), 14–25.

Reich, A. J., Claunch, K. D., Verdeja, M. A., Dungan, M. T., Anderson, S., Clayton, C. K., Goates, M. C., & Thacker, E. L. (2020). What does "successful Aging" mean to you? — Systematic review and cross-cultural comparison of lay perspectives of older adults in 13 countries, 2010–2020. *Journal of Cross-Cultural Gerontology, 35*(4), 455–478. https://doi.org/10.1007/s10823-020-09416-6

Riffenburgh, A., & Stableford, S. (2020). Health literacy and clear communication: Keys to engaging older adults and their families. *Gerontology for the health care professional* (4th ed., pp. 109–128). Jones & Bartlett.

Roche, M. L., Ambato, L., Sarsoza, J., & Kuhnlein, H. V. (2018). Mothers' groups enrich diet and culture through promoting traditional Quichua foods. *Maternal & Child Nutrition*, *13*(S3), e12530. https://doi.org/10.1111/mcn.12530

Ross, L. (1997). The nurse's role in assessing and responding to patients' spiritual needs. *International Journal of Palliative Nursing*, *3*(1), 37–42.

Samuels, C. (2022, December 13). *Portrait of Americans in assisted living, nursing homes, and skilled nursing facilities*. https://www.aplaceformom.com/caregiver-resources/articles/long-term-care-statistics

Santana, S., Brach, C., Harris, L., Ochiai, E., Blakey, C., Bevington, F., Kleinman, D., & Pronk, N. (2021). Updating health literacy for healthy people 2030: Defining its importance for a new decade in public health. *Journal of Public Health Management and Practice*, *27*(Supplement 6), S258. https://doi.org/10.1097/PHH.0000000000001324

Shaw, R. L., Gwyther, H., Holland, C., Bujnowska, M., Kurpas, D., Cano, A., Marcucci, M., Riva, S., & D'Avanzo, B. (2018). Understanding frailty: Meanings and beliefs about screening and prevention across key stakeholder groups in Europe. *Aging & Society*, *38*(5), 1223–1252.

Siddiq, H., Alemi, Q., & Lee, E. (2023). A qualitative inquiry of older Afghan refugee women's individual and sociocultural factors of health and health care experiences in the United States. *Journal of Transcultural Nursing*, *34*(2), 143–150. https://doi.org/10.1177/10436596221149692

Simpson, V., & Pedigo, L. (2018). Health risk appraisals with aging adults: An integrative review. *Western Journal of Nursing*, *40*(7), 1049–1068.

Søvde, B. E., Sandvoll, A. M., Natvik, E., & Drageset, J. (2022). Carrying on life at home or moving to a nursing home: Frail older people's experiences of at-homeness. *International Journal of Qualitative Studies on Health & Well-Being*, *17*(1), 1–11. https://doi.org/10.1080/17482631.2022.2082125

The Stern Center for Evidence-Based Policy. (n.d.). *Addressing the health needs of an aging America: New opportunities for evidence-based policy solutions*. University of Pittsburgh. https://www.healthpolicyinstitute.pitt.edu/sites/default/files/SternCtrAddressingNeeds.pdf

Strange, K. E., Troutman-Jordan, M., & Mixer, S. J. (2022). Influence of spiritual engagement on Appalachian older adults' health: A systematic review. *Journal of Psychosocial Nursing and Mental Health Services*, 1–8. https://doi.org/10.3928/02793695-20221026-02

Sudha, S. (2014). Intergenerational relations and elder care preferences of Asian Indians in North Carolina. *Journal of Cross Cultural Gerontology*, *29*(1), 87–107. https://doi.org/10.1007/s10823-013-9220-7

Taylor, H. O., Taylor, R. J., Nguyen, A. W., & Chatters, L. (2018). Social isolation, depression, and psychological distress among older adults. *Journal of Aging and Health*, *30*(2), 229–246.

Trinh, N.-H. T., Bernard-Negron, R., & Ahmed, I. I. (2019). Mental health issues in racial and ethnic minority elderly. *Current Psychiatry Reports*, *21*, 1–6.

United Health Foundation – America's Health Rankings. (2022). *Senior report*. https://www.americashealthrankings.org/learn/reports/2022-senior-report

Vespa, J. (2019, October 8). The U.S. joins other countries with large aging populations. *The Graying of America: More Older Adults than Kids by 2035*. https://www.census.gov/library/stories/2018/03/graying-america.html

Vespa, J., Medina, L., & Armstrong, D. M. (2020, February). *Demographic turning points for the United States: Population projections for 2020 to 2060* (Current Population Reports P25-1144). United States Census Bureau. https://www.census.gov/library/publications/2020/demo/p25-1144.html

Victor, C. G. P., & Treschuk, J. V. (2020). Critical literature review on the definition clarity of the concept of faith, religion, and spirituality. *Journal of Holistic Nursing*, *38*(1), 107–113. https://doi.org/10.1177/0898010119895368

Volkert, D., Beck, A. M., Cederholm, T., Cruz-Jentoft, A., Hooper, L., Kiesswetter, E., et al. (2022). ESPEN practical guideline: Clinical nutrition and hydration in geriatrics. *Clinical Nutrition*, *41*(4), 958–989. https://doi.org/10.1016/j.clnu.2022.01.024

Wehbe-Alamah, H. B. (2018). The ethnonursing research method: Major features and enablers. In M. R. McFarland & H. B. Wehbe-Alamah (Eds.), *Leininger's transcultural nursing: Concepts, theories, research & practice* (4th ed., pp. 57–84). McGraw-Hill Education.

Whitman, A., De Lew, N., Chappel, A., Aysola, V., Zuckerman, R., & Sommers, B. D. (2022, April 1). Addressing social determinants of health: Examples of successful evidence-based strategies and current federal efforts. Assistant Secretary for Planning and Evaluation: Office of Health Policy. https://aspe.hhs.gov/reports/sdoh-evidence-review

Wixwat, M., & Saucier, G. (2021). Being spiritual but not religious. *Current Opinion in Psychology*, *40*, 121–125. https://doi.org/10.1016/j.copsyc.2020.09.003

World Health Organization. (2022). *Ageing and health*. https://www.who.int/news-room/fact-sheets/detail/ageing-and-health

Zhao, I. Y., Holroyd, E., Garrett, N., Write-St Clair, V. A., & Neville, S. (2021). Chinese late-life immigrants' loneliness and social isolation in host countries: An integrative review. *Journal of Clinical Nursing*, *32*(9–10), 1615–1624. https://doi.org/10.1111/jocn.16134

Healthcare Systems

Creating Culturally Competent Healthcare Organizations

• Patti Ludwig-Beymer

Chapter 9

Key Terms

Community-based
  participatory research
Cultural competence
Cultural humility

Culturally congruent services
Limited English proficiency
  (LEP)
Magnet designation
Participatory action research

Racism
Transcultural nursing
  administration

Learning Objectives

1. Assess the need for culturally competent healthcare organizations.
2. Discuss how to achieve health equity, eliminate disparities, and improve the health of all groups.
3. Evaluate organizational cultures.
4. Describe how organizations can develop cultural competency.
5. Analyze culturally competent initiatives designed and implemented by healthcare organizations.

Introduction

An individual's culture affects access to healthcare and health-seeking behaviors, as well as perceived quality of care. In addition to understanding the culture of clients, however, it is also essential to examine the culture of healthcare organizations.

The interplay of client, provider, and organizational cultures may create barriers, lead to a client's lack of trust or reluctance to access services, cause cultural conflicts, and ultimately result in healthcare inequities. Conversely, organizational culture may facilitate access that decreases health disparities.

This chapter serves to augment the current dialogue on creating culturally competent organizations. It defines a culturally competent organization, explains the need for culturally competent organizations, describes mechanisms for assessing organizational culture, and provides strategies for developing culturally competent organizations.

Defining a Culturally Competent Healthcare Organization

Today, there is debate over the use of the phrase **cultural competence**, with some preferring to use the phrase **cultural humility**. According to the Office of Minority Health (2021b), cultural competence is a developmental process that results in increasing awareness, knowledge, and skills and results in an improved ability to effectively work with diverse populations. In contrast, cultural humility is a reflective process of understanding one's biases and privileges, managing power imbalances, and being open to the beliefs and values of others. While both are important, we will use cultural competence in this chapter as it refers to the ability of healthcare providers and organizations to understand and respond effectively to the cultural and linguistic needs of clients. Culturally competent organizations are respectful of and responsive to the health beliefs, practices, and needs of diverse patients (Office of Minority Health, 2021b). Cultural competence encompasses a variety of diversities, including age, biology, culture, disability status, ethnicity, sex, gender identity, geographic location, language, race, religion, sexual orientation, spirituality, socioeconomic status, and sociological characteristics. A culturally competent organization is one that acknowledges the importance of culture, incorporates the assessment of cross-cultural relations, recognizes the potential impact of cultural differences, expands cultural knowledge, and adapts services to meet culturally unique needs. Ultimately, cultural competence is recognized as an essential means

of reducing health disparities (Health Research and Educational Trust, 2013).

The Need for Culturally Competent Healthcare Organizations: External Motivation

Nursing has been at the forefront of cultural competence for individuals and organizations. The Transcultural Nursing Society was established in 1975; its mission is to enhance the quality of culturally congruent, competent, and equitable care that results in improved health and well-being for people worldwide (Transcultural Nursing Society, 2022). An expert panel identified 10 standards of practice for culturally competent nursing care. Salient to this chapter is Standard 6, Cultural Competence in Healthcare Systems and Organizations. The standard holds that "Healthcare organizations should provide structures and resources necessary to evaluate and meet the cultural and language needs of their diverse clients" (Douglas et al., 2014, p. 113).

The American Nurses Association has also been proactive in addressing discrimination and racism in healthcare and promoting justice in access and delivery of healthcare to all people. ANA (2016) revised a position statement on ethics and human rights to provide nurses with specific actions to protect and promote human rights in every practice setting. Box 9-1 contains a partial listing of their recommendations. In addition, they expanded the Nursing Social Policy Statement by creating Diversity Awareness materials that address nursing organizations; health insurance and healthcare access; the lesbian, gay, bisexual, transgender, and queer (or questioning), and other sexual and gender identities (LGBTQ+) communities; mental health; bariatric/obesity care; racial and ethnic minority communities; older adults, self-assessment; and culturally specific tools (ANA, 2018). As seen in Chapter 2, many other nursing organizations emphasize the need for culturally competent nurses.

BOX 9-1	American Nurses Association Recommendations Related to Cultural Competence

- Nurses promote the human rights of patients, colleagues, and communities.
- Healthcare agencies assess for human rights violations related to patients, nurses, healthcare workers, and others within their organizations.
- Nurses serve on ethics committees, discuss ethics and human rights with colleagues, and participate in policy development to increase care access and equality.
- Nurses collaborate to promote, protect, and sustain ethical practice and the human rights of all patients and providers.
- Nurse educators use the principles of justice and caring to teach students about ethics and human rights in healthcare delivery.
- Nurse educators help students identify nursing professional responsibilities to address unjust systems and structures. Educators demonstrate the profession's commitment to health and social justice through class content, critical thinking exercises, and clinical experiences.
- Nurse researchers conduct research that is relevant to communities of interest. They invite communities to identify research problems and work to benefit patients, society, and professional nursing practice.
- Nurse executives implement ethics and human rights principles by monitoring the practice environment for actual or potential human rights violations of patients, nurses, and other healthcare providers.
- Nurse executives analyze policies and practices and identify risks for reduced safety and quality that may result from unacknowledged violations of human rights.
- Nurse executives promote a caring, just, inclusive, and collaborative environment in their organizations and communities.

Source: American Nurses Association. (2016). *The nurse's role in ethics and human rights: Protecting and promoting individual worth, dignity, and human rights in practice settings*. https://www.nursingworld.org/globalassets/docs/ana/nursesrole-ethicshumanrights-positionstatement.pdf

Other professional organizations also express the need for culturally competent organizations. For example, the Health Research and Educational Trust (2013) offers recommendations for building more culturally competent organizations (see Box 9-2). The Institute for Diversity and Health Equity (IFDHE), part of AHA, works closely with health services organizations to advance health equity for all and to expand leadership opportunities for underrepresented ethnicities and races in health management. They believe that promoting diversity within healthcare leadership and tackling health disparities is critical to ensuring the highest quality of care for everyone (IFDHE, 2022).

Regulatory agencies address the need for culturally competent organizations by communicating standards and guidance to healthcare organizations. The Centers for Medicare and Medicaid Services (2012) issued guidance to help healthcare providers become more effective and culturally aware of how they provide care to diverse populations. The Joint Commission (2022) provides resources on effective communication, cultural competence, patient- and family-centered care, and innovative ways to eliminate health disparities. They include standards to ensure that clients receive care that respects their cultural, psychosocial, and spiritual values.

The U.S. government has also addressed culturally appropriate healthcare systems. The National Standards for Culturally and Linguistically Appropriate Services in Health Care (CLAS Standards), outlined in Box 9-3, were developed by the U.S. Department of Health and Human Services' Office of Minority Health (2021a) to advance health equity, improve quality, and help reduce health disparities, holding that

BOX 9-2	Recommendations for Building Culturally Competent Organizations

- Collect race, ethnicity and language preference data.
- Identify and report disparities.
- Provide culturally and linguistically competent care.
- Develop culturally competent disease management programs.

- Increase diversity and minority workforce pipelines.
- Involve the community.
- Make cultural competency an institutional priority

Source: Health Research and Educational Trust. (2013). *Becoming a culturally competent healthcare organization: Equity of Care*. https://www.aha.org/ahahret-guides/2013-06-18-becoming-culturally-competent-health-care-organization

all people entering the healthcare system should receive equitable and effective care in a culturally and linguistically appropriate manner. The CLAS standards are inclusive of all cultures and are especially designed to address the needs of racial, ethnic, and linguistic populations that experience unequal access to health services. Ultimately, the aim of the standards is to contribute to the elimination of racial and ethnic health disparities and to improve the health of all Americans.

The Need for Culturally Competent Organizations: Eliminating Health Disparities

Disparities in health have long been acknowledged; these disparities document the reality of unequal healthcare treatment. The Centers for Disease Control and Prevention (2022b) defines health disparities as "preventable differences in the burden of disease, injury, violence, or opportunities to achieve optimal health that are experienced by populations that have been disadvantaged by their social or economic status, geographic location, and environment" (July 1, 2022, para. 3). Health disparities adversely affect groups of people who have systematically experienced

greater obstacles to health based on their racial or ethnic group; religion; socioeconomic status; gender; age; mental health; cognitive, sensory, or physical disability; sexual orientation or gender identity; geographic location; or other characteristics historically linked to discrimination or exclusion.

At the most basic level, disparities are evident in life expectancies. For example, the Centers for Disease Control and Prevention (2022a) reported that the overall US life expectancy at birth in 2021 was 76.1 years, with decreases seen in both 2020 and 2021. The decreases in life expectancy were largely driven by the COVID pandemic, followed by accidents and unintentional injuries including drug overdoses. In addition, life expectancy varies by race, ethnicity, and gender. The shortest life expectancy is seen in the American Indian/Alaska Native population at 65.2 years, followed by Black (79.8 years), Non-Hispanic White (76.4 years), Hispanic (77.6 years), and Asian (83.5 years). Women continue to live longer than men, at 79.1 years and 74.2 years respectively. In Canada, the 2021 life expectancy was reported as 79.49 years for males and 83.96 years for females (Statistics Canada, 2022).

Annually, the Agency for Healthcare Research and Quality (AHRQ) tracks disparities in healthcare delivery as they relate to race, ethnicity,

BOX 9-3	National Standards for Culturally and Linguistically Appropriate Services (CLAS) in Health Care

Principal Standard

1. Provide effective, equitable, understandable, and respectful quality care and services that are responsive to diverse cultural health beliefs and practices, preferred languages, health literacy, and other communication needs.

Governance, Leadership, and Workforce

2. Advance and sustain organizational governance and leadership that promotes CLAS and health equity through policy, practices, and allocated resources.
3. Recruit, promote, and support a culturally and linguistically diverse governance, leadership, and workforce that are responsive to the population in the service area.
4. Educate and train governance, leadership, and workforce in culturally and linguistically appropriate policies and practices on an ongoing basis.

Communication and Language Assistance

5. Offer language assistance to individuals who have limited English proficiency and/or other communication needs, at no cost to them, to facilitate timely access to all healthcare and services.
6. Inform all individuals of the availability of language assistance services clearly and in their preferred language, verbally and in writing.
7. Ensure the competence of individuals providing language assistance, recognizing that the use of untrained individuals and/or minors as interpreters should be avoided.

8. Provide easy-to-understand print and multimedia materials and signage in the languages commonly used by the populations in the service area.

Engagement, Continuous Improvement, and Accountability

9. Establish culturally and linguistically appropriate goals, policies, and management accountability, and infuse them throughout the organization's planning and operations.
10. Conduct ongoing assessments of the organization's CLAS-related activities and integrate CLAS-related measures into assessment measurement and continuous quality improvement activities.
11. Collect and maintain accurate and reliable demographic data to monitor and evaluate the impact of CLAS on health equity and outcomes and to inform service delivery.
12. Conduct regular assessments of community health assets and needs and use the results to plan and implement services that respond to the cultural and linguistic diversity of populations in the service area.
13. Partner with the community to design, implement, and evaluate policies, practices, and services to ensure cultural and linguistic appropriateness.
14. Create conflict- and grievance-resolution processes that are culturally and linguistically appropriate to identify, prevent, and resolve conflicts or complaints.
15. Communicate the organization's progress in implementing and sustaining CLAS to all stakeholders, constituents, and the general public.

Source: Office of Minority Health, Department of Health and Human Services. (2021a). *Think cultural health: The national CLAS standards*. https://minorityhealth.hhs.gov/omh/browse.aspx?lvl=2&lvlid=53

geography, insurance, and socioeconomic status. These themes emerged from the 2021 National Healthcare Quality and Disparities Report (AHRQ, 2022):

1. Several areas in which the nation has invested in quality improvement and patient safety have shown improvements. For example:
   a. The death rate from HIV decreased from 5.2 to 1.5 deaths per 100,000 population (2000 to 2018 data).
   b. The rate of colon cancer deaths decreased 36%, from 20.8 to 13.4 deaths per 100,000 population (2000 to 2018 data).
2. The United States has seen significant gains in the number of people covered by health insurance and who have a usual source of healthcare. For example:
   a. The percentage of people under age 65 years who had any period of uninsurance decreased by 33% (2002 to 2018 data).
   b. The percentage of people under age 65 who were uninsured all year decreased by 42%.
   c. Concurrently, the percentage of Americans who have access to a usual source of care improved (2002 to 2018 data).
3. Personal spending on health insurance and healthcare services decreased for people under age 65 with public insurance and increased for people with private insurance (2002 to 2018 data).
4. Access to dental care and oral healthcare services remains low and has not substantially improved, particularly for people with low income or who live in rural areas. For example:
   a. The percentage of adults who received preventive dental care services in the calendar year showed no statistically significant change, going from 33.6% to 35.4% (2002 to 2018 data).
5. The opioid and mental health crisis worsened in the years leading up to COVID-19. Limited access to substance use and mental health treatment may have contributed to this crisis. For example:
   a. Opioid-related emergency department (ED) visits and hospitalizations more than doubled between 2005 and 2018.
   b. Suicide death rates rose 23%, going from 14.0 deaths to 17.2 deaths per 100,000 population (2008 to 2018 data).
   c. The percentage of adults with a major depressive episode who received depression treatment showed no statistically significant changes, going from 68.3% to 66.3% (2008 to 2019 data).
   d. The percentage of children aged 12 to 17 with a major depressive episode who received depression treatment showed no statistically significant changes, going from 37.7% to 43.3% (2008 to 2019 data).
6. While Black, Hispanic, and American Indian and Alaska Native communities all experienced substantial improvements in healthcare quality, significant disparities in all domains of healthcare quality persist. Even when rates of improvement in quality exceeded those experienced by White Americans, they have not been enough to eliminate disparities. For example:
   a. HIV deaths in Black populations decreased from 23.3 deaths to 6.2 deaths per 100,000 population. However, deaths in Black populations remain more than six times as high as HIV deaths in White populations (0.9 deaths per 100,000 population) (2000 to 2018 data).
   b. While the incident rates of end-stage kidney disease due to diabetes decreased in the populations, significant disparities persist among Non-Hispanic Black, Hispanic, and American Indian and Alaska Native populations compared to the Non-Hispanic White populations, with respective incident rates of 372.2, 292.7, 273.1, and 152.2 events per million population in 2018 (2001 to 2018 data).

The relationships between race/ethnicity, socioeconomic status, gender, age, and geography and health are complex and not easily summarized here. Access (getting into the healthcare system) and quality care (receiving appropriate, safe, and effective healthcare in a timely manner) are key factors in achieving good health outcomes. While many believe that access to high-quality care is a fundamental human right, those with low socioeconomic status and racial and ethnic minorities often face more barriers to care and receive poorer quality of care when they access care. The 2021 National Healthcare Quality and Disparities Report (AHRQ, 2022) reports access and quality measures based on race, ethnicity, socioeconomic status, geographic location, and other variables. Examples of these measures are presented in Box 9-4.

As discussed above, many populations experience health disparities, including people from many racial and ethnic minority groups, people with disabilities, women, people who are LGBTQ+, people with limited English proficiency, people with limited economic status, people in specific geographic areas, and other groups. The impact social determinants of health (SDOH) have on health disparities cannot be overlooked. *Healthy People 2030* (2022) identifies five key areas of SDOH: healthcare access and quality, education access and quality, social and community context, economic stability, and the neighborhood and built environment. Social and community context includes discrimination and racism, discussed in the upcoming Acknowledging Racism in Healthcare Organizations and Society section.

Canada's experience with universal access to care suggests that access may help to reduce health disparities between groups but does not eliminate them (Alter et al., 2011). Their longitudinal study followed nearly 15,000 people for over a decade and found that clients with lower incomes used more healthcare resources than did those with a higher socioeconomic status. Regardless, individuals with lower incomes had poorer health, including depression, hypertension, diabetes, cancer, and cataracts, and were more likely to die during the longitudinal study.

These findings imply that factors besides access account for some health disparities. Potential barriers that contribute to the disparities may be related to demographics, culture, and the healthcare system itself. Some of these are summarized in Box 9-5.

In contrast to health disparities, health equity is the state in which everyone has a fair and just opportunity to attain their highest level of health. Achieving this requires ongoing societal efforts. We must address historical and contemporary injustices; overcome economic, social, and other obstacles to health and healthcare; and eliminate preventable health disparities. In short, to achieve health equity, we must change the systems and policies that have caused generational injustices and resulted in racial and ethnic health disparities (CDC, July 1, 2022b). A necessary step is for culturally competent providers to deliver care within culturally competent healthcare organizations.

Acknowledging Racism in Healthcare Organizations and Society

Ethnocentrism, stereotyping, prejudice, discrimination, and racism are present in society and within healthcare settings. Racism has existed for more than 400 years in the United States and the precursor original colonies; it remains pervasive in structures and processes today. **Racism** is a system, supported and maintained through institutional structures and policies, cultural norms and values, and individual behaviors. Racism may be internalized, interpersonal, and/or structural. Internalized racism is the acceptance of negative messages about one's own abilities and worth by members of the stigmatized group. Interpersonal racism is prejudice and discrimination by individuals towards others. Structural racism is a system in which public policies, institutional practices, cultural representations, and other norms work to reinforce and perpetuate racial group inequity. It is a feature of our social, economic, and

BOX 9-4	Disparities by Race, Ethnicity, and Income, 2017 to 2019 Data				
Measures	Black Compared to White	Asian Compared to White	Native Hawaiian/ Pacific Islander Compared to White	American Indian/ Alaska Native Compared to White	Hispanic, All Races Compared to Non-Hispanic White	Individual at or Below the Poverty Level Compared to Those With High Income
Patient Safety	Better = 5 Same = 13 Worse = 11	Better = 8 Same = 14 Worse = 5	Better = 1 Same = 9 Worse = 2	Better = 1 Dame = 9 Worse = 3	Better = 5 Same = 13 Worse = 5	Better = 0 Same = 10 Worse = 6
Person Centered Care	Better = 3 Same = 17 Worse = 7	Better = 0 Same = 11 Worse = 18	Better = 2 Same = 9 Worse = 7	Better = 1 Same = 6 Worse = 12	Better = 2 Same = 10 Worse = 5	Better = 1 Same = 2 Worse = 7
Care Coordination	Better = 1 Same = 5 Worse = 16	Better = 16 Same = 1 Worse = 4	Better = 1 Same = 3 Worse = 3	Better = 0 Same = 3 Worse = 5	Better = 5 Same = 5 Worse = 8	Better = 0 Same = 0 Worse = 19
Effectiveness of Care	Better = 5 Same = 20 Worse = 18	Better = 10 Same = 18 Worse = 6	Better = 7 Same = 5 Worse = 2	Better = 5 Same = 11 Worse = 5	Better = 8 Same = 21 Worse = 13	Better = 2 Same = 19 Worse = 5
Healthy Living	Better = 6 Same = 34 Worse = 32	Better = 15 Same = 30 Worse = 15	Better = 4 Same = 17 Worse = 9	Better = 4 Same = 23 Worse = 18	Better = 13 Same = 27 Worse = 30	Better = 3 Same = 13 Worse = 28
Affordable Care	Better = 1 Same = 1 Worse = 0	Better = 1 Same = 1 Worse = 0	Not reported	Better = 0 Same = 1 Worse = 0	Better = 1 Same = 0 Worse = 1	Better = 0 Same = 0 Worse = 2

Examples of disparities					
• Cervical cancer diagnosed at advanced stage per 100,000 women aged 20 and over • Breast cancer diagnosed at advanced stage per 100,000 women aged 40 and over • Infant mortality per 1,000 live births, birth weight 2,500 g or more • Live-born infants with low birth weight (less than 2,500 g)	• Sepsis diagnoses per 1,000 elective-surgery admissions of length 4 or more days, adults • Deaths per 1,000 hospital admissions with percutaneous coronary intervention, aged 40 and over • Children ages 12–17 with a major depressive episode in the last 12 months • Live-born infants with low birth weight (less than 2,500 g)	• High-risk, long-stay nursing home patients with pressure ulcer • New HIV cases per 100,000 population age 13 and over • Hospital patients who received influenza vaccination	• High-risk, long-stay nursing home patients with pressure ulcer • Adjusted incident rates of end stage renal disease due to diabetes per million population • New HIV cases per 100,000 population aged 13 • Live-born infants with low birth weight (less than 2,500 g) • Infant mortality per 1,000 live births, birth weight 2,500 grams or more	• Postoperative respiratory failure per 1,000 elective surgical hospital discharges, adults • Hospital admissions for asthma per 100,000 population, children ages 2–17 • HIV infection deaths per 100,000 population • Live-born infants with low birth weight (less than 2,500 g)	• Deaths per 1,000 hospital admissions with expected low-mortality • Hospital admissions for lower extremity amputations per 1,000 population, aged 18 and over with diabetes • Emergency department visits involving opioid-related diagnoses per 100,000 population • Children ages 5–17 with untreated dental caries

Note: The Federal Poverty Level is established annually by the U.S. Bureau of the Census based on family size and composition. Overall, 11.6% of individuals were below the poverty level in 2021. Poverty rates differ by many variables. In terms of race and ethnicity, 24.3% of American Indian and Alaska Native, 19.5% of Black, 17.1% of Hispanic of any race, 14.2% of two or more races, 9.3% of Asian, and 8.1% of non-Hispanic White individuals were classified as living in poverty. Poverty affected 27.2% of those aged 24 and above without a high school diploma, 24.9% of those with a disability, 15.3% of those under the age of 18 years, 15% of those living outside a metropolitan statistical area, 13.2% of those living in the south, 12.6% of females, and 10.3% of those 65 years of age and older.

Sources: Agency for Healthcare Research and Quality. (2022). 2021 National Healthcare Quality and Disparities Report. https://www.ahrq.gov/research/findings/nhqrdr/nhqdr21/index.html; Creamer, J., Shrider, E.A., Burns, B. & Chen, F. (2022). Poverty in the United States: 2021. United States Census Bureau. https://www.census.gov/library/publications/2022/demo/p60-277.html

BOX 9-5 | Potential Demographic, Cultural, and Health System Barriers

Demographic Barriers

Age
Gender
Ethnicity
Primary language
Religion
Educational level and literacy level
Occupation, income, and health insurance
Area of residence
Transportation
Time and/or generation in the United States

Cultural Barriers

Age
Gender, class, and family dynamics
Worldview/perceptions of life
Time orientation
Primary language spoken
Religious beliefs and practices
Social customs, values, and norms
Traditional health beliefs and practices

Dietary preferences and practices
Communication patterns and customs

Health System Barriers

Differential access to high-quality care
Insurance and other financial resources
Orientation to preventive health services
Perception of need for healthcare services
Lack of knowledge and/or distrust of Western
    medical practices and procedures
Cultural insensitivity and incompetence in
    providers, including bias, stereotyping, and
    prejudice
Lack of diversity in providers
Western versus folk health beliefs and practices
Poor provider–client communication
Lack of bilingual and bicultural staff
Unfriendly and cold environment
Complex, fragmented, and uncoordinated health-
    care organizations
Physical barriers (such as excessive distances)
Information barriers

political systems and allows privileges associated with "Whiteness" and disadvantages associated with "color" to endure.

Structural racism, also called institutional or systemic racism, results in different access to goods, services, and opportunities based on race. This includes differential access to health insurance. The dominant subgroup is often ignorant of its own privilege. For example, services may be organized for the convenience of providers, and providers may be unaware that inconvenient hours or locations are affecting the community members who seek services. In contrast to individual behaviors, institutional racism occurs when systematic policies and practices disadvantage certain racial or ethnic groups. Institutions may be overtly racist, as when they specifically exclude certain groups from service. Institutions may also be unintentionally racist. For example, a dress code

that requires everyone to wear the same hat would institutionally discriminate against Sikh men, who are expected to wear turbans, and Muslim women, who wear the hijab or veil. Institutions do not necessarily adopt such policies with the intention of discriminating and often revise their practice once the discrimination is identified.

Institutional racism has been well documented in U.S. healthcare (Feagin & Bennefield, 2014; Metzl & Hansen, 2014) and is a major contributor to the growing health inequities between Americans with the highest and lowest incomes (Krisberg, 2017). Institutional racism is also an international concern. In England, institutional racism is defined as "the collective failure of an organisation to provide an appropriate and professional service to people because of their colour, culture, or ethnic origin" (McKenzie & Bhui, 2007, p. 649). Differences in the treatment of mental illness have been documented in England and Wales (McKenzie & Bhui, 2007). Reports in Sweden and the United Kingdom suggest continued concerns about discrimination and inequity in services (Bhopal, 2007). Contributing factors include the actions of individual staff members and policies that are based on the needs of the ethnic majority population rather than considering the needs of minority populations (Bhopal, 2007). Henry et al. (2004) suggest that healthcare in Australia is institutionally racist and that such racism represents one of the greatest barriers to improving the health of Aboriginal and Torres Strait Islander people. Examples include funding inequities, differences in performance criteria, and differences in treatment regimens.

Like structural racism, interpersonal racism continues to exist. In a survey of over 5,600 nurses, (ANA, 2022, January 25) 92% of Black, 73% of Asian, and 69% of Hispanic nurses reported that they had personally experienced racism in the workplace. Acts of racism were most often perpetrated by colleagues and those in positions of power. Perceptions of racism varied by race; 72% of Black nurses indicated there was a lot of racism in nursing compared to 29% of White nurse respondents. Over three fourths of Black nurses surveyed indicated that racism in the workplace had negatively impacted their professional well-being. Patients and families also commit racist acts. A common microaggression is the assumption that a nurse of color is an assistant, dietary staff, or housekeeper rather than a nurse. This occurs daily and must be addressed calmly and firmly. Patients sometimes request a White nurse. Such requests cannot be granted for both ethical and legal reasons (Ludwig-Beymer, 2018).

Racism has created most of the inequitable structures that exist in our society, has negatively impacted communities of color, and has resulted in today's health inequities (CDC, July 1, 2022b). To begin to address racism, Metzl et al. (2018) suggest using a structural competency framework to help health professionals understand how contextual factors such as racism shape health and illness. Healthcare organizations must be built upon the cultural values of the people they serve. The strategies outlined in this chapter and throughout this book are needed to overcome institutional and interpersonal racism and build culturally competent healthcare organizations. Individually and collectively, we must become antiracist.

Assessing Organizational Culture

Organizational culture has emerged as an important variable for behavior, performance, and outcome in the workplace. Leininger (1996) defined organizational culture as the goals, norms, values, and practices of an organization in which people have goals and try to achieve them in beneficial ways. Organizations are complex, with multiple and competing subcultures. The sub-cultural systems have inherent values and beliefs, folklore, and language; these systems are organized in a hierarchy of authority, responsibilities, obligations, and functional tasks that are understood by members of the organization.

Organizational culture has been studied as it relates to accountability, change, emotional intelligence, effectiveness, implementation of best practices and research, leadership and management, Magnet recognition status, mentoring, and patient safety. Organizational culture affects not only people working in the institution, such as employees, physicians, and volunteers, but also those who access the institution's services, such as clients, families, and community members. The social organization of hospitals and other healthcare facilities profoundly affects clients, both directly through the care provided and indirectly through organizational policies and philosophy.

Theories of Organizational Culture

A variety of definitions, methods of measurement, and theories for organizational culture exist. There is reasonable consensus on the following (Thomas & Winter, 2020):

- An organization's culture consists of shared values, beliefs, assumptions, perceptions, and norms leading to specific patterns of behaviors.
- Organizational culture is made up of many subcultures, including various professions and groups of staff, race and ethnicity of staff and leaders, original culture of the organization's founders, existing policies and procedures, religious sponsors, and ongoing governance cultures.
- An organization's culture results from an interaction among many variables, including mission, vision, values, strategy, structure, leadership, and staff.
- Culture is both constantly shifting and self-reinforcing; once in place, it provides stability, and organizational members may resist changes.

Bolman and Deal's Organizational Culture Perspective

Bolman and Deal (2017) describe four organizational culture perspectives or "frames" that affect the way in which an organization resolves conflicts: Human resources (HR), political, structural, and symbolic. The HR frame strives to facilitate the fit between person and organization. When conflict arises, the solution considers the needs of the individual or group as well as the needs of the organization. The political frame emphasizes power and politics. Problems are viewed as "turf" issues and are resolved by developing networks to increase the power base. The structural frame focuses on following an organization's rules or protocols. This culture relies on its policies and procedures to resolve conflict. The symbolic frame relies on rituals, ceremony, and myths in determining appropriate behaviors.

To understand how these four perspectives will result in different outcomes, consider typical responses to the following situation. Hospital

A is located on the border of two communities. One community is primarily African American. The other community is primarily Hispanic. The hospital has traditionally provided care to African Americans and is well regarded by that community. The hospital has noted, however, that few members of the Hispanic community use its services. The hospital's board of directors realizes that, to survive, the hospital must expand its client base. The approach to this challenge will vary based on the organization's culture.

Hospital leaders with an HR perspective are likely to approach the situation by assessing the needs of both communities and the staff. For example, the hospital may convene focus groups with members of the Hispanic community to identify why the hospital's services are not used by that community. At the same time, the hospital will assess the African American community's perspective on the hospital's plan to expand its services and become a more inclusive organization. The hospital will also encourage staff members to provide input and to express their feelings about the goals of the organization. In the end, the hospital with an HR perspective will reach a decision that balances the needs of all the groups while enhancing the goal of expanding the client base.

Hospital leaders in a political culture will take a different approach. They will identify key "power" leaders in the Hispanic community. Perhaps they will invite a Hispanic leader to join their board of directors or serve in another advisory capacity; or they may ask a priest from a Hispanic congregation to serve as a hospital chaplain. In addition, they will actively recruit Hispanic physicians and other clinicians. They will build a Hispanic power base within the hospital and use it to reach out to the larger Hispanic community and expand the client base.

Hospital leaders in a structural culture will develop policies and procedures to attract more Hispanic clients. For example, they may make certain that all signage appears in both English and Spanish or develop a policy that requires all client educational materials to be available in both Spanish and English. They may require all staff to attend a session on Hispanic cultures and may strongly encourage or mandate Spanish-language training for key personnel.

Hospital leaders in a symbolic culture will use ceremony to meet their goal. They will make physical changes to the environment to attract more Hispanic patients. For example, they may create or alter a chapel, inviting a priest from a Hispanic congregation to say mass. They may display other religious symbols, such as a crucifix or a statue of Our Lady of Guadalupe. They may alter their artwork to be more culturally inclusive. They may also include Hispanic stories and rituals in their internal communications. These leaders will draw on symbols and rituals that will help make persons of Hispanic cultures comfortable in the hospital environment, and doing so will attract a larger Hispanic client base.

None of these organizational cultures are inherently good or bad, just different. Each perspective presents both strengths and weaknesses, and more than one culture may exist in an organization. For example, an organization may be guided primarily by both HR and symbolic perspectives.

Schein's Organizational Culture

Schein (2016) describes organizational culture at three levels: (1) observable artifacts, (2) values, and (3) basic underlying assumptions. Artifacts are visible manifestations of values. Artifacts may include signage, statues and other decorations, pictures, décor, dress code, traffic flow, medical equipment, and visible interactions. Values are explicitly stated norms and social principles and are manifestations of assumptions. Underlying assumptions are shared beliefs and expectations that influence perceptions, thoughts, and feelings about the organization; they are the core of the organization's culture. Assumptions define the culture of the organization, but because they are invisible, they may not be recognized. At times, the assumptions of an institution are ambiguous and self-contradictory, especially when an institutional merger or acquisition has occurred.

A Framework for Describing Healthcare Delivery Organizations

Pina et al. (2015) developed a framework for describing healthcare delivery organizations. The framework includes six domains: capacity, organizational structure, finances, patients, care processes and infrastructure, and culture. The way in which they derived the domains and the contents of each domain are summarized in Evidence-Based Practice 9-1.

Organizational Culture, Employees, and the Community

Many organizations are aware of the impact of organizational culture on employees. When filling positions, recruiters consider the "fit" between the organization and the potential employee, because a good "fit" results in better retention and satisfied employees. Nurses and other healthcare professionals also learn how to determine whether an organization will match their personal values. For example, a nurse who wants to provide care in a culturally competent manner to individuals who are LGBTQ+ will not be happy in a critical care unit that restricts visitors to nuclear family members (traditionally defined as a married couple and their children).

Humans need care to survive, thrive, and grow. According to Leininger (1996), organizations need to incorporate universal care constructs, including respect and genuine concern for clients and staff. These caring organizations are needed for nurses and other staff members. Historically, however, organizations have made few attempts to nurture and nourish the human spirit. Research conducted during the COVID-19 pandemic found that effective and genuine leadership communication mitigated moral distress and enhanced longer-term mental health (Lake et al., 2022).

A caring organization embraces diversity, equity, and inclusion (The National Academies of Sciences, Engineering, and Medicine, 2021) with a further focus on fostering a sense of belonging.

Healthcare Delivery System Framework Domains and Elements

Pina et al. (2015) propose a framework for describing healthcare delivery systems that allows healthcare stakeholders to understand, evaluate, implement, and disseminate innovations to improve care and more easily compare health systems. For each step in the development of the framework, the researchers used two approaches: a review of the literature and the Delphi method with the Agency for Healthcare Research and Quality's Effective Health Care Stakeholders Group (SG). Nominations for the SG occurred via a public process. The group represented broad constituencies including patients, caregivers, and advocacy groups; clinicians and professional associations; hospital systems and medical clinics; government agencies; purchasers and payors; and healthcare industry representatives, policymakers, and researchers. The Delphi method consisted of facilitated group discussions and interactive rounds of individual written feedback on each draft of the framework. The process yielded six domains with 26 elements as summarized below.

1. Capacity

Size—The system's productive capacity

Capital assets—The property, facilities, physical plant, and the property's ownership, equipment, and other infrastructure used to provide and manage healthcare services

Comprehensiveness of services—The scope and depth of services available in terms of setting, specialty, ancillary services, and acuity of care

2. Organizational structure

Configuration—The arrangement of the functional units in the system in terms of workflow, hierarchy of authority, patterns of communication, and resource flows among them

Leadership structure and governance—The level of formal decision-making authority for an office holder in terms of scope of decisions that can be made independently and with concurrence of others

Research and innovation—The extent to which participation in clinical and basic scientific research and healthcare innovation is a feature of the mission and activities of the organization

Professional education—The extent to which professional education and training is a feature of the mission and activities of the organization

3. Finances

Payment received for services—The categorical types of payment received, the approach to accountability for services provided, the proportion of each payment type, and the degree of financial risk held

Provider payment systems—The categorical types of payment to individual providers for their services and the proportion of each payment type

Ownership—The corporate status and healthcare industry affiliation of the owner of the healthcare system

Financial solvency—The extent to which the organization's financial resources exceed the organization's current liabilities and long-term expenses

4. Patients

Patient characteristics—Proportion of patients with different characteristics, health conditions, and coverage types

Geographic characteristics—Geographic location, type of community in which the healthcare delivery system functions, and size of the catchment area

5. Care processes and infrastructure

Integration—The extent to which a network of organizations or units within one organization provides or arranges to provide a coordinated continuum of services to a population and is willing to be held clinically and fiscally accountable for the outcomes and health status of the population served

Standardization—The extent to which the healthcare delivery system reduces unnecessary variation

Healthcare Delivery System Framework Domains and Elements (continued)

while encouraging differences dictated by diversity among patients in their conditions and preferences

Performance measurement, public reporting, and quality improvement—The extent to which the organization conducts regular measurement of performance with public reporting, feedback, and a systematic process for improvement

Health information system—The extent to which clinical and administrative information is organized and available to those who need it in a timely way and the extent to which they have electronic support for those functions

Patient care team—The extent to which patient care is delivered by clinicians and staff who regularly work together in an integrated way to serve patients and families

Clinical decision support—The extent to which clinical guideline–based reminders and decision aids are incorporated in the process of patient care

Care coordination—The deliberate organization of patient care activities between two or more participants involved in a patient's care to facilitate and maximize the appropriate delivery of healthcare services to achieve optimal patient experience and outcomes

6. Culture

Patient centeredness—The degree to which healthcare delivery is designed to serve the interests of patients rather than providers

Cultural competence—Ability of systems to provide care to patients with diverse values, beliefs, and behaviors, including tailoring delivery to meet patients' social, cultural, and linguistic needs

Competition–collaboration continuum—Where the organization falls on a scale from competitive to collaborative in relation to other organizations in its locale

Community benefit—The extent to which the organization is concerned about the health of the local community and takes advantage of community services for its patients through collaboration

Innovation diffusion—The degree to which the healthcare delivery organization or system is focused on creating and adopting new ways to provide care and accomplish its mission

Working climate—The degree to which the organization's employees perceive an environment of openness and fair process

Clinical Implications

During a clinical rotation, consider the following questions related to a domain and element.

Patients: Patient characteristics. What are the demographics of patients, such as age, gender, race, ethnicity, disability, education, income, and insurance coverage?

Culture: Patient centeredness. How are patients and family members involved in decision-making and the provision of care? How do clinicians adjust care based on the personal preferences of patients? How do they coordinate care for patients?

Culture: Cultural competence. What informational materials are available in which languages? How are professional interpreters arranged? What cultural competence goals are included in the organization's strategic plan? What strategies are in place to recruit, retain, and promote diverse leadership and staff?

Culture: Community benefit. How much uncompensated care is provided? How does the organization assess and prioritize local healthcare needs? What formal community partnerships are in place? What have the partnerships accomplished?

Reference: Pina, I. L., Cohen, P. D., Larson, D. B., Marion, L. N., Sills, M. R., Solberg, L. I., & Zerzan, J. (2015). A framework for describing health care delivery organizations and systems. *American Journal of Public Health, 105*(4), 670–679.

Such a workplace is not satisfied simply by having a diverse workforce. Instead, the organization focuses on capitalizing on the unique perspectives of the diverse workforce. Culturally competent leaders must watch carefully for racism and microaggressions experienced by staff members. Racism, discrimination, and microaggression cannot be tolerated from any source.

A caring healthcare organization also reaches out beyond their facility by forming community coalitions to address SDOH and pervasive health inequities (The National Academies of Sciences, Engineering, and Medicine, 2021). Caring organizations also encourage members of the workforce to become active in the community and participate in state and federal programs, working with economically disadvantaged groups and with diverse cultural groups. Rather than espousing the golden rule (treat others as you wish to be treated), an inclusive workplace treats others as they wish to be treated, in what is sometimes called the platinum rule (Alessandra, 2010). Caring organizations with inclusive workplaces draw staff members who are committed to cultural competence and who value diversity and mutual respect for differences.

Although the impact of organizational culture on employees has been acknowledged, the impact of organizational culture on the community being served has received less attention. For years, hospitals and other healthcare organizations have espoused the view that "If we build it, they will come" (i.e., they need only offer the services). Now, there is a growing recognition that healthcare services should be structured in ways to appeal to and meet the needs of various members of the community. Healthcare leaders recognize that cultural competence in organizations is essential if organizations are to survive, grow, satisfy customers, and achieve their goals. Image is critically important for an organization's survival. A variety of factors are needed to move an organization toward cultural competence, including changes to structures, processes, knowledge, attitude, and skills.

Assessment Tools

Organizational culture may be assessed in numerous ways. The Magnet Hospital Recognition Program for Excellence in Nursing Services evaluates organizational climate or culture (American Nurses Credentialing Center, 2021) and is used by many organizations as a blueprint for achieving excellence (Schaffner & Ludwig-Beymer, 2003). Evidence-Based Practice 9-2 outlines the original research that resulted in the creation of **Magnet designation**. Evaluating the five key components of the Magnet model may be helpful in assessing the culture of an organization. These five key components are transformational leadership; structural empowerment; exemplary professional practice; new knowledge, innovations, and improvements; and empirical outcomes.

Leininger's (1991) theory of culture care diversity and universality is also helpful in assessing the culture of an institution. Leininger's culture care model may be used to conduct a cultural assessment of the organization, with dominant segments of the sunrise model identified. An example of such an assessment is provided in Box 9-6.

Other cultural care assessment tools are available to assess the culture of an institution. This assessment is then compared with the values and beliefs of the groups who use the healthcare organization. See Appendix C for an example assessment guide for healthcare organizations and facilities.

Building Culturally Competent Organizations

Cultural competence has been identified as a key strategy for eliminating racial and ethnic health disparities. However, the competence must extend beyond the provider, into the system of healthcare. It would be naive to assume that building culturally competent organizations will resolve all health disparities. However, when healthcare is delivered within a culturally competent organization, diverse healthcare consumers are more likely to access the services, return,

Magnet Research and the Magnet Model

The Magnet Recognition Program for Excellence in Nursing Services grew out of a 1982 descriptive study conducted by the American Academy of Nursing's Task Force on Nursing Practice (McClure et al., 1983). The study began by asking Fellows from the American Academy of Nursing to identify hospitals that attracted and retained professional nurses who experienced professional and personal satisfaction in their practice. The Fellows nominated 165 institutions. These institutions were viewed as "Magnets." The task force then began narrowing the list based on specific criteria and the hospitals' willingness and availability to participate in the study.

Data were then collected from staff nurses and nursing directors in 41 hospitals. Nurses identified and described variables that created an environment that attracted and retained well-qualified nurses and promoted quality patient care. Nurses were asked nine questions, which remain valuable for structuring nursing input even today:

1. What makes your hospital a good place to work?
2. Can you describe particular programs that you see leading to professional/personal satisfaction?
3. How is nursing viewed in your hospital, and why?
4. Can you describe nurse involvement in various ongoing programs/projects whose goals are quality of patient care?
5. Can you identify activities and programs calculated to enhance, both directly and indirectly, recruitment/retention of professional nurses in your hospital?
6. Could you tell us about nurse–physician relationships in your hospital?
7. Describe staff nurse–supervisor relationships in your hospital.
8. Are some areas in your hospital more successful than others in recruitment/retention? Why?
9. What single piece of advice would you give to a director of nursing who wishes to do something about high RN vacancy and turnover rates in their hospital?

Staff nurses identified a variety of conditions that made a hospital a good place for nurses to work, specifically related to administration, professional practice, and professional development. Clustered together, a very clear culture of nursing emerged from this descriptive study.

Based on findings from the original Magnet study, the Magnet Recognition Program was developed in 1990. The program was created to advance three goals:

- Promote quality in a milieu that supports professional practice
- Identify excellence in the delivery of nursing services to patients/residents
- Provide a mechanism for the dissemination of "best practices" in nursing services

Clinical Implications

During clinical rotations to different facilities, nursing students are in an ideal position to evaluate organizational climate. Consider the following dimensions:

- Transformational leadership—How do the nursing leaders stimulate and inspire followers to achieve extraordinary outcomes? How do nursing leaders help others to develop their own leadership capacity?
- Structural empowerment—How are nurses involved in decision-making structures and processes to establish standards of practice and address opportunities for improvement? How does information flow between the chief nursing officer and all professional nurses? How do nurses partner with the community to improve patient outcomes and advance the health of the community? How do nurses enhance their professional development?
- Exemplary professional practice—What is the professional practice model? How do nurses partner with patients, families, and interprofessional team members to provide effective and efficient care? How do nurses enhance safety, quality, and quality improvement? How is workplace advocacy supported within the organization?

(continued)

Magnet Research and the Magnet Model (continued)

- New knowledge, innovations, and improvements—How are evidence-based practice and research incorporated into clinical and operational processes? What infrastructure and resources are in place to support the advancement of evidence-based practices, research, and innovation in clinical settings?
- Empirical outcomes—What are the quantitative outcomes for the organization in terms of safety, quality, patient experience, and nurse satisfaction?

Nurses and nursing students are encouraged to use the Magnet framework to assess nursing subcultures and determine organizational fit.

References: McClure, M. L., Poulin, M. A., Sovie, M. D., Wandelt, M. A.; & For the American Academy Task Force on Nursing Practice in Hospitals. (1983). Magnet hospitals. Attraction and retention of professional nurses. American Nurses Association; American Nurses Credentialing Center. (2021). *2023 Magnet® application manual*. American Nurses Credentialing Center.

BOX 9-6	Example of Leininger's (1991) Culture Care Model Used to Conduct an Organizational Assessment

Factor: Environmental Context

Types of Questions: What is the general environment of the community that surrounds the organization? Socioeconomic status? Race/ethnicity? Emphasis on health? Living arrangements? Access to social services? Employment? Proximity to other health facilities?

Sample Findings: Hospital A is in a low-income urban setting. The neighborhood includes Black, White, and Hispanic residents. A public housing complex is located within a few blocks of the hospital. The economy is depressed, and many are out of jobs. Harmful drug use and substance use disorders are rampant. Families are challenged to survive, and they tend to view disease prevention as less important than their daily living. Health is defined as being able to participate in normal activities. Several social agencies nearby provide food pantries. There are no other hospitals within a 10-mile radius.

Factor: Language and Ethnohistory

Types of Questions: What languages are spoken within the institution? By employees? By patients and clients? How formal or informal are the lines of communication? How hierarchical? What communication strategies are used within the institution? Written? Poster? Electronic? Oral? "Grapevine"? How did the institution come to be? What was the original mission? How has it changed over the years?

Sample Findings: Clients primarily speak English or Spanish. While the most common languages spoken by employees are English, Spanish, or Polish, many other languages are heard throughout the organization. The grapevine is alive and well at Hospital A. Although memos and e-mails are circulated, verbal communication is prized throughout the institution. The president/chief executive officer, chief nursing officer, and chief medical officer all maintain an open-door policy in their offices. Posters are also used to communicate, especially in the elevators. Electronic communication to direct care staff via e-mail has not been successful because computer workstations are in short supply throughout the institution. Hospital A was founded by a Roman Catholic religious order of nuns in 1885. The original mission was to provide care

BOX 9-6 | **Example of Leininger's (1991) Culture Care Model Used to Conduct an Organizational Assessment (continued)**

to immigrants and low-income community members. Immigrants from many nations, including Ireland, Poland, Hungary, and Russia, originally inhabited the area. The mission is still to provide the highest quality of care to the economically disadvantaged and underserved, although that is becoming increasingly difficult financially.

Factor: Technology

Types of Questions: How is technology used in the institution? Who uses it? Is client documentation electronic? Is electronic order entry in place? Is cutting-edge technology in place in the ED, critical care units, labor and delivery, radiology, surgical suites, and similar units? Are instant messaging, text messaging, and tweets used? Is web-based technology embraced?

Sample Findings: There are a few computer workstations on each nursing unit. Nurses document electronically; physicians, Advanced Practice Registered Nurses, and Physician Assistants use computerized provider order entry. Hospital A received external funding several years ago to renovate their old ED. The new ED has state-of-the art equipment, as do the critical care units. The labor and delivery unit is cramped and overcrowded. Equipment is well worn. Similarly, the surgical suites are dated. The radiology department is scheduled for a major capital investment next year.

Factor: Religious/Philosophical

Types of Questions: Does the institution have a religious affiliation? Are religious symbols displayed within the facility? By clients? By staff? Is the institution private or public? For-profit or not-for-profit?

Sample Findings: Founded by a religious order, Hospital A is very clearly viewed as Roman Catholic. Outside, the hospital is marked with a large cross on its roof. Inside, a crucifix hangs in each client room. A large chapel is used for daily mass. A chaplain distributes communion to clients and staff every evening. Nurses demonstrate a variety of religious symbols. One nurse is seen wearing a cross; another wears a Star

of David. Clients adhere to a variety of faith traditions, including Roman Catholic, Southern Baptist, and Muslim. Chaplains come from a variety of faith traditions and attempt to meet the needs of diverse groups.

Factor: Kinship and Social Factors

Types of Questions: What are the working relationships within nursing? Between nursing and ancillary services? Between nursing and medicine? How closely are staff members aligned? Is the environment emotionally "warm" and close or "cold" and distant? How do employees relate to one another? Do they celebrate together? Rely on each other for support? Do employees get together outside of work?

Sample Findings: RNs at Hospital A are most often White, are frequently the children of immigrants, and are typically educated in associate degree programs. About 20% of the nurses are Filipino with a few Hispanic and Black nurses. Nursing assistants are most often African American. There is tension between the two groups especially as the role of the aide has expanded. Nurses tend to be somewhat intimidated by physicians. Physicians' attitudes toward nurses range from respect to disrespect. Many physicians are angry about the erosion of their autonomy and economic security and the required use of computerized provider order entry. Most units tend to be tight knit, with celebrations of monthly birthdays and recognition provided when staff members "go the extra mile." Nurses rarely socialize with one another outside of work. Staff nurses have a mean age of 45. Most of them commute from the suburbs to the hospital and return home after their shift. In contrast, many of the aides are from the immediate community, know each other, and socialize outside of work.

Factor: Cultural Values

Types of Questions: Are values explicitly stated? What is valued within the institution? What is viewed as good? What is viewed as right? What is seen as truth?

(continued)

BOX 9-6 | **Example of Leininger's (1991) Culture Care Model Used to Conduct an Organizational Assessment (continued)**

Sample Findings: The institution clearly identifies its mission and strives to fulfill it in economically difficult times. Its stated values are collaboration and diversity. Although diversity training has been provided to managers, tensions still exist between work groups, particularly because the workforce tends to be racially divided.

Factor: Political/Legal

Types of Questions: How politically charged is the institution? Where does the power rest within the institution? With medicine? With finance? With nursing? With information technology? Is power shared? What types of legal actions have been taken against the institution? On behalf of the institution?

Sample Findings: Historically, Hospital A has been politically naive. It has gone about its mission without regard to the external environment. Recently, the hospital has begun to lobby for better reimbursement for care provided under Medicaid. Institutional power rests with the department chairs and strong medical staff.

Factor: Economic

Types of Questions: What is the financial viability of the institution? Who makes the financial decisions? How do the salaries and benefits compare with those of competitors in the immediate environment?

Sample Findings: Hospital A has a very low profit margin, 0.5%, compared with an industry standard of about 3%. This means that little money is available for capital improvements, which results in less technology and some units being cramped. Community needs are considered when making all financial decisions. People are valued, and efforts are made to keep salaries competitive. Starting salaries are increasing

for new graduates, and experienced nurses are complaining of salary compression.

Factor: Educational

Types of Questions: How is education valued within the institution? What type of assistance (financial, scheduling, flexibility) is provided for staff seeking additional degrees? Does the institution provide education for medicine, nursing, and other professions? Are advanced practice nurses utilized? What is the educational background of staff nurses? Nurse managers? Nursing leaders? How does this compare with education of other professional groups? With competing organizations?

Sample Findings: Nurses are most often educated in associate degree programs. Although flexible scheduling and limited tuition reimbursement are provided, many nurses do not take advantage of the benefits because of competing personal and family priorities and the need to work extra shifts to ensure staffing. All nurse managers and directors are required to have a baccalaureate degree in nursing. Some high-performing nurses are encouraged to return to school to become nurse practitioners, as the hospital plans to expand the use of that role. Nursing students from five different programs rotate through the institution, with priority given to local programs. Medical education is provided at Hospital A, with 100 residents and many 3rd year and 4th year medical students rotating through the facility. The residents, while learning, also provide important service to the community, particularly through their clinic rotations. Respiratory, social work, dietitian, physical therapy, occupational therapy, speech therapy, and pastoral care students also have clinical rotations at Hospital A.

---

adhere to the plan of care, and make necessary lifestyle changes.

Weech-Maldonado et al. (2012) conducted research to examine the relationship between hospital cultural competence and satisfaction

with inpatient care. They found that inpatients reported higher satisfaction with hospitals that had greater cultural competency. The findings were particularly striking among under-represented individuals, who reported higher satisfaction with nurse communication, physician communication, staff responsiveness, pain control, and environmental factors in hospitals with greater cultural competency.

Guerrero (2012) examined the extent to which internal and external organizational pressures contributed to the degree of adoption of culturally and linguistically responsive practices in outpatient substance use treatment systems. Higher adoption of culturally competent practices was found in programs with more external funding and regulation and with managers who had higher levels of cultural sensitivity. Organizations with a large number of professional staff had lower adoption of culturally competent practices when compared to organizations with fewer professional staff members. Weech-Maldonado et al. (2012a) found that hospitals that were not for profit, served a more diverse inpatient population, and were located in more competitive and affluent markets exhibited a higher degree of cultural competency.

As with cultural competence in individuals, cultural competency in organizations develops over time as part of an ongoing journey. The process involves all aspects of the organization. For the sections below, concepts from many authors have been combined and consolidated. Seven specific areas critical to fostering culturally competent healthcare organizations are discussed: governance and administration, internal evaluation of adherence to cultural competence standards, staff competence, the physical environment of care, linguistic competence, community involvement, and **culturally congruent services** and programs. Cultural congruency refers to care that is compatible with the client's culture; it results in effective interactions between the provider and client in the context of the healthcare organization.

Governance and Administration

Governance is defined as members of the Board of Directors and any sub-boards, such as Board Finance or Board Quality. Administration is defined as those individuals who serve as department heads. Together, governance and administration are responsible for ensuring that the organization continually develops cultural competence. Douglas et al. (2014) recommend 10 practices by leaders to build cultural competence in healthcare organizations, summarized in Box 9-7. The Wellesley Institute in Ontario (Kouri, 2012) identifies key strategies and tools helpful for reducing health disparities; several strategies helpful for governance and administration to consider are summarized in Box 9-8.

Ideally, both board members and administrators reflect the ethnic and racial diversity of the community served. The board and administration set the strategic plan for the organization. The strategic plan sets the direction for an organization and is used to communicate organizational goals and the actions needed to achieve those goals. The strategic planning process should begin with an assessment of community strengths and needs (Castillo & Guo, 2011; HRET, 2013; Purnell et al., 2011). In a study designed to determine factors related to organizational cultural competence, Guerrero (2013) found that leadership skills and strategic climate in addiction health service settings resulted in a better understanding and responsiveness to community needs. Board members and administration also establish the mission, vision, and values for the organization. The mission statement describes the purpose of the organization, its reason for existing. The mission statement should be inclusive. The basic premises of an organization, reflected in its mission statement, provide insight into the presence or absence of a commitment to providing culturally competent care. Many organizations also establish a vision and values to guide their culture. The vision projects the future status of an organization and inspires and generates a shared purpose among organization members. Whether or not they are explicitly stated, all organizations have values. Values are sometimes called Pillars. Values are the standards that guide the perspective and action of the organization and help to define an organization's culture and beliefs. The strategic plan is based on the mission,

---

BOX 9-7 | The Role of Healthcare Organization Leaders in Developing Culturally Competent Healthcare Systems and Organizations

1. Develop systems to promote culturally competent care delivery.
2. Ensure that mission and organizational policies reflect respect and values related to diversity and inclusivity.
3. Assign a managerial-level task force to oversee and take responsibility for diversity-related issues within the organization.
4. Establish an internal budget for the provision of culturally appropriate care, such as for the hiring of interpreters, producing multilanguage client education materials, adding signage in different languages, and so on.
5. Include cultural competence requirements in job descriptions, performance measures, and promotion criteria.
6. Develop a data collection system to monitor demographic trends for the geographic area served by the agency.
7. Obtain patient satisfaction data to determine the appropriateness and effectiveness of services.
8. Collaborate with other health agencies to share ideas and resources for meeting the needs of culturally diverse populations.
9. Bring healthcare directly to the local ethnic populations.
10. Enlist community members to participate in the agency's program planning committees, for example, for smoking cessation or infant care programs.

Source: Douglas, M. K., Rosenkoetter, M., Pacquiao, D., Callister, L. C., Hattar-Pollara, M., Lauderdale, J., Milstead, J. & Nardi, D., Purnell, L. (2014). Guidelines for implementing culturally competent nursing care. *Journal of Transcultural Nursing, 25*(2), 109–121.

BOX 9-8 | Strategies and Tools for Reducing Health Disparities

- Conduct local research and analyze health disparities.
- Provide primary healthcare practices and resources.
  - Offer convenient locations and hours.
  - Deliver appropriate care.
- Form effective partnerships.
  - Collaborate to reduce poverty.
  - Provide opportunities for early childhood development.
  - Implement school-based strategies.
- Advocate for public education and policy changes.
- Participate in community development.

Source: Kouri, D. (2012, March). *Reducing health disparities: How can the structure of the health system contribute?* Wellesley Institute. http://www.wellesleyinstitute.com/wp-content/uploads/2012/09/Reducing-Health-Disparities-how-can-health-system-structure-contribute.pdf

---

vision, and values. The plan should include tactics for developing culturally congruent services and programs to meet community needs, partnering with key community organizations, and developing the organization's cultural competence. The mission, vision, and values may also include specific behaviors demonstrated toward both customers and colleagues.

Administration is responsible for developing the organization's budget, which is then approved by the board of directors. Financial resources, including funding for capital, staff, and programs for the delivery of care, must be allocated appropriately to foster organizational cultural competence. For example, the environment should be welcoming, with the space and décor appropriate for the cultural groups served. Funding for staff recruitment, orientation, and training is also essential. Funding for the delivery of care must always consider cultural components. For example, funding is needed to advertise new and existing programs, using the venues and languages appropriate to the community. Pictures on the advertising materials must reflect the client population.

Nurse executives can take the lead in developing culturally competent healthcare organizations. Leininger (1996) defined **transcultural nursing administration** as "a creative and knowledgeable process of assessing, planning, and making decisions and policies that will facilitate the provision of educational and clinical services that take into account the cultural caring values, beliefs, symbols, references and lifeways of people of diverse and similar cultures for beneficial or satisfying outcomes" (p. 30). Nurse administrators must ensure that organizational policies are culturally sensitive and appropriate and that they recognize the rights of individuals and families. Such policies should incorporate Leininger's (1991)

decisions and actions of culture care preservation/maintenance, culture care accommodation/negotiation, and culture care repatterning/restructuring.

Nurse leaders who recognize the importance of transculturally based administration are essential for culturally competent healthcare organizations. The American Organization for Nursing Leaders (AONL, 2015) identifies five nurse executive competencies: communication, knowledge, leadership, professionalism, and business skills. Nurse executive competencies related to diversity are summarized in Box 9-9. Nurse administrators must foster a climate in which nurses and other healthcare providers realize that provider–client encounters include the interaction of three cultural systems: the organization, the providers, and the client.

Nurse leaders must also ensure that the work environment is safe for patients, visitors, and staff. As discussed above, racism and microaggressions from any source must not be tolerated. Frontline leaders, such as charge nurses, assistant managers, and managers, must intervene immediately. Special training may be needed to foster these skills.

In culturally competent healthcare organizations, nurse leaders also recognize the relationship between a culturally diverse nursing

BOX 9-9	American Organization of Nurse Leaders (AONL) Nurse Executive Communication and Relationship Building Competencies Related to Diversity

Diversity

- Establish an environment that values diversity (e.g., age, gender, race, religion, ethnicity, sexual orientation, culture).
- Establish cultural competency in the workforce.
- Incorporate cultural beliefs into care delivery.

- Provide an environment conducive to opinion sharing, exploration of ideas, and achievement of outcomes.

Community Involvement

- Represent the community perspective (during organizational/system decision-making)

Source: American Organization for Nursing Leadership. (2015). *Nurse executive competencies*. https://www.aonl.org/system/files/media/file/2019/06/nec.pdf

workforce and the ability to provide culturally competent patient care. The need to attract students from underrepresented groups is gaining recognition (AACN, 2023) and calls for new partnerships between practice, community, and academic settings.

Administration and the board of directors must work together to ensure that the healthcare organization continues to grow in cultural competence. This includes setting strategic priorities and funding appropriate programs for staff and clients.

Internal Evaluation of Adherence to Cultural Competence Standards

In addition to recognizing and acknowledging the overall culture of a healthcare organization, organizations must also evaluate how they are adhering to cultural competence standards as an organization and determine how effectively the organization is meeting the needs of the populations they serve. Healthcare services may be evaluated based on their availability, accessibility, affordability, acceptability, and appropriateness by answering these questions:

- *Are the health services that are needed by the community readily available?* In a community with rampant illicit drug use, for example, one should expect to find a variety of types of drug use prevention and treatment programs offered that are readily available to the local population.
- *Are healthcare resources accessible?* A pediatrician's office, for example, might need to expand its hours of operation to accommodate the schedules of working parents. Geographic location should be considered in terms of proximity to public transportation, traffic patterns, and available parking. Structural changes may also be needed to accommodate specific types of clients, such as those who use wheelchairs.

- *Are the services affordable?* Partnerships between public and private organizations may be needed to ensure that services are affordable. A sliding scale might be developed to accommodate the needs of people with limited financial resources.
- *Are the services acceptable?* Providers need to carefully consider this question. Do community members who use the services perceive the services to be of high quality? Do community members value the services? Are the waiting rooms stark, dimly lit, or untidy? Is the furniture worn or the reading material frayed and outdated? Providers need to understand what makes services acceptable to the community they seek to serve. Community members may avoid a particular agency or institution because services are delivered in a noncaring and patronizing fashion.
- *Are the services appropriate?* Community members may shun services if they do not perceive that these services meet their needs. For example, community members who struggle with day-to-day survival with limited financial and social resources may not use fitness classes. Programs that are disconnected from the daily life of community members are likely to fail.

An organization may also compare their performance to standards provided by regulatory bodies, government agencies, and professional organizations. For example, the Cultural Competency Assessment Tool for Hospitals was created to assess adherence to the CLAS standards (Weech-Maldonado et al., 2012b). The instrument measures 12 composites: leadership and strategic planning, data collection on inpatient population, data collection on service area, performance management systems and quality improvement, HR practices, diversity training, community representation, availability of interpreter services, interpreter services policies, quality of interpreter services, translation of written materials, and clinical cultural competency practices.

To evaluate how effectively the healthcare organization is meeting community needs, a variety of data elements may be considered, including clinical data and patient satisfaction. Healthcare organizations should assess their own practices to determine if there are unknown disparities in care. As an example, Figure 9-1 presents data for long-bone fracture pain management from the ED of a community hospital. The mean and median turnaround time for pain medication is shorter than the national average for all groups but is slightly longer for Asian populations compared to all other populations at the author's hospital. Examination of the data helps the organization to determine the causes of the variations.

Focused interventions can help administrators to improve their cultural competence. Weech-Maldonado et al. (2018) provided a systematic, multifaceted, and organizational-level cultural competency intervention to executive leadership at two hospitals within a system, with a third hospital in the system serving as a control. Overall performance improvement was greater in each of the two intervention hospitals than in the control hospital. Statistically significant improvements were noted in the organizational-level competencies of diversity leadership and strategic HR management, in individual-level competencies for diversity attitudes and implicit bias, and in overall diversity climate.

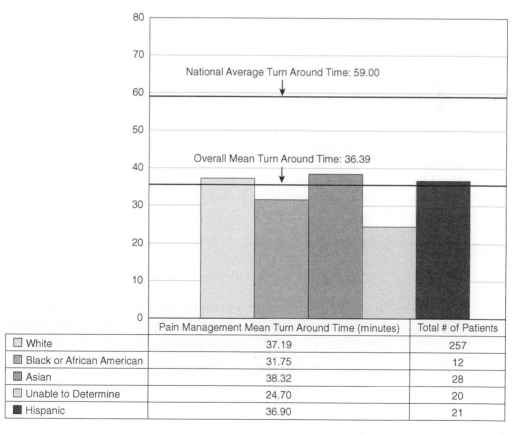

	Pain Management Mean Turn Around Time (minutes)	Total # of Patients
☐ White	37.19	257
▨ Black or African American	31.75	12
▨ Asian	38.32	28
☐ Unable to Determine	24.70	20
■ Hispanic	36.90	21

Figure 9-1. Example of emergency department turnaround time for pain medication in clients with long bone fracture by race/ethnicity, FY2013. (Data from Edward Hospital at Edward-Elmhurst Health.)

Staff Competence

Culturally competent individual healthcare providers are essential for building culturally competent organizations. All staff members must be competent; this is especially critical for direct care nurses and other staff members. Many times, nurses and other care providers interact based on their own cultural values, experience, and preferences. They need to be taught how to interact with patients from various cultures to provide patient-centered care and serve as patient advocates (Sherrod, 2013). Key processes, including organizational support, orientation, and ongoing education, are needed to enhance staff competence.

The HR department typically provides organizational support for staff. The department plays a key role in ensuring that recruitment and hiring activities reflect the diversity of the community served by the healthcare organization. HR can also prioritize recruitment of bilingual staff members and ensure appropriate compensation. Policies, position descriptions, and performance reviews, typically overseen by HRs, must reflect cultural competence.

Orientation and ongoing education are needed for employees at all levels to develop and foster cultural sensitivity and competence. Diversity in its broadest terms should be discussed in orientation. This should include race, ethnicity, religion, age, sex, sexual orientation, gender identity, socioeconomics, educational backgrounds, disabilities, and more for both clients and staff members. Education content should include the changing population of the United States, demographics of the healthcare organization, and how working with diverse cultures impact clinical encounters. Online education might be helpful but is never sufficient. Multiple educational methods should be used, including reviewing SDOH, conducting case study reviews, and including live interactions (Delphin-Rittmen, 2013; HRET, 2013; Purnell et al., 2011). Volunteers and medical staff members also need to be oriented to the organization's culture, strategy, and expectations.

Beyond orientation, ongoing education is needed to reinforce learning. While staff cannot learn about all diversity, they should be equipped with a general cultural framework and have specific knowledge about the cultural groups for whom they most often provide care. Cultural humility provides a first step. This includes awareness of personal beliefs, values, and implicit biases. Staff need to be aware of their own lack of knowledge, be open to learning, acknowledge patient expertise, and demonstrate empathy toward other life experiences (Office of Minority Health, 2021b). Cultural humility is facilitated through reflection and discussion and is a necessary precursor to cultural competence. By acknowledging their own beliefs, staff members may be helped to avoid stereotyping and cultural imposition. Ongoing education should incorporate reviewing patient satisfaction and quality indicators to determine continued opportunities to reduce healthcare disparities. Inviting members of a particular culture or religion to discuss their beliefs and practices is often engaging for both the community and staff. To help hold staff members accountable for their actions, performance reviews must reflect the organization's commitment to cultural competence.

Staff members must continue to enhance their cultural competence to help build culturally competent healthcare organizations. Staff members who lack competency may fail to take the client's culture seriously, misinterpret the client's value system, and elevate their own value systems. This posture is culturally destructive because it minimizes the other person's culture. Culturally competent staff members will take time to ask questions about what the client prefers and listen attentively. In the end, this will increase understanding, trust, collaboration, adherence, and satisfaction.

Nurses and other healthcare staff members also need training in obtaining accurate patient data. Research suggests that 80% of hospitals collect data on race and ethnicity, primarily in response to a law or regulatory requirement (Hasnain-Wynia et al., 2004). However, the information may not be accurate or valid. Gomez et al. (2003) found that while 85% of hospitals reported collecting data on race, approximately half of them obtained the data by observing a client's physical appearance. In addition, only 12% of the hospitals reported having a procedure for recording the race and/or ethnicity of a client with mixed ancestry, and 55% reported never collecting ethnicity data. Regenstein and Sickler (2006) found that 78.4% of hospitals collect race information, 50.4% collect data on client ethnicity, and 50.2% collect data on language preference. However, only 20% had formal data collection policies, and fewer than 20% used the data to assess and compare care quality, health services utilization, health outcomes, or patient satisfaction. The Institute of Medicine (2002) standardized the collection of race, ethnicity, and language data over 20 years ago. Unfortunately, this has not been consistently applied in practice.

Hospitals must standardize who provides the information, when it is collected, which racial and ethnic categories are used, how the data are stored, and how the data are used to improve health equity. The Agency for Healthcare Research and Quality (2018) has identified steps an organization can take to collect more accurate data. This includes how to ask patients and enrollees questions about race, ethnicity, and language and communication needs; how to train staff to elicit this information in a respectful and efficient manner; how to address the discomfort of registration/admission staff or call center staff about requesting this information; how to address potential patient or enrollee pushback respectfully; and how to address system-level issues, such as changes in patient registration screens and data flow.

Nurses and other healthcare providers can help the organization grow in cultural understanding. If they listen and attend carefully, healthcare providers have a valuable window directly into the world of their clients. They can take what they learn and share it with administrative leaders to improve the cultural responsiveness of their organization. Individuals and groups of clinicians can

also develop special programs to meet the needs of the specific populations they serve. Speaking the language is a definite advantage.

The Physical Environment of Care

As part of building a culturally competent organization, the physical environment should always be assessed. Approaching this assessment from the perspective of a potential client is helpful, and a variety of factors should be considered. What message does the organization send through its physical surroundings? How is the facility organized physically? How does the entryway present the culture of the organization to the public? Is the entrance warm and inviting? Is the signage prominent? What languages are included on the signs? Is information presented clearly and unambiguously? Are amenities available to clients and their family members? Are the doors open or closed? Do people talk with one another, and what languages are spoken? What is the traffic pattern, and what is the general flow of traffic? Does the environment appear calm or turbulent? Are the staff members attentive and courteous?

A physical environment may send unintentional messages. For example, consider the birthing center at a city hospital. The hospital's service area is undergoing change, with increased number of Black, Hispanic, Indian, Polish, and LGBTQ+ populations. The birthing unit is beautifully and tastefully decorated with oak furniture and pastel prints. Every picture on the walls, however, shows a White nuclear family: baby, mother and father. This clearly sends a message of exclusivity rather than inclusiveness. When this is brought to the attention of the nurse manager, she is completely dumbfounded and quickly takes steps to rectify the situation. Ethnocentrism and stereotyping are in play here, and it takes a degree of cultural competence to identify this and bring it to recognition and resolution.

Organizational leaders must also assess the physical environment of care to identify potential barriers. A flow chart is a helpful tool for determining such barriers. For example, to provide comprehensive women's health programs in a caring fashion, organizational leaders may examine the steps for admission to the labor and delivery unit for the delivery of a baby. To determine this, staff members walk through the care process and create a flow chart that outlines the steps. Staff members must be alert for possible sources of confusion for parents at this highly stressful time. The flow chart can then be used to design changes in the environment that can be implemented to decrease barriers and improve services.

Linguistic Competence

Limited English Proficiency (LEP) may become a major barrier to quality healthcare (Office of Minority Health, 2021a). The Institute of Medicine (2002) reports that 51% of providers believe that clients do not adhere to treatment because of culture or language. At the same time, nurses and other healthcare providers report having received no language or cultural competency training (Park et al., 2005). Twenty-two percent of medical residents feel unprepared to treat patients who have LEP (Weissman et al., 2005). Providing care to non–English-speaking patients presents a special challenge. Addressing this challenge begins when the nurse determines the preferred language for healthcare discussions with the patient. This information must be recorded and shared with all healthcare providers. Patients must be informed that an interpreter will be provided for them at no cost. Interpreter services may be provided in person, by videoconferencing, or by telephone.

Competent interpreter services are necessary when providing care and services. Because communication is a cornerstone of patient safety and quality care, all patients have the right to receive information in a manner they understand. Effective communication allows patients to participate more fully in their care, is critical to the informed consent process, and helps practitioners and healthcare organizations give the best possible care. For communication to be effective, the information provided must be complete, accurate, timely, unambiguous, and understood by the patient. Many patients of varying circumstances require alternative communication methods, including patients who speak and/or read languages other than English, patients who have limited literacy in any language, patients who have visual or hearing conditions, patients on ventilators, patients with cognitive disabilities, and children.

Healthcare organizations have many options to assist in communication with these individuals, such as interpreters, translated written materials, pen and paper, and communication boards. It is up to the hospital to determine which method is the best for each patient. Various laws, regulations, and guidelines are relevant to the use of interpreters. These include Title VI of the Civil Rights Act, 1964; Executive Order 13166; policy guidance from the Office of Civil Rights regarding compliance with Title VI, 2004; Title III of the Americans with Disabilities Act, 1990; state laws; and the National Council on Interpreting in Health Care (2005).

All healthcare organizations should have policies to address interpreter services, and staff members should be educated on them. Signage, consent forms, patient education, and other written materials should be translated and available in the most commonly spoken languages. Written materials should augment, not substitute for, discussion in the patient's language. The organization should evaluate written documents for cultural sensitivity. When collecting data, such as patient satisfaction or quality of life surveys, the organization should provide the surveys in the patient's preferred language. The organization should also work with the community to address health literacy and provide and encourage attendance at English as a Second Language classes.

Large healthcare organizations may have resources to secure trained professional interpreters and bilingual providers. Regardless of setting, however, Youdelman and Perkins (2005) suggest the following eight-step process for developing appropriate language services:

1. Designate responsibility
2. Conduct an analysis of language needs
3. Identify resources in the community
4. Determine what language services will be provided
5. Determine how to respond to LEP patients
6. Train staff
7. Notify LEP patients of available language services
8. Revise activities after periodic review

Community Involvement

Understanding what culturally competent healthcare means from the standpoint of patients is an important step in building culturally competent organizations. Napoles-Springer et al. (2005) conducted 19 community focus groups to determine the meaning of culture and what cultural factors influenced the quality of their medical visits. Culture was defined in terms of value systems, customs, self-identified ethnicity, and nationality. Black, Latino, and non-Latino White participants all agreed that the quality of healthcare encounters was influenced by clinicians' sensitivity to complementary/alternative medicine, health insurance discrimination, social class discrimination, ethnic concordance between patient and provider, and age-based discrimination. Ethnicity-based discrimination was identified as a factor for Latino and Black participants. Latino participants also described language issues and immigration status factors. Overall, participants indicated greater satisfaction with clinicians who demonstrated cultural flexibility, defined as the ability to elicit, adapt, and respond to patients' cultural characteristics.

Healthcare institutions exist to provide care. Many factors, such as tobacco, alcohol, and drug use; poor diet; and physical inactivity, contribute to mortality in the United States and Canada. Addressing these factors requires individual behavioral change, community change, social change, and economic change. Healthcare organizations cannot confront these complex factors in isolation; they must partner with their communities to build trust in their institutions and meet the needs of their local communities.

Community partnerships may be configured in a variety of ways. Hospitals and healthcare systems often articulate their desire to improve the health of the communities they serve as part of their mission. Historically, hospitals have fulfilled this mission through charity care, healthcare provider education, healthcare research, community education programming, and community outreach (Pelfrey & Theisen, 1993). However, true improvements in the health of a community require the focused efforts of the entire community. Such improvements may occur only in partnerships with community members and community organizations.

An ethnographic study of community (Davis, 1997) revealed five themes related to the experience of community caring. Three of these themes are particularly significant to this discussion: (1) Reciprocal relationships and teams working together are central to building healthy communities, (2) education with a focus on prevention is key to enhancing health, and (3) understanding community needs is a primary catalyst for healthcare reform and change.

Healthcare professionals in culturally competent organizations collaborate with surrounding communities to conduct community health assessments. In community mapping, staff collect a variety of data, including demographics, health status, community resources, barriers, and enablers. Both strengths and needs are identified from the perspective of the community. Data are then used collaboratively with communities to set priorities. An example of such a community assessment is provided in Box 9-10. The community assessment process guides the planning and implementation of key initiatives. These initiatives are most well accepted when they are sponsored by a variety of community organizations rather than by a single healthcare organization. Findings from the community assessment may also help to frame staff education (HRET, 2013).

Community-based participatory research or **participatory action research** is helpful in

BOX 9-10 | Community Assessment Example

As part of an assessment of the communities it serves, the hospital realized that Hispanic residents made up an increasing proportion of the population and were the most frequently underserved population. As a result, an interprofessional team led by a family practice physician proposed the idea of a community center for health and empowerment. A coalition composed of individuals from social services, healthcare agencies, schools, police, churches, businesses, city government, and other community services also identified the Hispanic community as underserved. This coalition provided an etic, or outsider, view of the Hispanic community.

To provide a local, or emic (insider) view, community members worked with healthcare personnel to design and conduct a door-to-door community assessment. Leininger's theory of cultural diversity and universality served to guide the assessment. The assessment process involved two focus groups, 15 community interviewers, and 220 door-to-door interviews. In addition, five meetings, attended by 180 community members, were held to report the findings to community members and solicit their input on how to maintain strengths and address needs. As a result, numerous task forces were formed to preserve strengths or mediate needs.

Major strengths identified were access to friends and families to socialize and get support; prenatal and postnatal care; and pediatric care. Major needs identified were affordable housing; programs to help immigrants; Spanish-speaking dentists; and activities for youth.

The community was involved in key decisions from the beginning, including selecting the site for the center, choosing the name for the center, and establishing a sliding scale for fees. The bilingual center includes primary healthcare services, a Women–Infant–Children program run by the county health department, and a community empowerment program. A salaried community outreach worker coordinates the community empowerment program. In collaboration with businesses, churches, and city services, community members received training in group work and priority setting.

Because of the identified need for dental care, the center arranged for monthly dental services through a dental van. To address the concern about activities for youth, community members and center personnel actively partnered with the park district, schools, churches, and the police to provide recreational activities for the youth. The community uses this as an opportunity to celebrate their cultural heritage. Health promotion materials and activities are also provided through collaboration.

Source: Ludwig-Beymer, P., Blankemeier, J. R., Casas-Byots, C., & Suarez-Balcazar, Y. (1996). Community assessment in a suburban Hispanic community: A description of methods. *Journal of Transcultural Nursing*, *8*(1), 19–27.

understanding a community and developing health improvement initiatives with community members. The method uses collaborative, participatory approaches to develop sustainable services (Koch & Kralik, 2006). Reese (2011) described a participatory action research project that addresses organizational barriers to cultural competence in hospice care through a university–community–hospice partnership. In addition, the National Institute on Minority Health and Health Disparities (NIMHD), located within the National Institutes of Health, funds disease intervention research to reduce and eliminate health disparities using community-based participation research that is jointly conducted by health disparity communities and researchers (NIMHD, 2022). Focus groups may also assist an organization in assessing how well they are meeting the needs of the populations they serve.

Working with communities requires cultural awareness, sensitivity, humility, and competence. It involves working with other professions and sectors, such as community members, housing, education, criminal justice, faith communities, employers, social services, other healthcare organizations, and government agencies. This work is addressed in the *Future of Nursing 2020 to 2030* report (The National Academies of Sciences, Engineering, and Medicine, 2021). Interpreting the data requires knowledge of the cultural dimensions of health and illness. Using the data to develop and implement programs in conjunction with the community requires the ability to plan and implement culturally competent services. Guided by Leininger's Sunrise Enabler (McFarland & Wehbe-Alamah, 2019) and other transcultural models, transcultural nurses have long partnered with community and government agencies to obtain housing, food, water, transportation, and other services for their clients. The skill of a transcultural nurse or other culturally competent healthcare professional is invaluable in these situations.

Culturally Congruent Services and Programs

Culturally competent nurses and other healthcare providers develop and evaluate culturally competent initiatives. Many important factors must be considered in planning programs across cultural groups. In many cases, cultural competence must be demonstrated with multiple cultures simultaneously. For example, one hospital in the Chicago area provides care for individuals who, collectively, speak 64 different languages. This calls for much effort and creativity on the part of patients, healthcare providers, and interpreters. Case Study 9-1 describes the development and implementation of one culturally competent program provided to a community; however, additional programs, targeting the needs of other groups, may also be envisioned. For example, adult immunizations are a challenge for many communities, so a program might be developed that focuses specifically on older adults and their immunization needs. Similarly, programs might be instituted to deal with other health issues of concern to community members. The case study demonstrates the importance of incorporating an understanding of culture in every aspect of an initiative. To design and implement an effective program, the cultural values of patients must be understood and addressed.

CASE STUDY 9-1

Caring Hospital, a not-for-profit hospital, serves clients who differ in multiple ways, including but not limited to socioeconomic status, education, race, ethnicity, religion, language, sexual orientation, gender identity, and culture. Organizational leaders embrace Leininger's theory of culture care. Nursing leaders believe that nursing care must be congruent with the client's culture in order to promote the client's health and satisfaction.

Through a healthy community program, the hospital remains grounded in the reality of its clients. The healthy community program, developed and staffed by two nurses with community health backgrounds, is responsible for broadly defining community-based health promotion initiatives that address individual, social, and community factors. Their goal is to establish partnerships with community members and governmental and community organizations to ensure that everyone has access to the basics needed for health; that the physical environment supports healthy living; and that communities control, define, and direct action for health.

The nurses in the healthy community program bring together resources from settings both within and outside their hospital. For example, they work closely with other community-focused staff members, such as home care and faith-based nurses. They also work with multiple external organizations, such as local health departments and other government agencies, religious institutions, community businesses, schools, and other healthcare entities. These nurses work specifically with the communities surrounding their facility. In this way, they acknowledge the specific needs of diverse groups.

(continued)

The healthy community nurses use Leininger's culture care diversity and universality model in their practice. They use data gathered from cultural assessments to assist them in understanding the communities they serve. They consider environmental context, ethnohistory, language, kinship, cultural values and lifeways, the political and legal system, and technologic, economic, religious, philosophic, and educational factors. They understand the interactions among the folk system, nursing care, and the professional systems. They also understand the importance of using the three culture care modalities: preservation/maintenance, accommodation/negotiation, and repatterning/restructuring.

Because of their community health backgrounds, the nurses are knowledgeable about SDOH and health disparities. The nurses use data from a variety of sources, including hospital-specific data, census tract data, and health department data, to help them understand health and assess disparities in their area. They also talk to community members and to healthcare providers to identify competing priorities. Using these processes, they discover that their communities have not achieved the *Healthy People 2030* immunization goals for children by the age of 2 years.

To address the delay in immunizations, the nurses acknowledge that the issues that affect immunizations are multifaceted. The immunization schedule changes frequently and is quite complex. Even healthcare providers have difficulty interpreting it. Communication with parents has been inconsistent and has been complicated by controversy. Immunizations are sometimes seen by parents as nonessential for young children until they enter elementary school. Immunizations may not be easily accessible, available, and affordable. Parents may make decisions based on misinformation, rumor, or hearsay. The nurses know, however, that community members want to keep their children healthy and that immunizations have contributed greatly to reducing illnesses in individuals and improving overall health for the community. They also know that community members prefer their children receive immunizations in a consistent place, as part of an overall medical home.

Because the childhood immunization levels are suboptimal in the communities served by the hospital, childhood immunization is selected as a quality initiative. A group of consumers and clinicians is convened to implement a program with the goal of increasing immunization to the *Healthy People 2030* goals. There is much discussion on the best way to increase immunization rates through a broad-based program. The group considers mailed, telephoned, e-mailed, and texted reminders and opts to combine texted reminders with follow-up mailed reminders.

Various materials are developed in both English and Spanish, and incentives are put into place to assist parents. Babies are automatically enrolled in the program when they are born at the hospital; recognizing the increase in home births, the group develops and posts flyers to encourage parents to enroll children born at home. Mailings occur at regular intervals and include a personalized letter indicating what vaccines are due, a vaccine record, vaccine information statements, and a growth and development newsletter. Additionally, incentives are mailed to help keep the parents motivated to use preventive services. Materials are written at a sixth-grade level. All materials are reviewed for cultural congruity, and the illustrations include babies from various ethnic groups.

New materials are developed as needed based on a continuous assessment of the needs of the parents. For example, reproducing all the materials in all the languages used by clients is found to be too expensive, so a multiple-language brochure is developed in the 11 most common languages spoken in the community. The brochure explains the program and asks that non–English-speaking and non–Spanish-speaking families obtain help in translating the materials. A "calming strategies" flyer is developed based on family concerns about the multiple injections required to keep their babies fully immunized and their babies' resultant distress and crying.

Because financial barriers still exist among parents seeking immunizations for their children, the healthy community nurses implement several additional strategies. First, they work with physicians and help them enroll in the Vaccines for Children program, making vaccines available at no cost. They also work with the staff in physicians' offices to enhance their role in encouraging childhood immunizations. In addition, they work with the health department to provide monthly immunizations on-site at the hospital.

Summary

As with individuals, the quest for organizational cultural competence is a continuous journey. There is always more to learn. To be truly effective in improving patient care for all, healthcare services and social services must make an organizational commitment to cultural competence. Cultural competence cannot live in one or two nurses; it must be systemic. It must involve individuals at all levels of the organization: governance members, administrators, managers, providers, and support staff. In addition, an organization must have a mutually beneficial relationship with the community it serves and must involve community members in its quest for cultural competence.

REVIEW QUESTIONS

1. What types of access, healthcare, and health outcome disparities exist nationally? In your community?
2. How does the culture of an organization affect the quality of care provided?
3. What tools or models are helpful for assessing organizational culture?
4. How does an organization's culture influence or affect its employees?
5. What specific areas must receive attention when building culturally competent healthcare organizations?

CRITICAL THINKING ACTIVITIES

1. With some of your classmates, evaluate the availability, accessibility, affordability, acceptability, and appropriateness of the care provided at one healthcare organization. Discuss what actions could be taken by the organization to increase its cultural competency.
2. Use Leininger's (Leininger, 1991) theory of culture care diversity and universality to assess the culture of the same organization. Box 9-6 provides an example of how Leininger's culture care model can be used. Compare and contrast the values and beliefs of the organization with the values and beliefs of the groups using the healthcare organization's services. What areas would be most problematic, and why?
3. Lacking other access to care, some individuals use EDs for episodic care. Visit a busy ED. What languages do you hear? Assess the physical environment to determine potential barriers to culturally competent care. Develop a flow chart that outlines the steps clients take when they seek care in an emergency room. Identify changes that would decrease barriers and improve services if they were implemented.

REFERENCES

Agency for Healthcare Research and Quality. (2018). *Race, ethnicity, and language data: Standardization for health care quality improvement.* http://www.ahrq.gov/research/findings/final-reports/iomracereport/index.html

Agency for Healthcare Research and Quality. (2022). *2021 National healthcare quality and disparities report.* https://www.ahrq.gov/research/findings/nhqrdr/nhqdr21/index.html

Alessandra, T. (2010). *The platinum rule.* http://www.alessandra.com/abouttony/aboutpr.asp

Alter, D. A., Stukel, T., Chong, A., & Henry, D. (2011). Lessons from Canada's Universal Care: Socially disadvantaged patients use more health services, still have poorer health. *Health Affairs, 30*(2), 274–283.

American Association of Colleges of Nursing (AACN). (2023). *Fact sheet: Enhancing diversity in the nursing workforce.* AACN. https://www.aacnnursing.org/Portals/0/PDFs/FactSheets/Enhancing-Diversity-Factsheet.pdf

American Nurses Association. (2016). *The nurse's role in ethics and human rights: Protecting and promoting individual worth, dignity, and human rights in practice settings.* https://www.nursingworld.org/globalassets/docs/ana/nursesrole-ethicshumanrights-positionstatement.pdf

American Nurses Association. (2018). *Diversity awareness.* https://www.nursingworld.org/practice-policy/innovation-evidence/clinical-practice-material/diversity-awareness/

American Nurses Association. (2022). *New survey data: Racism within the nursing profession is a substantial problem.* https://www.nursingworld.org/news/news-releases/2021/new-survey-data-racism-in-nursing/

American Nurses Credentialing Center. (2021). *2023 Magnet® application manual.* American Nurses Credentialing Center.

American Organization for Nursing Leadership. (2015). *Nurse executive competencies.* https://www.aonl.org/system/files/media/file/2019/06/nec.pdf

Bhopal, R. S. (2007). Racism in health and health care in Europe: Reality or mirage? *European Journal of Public Health, 17*(3), 238–241.

Bolman, L. G., & Deal, T. E. (2017). *Reframing organizations: Artistry, choice, and leadership* (6th ed.). Jossey-Bass.

Castillo, R. J., & Guo, K. L. (2011). A framework for cultural competence in health care organizations. *The Health Care Manager, 30*(3), 205–214.

Centers for Disease Control and Prevention. (2022a, August 31). *Life expectancy in the U.S. dropped for the second year in a row in 2021.* https://www.cdc.gov/nchs/pressroom/nchs_press_releases/2022/20220831.htm

Centers for Disease Control and Prevention. (2022b, July 1). *What is health equity?* https://www.cdc.gov/healthequity/whatis/index.html

Centers for Medicare and Medicaid Services. (2012). *Cultural competence: A national health concern.* https://www.cms.gov/Outreach-and-Education/Medicare-Learning-Network-MLN/MLNMattersArticles/downloads/SE0621.pdf

Creamer, J., Shrider, E. A., Burns, B., & Chen, F. (2022). *Poverty in the United States: 2021.* United States Census Bureau. https://www.census.gov/library/publications/2022/demo/p60-277.html

Davis, R. N. (1997). Community caring: An ethnographic study within an organizational culture. *Public Health Nursing, 14*(2), 92–100.

Delphin-Rittmon, M. E. (2013). Seven essential strategies for promoting and sustaining systemic cultural competence. *Psychiatric Quarterly, 84*(1), 53–64.

Douglas, M. K., Rosenkoetter, M., Pacquiao, D., Callister, L. C., Hattar-Pollara, M., Lauderdale, J., Milstead, J., Nardi, D., & Purnell, L. (2014). Guidelines for implementing culturally competent nursing care. *Journal of Transcultural Nursing, 25*(2), 109–121.

Feagin, J., & Bennefield, Z. (2014). Systemic racism and U.S. health care. *Social Science & Medicine, 103*, 7–14.

Gomez, S. L., Le, G. M., West, D. W., Santariano, W. A., & O'Connor, L. (2003). Hospital policy and practice regarding the collection of data on race, ethnicity, and birthplace. *Journal of Public Health, 93*(10), 1685–1688.

Guerrero, E. (2012). Organizational characteristics that foster early adoption of cultural and linguistic competence in outpatient substance abuse treatment in the United States. *Evaluation and Program Planning, 35*(1), 9–15.

Guerrero, E. G. (2013). Organizational structure, leadership and readiness for change and the implementation of organizational cultural competence in addiction services. *Evaluation and Program Planning, 40*, 74–81.

Hasnain-Wynia, R., Pierce, D., & Pittman, M. A. (2004). *Who, when, and how: The current state of race, ethnicity, and primary language data collection in hospitals.* The Commonwealth Fund and the American Hospital Association's Health Research and Educational Trust. http://www.commonwealthfund.org/usr_doc/hasnain-wynia_whowhenhow_726.pdf

Health Research and Educational Trust. (2013). *Becoming a culturally competent health care organization: Equity of care.* https://www.aha.org/ahahret-guides/2013-06-18-becoming-culturally-competent-health-care-organization

Henry, B. R., Houston, S., & Mooney, G. H. (2004). Institutional racism in Australian healthcare: A plea for decency. *Medical Journal of Australia, 180*(10), 517–520.

Institute for Diversity and Health Equity. (2022). *The health equity road map.* https://ifdhe.aha.org/

Institute of Medicine. (2002). *Unequal treatment: Confronting racial and ethnic disparities in health care.* National Academies Press.

The Joint Commission. (2022). *Health care equity resource center.* https://www.jointcommission.org/our-priorities/health-care-equity/accreditation-standards-and-resource-center/

Koch, T., & Kralik, D. (2006). *Participatory action research in health care.* Wiley-Blackwell.

Kouri, D. (2012). *Reducing health disparities: How can the structure of the health system contribute?* Wellesley Institute. Retrieved May 30, 2018 from http://www.wellesleyinstitute.com/wp-content/uploads/2012/09/Reducing-Health-Disparities-how-can-health-system-structure-contribute.pdf

Krisberg, K. (2017). Economic, social inequities growing between richest, poorest Americans. *The Nation's Health, 47*(4), 6.

Lake, E. T., Narva, A. M., Holland, S., Smith, J. G., Cramer, E., Fitzpatrick Rosenbaum, K. E., French, R., Clark, R. R. S., & Rogowski, J. A. (2022). Hospital nurses' moral distress and mental health during COVID-19. *Journal of Advanced Nursing, 78*(3), 799–809.

Leininger, M. (1991). *Culture care diversity and universality: A theory of nursing care.* National League for Nursing Press.

Leininger, M. (1996). Founder's focus: Transcultural nursing administration: An imperative worldwide. *Journal of Transcultural Nursing, 8*(1), 28–33.

Ludwig-Beymer, P. (2018). Respect and Racism. *Journal of Transcultural Nursing, 129*(2), 121–122. doi:10.1177/1043659617747687

Ludwig-Beymer, P., Blankemeier, J. R., Casas-Byots, C., & Suarez-Balcazar, Y. (1996). Community assessment in a suburban hispanic community: A description of methods. *Journal of Transcultural Nursing, 8*(1), 19–27.

McClure, M. L., Poulin, M. A., Sovie, M. D., & Wandelt, M. A.; For the American Academy Task Force on Nursing Practice in Hospitals. (1983). *Magnet hospitals. Attraction and retention of professional nurses.* American Nurses Association.

McFarland, M. R., & Wehbe-Alamah, H. B. (2019). *Leininger's transcultural nursing: Concepts, theories, research and practice* (4th ed.). McGraw Hill.

McKenzie, K., & Bhui, K. (2007). Institutional racism in mental health care. *BMJ, 334*(7595), 649–650.

Metzl, J. M., & Hansen, H. (2014). Structural competency: Theorizing a new medical engagement with stigma and inequality. *Social Science & Medicine, 103*, 126–133.

Metzl, J. M., Petty, J., & Olowojoba, O. V. (2018). Using a structural competency framework to teach structural racism in pre-health education. *Social Science & Medicine, 11*, 189–201.

Napoles-Springer, A. M., Santoyo, J., Houston, K., Perez-Stable, E. J., & Stewart, A. L. (2005). Patients' perceptions of cultural factors affecting the quality of their medical encounters. *Health Expectations, 8*, 4–17.

The National Academies of Sciences, Engineering, and Medicine. (2021). *The future of nursing 2020-2030: Charting a path to achieve health equity.* The National Academies Press. https://nap.nationalacademies.org/login.php?record_id=25982

National Council on Interpreting in Health Care. (2005). *National standards of practice for interpreters in health care.* https://www.ncihc.org/assets/documents/publications/NCIHC%20National%20Standards%20of%20Practice.pdf

National Institute on Minority Health and Health Disparities. (2022). *Active NIMHD funding opportunities.* https://www.nimhd.nih.gov/funding/nimhd-funding/active_foa.html

Office of Minority Health, Department of Health and Human Services. (2021a). *Think cultural health: The national CLAS standards.* https://minorityhealth.hhs.gov/omh/browse.aspx?lvl=2&lvlid=53

Office of Minority Health, Department of Health and Human Services. (2021b). *Think cultural health.* https://minorityhealth.hhs.gov/omh/browse.aspx?lvl=2&lvlid=53

Park, E. R., Betancourts, J. R., Kim, M. K., Maina, A. W., Blumenthal, D., & Weissman, J. S. (2005). Mixed messages: Residents' experiences learning cross-cultural care. *Academic Medicine, 80*(9), 874–880.

Pelfrey, S., & Theisen, B. A. (1993). Valuing the community benefits provided by nonprofit hospitals. *Journal of Nursing Administration, 23*(6), 16–21.

Pina, I. L., Cohen, P. D., Larson, D. B., Marion, L. N., Sills, M. R., Solberg, L. I., & Zerzan, J. (2015). A framework for describing health care delivery organizations and systems. *American Journal of Public Health, 105*(4), 670–679.

Purnell, L., Davidhizar, R. E., Giger, J. N., Strickland, O. L., Fishman, D., & Allison, D. M. (2011). A guide to developing a culturally competent organization. *Journal of Transcultural Nursing, 22*(1), 7–14.

Reese, D. J. (2011). Proposal for a university-community-hospice partnership to address organizational barriers to cultural competence. *The American Journal of Hospital & Palliative Care, 28*(1), 22–26.

Regenstein, M., & Sickler, D. (2006). *Race, ethnicity, and language of patients.* National Public Health and Hospital Institute. https://publichealth.gwu.edu/departments/healthpolicy/DHP_Publications/pub_uploads/dhpPublication_3BD811C8-5056-9D20-3D8EFC1026A1B8A5.pdf

Schaffner, J. W., & Ludwig-Beymer, P. (2003). *Rx for the nursing shortage.* Health Administration Press.

Schein, E. H. (2016). *Organizational culture and leadership* (5th ed.). Jossey-Bass.

Sherrod, D. (2013). Ask, listen, respect. Nursing Management, *44*(11), 6.

Statistics Canada. (2022). *Life expectancy and deaths.* https://www.statcan.gc.ca/en/subjects-start/health/life_expectancy_and_deaths

Thomas, P. L., & Winter, J. (2020). Strategic practices in achieving organizational effectiveness. In L. Roussel, P. L. Thomas & J. L. Harris (Eds.), *Management and leadership for nurse administrators* (8th ed.). Jones & Bartlett Learning.

Transcultural Nursing Society. (2022). Transcultural Nursing Society Mission. https://tcns.org/

U.S. Health and Human Services Office of Disease Prevention and Health Promotion. (2022). *Healthy People 2030: Building a healthier future for all.* https://health.gov/healthypeople

Weech-Maldonado, R., Dreachslin, J. L., Brown, J., Pradhan, R., Rubin, K. L., Schiller, C., & Hays, R. D. (2012). Cultural competency assessment tool for hospitals: Evaluating hospitals' adherence to the culturally and linguistically appropriate services standards. *Health Care Management Review, 37*(1), 54–66.

Weech-Maldonado, R., Drecahskin, J. L., Epane, J. P., Gail, J., Gupta, S., & Wainio, J. A. (2018). Hospital cultural competency as a systematic organizational intervention: Key findings from the national center for healthcare leadership diversity demonstration project. *Health Care Management Review, 43*(1), 30–41.

Weech-Maldonado, R., Elliott, M. N., Pradhan, R., Schiller, C., Dreachslin, J., & Hays, R. D. (2012a). Moving toward culturally competent health systems: Organizational and market factors. *Social Science & Medicine, 75*(5), 815–822.

Weech-Maldonado, R., Elliott, M., Pradhan, R., Schiller, C., Hall, A., & Hays, R. D. (2012b). Can hospital cultural competency reduce disparities in patient experiences with care? *Medical Care, 50*, S48–S55.

Weissman, J. S., Betancourt, J. R., Campbell, E. G., Park, E. R., Kim, M., Clarridge, B., & Maina, A. W. (2005). Resident physicians' preparedness to provide cross-cultural care. *Journal of the American Medical Association, 294*(9), 1058–1067.

Youdelman, M., & Perkins, J. (2005). *Providing language services in small health care provider settings: Examples from the field*. The Commonwealth Fund. http://www.commonwealthfund.org/usr_doc/810_Youdelman_providing_language_services.pdf

Transcultural Perspectives in Mental Health Nursing

• Linda Sue Hammonds

Chapter 19

Key Terms

Culture care
Cultural safety
Culturally sensitive
   communication

Mental health continuum
Mental health vulnerabilities
Displacement and forced
   immigration
Immigration continuum

Microaggressions
Stigma
Trauma-informed care

Learning Objectives

1. Describe mental health and mental illness as a continuum.
2. Apply concepts and theories related to transcultural nursing and culture care to mental health vulnerabilities of the COVID-19 pandemic.
3. Describe immigration as a continuum.
4. Apply concepts and theories related to transcultural nursing and culture care to mental health vulnerabilities of displacement and forced immigration.

Transcultural Nursing and Culture Care for Managing Mental Health Vulnerabilities

Mental health and mental illness can be described as a continuum from no mental health symptoms to severe mental health symptoms with varying states in between (Peter et al., 2021). Mental health is a priority for the World Health Organization (WHO). The WHO describes mental health as a state of well-being in which individuals cope with normal daily stressors, function productively, and contribute to the community. Mental disorders, such as depression and schizophrenia, are those recognized in the *International Statistical Classification of Diseases and Health Related Problems, Tenth revision* (ICD-10). Research has demonstrated that **mental health vulnerabilities**, situations beyond the individual's control, may impact the individual's state of mental health and mental illness as located on the continuum (World Health Organization, 2021).

Recent devastating vulnerabilities include the COVID-19 pandemic and trauma related to **displacement and forced immigration**. This chapter presents knowledge for developing skills to improve mental health on the continuum for individuals from diverse cultural backgrounds, and the evidence-based methods presented in this chapter are applicable for all cultural situations.

Mental Health Vulnerabilities: The COVID-19 Pandemic

A coronavirus, SARS-CoV-2, was detected in China in December 2019. The virulence of the SARS-CoV-2 virus caused COVID-19 to be declared a global pandemic by WHO in March 2020 (Habas et al., 2020). In the beginning, treatment was supportive and aimed at preventing and managing respiratory failure (Habas et al., 2020; Ochani et al., 2021). Although the illness could be mild, many patients developed severe hypoxia requiring hospitalization and mechanical ventilation. Global healthcare systems were overburdened and near collapse.

Transmitted by respiratory droplets, the pandemic was influenced by logistical problems related to mass testing, lack of effective contact tracing, noncompliance with universal masking, and low efficacy of existing antiviral agents (Ochani et al., 2021). Effective treatments and vaccinations have been developed, but COVID-19 pandemic–related trauma continues to have far-reaching impact on diverse cultures at the time of this writing. The trauma from the COVID-19 pandemic is a shared trauma, trauma that has been experienced not only by patients but also by their care providers. Accordingly, shared trauma impacts the collective mental health of the world (Ali et al., 2021). COVID-19 has impacted the mental health similarly among the public, COVID-19 patients, and providers (Hossain et al., 2020). Specifically, mental health and psychological well-being worsened during the pandemic, with the most impact among those with family financial distress (Ozlu-Erkilik et al., 2020).

Co-Occurring Pandemics

The COVID-19 pandemic's global impact on mental health has yielded extensive research and publications concerning healthcare providers, including nurses, and managing what is regarded as a mental health pandemic co-occurring with the COVID-19 pandemic (Hossain et al., 2020). **Culture care** concerns include a lack of understanding about the risk factors and transmissibility of the virus, cultural diversity, and the problems associated with promoting adherence to health recommendations (de Almeida et al., 2021). Figure 10-1 shows a person demonstrating understanding of the transmissibility of the virus while maintaining mental health.

Disparities

Culture care necessarily acknowledges the disparities associated with the COVID-19 pandemic. The Centers for Disease Control describes disparities as greater disease levels among certain populations over others. These are populations that are impacted by socioeconomic status, unequal access to care, lack of education, racism, and stigma (2020). Carethers (2021) discussed four disparities increasing risk with COVID-19: (1) age, (2) comorbidities, (3) race/ethnicity, and (4) gender.

Disparity increases with advancing age among the older adult population, evident in the accumulation of significant comorbid health

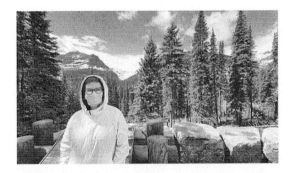

Figure 10-1. Maintaining mental health during the COVID-19 pandemic.

problems. Underlying socioeconomic factors in the United States contribute to the development of comorbidities among older adults (Carethers, 2021). Another factor is immunologic decline associated with aging (Chen et al., 2021). Older adults may have a delayed return to negative virological testing and prolonged shedding of the virus after symptoms have resolved, increasing the risk for transmission to others (Meyer et al., 2021). This is concerning when older adults live with a partner who is an older adult or live in institutional settings such as adult care facilities. Older adults are at risk for delirium with COVID-19, and delirium can be a presenting symptom (Zazzara et al., 2021). A meta-analysis found that vaccines are effective for preventing hospitalization, the need for intensive care, and death among older adults (Zheng et al., 2022). In the United States, the population aged 65 years and older has had the strongest response to efforts to vaccinate eligible individuals (USAFacts, 2022). However, advocacy is needed to counter hostile ageism, which may negatively impact societal management of COVID-19 in older adults (Apricino et al., 2021). In addition to older adults, children and adolescents are in a group with unique impacts from COVID-19 that are discussed in Box 10-1.

BOX 10-1   COVID-19 and Mental Health in Children and Adolescents

The COVID-19 pandemic carried risk for children and adolescents. A meta-analysis showed that approximately 51% of children and adolescents with COVID-19 experienced moderate disease. Among those under age 1 year, 14% were critically ill who had the virus (Cui et al., 2021). There were deaths among children and adolescents, though fewer than among adults (Ladhani et al., 2020). Children and adolescents contracting the disease were likely to be older, have a personal history of obesity, and have contact with someone who had COVID-19 (Murillo-Zamora et al., 2020). U.S. immunization rates of children and adolescents have been low. As of October 2022, only 31% of those aged 5 to 11 years have received two doses. The rate is higher among adolescents with 58% having received two doses (American Academy of Pediatrics, 2022). There were anxiety-producing reports of perimyocarditis among adolescents after immunization. However, the vaccines have been shown to be safe and effective in children and adolescents (Kildegaard et al., 2022). Long COVID is a concern for children and adolescents ranging from symptoms of COVID-19 continuing or resuming from 60 days after infection to over 6 months, to serious problems related to multisymptom inflammatory syndrome (Gupta et al., 2022).

The pandemic had a profound impact on lifestyle and mental health risk factors for children and adolescents. Experiences included an unbalanced diet increasing risk for excess weight and nutritional deficiencies, increases in sedentary behavior, disruptions in education, increased social isolation, and domestic violence (Scapaticci et al., 2022). Educational declines are beginning to be reported by organizations such as National Assessment of Educational Progress (NAEP) at the time of this writing. For example, U.S. fourth graders and eighth graders have had declines in scores for reading, mathematics, and confidence (NAEP, 2022). Mental health problems include symptoms on the **mental health continuum** ranging from worry and feelings of helplessness to suicidal thoughts. A meta-analysis of 16 studies that examined the impact of the pandemic reported depression, anxiety, post-traumatic symptoms, behavioral problems, and substance misuse (Meherali et al., 2021). Protecting factors for mental health include social support, positive social skills, parent–child discussions about the pandemic, and quarantining at home (instead of some other place) (Jones et al., 2021).

People with comorbidities including obesity, diabetes, cardiovascular disease, and chronic kidney disease also experience disparities as compared to individuals without these comorbid conditions (Carethers, 2021). In their meta-analysis, Gold et al., (2020) reported that over 40% of cases were among individuals with comorbidities, and among those who died, nearly 75% had comorbidities. The mortality rate was higher for those with two or more comorbidities (Djaharuddin et al., 2021). Of interest for mental health, anxiety disorders have been identified as comorbidities with greater COVID-19 risk (Kompaniyets et al., 2021).

In the United States, the Black American, Hispanic/Latino, and Native American/Native Alaskan populations carry increased risk from COVID-19 with higher rates of infection, hospitalization, and mortality (Carethers, 2021; Mackey et al., 2021). Contributing factors include a higher prevalence of underlying health problems, socioeconomic status, and racism spanning hundreds of years (Carethers, 2021; Hill et al., 2021; Kumar et al., 2021). To date, the Black American population was vaccinated at lower rates than the non-Hispanic White population (USAFacts, 2022). Likewise, the greatest vaccine hesitancy was in the Black American population (Willis et al., 2021). The Hispanic/Latino, Native Hawaiian/Pacific Islander, American Indian/Native Alaskan, and Asian populations have been vaccinated more than the non-Hispanic White population (USAFacts, 2022). The Asian and non-Hispanic White populations have had similar COVID-19 burdens (Mackey et al., 2021).

Stigma

The impact of the COVID-19 pandemic on global mental health raises the culture care concern of **stigma** as a barrier to seeking care. Stigma is frequently represented by microaggressions toward individuals with some level of mental health symptoms on the continuum. **Microaggressions** were first noted in reference to Black Americans and are defined as "brief and commonplace daily verbal, behavioural, or environmental indignities, whether intentional or unintentional, that communicate hostile, derogatory, or negative racial slights and insults to people of color" (Sue et al., 2007, p. 271). Microaggressions toward individuals with mental health problems have been more recently identified. Most microaggressions targeting individuals with mental health problems are from friends, family, and healthcare providers, people who might not be aware of the microaggressions that they inflict (Barber et al., 2019; Sue et al., 2007). Microaggressions can cause shame, a barrier to recovery (Yakely et al., 2019). "Shame is a sense of falling short of the standards and ideals of oneself or others, making the person feel small, inferior, or worthless" (Yakeley, 2018, p. s20). Guilt is a related, but different concept: "Guilt is the awareness of having done something bad, a feeling of responsibility or remorse for an offence, crime or wrong that the person has committed, whether real or imagined" (Yakeley, 2018, p. s20).

Cultural understandings of guilt and shame are important for providing culture care. In some cultures, the collective good is prioritized over the individual. Social order, moreover, may be maintained by shame and ostracism, a common practice in India, China, and Japan among others. In individualistic countries, such as the United States, Canada, and Australia, social order may be maintained by guilt and punishment. Stigma decreases when shame is mitigated as part of culture care for individuals with mental disorders and with understanding mental health and mental illness as a continuum (Peter et al., 2021; Yakeley, 2018).

Stigma has increased during the pandemic, including stigma directly related to COVID-19. Social distancing has had a significant role in containing the virus and preventing transmission. The result is stigma against and exclusion of others who are potential sources of COVID-19 creating disruption of normal socialization. In addition to stigma against those who are suspected of having the virus and individuals who have the virus, there has been stigma based on race, stigma toward healthcare professionals and other authorities, as well as stigma related to cause of death, related to religious beliefs, and against immigrants and refugees. These stigmas have impacted mental health (Bhanot et al., 2020). Culture care requires providers to address stigma.

Cultural Safety

Healthcare providers cannot be aware of all cultural beliefs related to mental health and stigma. These individual gaps in knowledge can be mitigated by providing care informed by the concept of **cultural safety**. As Curtis et al. (2019) explain:

> Cultural safety requires healthcare professionals and their associated healthcare organisations to examine themselves and the potential impact of their own culture on clinical interactions and healthcare service delivery. This requires individual healthcare professionals and healthcare organisations to acknowledge and address their own biases, attitudes, assumptions, stereotypes, prejudices, structures and characteristics that may affect the quality of care provided. In doing so, cultural safety encompasses a critical consciousness where healthcare professionals and healthcare organisations engage in ongoing self-reflection and self-awareness and hold themselves accountable for providing culturally safe care, as defined by the patient and their communities, and as measured by progress towards achieving health equity. Cultural safety requires healthcare professionals and their associated healthcare organisations to influence healthcare to reduce bias and achieve equity within the workforce and working environment. (p. 15)

Culturally Sensitive Communication

Providing culturally safe care is frequently inhibited by unsuccessful communication and failure to adapt to patient needs. These concerns of culture care require improving intercultural communication and intercultural interaction. **Culturally sensitive communication** is essential (Babitsch et al., 2020). Culturally sensitive communication includes language, symbols, signs, and behavior. Challenges to culturally sensitive communication are related to lack of familiarity with the communication of the other culture. Teach back methods, where the healthcare provider teaches and the patient teaches back, in combination with a qualified interpreter, are helpful for safety and culturally sensitive communication (Zeger & Auron, 2021). Qualified interpreters are trained to provide the services and use of untrained interpreters or minors should be avoided (U. S. Department of Health and Human Services, n.d.).

CASE STUDY 10-1

Aiyana is a Native American and young adult in their late 20s who resides in their own home, a double-wide trailer just off of the reservation. Aiyana has reported to the clinic on the reservation with shortness of breath, cough, and headache. Supplemental oxygen is in place, and testing shows that Aiyana is positive for SARS-CoV-2. Aiyana is admitted to the hospital on the reservation for supportive care and an Asian American nurse begins to help Aiyana settle into their room.

Which type of trauma has been experienced by Aiyana and the nurse that is shared and may impact culture care? (Choose the most appropriate answer.)

a. Racial trauma
b. Historical trauma
c. Shared trauma
d. Immigration trauma

Answer: C. Shared trauma is trauma that is shared by patients and their providers. An example is shared trauma from the COVID-19 pandemic. Racial trauma, the result of encounters with racial bias, may have been experienced by Aiyana and the nurse, but it is not shared trauma. Historical trauma, a trauma impacting multiple generations, might have been experienced by Aiyana and the nurse, but it is not shared trauma. Immigration trauma occurs on the immigration continuum. It has not been stated that Aiyana or the nurse have immigrated.

The nurse has graduated from their nursing program within the past 6 months and recently started working on the reservation. The culture on the reservation is new to the nurse.

What did the nurse learn in their nursing program that will most guide the nurse in the provision of culture care? (Choose the most appropriate answer.)

a. Cultural safety can mitigate gaps in cultural understanding.
b. Cultural understanding can facilitate competent provision of culture care.
c. Native Americans prefer nontraditional methods.
d. Native Americans prefer family involvement.

Answer: A. Cultural safety is an environment where patients feel safe and respected regarding their cultural concerns. Cultural safety is practiced even when the nurse is not familiar with the culture of the patient and it can mitigate gaps in cultural understanding. Cultural understanding can facilitate competent provision of culture care, but it is impossible for the nurse to know everything about the culture. Native Americans may prefer nontraditional methods and may prefer family involvement, but this knowledge does not mitigate what the nurse does not understand about the culture.

On the second day, the nurse notices that Aiyana seems sad. Aiyana hasn't smiled, and they don't seem interested in going home even though their status is improved and they are scheduled for discharge in the afternoon. The nurse wants to assess for depression.

What does the nurse consider regarding barriers to care while providing culture care in the COVID-19 pandemic? (Choose the most appropriate answer.)

a. Aiyana needs to be around nature for mental health.
b. Aiyana may be impacted by stigma from mental health problems and stigma from COVID-19.
c. Aiyana may be impacted by stigma from mental health problems and stigma from their racial/ethnic identification.
d. Aiyana may have mistrust for healthcare providers.

Answer: B. Stigma is a barrier to care. Culture care requires management of stigma. During the COVID-19 pandemic, stigma increased and included COVID-19-related stigma. Many Native Americans are culturally tied to nature and the earth. It may enhance mental health to be around nature, but this is not a barrier to care. Aiyana may experience stigma from their racial/ethnic identification, but not significantly within their racial/ethnic community. Aiyana may experience stigma from mental health problems and from COVID-19 within their own cultural community. Mistrust for healthcare providers is a barrier to care, but it is not unique to the COVID-19 pandemic.

Mental Health Vulnerabilities: Displacement and Forced Immigration

The COVID-19 pandemic expanded the vulnerabilities of the immigrant population, which is already burdened with mental health impacts related to immigration. With or without COVID-19, government policies create stressors for immigrants that affect mental health. The strategies used to cope with the stressors might worsen mental health, or they might mitigate mental health outcomes through resilience (Payan, 2022). This section presents problems associated with mental health outcomes of displacement and forced immigration, alone and in association with the COVID-19 pandemic, and culture care concerns for transcultural nursing.

Immigration and Stigma

Immigrants living in the United States include naturalized citizens, lawful permanent residents, refugees, asylees, and unauthorized immigrants

(U.S. Department of Homeland Security, 2022). Research demonstrates that governmental policies concerning immigration are social determinants of mental health and anti-immigration policies significantly and negatively impact immigrants. This impact extends beyond unauthorized immigrants to other immigrant statuses and even communities of color (Kiehne & Baca-Atlas, 2020). In the United States, news coverage of anti-immigration policies is associated with stigma. Reporting has focused on anti-immigration policies, despite integration policies enacted in 2017 to 2019. Immigration news from 2010 to 2013 emphasized the deficit of available resources and the economic drain associated with immigrants. From years 2017 to 2019, negative messages characterized immigrants as criminal, though there were some positive messages about how immigrants provide economic support to their families in the country of origin (Young et al., 2022). Culture care is helpful for immigrants of various statuses who are in an environment that affects their mental health negatively.

Reasons for Immigration and Stressors

Given the stressors associated with immigration, culture care must explore and understand the reasons for immigration. While immigration might occur for seemingly positive reasons, such as professional opportunities (Gea-Caballero et al., 2019; Kabbash et al., 2021), displacement and forced immigration occur from extreme stressors such as sociopolitical threats (Bhugra et al., 2021), war (UNICAN Immigration Office, 2022), civil unrest and violence (Jampaklay et al., 2020), and climate-related hazards (Oakes, 2019). Many immigrants needing culture care have left extremely distressing situations before facing the

stressors of immigration. Immigration may be conceptualized as a continuum including the time before immigration, the immigration journey, and the time after immigration with complex layers of trauma (Grafft et al., 2022). Immigrants might experience trauma at any time in or throughout the continuum (see Fig. 10-2). This trauma is often the result of physical and sexual violence (Fortuna et al., 2019; Jolie et al., 2021). After arrival in the new country, immigrants may experience structural violence in anti-immigration policies along with the threatening verbal assaults of politicians. Immigrants also face discrimination and often experience poverty due to low-income employment in the new country (Barajas-Gonzales, 2021; Cariello et al., 2020). Fear is pervasive throughout the **immigration continuum** (Jolie et al., 2021). Immigrants must cope with other threats such as immigration detention (von Werthern et al., 2018), family separation (Barajas-Gonzales et al., 2022), and acculturation stress in the new country (Cariello et al., 2020). In addition to the trauma associated with immigration, trauma related to historical discrimination, prejudice, mistreatment, and genocide can impact mental health (Guenzel & Struwe, 2020).

Trauma and Mental Health

The result of trauma experienced through the immigration continuum is the prevalence of increasing severity of symptoms on the continuum for mental health and mental illness. The most commonly reported symptoms are related to thinking too much, crying easily, and somatic concerns (Baird et al., 2020). Some cultures, such as Hispanic/Latinx/Latino, express mental distress more frequently in somatic symptoms (Bucay-Harari et al., 2020). Mental health disorders

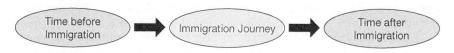

Figure 10-2. The immigration continuum.

commonly include mood disorders, anxiety disorders, and trauma-related disorders (Gearing et al., 2021; Lee et al., 2020; von Werthern et al., 2018). Acute mental health crises are common and have been found to be increased among those who spent time in refugee camps (van de Weil et al., 2021). The trauma and negatively impacted mental health were greatly increased from the COVID-19 pandemic. Many of those in immigration detention were kept in isolation as authorities sought to control the spread of the virus (Bingham & Pickles, 2021). It was reported that among Hispanic/Latinx/Latino immigrants knowing an undocumented immigrant, or knowing someone with COVID-19, increased severe mental health outcomes by 52% (Gomez-Aguinaga et al., 2021). Children and adolescents are impacted by the same stressors related to immigration and mental health as adults during developmental years. Box 10-2 discusses the experiences of displacement and forced immigration among children and adolescents.

BOX 10-2   **Children and Adolescents Experiencing Displacement and Forced Immigration**

Among those experiencing displacement and forced immigration, children and adolescents are particularly vulnerable to impacts of the complex layers of trauma that have been described elsewhere in this chapter. Due to their developmental life stages, there are unique risks and problems related to mental health, development, and education. Many are at a developmental stage where they do not understand their own immigration or detention in an immigration camp or facility (Kronick et al., 2018). Children and adolescents frequently must cope with the knowledge of deceased or missing relatives, forced separation from parents (Oldroyd et al., 2022), or knowledge that their parents are missing or deceased (Barajas-Gonzales et al., 2022). Those traveling as unaccompanied minors are at greater risk for victimization and child labor (Meyer et al., 2020). There are higher rates of posttraumatic stress disorder (PTSD), suicide attempts, and completed suicides among unaccompanied minors compared to accompanied minors (Daniel-Calveras et al., 2022). Over 50% of children and adolescents experience victimization and bullying as a result of being a refugee (Yilmaz et al., 2020).

Scharpf et al. reported that the risk factors for the mental health of children experiencing displacement and forced immigration include exposure to trauma, mental health problems of parents, impaired parenting, female gender, discrimination, acculturation stress (2021). They reported the following protective factors: family cohesion, support by peers, school connectedness, and experiences with integrative acculturation (as opposed to discriminatory acculturation) (Scharpf et al., 2021). In addition to other mental health problems, children and adolescents are at risk for pervasive refusal syndrome with symptoms that do not match convincingly with a *Diagnostic and Statistical Manual of Mental Disorders*, 5th edition diagnosis (Otasowie, et al., 2020). Symptoms include refusal to eat, move, walk, talk, or engage in personal care activities such as bathing. Social withdrawal and refusal to go to school are common. Encouraging the child to do these things leads to physical resistance and anger (Jaspers et al., 2009).

These children and adolescents experience disruptions in their developmental progress. They have increased disruptive behaviors compared to nonimmigrant children and adolescents (Kim et al., 2018). Conduct problems are increased (Duinhof et al., 2020). Adolescents may engage in sexual behaviors that increase their risk of pregnancy or sexually transmitted infections due to inaccurate sexual knowledge or as a conduct problem (Kronick et al., 2018). Adolescents might develop a negative view of their futures at a time when they are beginning to consider adulthood (Subasi et al., 2021). Closely linked to the disruptions in developmental

(continued)

BOX 10-2	Children and Adolescents Experiencing Displacement and Forced Immigration (continued)

progress are the disruptions in educational progress. Nearly half of child and adolescent refugees were not attending school (USA for UNHCR The UN Refugee Agency, 2022). Frequently, there is poor school performance after resettlement (Berg et al., 2022).

The COVID-19 pandemic was especially risky for children and adolescents experiencing displacement and forced migration. The availability and follow-through for immunization was negatively impacted. For example, in Germany, a study of refugee camps showed that among the camps 27.8% to 75% of children under age 5 years was fully vaccinated, once the vaccine became available to them. Also, among those younger than 18 years, up to 93% were partially vaccinated, and at least 5% had received no doses of an effective vaccination for COVID-19 (Fozouni et al., 2019).

Barriers to care for immigrants negatively impact the course and management of mental health problems, and there are many barriers. Immigrants might not seek mental healthcare due to unfamiliarity and mistrust of healthcare providers and the healthcare system, negative previous experiences with mental healthcare, mental health illiteracy, previous experiences with culturally inappropriate care, privacy and confidentiality concerns, unaffordability of care, fear of deportation (Place et al., 2021), lack of proficiency in the language of the host country, and lack of connection to the community (Wylie et al., 2020). Other barriers are due to the healthcare system and other structures. Care might not be available in an accessible location, or it might be available only to a particular group of patients such as children and adolescents (Place et al., 2021). A lack of preparation for immigrants and refugees is a barrier. This is demonstrated by a lack of interpreters, a lack of mental health providers with training specific to immigrants and refugees, providers feeling helpless or becoming over-involved (Duden & Martins-Bogen, 2021), a lack of coordination among healthcare providers, and culturally inappropriate policies and procedures (Wylie et al., 2020).

An Evidence-based Transcultural Approach to Care of Immigrants

A transcultural approach to care of people with a history of trauma, along with trauma-informed care, has been shown to improve screening, assessment, and quality of care (Wylie et al., 2020). Im et al. (2021) recommended a Multitier Mental Health and Psychosocial Support (MMHPS) model for the management of displaced patients who have experienced forced immigration. The model includes both culture-informed care and trauma-informed care in four tiers. **Trauma-informed care** is grounded in four principles: (1) understanding that trauma is widespread and has far reaching consequences, (2) recognition of the signs and symptoms of trauma, (3) integration of that understanding and recognition into care, and (4) using care to avoid retraumatization (Agency for Healthcare Research and Quality, 2022). The first tier includes basic services such as food, shelter, protection, and advocacy that are needed by this population. The second tier is focused on the development and strengthening of supports in the family and community. The third tier involves nonspecialized mental health services directly related to the trauma and provided by mental health professionals or para-professionals. The fourth tier involves specialized psychological and psychiatric treatments focused on severe mental illness and severe problems with daily functioning (Im et al., 2021). Supportive mental healthcare is promoted by the inclusion of the patients in society, competency of the mental healthcare system, cultural humility by providers, and development of a trusting therapeutic relationship between providers and patients (Duden & Martins-Bogen, 2021). Provider management of the needs of displaced patients who have experienced forced immigration is facilitated by knowledge of those needs, development of the skills to address them, and appropriate cultural attitudes for care (Baarnhielm & Schouler-Ocak, 2022). The patient benefits from a cultural desire among mental health providers for the recovery of the patient through nurses, other healthcare providers, an environment of culture care, and the patient's own methods for recovery (Kallakorpi et al., 2019).

CASE STUDY 10-2

Adoncia is a 36-year-old undocumented immigrant from Mexico living in the United States. She has come to the clinic with symptoms of anxiety and depression. Adoncia speaks little English, and she is accompanied by a friend, also an unauthorized immigrant, who speaks English and Spanish and is willing to translate during the encounter.

Who is the most appropriate translator for the encounter to promote cultural safety?

a. Adoncia's friend for her comfort
b. The receptionist at the clinic who speaks Spanish
c. A professional interpreter trained for healthcare
d. An online interpreting service

Answer: C. For cultural safety, a professional interpreter trained for healthcare provides competent and accurate translation services. Adoncia's friend may provide comfort, but safety may be compromised by information omitted or changed due to cultural expectations or misunderstandings of the healthcare information. The receptionist at the clinic speaks Spanish, but may not be trained for interpretation in healthcare. An online interpreting service may be used if a professional interpreter trained for healthcare is not available, but a professional interpreter is preferable due to nuances in communication.

Adoncia quickly becomes tearful during the encounter while explaining that she is fearful for her brother, who told her he was en route to the United States after paying someone to help him cross the border. Another unauthorized immigrant, who had crossed with her brother, has told her that her brother had gone missing in the Chihuahuan Desert not long after crossing. It is summer with temperatures reaching 115°F in the desert. After her first crossing, Adoncia spent 6 months in immigration detention before being deported to Mexico. She kept trying because she is fleeing terrorism from the drug cartel and seeking a better life.

Which evidence-based model, along with culture care, is most appropriate to help Adoncia?

a. Trauma-informed care
b. Shared decision-making
c. Motivational interviewing
d. Solution-focused therapy

Answer: A. Trauma-informed care involves understanding of the consequences of trauma, recognizes the impact of trauma, integrates understanding into care, and avoids retraumatization. It is the most appropriate for the trauma described over the immigration continuum. Shared decision-making increases the likelihood of a patient collaborating in care. It might be helpful, but it does not address the trauma described in the information. Motivational interviewing is used to assist patients to make healthy changes to reach their own goals. Solution-focused therapy assists patients to solve their own problems by focusing on desired personal objectives.

Adoncia is living in a situation where food, shelter, protection, and advocacy are provided while she seeks legal refugee status in the United States. She is in a community where she has friends, such as the friend who came to the appointment, and Adoncia is in contact with family remaining in Mexico. Volunteers who are trained to provide emotional support to immigrants are available there. After a complete psychiatric evaluation, Adoncia has a DSM-V diagnosis of PTSD. Adoncia is prescribed psychoactive medication, and an appointment is made with a therapist in the clinic.

Using MMHPS, which tiers of care have been provided for Adoncia?

a. Tier 1 and Tier 4
b. All tiers
c. No tiers
d. Tier 2 and Tier 4

Answer: B. All tiers have been provided to Adoncia. The description includes basic support (food, shelter, protection, advocacy), strengthening of support from family and community, mental health support related to immigration, and specialized mental health support provided by professionals. The other answers do not include all of the tiers of support that have been provided for Adoncia.

Summary

This chapter began by describing mental health and mental illness on a continuum. Vulnerabilities were described as having impact on the mental health of individuals on the continuum. Transcultural nursing and culture care were discussed in terms of two vulnerabilities impacting mental health: (1) the COVID-19 pandemic and (2) displacement and forced immigration. Evidence-based methods were included for maintaining and improving mental health: (1) culture care theory, (2) other culture theories, (3) acknowledgment of disparities, (4) acknowledgment of stigma, (5) cultural safety, (6) culturally sensitive communication, and (7) trauma-informed care. Readers practiced these evidence-based methods in a case representation involving COVID-19 and case representation involving forced displacement and immigration.

REVIEW QUESTIONS

1. Describe mental health and mental illness on a continuum.
2. Define "mental health vulnerability."
3. Discuss shared trauma as a feature of the COVID-19 pandemic.
4. List four disparities of the COVID-19 pandemic.
5. Discuss stigma as a barrier to care.
6. Explain how culturally sensitive communication promotes cultural safety.
7. List U.S. immigration statuses.
8. Describe the immigration continuum.
9. Discuss acculturation stress.
10. Describe trauma-informed care.

CRITICAL THINKING ACTIVITIES

1. Create a group to discuss mental health vulnerabilities and culture care. Over the past few years, a large number of articles have been published about mental health and the COVID-19 pandemic. Look up and discuss several of these articles at group meetings. What are the mental health vulnerabilities of the COVID-19 pandemic? What is the impact on mental health related to the COVID-19 pandemic? How was mental health maintained during the COVID-19 pandemic? What did you learn about the impact of transcultural nursing and culture care on mental health during the COVID-19 pandemic?

2. The COVID-19 pandemic is a global event that has impacted every place and every person in some way. Talk to nearly anyone about the COVID-19 pandemic. Ask about mental health vulnerabilities that person may have experienced or observed in the COVID-19 pandemic. Ask about the impact of the COVID-19 pandemic on their emotional and mental health, and the impact on others around them. Ask how they maintained their mental health during the COVID-19 pandemic. Ask about cultural concerns that they may have had during the COVID-19 pandemic.

3. Create a group to discuss mental health vulnerabilities and culture care. Over the past few years, a large number of articles have been published about mental health, displacement, and forced immigration. Discuss several of these articles at group meetings. What are the mental health vulnerabilities of displacement and forced immigration? What is the impact on mental health related to displacement and forced immigration? How is mental health maintained during displacement and forced immigration? What did you learn about the impact of transcultural nursing and culture care on mental health during displacement and forced immigration?

4. Alone, or with the group created to discuss mental health vulnerabilities and culture care, visit with someone who has immigrated to your area. This may be someone who immigrated voluntarily, or someone who experienced displacement and forced immigration. Ask about mental health vulnerabilities that they may have experienced or observed related to their immigration experience. Ask about the impact of immigration on their emotional and mental health, and the impact on others around them. Ask how they maintained their mental health during and after immigration. Ask about cultural concerns that they experienced during and after immigration.

5. Create a group to discuss mental health vulnerabilities and culture care. Explore journal articles to discover mental health vulnerabilities, other than the COVID-19 pandemic and other than displacement and forced immigration. An example is the vulnerabilities related to the experience of natural disasters. What mental health vulnerabilities were discovered? What is the impact of these vulnerabilities on mental health? How was mental health maintained during the vulnerabilities that were discovered? What did you learn about the impact of transcultural nursing and culture care on mental health related to the vulnerabilities that were discovered?

6. Create a group to discuss mental health vulnerabilities and culture care. It is impossible to understand every cultural concern in every situation. Explore journal articles to discover evidence-based information to assist you in providing culture care in situations where you may know little or nothing about the culture. An example from this chapter is cultural safety. What other evidence-based information was discovered as you explored the journals? Role play examples of implementing the evidence-based information to provide culture care.

REFERENCES

Agency for Healthcare Research and Quality. (2022). *Trauma-informed care.*

Ali, D. A., Figley, C. R., Tedeschi, R. G., Galarneu, D., & Amara, S. (2021). Shared trauma, resilience, and growth: A roadmap toward transcultural conceptualization. *Psychological Trauma: Theory, Research, Practice, and Policy, 15*(1), 45–55. Advance Online Publication. https://doi.org/10.1037/tra0001044.

American Academy of Pediatrics. (2022). *Summary of data publicly reported by the Centers for Disease Control and Prevention.* Children and COVID-19 Vaccination Trends (aap.org).

Apricino, M., Lytle, A., Monahan, C., Macdonald, J., & Levy, S. R. (2021). Prioritizing health care and employment resources during COVID-19: Roles of benevolent and hostile ageism. *The Gerontologist, 61,* 98–102. https://doi.org/10.1093/geront/gnaa165.

Baarnhielm, S., & Schouler-Ocak, M. (2022). Training in cultural psychiatry: Translating research into improvements in mental health care for migrants. *Transcultural Psychiatry, 59,* 111–115. https://doi.org/10.1177/13634615221089384.

Babitsch, B., Bretz, L., Mansholt, H., & Gotz, N.-A. (2020). The relevance of cultural diversity on safety culture: A CIRS data analysis to identify problem areas and competency requirements of professionals in healthcare institutions. *GMS Journal for Medical Education, 37,* Doc14. https://doi.org/10.3205/zma001307.

Bai, F., Tomasoni, D., Falcinella, C., Barbanotti, D., Castoldi, R., Mule, G., Augello, M., Mondatore, D., Allegrini, M., Cona, A., Tesoro, D., Tagliaferri, G., Vigano, O., Suardi, E., Tincati, C., Beringheli, T., Varisco, B., Battistini, C. L., Piscopo, K., ... Monforte, A. d'. A. (2022). Female gender is associated with long COVID syndrome: A prospective cohort study. *Clinical Microbiology and Infection, 28,* 611. https://doi.org/10.1016/j.cmi.2021.

Baird, M. B., Cates, R., Bott, M. J., & Buller, C. (2020). Assessing the mental health of refugees using the Refugee Health Screener-15. *Western Journal of Nursing Research*, *42*, 910–917. https://doi.org/10.1177/0193945920906210.

Barajas-Gonzales, R. G. (2021). *Early care and education workforce stress and needs in a restrictive anti-immigration climate*. Research Report in Urban Institute.

Barajas-Gonzales, R. G., Ursache, A., Kamboukos, D., Huang, K.-Y., Dawson-McClure, S., Urcuyo, A., Huang, T. J. J., & Brotman, L. M. (2022). Parental perceived immigration threat and children's mental health, self-regulation, and executive functioning in pre-kindergarten. *American Journal of Orthopsychiatry*, *92*, 176–189. https://doi.org/10.1037/ort0000591.

Barber, S., Gronholm, P. C., Ahuja, S., Rusch, N., & Thornicroft, G. (2019). Microaggressions towards people affected by mental health problems: A scoping review. *Epidemiology and Psychiatric Sciences*, *16*, 29. https://doi.org/10.1017/S2045796019000763.

Berg, L., Brendler-Lindquist, M., de Montgomery, E., Mittendorfer-Rutz, A., & Hjern, A. (2022). Parental post-traumatic stress and school performance in children. *Journal of Traumatic Stress*, *35*, 138–147. https://doi.org/10.1002/jts.22708.

Bhanot, D., Singh, T., Verma, S. K., & Sharad, S. (2020). Stigma and discrimination during the COVID-19 pandemic. *Frontiers in Public Health*, *8*, 577018. https://doi.org/10.3389/fpubh.2020.577018.

Bhugra, D., Watson, C., & Ventriglio, A. (2021). Migration, cultural capital, and acculturation. *International Review of Psychiatry*, *33*, 126–131. https://doi.org/10.1080/09540261.2020.1733786.

Bienvenu, L. A., Noonan, J., Wang, X., & Peter, K. (2020). Higher mortality of COVID-19 in males: Sex differences in immune response and cardiovascular comorbidities. *Cardiovascular Research*, *116*, 2197–2206. https://doi.org/10.1093/cvr/cvaa284.

Bingham, R., & Pickles, H. (2021). Prolonged solitary confinement of UK immigration detainees during the pandemic. *BMJ*, *16*, 374. https://doi.org/10.1136/bmj.n2016.

Botelho, M. J., & Lima, C. A. (2020). From cultural competence to cultural respect: A critical review of six models. *Journal of Nursing Education*, *59*, 311–318. https://doi.org/10.3928/01484834-20200520-03.

Bucay-Harari, L., Page, K. R., Krawczyk, N., Robles, Y. P., & Castillo-Salgado, C. (2020). Mental health needs of an emerging Latino community. *Journal of Behavioral Health Services and Research*, *47*, 388–398. https://doi.org/10.1007/s11414-020-09688-3.

Carethers, J. M. (2021). Insights into disparities with COVID-19. *Journal of Internal Medicine*, *289*, 463–473. https://doi.org/10.1111/joim.13199.

Cariello, A. N., Perrin, P. B., Williams, C. D., Espinoza, G. A., Morlett-Paredes, A., Moreno, O. A., & Trujillo, M. A. (2020). Moderating influence of enculturation on the relations between minority stressors and physical health via anxiety in Latinx immigrants. *Cultural Diversity and Ethnic Minority Psychology*, *26*, 356–366. https://doi.org/10.1037/t05154-000.

Centers for Disease Control. (2020). *Defining health disparities*.

Chen, Y., Klein, S. B., Garibaldi, B. T., Li, H., Wu, C., Osevala, N. M., Li, T., Margolick, J. B., Pawelec, G., & Leng, S. X. (2021). Aging in COVID-19: Vulnerability, immunity, and intervention. *Ageing Research Reviews*, *65*, 101204. https://doi.org/10.1016/j.arr.2020.101205.

Cui, X., Zhao, Z., Zhange, T., Guo, W., Guo, W., Zheng, J., Zhang, J., Dong, C., Na, R., Zheng, L., Li, W., Liu, Z., Ma, J., Wang, J., He, S., Xu, Y., Si, P., Shen, Y., & Cai, C. (2021). A systematic review and meta-analysis of children with coronavirus disease 2019 (COVID-19). *Journal of Medical Virology*, *93*, 1057–1069. https://doi.org/10.1002/jmv.26398.

Curtis, E., Jones, R., Tipene-Leach, D., Walker, C., Loring, B., Paine, S.-J., & Reid, P. (2019). Why cultural safety rather than cultural competency is needed to achieve health equity: A literature review and recommended definition. *International Journal for Equity in Health*, *18*, 174. https://doi.org/10.1186/s12939-019-1082-3.

Daniel-Calveras, A., Baldaqui, N., & Baeza, I. (2022). Mental health of unaccompanied refugee minors in Europe: A systematic review. *Child Abuse and Neglect*, *133*, 105865. https://doi.org/10.1016/j.chiabu.2022.105865.

de Almeida, G. M. F., Nascimento, T. F., da Silva, R. P. L., Bello, M. P., & Fontes, C. M. B. (2021). Theoretical reflections of Leininger's cross-cultural care in the context of Covid-19. *Revista Gauche de Enfermagem*, *42*. https://doi.org/10.1590/1983-1447.2021.20200209.

Djaharuddin, I., Munawwarah, S., Nurulita, A., Llyas, M., Tabri, M. U., & Lihawa, N. (2021). Comorbidities and mortality in COVID-19 patients. *Gacita Sanitaria*, *35*(Suppl), S530–S532. https://doi.org/10.1016/j.gaceta.2021.10.085.

Duden, G. S., & Martins-Bogen, L. (2021). Psychotherapy with refugees-supportive and hindering elements. *Psychotherapy Research*, *21*, 386–401. https://doi.org/10.1080/10503307.2020.1820596.

Duinhof, H. L., Smid, S. C., Vollenbergh, W. A. M., & Stevens, G. W. J. M. (2020). Immigration background and adolescent mental health problems: The role of family affluence, adolescent education level and gender. *Social Psychiatry and Psychiatric Epidemiology*, *55*, 435–445. https://doi.org/10.1007/s00127-019-01821-8.

Fortuna, L. R., Norona, C. R., Porche, M. V., Tillman, C., Patil, P. A., Wang, Y., Markle, S. L., & Alegria, M. (2019). Trauma, immigration and sexual health among Latina women: Implications for maternal-child well-being and reproductive justice. *Infant Mental Health Journal*, *40*, 640–658. https://doi.org/10.1002/imhj.21805.

Fozouni, L., Weber, C., Lindner, A. K., & Rutherford, G. W. (2019). Immunization coverage among refugee children in Berlin. *Journal of Global Health*, *9*, 010432. https://doi.org/10.7189/jogh.09.010432.

Gea-Caballero, V., Castro-Sanchez, E., Diaz-Herrera, M. A., Sarabia-Cobo, C., Juarez-Vela, R., & Zabaleta-Del Olmo, E. (2019). Motivations, beliefs, and expectations of Spanish nurses planning migration for economic reasons: A cross-sectional, web-based survey. *Journal of Nursing Scholarship*, *51*, 178–186. https://doi.org/10.1111/jnu.12455.

Gearing, R. E., Washburn, M., Torres, L. R., Carr, L. C., Cabrera, A., & Olivares, R. (2021). Immigration policy changes and mental health of Mexican-American immigrants. *Journal of Racial and Ethnic Health Disparities*, *8*, 579–588. https://doi.org/10.1007/s40615-020-00816-5.

Glittenberg, J. (2004). A transdisciplinary transcultural model for healthcare. *Journal of Transcultural Nursing*, *15*, 6–10. https://doi.org/10.1177/1043659603260037.

Gold, M. S., Sehayek, D., Gabrielli, S., Zhang, X., McCusker, C., & Ben-Shoshan, M. (2020). COVID-19 and comorbidities: A systematic review and meta-analysis. *Postgraduate Medicine*, *132*, 749–755. https://doi.org/10.1080/0032548 1.2020.1786964.

Gomez-Aguinaga, B., Dominquez, M. S., & Manzano, S. (2021). Immigration and gender as social determinants of mental health during the COVID-19 outbreak: The case of US Latina/os. *International Journal of Environmental Research and Public Health*, *18*, 6065. https://doi. org/10.3390/ijerph18116065.

Grafft, N., Rodriguez, K., Costas-Rodriquez, B., & Pineros-Leano, M. (2022). Latinx immigrants and complex layers of trauma: Providers' perspectives. *Journal of Latinx Psychology*, *10*, 291–303. https://doi.org/10.1037/lat0000210.

Guenzel, N., & Struwe, L. (2020). Historical trauma, ethnic experience, and mental health in a sample of urban American Indians. *Journal of the American Psychiatric Nurses Association*, *26*, 145–156. https://doi. org/10.1177/1078390319888266.

Gupta, M., Gupta, N., & Esang, M. (2022). Long COVID in children and adolescents. *The Primary Care Companion for CNS Disorders*, *24*, 21r03218. https://doi.org/10.4088/ PCC.21r03218.

Habas, K., Nganwuchu, C., Shahzad, F., Gopalan, R., Haque, M., Rahman, S., Majumder, A. A., & Nasim, T. (2020). Resolution of coronavirus disease 2019 (COVID-19). *Expert Review of Anti-Infective Therapy*, *18*, 1201–1211. https://doi.org/10.1080/14787210.202 0.1797487.

Hill, M., Houghton, F., & Hoss, M. A. K. (2021). The inequitable impact of COVID-19 among American Indian/ Alaskan Native (AI/AN) communities is the direct result of centuries of persecution and racism. *Journal of the Royal Society of Medicine*, *114*, 549–551. https://doi. org/10.1177/01410768211051710.

Hossain, M. M., Tasnim, S., Sultana, A., Faizah, F., Mazumder, H., Zou, L., McKyer, E. L. J., Ahmed, H. U., & Ma, P. (2020). Epidemiology of mental health problems in COVID-19: A review. *F1000 Research*, *9*, 636. https://doi.org/10.12688/ f1000research.24457.1.

Im, H., Rodriguez, C., & Grumbine, J. M. (2021). A multitier model of refugee mental health and psychosocial support in resettlement: Toward trauma-informed and culture-informed systems of care. *Psychological Services*, *18*, 345–364. https://doi.org/10.1037/ser0000412.

Jampaklay, A., Ford, K., & Chamratrithirong, A. (2020). Migration and unrest in the deep south Thailand: A multilevel analysis of a longitudinal study. *Demography*, *57*, 727–745. https://doi.org/10.1007/s13524-020-00856-w.

Jaspers T., Hanssen G. M., van der Valk J. A., Hanekom J. H., van Well G. T., Schieveld J. N. H. G. (2009). Pervasive refusal syndrome as part of the refusal–withdrawal–regression spectrum: Critical review of the literature illustrated by a case report. *European Child & Adolescent Psychiatry*, *18*, 645–651. https://doi.org/10.1007/s00787-009-0027-6.

Jolie, S. A., Onyeka, O. C., Torres, S., DiClemente, C., Richards, M., & Santiago, C. D. (2021). Violence, place, and strengthened space: A review of immigration stress, violence exposure, and intervention for Latinx youth and families. *Annual Review of Clinical Psychology*, *7*, 127–151. https://doi.org/10.1146/annurev-clinpsy-081219-100217.

Jones, E. A. K., Mitra, A. K., & Bhuiyan, A. R. (2021). Impact of COVID-19 on mental health in adolescents: A systematic review. *International Journal of Environmental Research and Public Health*, *18*, 2470. https://doi.org/10.3390/ ijerph18052470.

Kabbash, I., El-Sallamy, R., Zayed, H., Alkhyate, I., Omar, A., & Abdo, S. (2021). The brain drain: Why medical students and young physicians want to leave Egypt. *Eastern Mediterranean Health Journal*, *27*, 1102–1108. https:// doi.org/10.26719/emhj.21.050.

Kallakorpi, S., Haatainen, K., & Kankkunen, P. (2019). Psychiatric nursing care experiences of immigrant patients: A focused ethnographic study. *International Journal of Mental Health Nursing*, *28*, 117–127. https:// doi.org/10.1111/inm.12500.

Kiehne, E., & Baca-Atlas, S. N. (2020). Immigration policy as a social determinant of health: Development and initial validation of a measure to assess attitudes toward immigrant integration. *Social Work in Public Health*, *35*, 293–307. https://doi.org/10.1080/19371918.2020.1781014.

Kildegaard, H., Lund, L. C., Hojlund, M., Stensballe, L. G., & Pottegard, A. (2022). Risk of adverse events after COVID-19 in Danish children and adolescents and effectiveness of BNT162b2 in adolescents: Cohort study. *BMJ*, *11*, e068898. https://doi.org/10.1136/bmj-2021-068898.

Kim, J., Nicodimos, S., Kushner, S. E., Rhew, I. C., McCauley, E., & Stoep, A. V. (2018). Comparing mental health of US children of immigrants and non-immigrants in 4 racial/ethnic groups. *Journal of School Health*, *88*, 167–175. https://doi. org/10.1111/josh.12586.

Kompaniyets, L., Pennington, A. F., Goodman, A. B., Rosenblum, H. G., Belay, B., Ko, J. Y., Chevinsky, J. R., Scheiber, L. Z., Summers, A. D., Lavery, A. M., Preston, L. E., Danielson, M. L., Cui, Z., Namulanda, G., Yusuf, H.,

Kenzie, W. R. M., Wong, K. K., Baggs, J., Boehmer, T. K., & Gundlapalli, A. V. (2021). Underlying medical conditions and severe illness among 540,667 adults hospitalized with COVID-19, March 2020-March 2021. *Preventing Chronic Disease, 18*, E66. https://doi.org/10.5888/pcd18.210123.

Kronick, R., Rousseau, C., & Cleveland, J. (2018). Refugee children's sand play narratives in immigration detention in Canada. *European Child and Adolescent Psychiatry, 27*, 423–437. https://doi.org/10.1007/s00787-017-1012-0.

Kumar, S., Kumar, P., Kodidela, S., Duhart, B., Cernsev, A., Nookala, A., Kumar, A., Singh, U. P., & Bissler, J. (2021). Racial health disparity and COVID-19. *Journal of Neuroimmune Pharmacology, 16*, 729–742. https://doi.org/10.1007/s11481-021-10014-7.

Ladhani, S. N., Amin-Chowdhury, Z., Davies, H. G., Aiano, F., Hayden, I., Lacy, J., Sinnathamby, M., de Lusignan, S., Demirjian, A., Whittaker, H., Andrews, N., Zambon, M., Hopkins, S., & Ramsay, M. E. (2020). COVID-19 in children: Analysis of the first pandemic peak in England. *Archives of Disease in Childhood, 105*, 1180–1185. https://doi.org/10.1136/archdischild-2020-320042.

Lee, M., Bhimla, A., & Ma, G. X. (2020). Depressive symptom severity and immigration-related characteristics in Asian American immigrants. *Journal of Immigration and Minority Health, 22*, 935–945. https://doi.org/10.1007/s10903-020-01004-7.

Mackey, K., Ayers, C. K., Kondo, K. K., Saha, S., Advani, S. M., Young, S., Spencer, H., Rusek, M., Anderson, J., Veazie, S., Smith, M., & Kansagara, D. (2021). Racial and ethnic disparities in COVID-19-related infections, hospitalizations, and deaths: A systematic review. *Annals of Internal Medicine, 174*, 362–373. https://doi.org/10.7326/M20-6306.

Meherali, S., Punjani, N., Louie-Poon, S., Rahim, K. A., Das, J. K., Salam, R. A., & Lassi, Z. S. (2021). Mental health for children and adolescents amidst COVID-19 and past pandemics: A rapid systematic review. *International Journal of Environmental Research and Public Health, 18*, 3432. https://doi.org/10.3390/ijerph18073432.

Meyer, S. R., Yu, G., Reiders, E., & Stark, L. (2020). Child labor, sex and mental health outcomes amongst adolescent refugees. *Journal of Adolescence, 81*, 52–60. https://doi.org/10.1016/j.adolescence.2020.04.002.

Meyer, M., Calabrese, L., Meyer, A., Constancias, F., Porter, L. F., Muller, M., Leitner, M., Leitner, A., Michaud, A., Kaltenbach, G., Schmitt, E., Karcher, P., Sauleau, E., Chayer, S., Zeyons, F., Riou, M., Ado, S. E. G., Blanc, F., Fafi-Kramer, S., ... Vogel, T. (2021). Clinical and virological follow-up of a cohort of 76 COVID-19 older hospitalized adults. *Journal of the American Geriatrics Society, 69*, 1167–1170. https://doi.org/10.1111/jgs.17023.

Molloy, L., Beckett, P., Chidarikire, S., Merrick, T. T., Guha, M., & Patton, D. (2020). Culture, stigma of mental illness, and young people. *Journal of Psychosocial Nursing and Mental Health Services, 58*, 15–18. https://doi.org/10.3928/02793695-20201013-03.

Murillo-Zamora, E., Aguilar-Sollano, F., Delgado-Enciso, I., & Hernandez-Suarez, C. M. (2020). Predictors of laboratory-positive COVID-19 in children and teenagers. *Public Health, 189*, 153–157. https://doi.org/10.1016/j.puhe.2020.

National Institutes of Health. (2021). *Cultural respect.*

National Assessment of Educational Progress. (2022). *2022 mathematics and reading report cards at grades 4 and 8.* The Nation's Report Card (nationsreportcard.gov).

O'Donovan, R. O., Ward, M., Brun, A. D., & McAuliffe, E. (2018). Safety culture in health care teams: A narrative review of the literature. *Journal of Nursing Management, 27*, 871–883. https://doi.org/10.1111/jonm.12740.

Oakes, R. (2019). Culture, climate change and mobility decisions in Pacific small island developing states. *Population and Environment, 40*, 480–503. https://doi.org/10.1007/s11111-019-00321-w.

Ochani, R. K., Asad, A., Yasmin, F., Shaikh, S., Khalid, H., Batra, S., Sohail, M. R., Mahmood, S. F., Ochani, R., Arshad, M. H., Kumar, A., & Surani, S. (2021). COVID-19 pandemic: From origins to outcomes. A comprehensive review of viral pathogenesis, clinical manifestations, diagnostic evaluation, and management. *Le Infezioni in Medicina, 29*, 20–36.

Oldroyd, J. C., Kabir, A., Dzakpasu, F. Q. S., Mahmud, H., Rana, J., & Islam, R. M. (2022). The experiences of children and adolescents undergoing forced separation from their parents during migration: A systematic review. *Health and Social Care in Community, 30*, 888–898. https://doi.org/10.1111/hsc.13595.

Otasowie, J., Paraiso, A., & Bates, G. (2020). Pervasive refusal syndrome: Systematic review of case reports. *European Child and Adolescent Psychiatry, 30*, 41–53. https://doi.org/10.1007/s00787-020-01536-1.

Ozlu-Erkilik, Z., Wenzel, T., Kothgassner, O. D., & Akkaya-Kalayci, T. (2020). Transcultural differences in risk factors and in triggering reasons of suicidal and self-harming behaviour in young people with and without a migration background. *International Journal of Environmental Research and Public Health, 17*, 6498. https://doi.org/10.3390/ijerph17186498.

Payan, T. (2022). Understanding the nexus between undocumented immigration and mental health. *Current Opinion in Psychology, 47*, 101414. https://doi.org/10.1016/j.copsyc.2022.101414.

Peter, L.-J., Schindler, S., Sander, C., Schmidt, S., Muehlan, H., McLaren, T., Tomczyk, S., Speerforck, S., & Schomerus, G. (2021). Continuum beliefs and mental illness stigma: A systematic review and meta-analysis of correlation and intervention studies. *European Journal of Public Health, 31*, 283. https://doi.org/10.1017/S0033291721000854.

Place, V., Nabb, B., Gubi, E., Assel, K., Ahlen, J., Hagstrom, A., Baarnhielm, S., Dalman, C., & Hollander, A- C. (2021). Perceived barriers to care for migrant children and young people with mental health problems and/or neurodevelopmental differences in high-income countries: a meta-ethnography. *BMJ Open*, *11*(9):e045923. https://doi.org/10.1136/bmjopen-2020-045923.

Scapaticci, S., Neri, C. R., Marseglia, G. L., Staiano, A., Chiarelli, F., & Verduci, E. (2022). The impact of COVID-19 on lifestyle behaviors in children and adolescents: An international overview. *Italian Journal of Pediatrics*, *48*, 22. https://doi.org/10.1186/s13052-022-01211-y.

Scharpf, F., Kaltenbach, E., Nickerson, A., & Hecker, T. (2021). A systematic review of socio-ecological factors contributing to risk and protection of the mental health of refugee children and adolescents. *Clinical Psychology Review*, *83*, 101930. https://doi.org/10.1016/j.cpr.2020.101930.

Subasi, D. M., Sumengen, A. A., Ekim, A., Ocakci, A. F., & Beser, A. (2021). The relation between quality of life and future expectations for refugee adolescents. *Journal of Child and Adolescent Psychiatric Nursing*, *34*, 206–211. https://doi.org/10.1111/jcap.12314.

Sue, D. W., Capodilupo, C. M., Torino, G. C., Bucceri, J. M., Holder, A. M. B., Nadal, K. L., & Esquilin, M. (2007). Racial microaggressions in everyday life implications for clinical practice. *American Psychologist*, *62*, 271–286. https://doi.org/10.1037/0003-066X.62.4.271.

U.S. Department of Health and Human Services. (n.d.). *National culturally and linguistically appropriate service standards*.

U.S. Department of Homeland Security. (2022). *Immigration data and statistics*.

UNICAN Immigration Office. (2022). *What is the biggest reasons for Immigration: 2022*.

USA for UNHCR The UN Refugee Agency. (2022). *Refugee statistics*.

USAFacts. (2022). *US Coronavirus Vaccine Tracker: Each state has a different plan-and different challenges-in distributing vaccines. Learn more about who is getting vaccinated by parsing the data by age, sex and race.*

van de Weil, W., Castillo-Laborde, C., Uruza, I. F., Fish, M., & Scholte, W. F. (2021). Mental health consequences of long-term stays in refugee camps: Evidence from Moria. *BMC Public Health*, *21*, 1290. https://doi.org/10.1186/s12889-021-11301-x.

von Werthern, M., Robjant, K., Chui, Z., Schon, R., Ottisova, L., Mason, C., & Katona, C. (2018). The impact of immigration detention on mental health: A systematic review. *BMC Psychiatry*, *18*(1):382 https://doi.org/10.1186/s12888-018-1945-y.

Willey, S., Desmyth, K., & Truong, M. (2022). Racism, healthcare access and health equity for people seeking asylum. *Nursing Inquiry*, *1*, 1–9. https://doi.org/10.1111/nin.12240.

Willis, D. E., Andersen, J. A., Bryant-Moore, K., Selig, J. P., Long, C. R., Felix, H. C., Curran, G. M., & McElfish, P. A. (2021). COVID-19 vaccine hesitancy: Race/ethnicity, trust, and fear. *Clinical and Translational Science*, *14*, 2200–2207. https://doi.org/10.1111/cts.13077.

World Health Organization. (2021). *Comprehensive mental health action plan 2013-2030*.

Wright, N., Jordan, M., & Lazzarino, R. (2021). Interventions to support the mental health of survivors of modern slavery and human trafficking: A systematic review. *The International Journal of Social Psychiatry*, *67*, 1026–1034. https://doi.org/10.1177/00207640211039245.

Wylie, L., Corrado, A. M., Edwards, N., Benlamri, M., & Murcia Monroy, D. E. (2020). Reframing resilience: Strengthening continuity of patient care to improve the mental health of immigrants and refugees. *International Journal of Mental Health Nursing*, *29*, 69–79. https://doi.org/10.1111/inm.12650.

Yakeley, J. (2018). Shame, culture, and mental health. *Nordic Journal of Psychiatry*, *72*, S20–S22. https://doi.org/10.1080/08039488.2018.1525641.

Yakely, A. E., Avni-Singer, L., Oliveira, C. R., & Niccolai, L. M. (2019). Human Papillomavirus Vaccination and Anogenital Warts: A Systematic Review of Impact and Effectiveness in the United States. *Sexually transmitted diseases*, *46*(4), 213–220. https://doi.org/10.1097/OLQ.0000000000000948.

Yilmaz, R., & Uytun, M. C. (2020). What do we know about bullying in Syrian adolescent refugees? A cross-sectional study from Turkey: (Bullying in Syrian adolescent refugees). *The Psychiatric Quarterly*, *91*, 1395–1406. https://doi.org/10.1007/s11126-020-09776-9.

Young, M.-E. D. E. T., Sarnoff, H., Lang, D., & Ramirez, A. S. (2022). Coverage and framing of immigration policy in US newspapers. *The Milbank Quarterly*, *100*, 78–101. https://doi.org/10.1111/1468-0009.12547.

Zazzara, M. B., Penfold, R. S., Roberts, A. L., Lee, K. A., Dooley, H., Sudre, C. H., Welch, C., Bowyer, R. C. E., Visconti, A., Mangino, M., Freidin, M. B., Moustafa, J. S. E.-S., Small, K. S., Murray, B., Modat, M., Graham, M. S., Wolf, J., Ourselin, S., Martin, F. C., ... Lochlainn, M. N. (2021). Probable delirium is a presenting symptom of COVID-19 in frail, older adults: A cohort of 322 hospitalised and 535 community-based older adults. *Age and Ageing*, *50*, 40–48. https://doi.org/10.1093/ageing/afaa223.

Zeger, C., & Auron, M. (2021). Addressing the challenges of cross-cultural communication. *The Medical Clinics of North America*, *106*, 577–588. https://doi.org/10.1016/j.mcna.2022.02.006.

Zheng, C., Shao, W., Chen, X., Zhang, B., Wang, G., & Zhang, W. (2022). Real-world effectiveness of COVID-19 vaccines: A literature review and meta-analysis. *International Journal of Infectious Diseases*, *114*, 252–260. https://doi.org/10.1016/j.ijid.2021.11.009

Culture, Family, and Community

Chapter 11

• Joyceen S. Boyle, Martha B. Baird, and John W. Collins

Key Terms

Acculturation
Aggregates
Assimilation
Asylees
Community-based nursing
Community-based setting
Community health nursing
Community nursing
Community settings

COVID-19
Cultural assessment
Cultural knowledge
Cultural sensitivity
Culturally competent care
Disaster preparedness
Emergency response plans
Immigrants
Integration
Medically underserved

Pandemic
Public health nursing
Refugees
Social determinants of health
Subcultures
Traditional health beliefs and
    practices
Vulnerable populations

Learning Objectives

1. Use cultural concepts to provide transcultural nursing care to families, communities, and aggregates.
2. Understand the necessary components of a cultural assessment of an aggregate group. See Appendix B.
3. Explore interactions of community and culture as they relate to concepts of community-based nursing practice and specialized community interventions.
4. Analyze how cultural factors influence health and illness of groups as well as social equity.
5. Assess factors that influence the health of diverse groups within the community.
6. Evaluate potential health problems and solutions in refugee and immigrant populations.
7. Identify interventions that are culturally sensitive and relevant to address health concerns of refugee and immigrant populations.
8. Analyze various strategies for emergency and disaster planning in community settings.

Introduction

An understanding of culture and cultural concepts contributes to the nurse's knowledge and facilitates culturally competent nursing care in community-based settings. Currently, many nurses practice in **community settings** with clients from a wide variety of cultural backgrounds; this trend is expected to increase with more nurses moving from acute care institutions to community settings (Institute of Medicine, 2011). The care of clients in the community can be extremely complex, calling for a high level of nursing skill. Cultural diversity is also expected to increase in the United States. Significant changes in the healthcare system, including an increased emphasis on health promotion and disease prevention, have influenced nurses to make changes in their practice and the settings in which care is delivered. Concepts such as health equity, diversity, partnership, empowerment, and facilitation now form the basis for community-based nursing practice with individuals, families, and aggregates in the community. An **aggregate** is a collection of people who can be thought of as a whole because they happen to be in the same place at the same time. For some time, national nursing associations, including the National Institute of Nursing Research, have urged an aggregated community and population focus in both nursing research and practice. Involving clients in planning for and providing community nursing services is the foundation of **culturally competent care** and involves learning individual and community perspectives to plan and provide community-aggregated services.

Specialized community interventions that are culturally relevant to the people served are built on collaboration and partnerships between community leaders, health consumers, and healthcare providers. When community residents or health consumers are involved as partners, community-based services are more likely to be responsive to locally defined needs, are better used, and are sustained through local actions. Specialized community interventions are complex and often very time-consuming. They require a high level of nursing knowledge and skill in working with and relating to different individuals and groups. In many instances, the complexity is increased when clients and nurses are from different cultures. Nurses must understand how to help community members from various cultural groups to work with community leaders and healthcare providers forming partnerships that are responsive and structure nursing and healthcare in ways that are culturally sensitive and appropriate. It is often the cultural factors that influence whether a particular population will choose to participate in community-based health services. For example, if the healthcare providers speak Spanish, a Spanish-speaking population might be more inclined to participate in the health program. There is always a need for continuing communication among healthcare providers and community residents that is characterized by mutual understanding and respect. This understanding and respect form the basis for culturally relevant and competent nursing care.

In this chapter, the terms **community nursing**, **community-based nursing**, **community health nursing**, and **public health nursing** are used interchangeably, even though they have different meanings in some settings and in different contexts (Rector, 2022). Whether the nurse is employed as a public health nurse or a community health nurse in a health department or practices in a community-based setting, they need the knowledge and skills to provide culturally competent care. The practice of nursing in a community setting requires that nurses be comfortable with clients from diverse cultures and the broader socioeconomic context in which nurses personally live. As the population continues to grow in diversity, health disparities have become more apparent in diverse populations and are now a vital area of focus for researchers and practitioners. Care that is not congruent with the client's value system is likely to increase the cost of care because it compromises quality and inhibits access to services (Gainsbury, 2017). Furthermore, members of diverse cultural groups, such as the officially designated minority groups in the United States, tend to experience greater health inequalities than do members of the general population. This was the impetus for targeting federally defined population categories, that is, White, Black, Hispanic, Asian/Pacific Islander, and American Indian/Alaska Native in the first *Healthy People 2000* (National Health Promotion and Disease Prevention Objectives, 1991). Cultural diversities must be respected and taken into account by healthcare professionals and the unique characteristics and individual differences recognized as well. Equally important, we must address the stark inequalities that exist in health status between minority groups and the wider American society. *Healthy People 2030* is a set of goals and objectives with 10-year targets designed to guide national health promotion and disease prevention efforts to improve the health of all people in the United States (*Healthy People 2030*). Box 11-1 shows what is new in *Healthy People 2030*.

Overview of Culturally Competent Nursing Care in Community Settings

Nurses practice in many different settings within the community, including worksites, schools, physicians' offices, healthcare program sites, clinics, churches, and public health departments. The use of **cultural knowledge** in community-based nursing practice begins with a careful assessment of clients and families in their own environments. Cultural data that have implications for nursing care are selected from clients, families, and the environment during the assessment phase and are discussed with the client and family to develop mutually shared goals. The Andrews/Boyle Transcultural Nursing Assessment Guide for Individuals and Families (Appendix A) and the Andrews/Boyle Transcultural Nursing Assessment Guide for Groups and Communities (Appendix B) are helpful when assessing clients, families, groups, and communities.

Cultural data are important in the care of all clients; however, in community nursing, they are a prerequisite to successful nursing interventions. Community nursing is practiced in a community setting, often in the home of the client, and frequently requires more active participation by the client and family. Frequently, the client and family must consider making basic changes in lifestyle, such as changes in diet and exercise patterns. Cultural competence requires that the nurse understand the family lifestyle and value system as well as those cultural forces that are powerful determinants of health-related behaviors. Nurses often work closely with clients with chronic diseases or those who have other health problems, and nursing interventions must include aspects of counseling and education as well as anticipatory guidance directed toward helping clients and families adjust to what may be lifelong conditions. Nurses must take into account the diverse cultural factors

---

BOX 11-1 What's New in *Healthy People 2030*?

1. Emphasizing ideas of health equity that address social determinants of health and promote health across all stages of life.
2. *Healthy People 2030* objectives are organized into intuitive topics so you can easily find the information and data you are looking for and explore the relevant topics such as Health Conditions, Health Behaviors, Populations, Settings and Systems, and Social Determinants of Health.

Reference: https://www.healthypeople.gov/

that may motivate clients to make successful changes in behavior because improvement in health status requires lifestyle and behavioral modifications. Transcultural nursing practice has the potential to improve the health of the community as well as the health of individual clients and families. An additional consideration of nurses who practice in community settings are the needs of populations at risk. Special at-risk groups can be found in all communities: people experiencing homelessness, those with low incomes, those engaging in harmful drug use, migrants, refugees, prison populations, and older adults are groups at risk for decreased health status.

Consider the difficulty of designing a health program for a community composed primarily of refugees who recently arrived in the United States. By definition, **refugees** are individuals who have been forced to leave their home country due to war, violence, or persecution. They may have spent years in refugee camps in other countries, may have lost family members, or may have family members still living in their home country, and yet the refugees are now making a life for themselves in a strange country. While refugees may come from all levels of the socioeconomic status in their homeland, many refugees will have not had access to medical, dental, and other healthcare services while in refugee status, even if they may have had healthcare access prior to fleeing their native country. Certainly, language barriers would be a major problem, but so could many other cultural differences, from nuances in communication to differences in beliefs of what constitutes health and illness as well as treatment and cure. A failure to understand and deal with these differences would have serious implications for the success of any health or nursing intervention. Nurses who have knowledge of, and an ability to work with, diverse cultures can devise effective community interventions to reduce risks in a manner that is consistent with the community and group, as well as individual values and beliefs of community members.

A Transcultural Framework

A distinguishing and important aspect of community-based nursing practice is the nursing focus on the community as the client (Rector & Stanley, 2022). Effective community nursing practice must reflect accurate knowledge of the causes and distribution of health problems and of effective interventions that are congruent with the values and goals of the community. A transcultural approach can be used by the community nurse to collect, organize, and analyze information about high-risk and vulnerable groups from different cultural backgrounds that are encountered in community practice.

Identifying Subcultures and Devising Specialized Community-Based Interventions

A transcultural framework for nursing care helps the nurse to identify **subcultures** within the larger community and to devise community-based interventions that are specific to community health and nursing goals. For example, in the multicultural society of the United States, it is common to speak of "the Black community," "the Hispanic community," or "the Francophone community." We might also speak more broadly of "the immigrant community" or the "refugee community," or of other unique groups within or near a local community. A cultural focus allows this variety and facilitates data collection about specific groups based on their health risks. A transcultural framework facilitates a view of the community as a complex collective yet allows for diversity within the whole. Interventions that are successful in one subgroup may fail with another subgroup of the same community, and often, the failure can be attributed to cultural differences or barriers that arise because of these differences. Often, the community location of a diverse subculture reflects distinctive aspects of the cultural group. Figure 11-1 shows murals on the wall of a library in El Rio, a Mexican American barrio in Tucson, AZ.

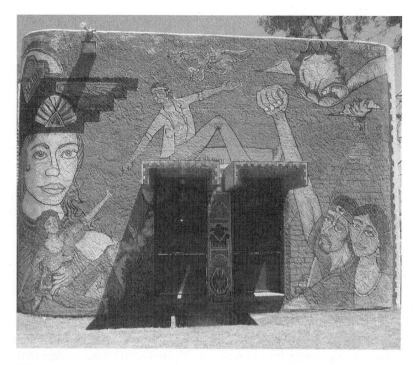

Figure 11-1. These murals reflect the Mexican American culture of the El Rio barrio in Tucson, AZ. They were painted by community residents.

Identifying the Values and Cultural Norms of a Community

A transcultural framework is essential for the community health nurse to identify the values and cultural norms of a community. Although values are universal features of all cultures, their types and expressions vary widely, even within the same community. Values often serve as the foundation for a community's acceptance and use of health resources or a group's participation in community-based intervention programs to promote health and wellness. Just as nurses share data and collaborate with clients and families to establish mutually acceptable goals for nursing care, the community-based nurse works with the community or aggregates within the community to plan community-focused health programs. Identifying values and cultural norms within a community or aggregate correctly often requires community nurses to spend time interacting with

and learning from members of those populations. In addition to forming partnerships with communities, the community nurse considers the influences of social, economic, ecological, and political issues. Larger policy issues directly and profoundly affect many, if not all, community health issues. These larger policy issues are, in turn, influenced by the wider national and/or international culture.

Cultural Issues in Community Nursing Practice

The need for nurses to be sensitive to clients who are culturally different is increasing as we become more aware of the complex interactions between healthcare providers and clients and how these interactions might affect the client's health. Different cultural groups who have limited access to health services, along with barriers resulting from language, economic difficulties, and cultural differences, often suffer from a variety of health disparities (Weech-Maldonado et al., 2018). The information in this chapter will assist nurses to become aware of cultural factors that affect health, illness, and the practice of nursing in community settings.

Purnell and Fenkl (2021) as well as Andrews and Boyle (2016) have provided models or frameworks to guide the nurse in the assessment of cultural factors in patient care. The Andrews/Boyle Transcultural Nursing Assessment Guides (see Appendices A, B, and D) provide outlines for the nurse to collect and assess cultural data relevant to individuals, families, and communities. Most cultural assessment guides are oriented toward individual clients and occasionally toward families. The Andrews/Boyle assessment guides have the comprehensive view necessary for assessing cultural factors for intervention at the individual, family, and community levels. Because individual clients and their families constitute larger communities, nurses who work in community settings must understand cultural issues as they relate to individuals and families as well as the context in which they live.

Cultural Influences on Individuals and Families

Cultural influences—values, norms, beliefs, and behaviors—have a profound effect on health. When assessing individuals and families, the community health nurse should carefully examine the following:

1. Family structure and makeup (multigenerational, nuclear, extended family, significant others, etc.), individual roles and responsibilities, and dynamics in the family, particularly communication patterns and decision-making.
2. Health beliefs and practices related to disease causation, treatment of illness, and the use of indigenous healers or folk practitioners and other alternative/complementary therapies.
3. Patterns of daily living, including work, school, and leisure activities.
4. Social networks, including friends, neighbors, kin, and significant others, and how they influence health and illness.
5. Ethnic, cultural, or national identity of client and family, for example, identification with a particular group, including language.
6. Nutritional practices and how they relate to cultural factors and health.
7. Religious preferences and influences on well-being, health maintenance, and illness as well as the impact religion might have on daily living and taboos or restrictions arising from religious beliefs that might influence health status or care.
8. Culturally appropriate behavior styles, including what is manifested during anger, competition, and cooperation, as well as relationships with healthcare professionals, relationships between genders, and relations with other groups in the community.
9. Health professionals should always be aware of their own personal beliefs and biases and how those can impact the client's health.

A cultural assessment of individuals and families includes all of the preceding factors. This list is a starting point for community nurses to use when assessing individuals and families in everyday practice. Cultural values shape human health behaviors and determine what individuals and families will do to maintain their health status, how they will care for themselves and others who become ill, and where and from whom they will seek healthcare. Most importantly, family members are often the ones who decide on the course of treatment. Families have an important role in the transmission of cultural values and learned behaviors that relate to both health and illness. It is within the family context that individuals learn basic ways to stay healthy and to ensure their own well-being and that of their family members.

One commonality shared by members of healthy families is a concern for the health and wellness of each individual within the family. The nurse must not only assess the health of each family member but also determine how well the family can meet family health needs. Just how well families can meet the needs of each family member will determine how, when, and where interventions will take place. A cultural orientation assists the nurse in understanding cultural values and interactions, the roles that family members assume, and the support systems available to the family to help them when health needs are identified.

The family is usually an individual's most important social unit and provides the social context within which illness occurs and is resolved. Health promotion and maintenance also occur within the family group. Some **traditional health beliefs and practices** promote the health of the family because they are generally family and socially oriented. Frequently, traditional beliefs and practices reinforce family cohesion. Some values are more central and influential than others; given a competing set of demands, these central values will typically determine a family's priorities. In families that adhere to traditional cultural values, the families' (or tribe's and/or community's) needs and goals often will take precedence over an individual's needs and goals. The culturally competent nurse can recognize and use the family's role in promoting and maintaining health. This requires an appreciation of the family context in health and illness and how this varies among cultures (Leininger, 1978).

Cultural Factors Within Communities

In addition to identifying and meeting the cultural needs of clients and families, the community health nurse must consider social and cultural factors on a community level to understand and respect cultural values, mobilize local resources, and develop culturally appropriate health programs and services. Important factors to consider include the influence of demographics on healthcare, subcultures within refugee and immigrant populations, degree of acculturation and/or maintenance of traditional values and practices,

and access to health and nursing care for these population groups.

In addition, new and important areas of nursing practice are incorporating transcultural concepts to reach underserved or **vulnerable populations** that are at high risk in our rapidly changing society.

Demographics and Healthcare

During the 21st century, the United States and many other countries will face enormous demographic, social, cultural, and environmental changes. The United States is becoming more diverse, and it is incumbent on nurses to be prepared to respond appropriately as the health status of individuals differs dramatically across cultural/ethnic groups and social classes. Certain groups in the United States face greater challenges than does the general population in accessing timely and needed healthcare services. Major indicators such as morbidity and mortality rates for adults and infants show that the health status of many racial/ethnic minority Americans in the United States is substantially worse than that of White Americans. Health status is worse among those who are **medically underserved**—those populations who have inadequate access to quality healthcare. Community nurses must assess groups within the community in a very sensitive manner; often those characteristics that we assume are related to the group's culture may be influenced by other factors such as economic factors, trauma experienced in the migration experience, or racism.

Subcultures or Diversity Within Communities

Caring for diverse groups within the community has been a focus of public health nursing since the days of Lillian Wald, an early nurse leader. Home care was provided to residents of low-income areas of cities, particularly recently arrived immigrants. Because nurses were not from the same cultural background as their clients, they had to deal with cultural differences between themselves and the clients in their care. Today, the need for nurses to provide culturally relevant care is greater than ever. Currently, the focus of community nursing is on efforts aimed at the promotion, protection, and preservation of the public's health (Rector, 2022). This often involves health education to individuals, families, and community groups. Health education should be structured in such a way to appeal to people from different subcultures. Subcultures are aggregates of people who establish certain rules of behavior, values, and living patterns that are different from mainstream culture. Leininger described subcultures as having "distinctive patterns of living with sets of rules, special values and practices that are different from the dominant culture" (Leininger, 1995, p. 60). There can also be diversity within each subculture. Hispanic culture as a group is very broad and includes Mexican Americans, Puerto Ricans, Dominicans, Cubans, and Central and South Americans. There is diversity within each of these groups as well.

Certain geographic areas of the country, such as Appalachia, are examples of areas where distinct subcultures can be identified. Persons born and reared in the southern states or in New York City can often be identified as members of a distinct subculture by their dialect and mannerisms.

The United States used to be described as a "melting pot" culture, indicating that new arrivals gave up their former languages, customs, and values to become Americans. This concept may not be appropriate, however. A more accurate metaphor for the American population is a rich and complex tapestry of colors, backgrounds, and interests. One subculture that has retained many aspects of their traditional culture is the Hmong people from Southeast Asia. They came to the United States in the 1970s as refugees after the Vietnam War. The large Hmong community in Fresno, CA, sponsors a New Year's Day Celebration that is attended by as many as 100,000 Hmong from all over the United States (Fig. 11-2).

Refugee and Immigrant Populations

Migration affects the health and well-being of communities, regardless of the cause (weather, war, or lack of resources). The United Nations reports global displacement at an all-time high, representing 1% of the world's population, over 100 million people (United Nations, 2022). Communities from which individuals emigrate as well as those communities that accept immigrants are profoundly affected by human migration patterns. Therefore, it is important for

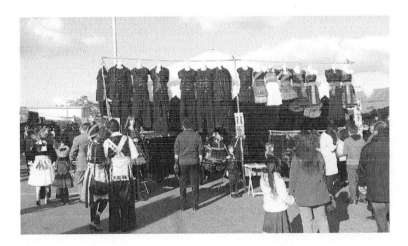

Figure 11-2. The Hmong New Year's Celebration in Fresno, CA, is attended by 100,000 Hmong. In this photo, several Hmong admire the merchandise in a booth selling traditional clothes.

community health providers to understand the makeup of community members in order to provide services.

The term "immigrant" is a broad designation and refers to an individual who leaves their country of origin or residence to relocate to another country. There are many subcategories of immigrants including refugees, **asylees**, and those with temporary protected status. The various types of immigrants are divided into those that have documentation, as a legal entrant, or those that are undocumented as an illegal entrant.

Immigrants are persons who voluntarily enter another country with the intention to stay. Immigrants come of their own choice, and most hope to eventually become citizens of their new host country. Persons who enter another country without the proper documentation are often referred to as "undocumented" migrants, "illegal immigrants," or "illegal aliens." The terms illegal and alien should be avoided in nursing discourse and the professional literature to show respect for the undocumented immigrant as a human being (McGuire, 2014). Currently, immigration of undocumented individuals, or those who do not have the appropriate documentation to immigrate, can be a contentious issue. Many of the key issues in the debate about immigration policies in the United States are based on economic and political factors (Ayón, 2018).

Under international law, refugee is a special type of documented immigrant who is outside of their country of nationality or habitual residence and who has a well-founded fear of persecution if they return to their own country. By definition, refugees are persons escaping persecution based on race, religion, nationality, or political stance (UNHCR, 2010). Most countries allow a certain number of refugees for resettlement each year.

Another classification of immigrant is an asylee. These are persons who come to a particular country seeking political asylum from some sort of persecution in their home country. These various types of classification—immigrant, undocumented immigrant, refugee, and asylee—often determine the rights allotted to individuals. The legal designation will determine eligibility for work permits, residency status, and the entitlement to social and health services. In addition, those who are undocumented, or without appropriate residency status, may face arrest and deportation to their country of origin. Table 11-1 lists some of the more common terms for individuals residing in a country who are not citizens.

Studies have suggested that there is a need for research about refugees who are distinct from other categories of immigrants (Betancourt et al., 2017; Golub et al., 2018). The circumstances that lead to forced migration of refugees are very different from those that influence a voluntary

Table 11-1	Terms Used for Individuals Residing in a Country Who Are Not Citizens
Term	**Description**
Immigrant	A person who comes to a country to take up permanent residence
Refugee	A person who is escaping persecution based on race, religion, nationality, or political persuasion
Emigrant	A person departing from a country to settle elsewhere
Émigré	A person forced to emigrate for political reasons
Asylee	A person seeking political asylum from persecution in their home country
Temporary stay migrant	A person who moves to another country with the intention of staying there for only a limited time, usually for occupational reasons
Undocumented	A person without the required documents that provide evidence of status or qualification, such as nationality or specified length of time a person may legally reside within a country

immigrant to relocate, and these differences can have distinct health implications. In recent times, refugees fleeing war, famine, and other social upheavals have come to the United States from all continents including the Middle Eastern countries of Afghanistan, Iraq, and Syria, as well as Myanmar (Burma); the African nations of Sudan, Somalia, the Democratic Republic of the Congo; and most recently European country of Ukraine. Most refugees arrive from countries undergoing violent political and social conflicts (Igielnik & Krogstad, 2017; Krogstad, 2017).

Evidence-Based Practice 11-1 presents a study about the consequences of forced migration among Syrian refugee families resettled to Jordan. The United Nations High Commissioner for Refugees (UNHCR) has suggested that violence against displaced women and children is considered the most pervasive human rights violation in the world (Gaynor, 2015). Intimate partner violence is exacerbated in war-torn countries, with a high incidence of rape and other physical/sexual abuse during armed conflicts. Women and girls, often unaccompanied by family members, are particularly at high risk. Many refugees who come to the United States have experienced these human rights violations (Meffert et al., 2016; Musalo & Lee, 2017).

Many immigrants and refugees face challenges integrating into countries of resettlement. There is pressure to acculturate into societies that may have very different cultural values and social structures. In addition, immigrants may experience prejudice or racism in their new community and feel unwelcome. Many arrive with scant economic resources and must learn English and become economically self-sufficient as quickly as possible. Certain factors, such as settlement patterns, that is, living near family, friends, or others from their home region, communication networks, social class, and education, have helped many immigrants maintain their cultural traditions. Immigrant or refugee communities provide support for newcomers and opportunities for cultural continuity because these ethnic communities reflect the identities of the home countries. At the same time, belonging to such a community tends to set immigrants and refugees apart and isolate them from the larger community. For example, newcomers from Mexico realize that they need to learn English to get better jobs, but they often join expanding Latino communities where most residents speak Spanish. Learning English well enough to obtain employment in the English-speaking world is difficult and takes time.

In addition to the legal entrance of immigrants and refugees, other persons seeking political asylum have entered the United States from all over the world. Regardless, those seeking asylum or those who enter the country legally or illegally are at considerable risk for health and social problems. In particular, healthcare along the United States–Mexico border, where many individuals are undocumented, poses special problems and challenges for healthcare providers (Ayón, 2018; McEwen et al., 2015). Immigrants, refugees, and asylees face language and employment barriers, often with little or no economic reserve to draw from. Some have experienced rapid change and traumatic life events with few resources available to assist them. Refugees, asylees, and immigrants in general have special health risks that healthcare clinicians must be aware of and sensitive to so that appropriate care can be provided.

Planning Nursing Care for Refugee Families and Communities

Before being admitted to the United States, refugees undergo extensive background checks and are mandated to receive both physical and mental health screenings within 30 days of arrival through a public health department or a primary care agency contracted with the Office of Refugee Resettlement (2013, 2022). Many refugees experience mental health issues as a result of the trauma they experience during their relocation journey, including anxiety, depression, and posttraumatic stress disorder (PTSD) (Shawyer et al., 2017; Wong et al., 2017).

To address these issues, careful assessment of cultural backgrounds and individual factors can

Through Her Eyes: The Impact of War on Syrian Refugee Families

This descriptive phenomenological study that explores the impact of the civil war and displacement of Syrian families from a cultural perspective. The study highlights the experiences of Syrian war-refugee families who have sought shelter in a host country. It was conducted with 16 Syrian women who were seeking care at a health center in Jordan. Three major themes emerged from the data.

Theme 1: War as a Source of Final and Social Stress

Men lost employment because they had fled their country. Losing employment meant women and children also lost their familiar lifestyles. Social stressors were being displaced in a new country, different culture, fear for safety, being isolated from family members, and significant financial stressors.

Theme 2: Family Violence Was a Consequence of War

Study participants reported the harmful effects of war on their husbands' attitudes and behaviors, which led to an increase in family violence. Anxiety, nervousness, and becoming easily stressed led to abusive interactions with wives and children. Social media and television news programs reporting on the conditions in Syria influenced the men's violent outbursts. The increase in family violence negatively affected all members of the family.

Theme 3: The Adverse Effects of the War on the Health and Well-being of Women and Children

The higher cost of living in the host country, the husband's unemployment, refugee status, and the disruption of traditional family roles resulted in hypertension and depression. Chronic illnesses were compounded by the lack of access to healthcare and the high cost of medications. The education of Syrian children was disrupted and many of them were required to work and contribute to expenses of daily living. The children exhibited intensified emotions, including sadness, depression, anxiety, and crying episodes. Syrian men used physical abuse toward their wives and children for minor infractions to reestablish their place as head of the family. This affected the patterns of family communication leading to more anxiety, depression, and family violence.

Clinical Implications

Nurses should be aware of the everyday struggles for justice and human dignity that refugees experience when war impacts their daily lives. Nurses can be culturally sensitive and refer refugees to social, mental, and physical health/humanitarian care agencies that are equipped to meet their needs. Teaching culturally congruent care in nursing programs throughout host countries is essential to ensure that new graduates are aware of and can deal with the cultural issues they will face as providers. International aid agencies can provide their staff with training to deal with war-related stressors. Providing educational seminars, which include reviews on culture, health, and implicit bias training, are essential for healthcare providers to maintain cultural competency in the day-to-day of refugees. Research studies that explore the relationship of cultural beliefs and values to mental and physical health are important to help providers continue to understand how to best serve displaced refugees. These studies provide transcultural nursing knowledge, allowing nurses to be grounded in individualized culturally specific care.

Reference: Al-Natour, A., Morris, E. J., & Al-Ostaz, S. M. (2022). Through her eyes: The impact of war on Syrian refugee families. *Journal of Transcultural Nursing, 33*(1), 26–32. https://doi.org/10.1177/10436596211026367

help nurses anticipate and work with challenges experienced by refugees and immigrants seeking healthcare. The Baird/Boyle Assessment Guide for Refugees (Appendix D) is recommended for use with refugee clients and their families.

Assessment of these factors will assist the nurse in planning healthcare for refugee and/or immigrant families. Health services, preventive care, and health education have repeatedly been identified as important needs in health surveys that have been conducted in refugee communities. Conflicts worldwide continue to generate refugees fleeing violence and war.

The stress of resettlement is often a significant problem of refugees. Stress is related to the refugee experience and also to inadequate income, work-related problems, and loss of culture and traditions. The lack of mental health services is a real concern in refugee and immigrant communities and requires creative and innovative solutions. In refugee communities, a church, synagogue, or mosque can play a positive and important role—religion is often identified as a protective factor by refugees in facilitating wellness and increasing quality of life. Refugees from some cultures may be reluctant to seek mental health services because of the stigma of mental illness (Xin, 2020). Postmigration stress may be exacerbated by unemployment or underemployment and may contribute to depression, PTSD, alcohol and substance misuse, and poor general health status.

Refugee families need particular support to raise their children in a new country and culture. The children are often exposed to different values and norms in a new society that clash with traditions of the parents and elders. This can create conflict and may result in a breakdown of the family structure. Community-based interventions such as A Family Strengthening Program for Refugees (see Evidence-Based Practice 11-2) can help newly resettled refugee families adjust to strain of facing families in a new environment.

Many refugees come from resource-constrained countries with limited availability of healthcare services, and the idea of preventive care is foreign to them. Preventive health practices such as dental care, breast self-examination, mammography, and Papanicolaou (Pap) smears, and regular prostate and testicular examinations are important for refugees. Many barriers to good preventive care for newcomers to the United States are environmental and social rather than cultural. Constraints are based on the refugee's individual situations as well as language, economic, occupational, and transportation problems. Cultural groups differ in regard to the priority given to individual goals versus those of the larger group. For example, many refugee communities are collectivist societies that value the good of the group, traditional values, and group loyalty. This often conflicts with the individualistic American society. Many refugees, such as those from African countries, may suffer from racism and discrimination when they resettle in the United States, and this too impacts mental health and successful resettlement.

Health education, including information about access to care, is always important in planning services for refugee and immigrant communities. Many refugees and immigrants do not use health education services, not necessarily because of cultural barriers but because of difficulties with language and access, the need for translation and transportation, the desire for same-sex healthcare providers, and other barriers such as child care.

Healthcare institutions and agencies serving refugee and immigrant communities should include multicultural healthcare providers on their staff. Further, community health workers should be trained to serve as interpreters and translators, as it is often problematic for healthcare providers to use family members as interpreters because of divisions along age and gender lines. Children learn English more quickly than do their parents and could conceivably serve as interpreters, but it would be inappropriate to expect a young boy to interpret a conversation about his mother's Pap smear. The healthcare provider's gender is also important, as many refugee women are not comfortable with male doctors or nurses and might avoid

A Family Strengthening Intervention for Refugees

This community-based participatory mixed-method study examined outcomes from The Family Strengthening Intervention for Refugees program. This peer-delivered preventative home visiting program was designed to improve family communication, positive parenting, and caregiver–child relationships with the goal of reducing children's risk of mental health problems. The intervention study was carried out in New England, with 40 resettled Bhutanese and Somali Bantu refugee families.

The evidenced-based intervention included five components:

1. Psychoeducation: self-regulation strategies for children and caregivers
2. Family narrative to identify strengths and build sense of future
3. Positive parenting
4. Resource navigation for formal and nonformal supports
5. Positive parenting skills, alternative to violence, and family problem-solving skills

Results of this community-based participatory research study found positive patterns in improved parenting skills and child mental health. The parents described meaningful change from participation in the program in both their parenting skills and their children's responses. In addition, those who participated in the program reported improvements in depression and PTSD symptoms.

Clinical Implications

- As the refugee crisis continues to grow globally, nurses should be aware of the toll of migration and resettlement on the mental health of family members, including children.
- Interventions should be culturally tailored for different refugee populations and incorporate cultural values, beliefs, and practices.
- Members of the refugee community should be included in the planning, implementation, and evaluation of studies.

Reference: Neville, S. E., DiClemente-Bosco, K., Chamlagai, L.K., Bunn, M., Freeman, J., Berent, J. M., Gautam B., Abdi, A., & Betancourt, T. S. (2022). Investigating outcomes of a family strengthening intervention or resettled Somali Bantu and Bhutanese refugees: An explanatory sequential mixed methods study. *International Journal of Environmental Research and Public Health, 19,* 12415. https://doi.org/10.3390/ijerph191912415

healthcare altogether if female care providers are not available. Healthcare providers must be knowledgeable about the refugees' or immigrants' experiences and background, cultural and social factors, and other unique aspects of the population they serve. Refugees and new immigrants need access to language-appropriate and culturally relevant healthcare. Many refugees from community-oriented societies may prefer to receive such information in a group or social setting rather than a one-to-one basis that is common in many U.S. healthcare settings. For many refugee and/or immigrant communities, churches, mosques, and synagogues are appropriate settings for health education. Health fairs sponsored by community nurses and held within the refugee or immigrant communities have been very successful. Often, health fairs have been cosponsored by churches that serve immigrant or refugee communities.

Refugee women may have experienced gender-based violence (GBV) including torture, rape, and human rights abuses. Nurses and other health professionals, especially women physicians and nurses, must learn sensitive ways of broaching these subjects and helping refugee women access culturally appropriate care. Clinicians must be cognizant to design programs that address challenges in healthcare access, delivery of services in appropriate dialect, and provision of culturally sensitive healthcare for women who have experienced GBV.

The classic definition of community uses a geographic boundary such as a village, town, or urban settlement/city to provide parameters for and context of the population being described. This sense may be conveyed somewhat by terms for neighborhoods such as Little Havana, Little Kabul, and Little Saigon, but such designations do not really convey the nature or quality of the refugee or immigrant experience, which tends to cross geographic boundaries. Although refugees from certain geographical areas such as Sudan tend to be resettled in common locations when they arrive in the United States, they may later move to be closer to relatives or families who came from the same village or region of their homeland. The sense of shared displacement or "uprootedness" that serves to unite and distinguish immigrant or refugee communities from other groups or communities is quite profound and cannot be ignored when planning for community-based health services.

Immigrants and refugees are often seen by health professionals as dominated by psycho-emotional experiences and consequences of relocation. In other words, we focus on the effects of stress, relocation, and human rights violations. Indeed, much of the literature on immigrants and refugees focuses on PTSD. Although many immigrants and refugees have endured horrific experiences, this focus alone is not holistic. This view, according to McEwen et al. (2015), focuses on the primacy of the individual (an American value) rather than the community and thus prescribes psychiatric treatment instead of addressing the sociocultural and economic barriers at the macro level. It is at the macro level that transcultural healthcare providers must be engaged if they are to be effective participants in building healthy refugee and immigrant communities. This does not mean that individual health concerns should be ignored; it simply acknowledges that healthcare can be more effective when incorporated within a community focus, especially when dealing with immigrant or refugee communities.

Maintenance of Traditional Cultural Values and Practices

An important aspect of community nursing is the collection of cultural data and the assessment of traditional values and practices and how they are maintained over time. The terms **assimilation** and **acculturation** are often used to describe how immigrants and refugees adapt and change over time in a new country. Both of these terms imply that newcomers modify their traditional cultural traditions to adapt to the dominant culture. **Integration** may be a better term to describe the experience: it implies that an immigrant or refugee incorporates certain aspects of the new culture into their lifestyle, such as language and food, while still maintaining their cultural traditions and values. Both individuals and groups may be resistant to some changes and retain many traditional cultural traits, and the nurse should not expect that any client must or should integrate into American culture. For example, Hispanics are the largest cultural/ethnic group in the United States, and in several large American cities, they constitute a large percentage of the population (U.S. Department of Health and Human Services, Office of Minority Health, n.d.). In some Hispanic communities, it is easier to speak Spanish and to maintain traditional cultural practices. Because traditional health beliefs and practices influence health and wellness, it is important for the nurse to understand the degree to which clients, families, and communities adhere to traditional health values and how nursing practice should reflect those values. Spector (2013), an early transcultural scholar, suggested that a person's healthcare and behavior during illness may well have roots in that person's traditional belief system. Unless community nurses understand the traditional health beliefs and practices of their clients and communities, they may intervene at the wrong time or in an inappropriate way. Evidence-Based Practice 11-3 describes the patient care experience of Hispanic patients who are undergoing a transplant procedure. Patients told the researchers that they valued four interdependent

The Patient Care Experience as Perceived by Hispanic Patients With Chronic Illness Undergoing Transplant: A Grounded Theory

Hispanic people make up one of the largest-growing minority groups, yet little is understood of the patient experience from their perspective. As of 2019, 60.6 million persons identifying as Hispanic reside in the United States. While Spanish-speaking populations in the United States can be very diverse, as a general statement, Hispanic people face economic, social, and political barriers limiting access to healthcare services. Historically, "patient experience" has been measured through a survey known as the Hospital Consumer Assessment of Healthcare Providers and Systems (HCAHPS). Currently, hospitals that participate in the Hospital Value-Based Purchasing programs are required by the Centers for Medicare & Medicaid Services to administer the HCAHPS survey at discharge. Inadequate representation of diverse cultures such as Hispanic communities are often not represented in the development of research instruments and perceptions of care might be influenced by elements not currently assessed by this instrument. This study provides information on which factors are necessary and which should be avoided to promote a positive hospital experience for Hispanic transplant patients. Twenty participants were interviewed for the study. A theoretical model was developed with four interdependent and co-occurring concepts: they are Comfort, Communication, Connection, and Care.

- *Comfort* represented a state of ease. Participants described efforts by providers to ease their angst, distress, or pain as key to a positive hospital experience. Providers acted in certain ways or stated certain things that imbued consolation in the moment, which was expressed as physical or emotional comfort. One participant said, "Everyone is very, very cordial, very very attentive, just kindness."
- *Communication* was the process of exchanging information through use of shared verbal and nonverbal symbols. The role of communication in the nurse–patient relationship dominated the discourse of each interview. It included having questions answered and having the diagnosis and treatment explained in familiar and understandable terms. Participants considered the provider's nonverbal communication such as tone, attitude, and body language as important components of the encounter.
- *Connection* represents a link, a relationship between persons that remedied patient feelings of being alone. Connection invited expressions of faith and shared prayer and served as an acknowledgment that the patient was worthy of attention and respect. One patient described how nurses and doctors would pray with her—they wanted her to recover and not be sad.
- *Care* that is authentic along with the perception of attentiveness of staff and behaviors that build trust have long been components of a nurse–patient relationship. Mexican-born (traditional) participants had more trust in their providers when patient–provider dialogues with personable discussions occurring before clinical affairs were discussed. The friendliness and the way in which the women were talked to by their provider were considered the most important components of patient-centered care.

Clinical Implications

- When patients have positive hospital experiences with their providers, they leave the hospital receptive to clinical guidance, which leads to better quality health outcomes and decreased morbidity and mortality.
- Many hospitals and educational staff focus their efforts on the clinical aspects of care but neglect the communication competencies that establish and enhance the nurse–patient relationship. Focusing on the emotional needs of patients, customer service, and communication skills will support nurse–patient relationships.
- Concerted efforts to understand the healthcare experience of patients can affect clinical practice, research, and policy and improve care delivery for historically marginalized populations.

Reference: Cuizon, S. G. & Fry-Bowers, E. K. (2022). The patient care experience as perceived by Hispanic Patients with chronic illness undergoing transplant: A grounded theory. *Advances in Nursing Science, 45*(4),335–350. https://doi.org/10.1097/ANS.0000000000000429

and co-occurring concepts. These concepts are Comfort, Communication, Connection, and Care. Hispanic patients had more trust in their providers when patient–provider dialogues with personable discussions (omit occurred) before clinical affairs were discussed. This study was conducted with Hispanic patients and cannot be generalized to other populations.

Many factors influence the likelihood that clients, families, and communities will maintain traditional health beliefs and practices. For example, the length of time a person lives in the new host country will influence factors such as language and the use of media (e.g., radio, television, and computers). Teenagers may quickly adjust to American culture and begin to use a smartphone or an iPad and use the translation services on these devices to communicate with each other or their new American friends. The ability to understand and communicate with members of the majority culture is crucial to beginning to feel comfortable.

Generally, children acculturate more quickly because they are exposed to their peer group at school and they learn cultural characteristics through that association. The need to work outside the household often exposes women from traditional cultures to others of the majority culture; thus, they learn English more quickly than if they remain isolated at home. When individuals from other cultures seek healthcare in their host country, they become familiar with its healthcare system. This does not necessarily mean that they adhere to all health advice, but contact with the system decreases anxiety and confusion, and individuals are more likely to seek care again. In addition, if individuals or groups have distinguishing ethnic characteristics, such as skin color, they may be more isolated because of discrimination and thus retain traditional values, beliefs, and practices over a longer time. Some factors that influence the likelihood that clients, families, and communities will maintain traditional health beliefs and practices are shown in Box 11-2.

BOX 11-2 | Some Factors Influencing Traditional Beliefs and Practices

1. Length of time in the new host country.
2. Size of the ethnic or cultural group with which an individual identifies and interacts.
3. Age of the individual. As a general rule, children acculturate more rapidly than do adults or seniors.
4. Ability to speak English and communicate with members of the majority culture. Language spoken in the home among family members.
5. Economic status. For example, if an immigrant woman who has a work visa works outside the home, she may learn English more quickly than if she remains within the household and speaks only Spanish with her family members.
6. Educational status. In general, higher levels of education lead to faster acculturation.
7. Health status of family members. If individuals and their families seek healthcare in their host country, they begin to "learn the system." This does not mean that they accept all of the health advice, but contacts with the system should decrease anxiety and confusion.
8. Distinguishing ethnic characteristics, such as skin color. These individuals may be more isolated because of discrimination and thus may retain traditional values related to health beliefs and behavior.
9. Rigidity or flexibility of the host society. This refers to the extent to which the host society is willing to allow members of different ethnic groups, along with their traditions, beliefs, and practices, into their structure, culture, and identity.

Access to Health and Nursing Care for Diverse Cultural Groups

Members of diverse cultural groups, especially those with low incomes and without health insurance, face special problems in accessing health and nursing care. Access to care is often determined by economic and geographic factors. Certain cultural groups have faced discrimination and poverty, and their ability to access care has been compromised. Sensitivity to cultural factors has often been lacking in the healthcare of traditional communities and identified minority groups.

In addition to economic status and discriminatory factors that limit access to care, geographic location plays an important role in healthcare. Many medically underserved areas lack medical personnel and the variety of health facilities and services that are available to urban populations. For example, Native Americans living in sparsely settled and isolated reservations in the western part of the United States must travel long distances, sometimes over primitive roads, to obtain healthcare services. Individuals who live on the Navajo or Hopi reservations in northern Arizona and have type 2 diabetes or kidney failure requiring dialysis must travel long distances for care. They may be picked up as early as 4 a.m. by a shuttle van that takes them into Tuba City, AZ, for renal dialysis; the van takes them home later in the afternoon. Depending on the route and weather conditions, some individuals may arrive home as late as 5 or 6 p.m. having spent up to 8 hours per day in travel time plus the time required for dialysis. This arduous routine may take place as often as 3 days each week.

Other factors that may also limit access and use of healthcare services include the following:

- Clients from may be hesitant to seek the services of healthcare professionals who do not speak their language.
- Undocumented persons may be reluctant to seek healthcare because they are afraid of revealing their immigration status.
- Women from traditional Muslim cultures may be reluctant to seek care from male healthcare providers.
- Lack of understanding by clients of how to use health resources may deter them from seeking care.

Nurses can develop sensitivity to diverse groups within communities and reach out to them with culturally specific health programs. Box 11-3 lists some important factors that nurses

---

BOX 11-3   Factors to Consider in the Nursing Care of Culturally Diverse Groups

1. Employment opportunities and insurance coverage or the financial ability to pay for healthcare services.
2. Different traditional belief systems as well as different norms and values.
3. Lack of understanding, provider bias, and lack of trust on the part of social service and healthcare workers.
4. Lack of bilingual personnel or staff members or the lack of interpreters to assist clients and care providers.
5. Rapid changes in the U.S. healthcare system, where clients are "lost" in the gaps between agencies and services.
6. Inconvenient locations or hours of health and social services that preclude clients from accessing care.
7. Lack of understanding, trust, and commitment on the part of healthcare providers.
8. The Social Determinants of Health as defined by *Healthy People 2030*. They are economic stability, educational access and quality, healthcare access and quality, neighborhood and built environment, and social and community context (Office of Disease Prevention and Health Promotion (gov), n.d.).

must take into account for culturally appropriate community-based care.

Cultural Concepts in Disaster Preparedness

The roles and responsibilities of nurses in global and domestic crises are increasingly diverse. Since September 11, 2001, and the **COVID-19** pandemic, there has been an increased interest on the part of health professionals in **disaster preparedness**: examining how well we are prepared to function when faced with terrorism, pandemics, and other emergencies. This interest has only increased with the now frequent climate-related wildfires, floods, hurricanes, and droughts. Nurses, like other healthcare professionals, can make certain that **emergency response plans** in healthcare agencies and community settings are in order, are updated regularly, and that appropriate staff and community members know the emergency and disaster protocols.

The COVID-19 pandemic has revealed in stark detail the critical importance of having a national nursing workforce prepared with the knowledge, skills, and abilities to respond to these events. COVID-19 has revealed shocking chasms within our healthcare system, resulting in excess morbidity and mortality, glaring health inequities, and the inability to contain a rapidly escalating **pandemic**. Individuals and communities of color suffered from the disadvantages of racism, poverty, workplace hazards, limited healthcare access, and other factors that severely restricted their abilities to respond to the pandemic. Knowing in advance what is expected of us will provide an opportunity to acquire pertinent knowledge to practice the skills beforehand. There are four areas of emergency and disaster management defined by Shoaf and Rottman (2000). They are preparedness, mitigation, response, and recovery.

Preparedness

As Benjamin Franklin once said, "By failing to prepare, you are preparing to fail." Community-based nurses can demonstrate readiness to apply their skills from early planning stages for emergency events through long-term recovery, effectively responding to the needs of the population with culturally appropriate interventions. Nurses who work in community settings are familiar with the communities they serve; they know the community leaders, the church networks, and the healthcare providers who provide care to underserved communities. Nurses can use cultural concepts to work within community networks helping clients, families, and communities prepare for disasters and/or other emergencies.

Community-based nurses can begin by talking with clients and their families about developing an emergency plan for an evacuation from natural disasters, public health emergencies, or other crises. For example, it is always good idea for an identified family member to make certain that the family car always has at least half a tank of gas. Families should have a list of items to take with them if they must leave their home quickly. All family members should know where this list is kept and who is responsible for retrieving each item on that list. The emergency plan should be developed and discussed with consideration of the needs of each family. Each family member should have an opportunity to practice or describe their role in the emergency plan. Community nurses are the health professionals who frequently interact with underserved or high-risk communities in homes, health clinics, or other healthcare settings. For example, it is estimated that 12 million undocumented persons are living in the United States. Do migrant or mixed status families have a plan to respond if parents or other main caregivers are arrested at work by immigration officials? Who should the children contact? A neighbor? A pastor? Another relative? Talking about and planning for this possibility will decrease the anxiety and untoward effects of such an event.

Community-based nurses also know the high-risk groups in the community. For example, they can contact staff in assisted care facilities to discuss evacuation plans for patients with functional needs who live in care facilities. Nurses can work with refugee agencies to provide classes for emergency evacuation for recently arrived refugees as well as protecting the well-being of other underserved populations, striving for health equity, and advocating for those who are at risk when responding to a crises, natural disasters, or other health emergencies.

Mitigation

Community nurses can help to assure that plans for all major categories of emergencies respect the culture of the community and/or populations involved. They can identify and plan for ethical and cultural issues that may arise during a disaster. During the COVID pandemic, some families were unable to be at the bedside of a dying family member who was confined to an assisted care facility. Photos of grieving family members holding cell phones for a videoconference with a dying family member were widely circulated during this time. Caring appropriately for a patient who is dying in a care facility and their family during a pandemic or any other crisis that calls for an evacuation is a discussion that should be ongoing. In addition, community nurses can help to educate those persons who might be "vaccine hesitant," thus decreasing the risk for infections as well as counseling and supporting clients to alleviate fear and anxiety during a pandemic (Veenema et al., 2020).

Response

Nurses demonstrate leadership by working with leaders, both formal and informal, in diverse communities. Leadership means reaching out and building relationships with individuals of diverse cultures. Different cultural groups may have different ways of negotiation and resolving conflict. It is imperative that nurses discuss, understand, and build these relationships before a disaster or mass casualty event occurs. Nurses can identify cultural issues that may affect an individual's or community response to disasters or other emergencies. They are at the forefront in providing clinical care and medications; they

can assess and triage victims; allocate scarce resources; and monitor ongoing physical and mental health needs. In a community setting, nurses can work with community leaders to open and manage shelters, organize blood drives, and provide outreach to underserved populations (Heagele, 2017). They may also assist with the care of older adults with health needs (Heagele & Pacqiao, 2018; Kleier et al., 2018), assist with childbirth to ensure that pregnant people have healthy babies during a disaster (Badakhsh et al., 2010), and work to reunite families who have been separated during the disaster or other crises.

As an example, leaders of the Navajo Nation say their strategies have become a model for fighting the COVID-19 pandemic. At the beginning of the pandemic, the Navajo Nation made national news, first because of how hard it was hit, then because of how seriously leaders took the threat of COVID-19. The infection rate among Diné (Navajo people) was aggravated by several issues, including chronic illnesses, food and water insecurity, and a lack of electricity among a third of households. Many Diné live in homes with extended families where COVID-19 can spread quickly. Diné families had to endure more curfews than any other group of people in the United States. The Navajo Nation instituted a 57-hour weekend lockdown from Friday evening to Monday morning, as well as nightly curfews beginning at 8 p.m. or 9 p.m. and ending at 5 a.m. (Becenti, 2022).

Tribal officials worked to give out food and supply boxes and kept everyone informed through weekly town hall sessions broadcast on the Nation's radio stations. Involving tribal outreach organizations was a critical strategy. *Chizh for Cheii* is a reservation-based organization that has been delivering wood to native elders in need during the winters for years. Its workers are recognized and trusted by the people they serve. Tribal officials decided to use *Chizh for Cheii* to deliver emergency food and other supplies to elderly Diné and tribal members who lived in remote areas. To ensure that each of the *Chizh for Cheii* crew members were responsible and did not take any chances, they made a pact with one another to be extra careful, to avoid traveling or going to gatherings, and to stay within their own group. Being extra cautious worked. The Tribal Government emphasized the importance of working closely with public health officials. Early testing and vaccines were emphasized, and this unified response and efforts to keep everyone informed has made a remarkable difference (COVID-19: Disproportionate Impact on Navajo Nation and Tribal Communities, 2020).

Recovery

The recovery period from a disaster or emergency can be prolonged. Examples of recovery activities include preventing or reducing stress-related illnesses and excessive financial burdens, and rebuilding damaged structures. A priority in a disaster such as Hurricane Ian that struck the Ft. Myers area of Florida with such a vengeance in October 2022 was the reestablishment of electricity and water. Damages to homes and structures was substantial and finding shelter was essential in the immediate aftermath. Nurses are often needed at the initial rescue and in the immediate aftermath of a disaster or emergency to administer first aid to injured survivors. In terms of long-term recovery after a disaster or emergency, community nurses have trust and relationships with individuals and local leaders. They also develop a strong understanding of people's experiences, backgrounds, and the social factors that influence health, helping them to incorporate cultural knowledge in their nursing practice. Nurses who have experience in working with vulnerable communities and/or high-risk individuals will be critical to improving health equity and population health (*The Future of Nursing 2020-2030*).

Assessment of Culturally Diverse Communities

A **cultural assessment** is the process used by nurses to assess cultural needs of individual clients (Leininger, 1991, 1995) (see Appendix A). In general, the purpose of all successful cultural

assessments is to collect information that helps health professionals better understand and address the specific health needs and interests of their target populations. Individual cultural assessments are accomplished through the use of a systematic process. In community health nursing, the community is considered the client, and several models have been proposed to help nurses assess the community (Rector, 2022), including the Andrews/Boyle Transcultural Nursing Assessment Guide for Groups and Communities (Appendix B). A community nursing assessment requires gathering relevant data, interpreting the data (including problem analysis and prioritization), and identifying and implementing intervention activities for community health (Rector & Stanley, 2022). The community nursing assessment often focuses on a broad goal, such as improvement in the health status of a group of people. It is often the characteristics of people that give each community its uniqueness, and these common characteristics, which influence norms, values, religious practices, educational aspirations, and health and illness behaviors, are frequently determined by shared cultural experiences. Thus, including the cultural component to a community nursing assessment strengthens the assessment base. Box 11-4 provides basic principles underlying all cultural assessments.

Cultural Competence in Health Maintenance and Health Promotion

Leininger (1978, 1995) suggested that cultural groups have their own culturally defined ways of maintaining and promoting health. Nursing interventions to improve the health of individuals, groups, and communities can best be planned and implemented by evaluating persons within their social, cultural, and environmental contexts (Adams-Leander, 2022).

Community nurses, who have direct access to clients in the context of their daily lives, should be especially aware of the importance of cultural knowledge in promoting and maintaining health, because the promotion and maintenance

BOX 11-4	Basic Principles of Cultural Assessments

1. All cultures must be viewed in the context in which they have developed. Cultural practices develop as a "logical" or understandable response to a particular human problem, and the setting as well as the problem must be considered. This is one reason why environmental and/or contextual data are so important.

2. The meaning and purpose of the behavior must be interpreted within the context of the specific culture. For example, a Guatemalan client's refusal to take a "hot" medication with a cold liquid is understandable if the nurse is aware that many Central American and Mexican American clients adhere to hot/cold theories of illness causation. There is often a range or spectrum of illness beliefs, with one end encompassing illnesses defined within the biomedical model and the other end firmly anchored within the individual culture. The more widely disparate the differences between the biomedical model and the beliefs within the cultural group, the greater the potential for encountering resistance to biomedical interventions.

3. There is such a phenomenon as intracultural variation. Not every member of a cultural group displays all the behaviors that are associated with that group. For instance, not every Central American or Mexican American client will adhere to hot/cold theories of illness or disease. It is only by careful appraisal of the assessment data, and validation of the nurse's assessment with the client and family, that culturally competent care can be provided (Ellis & Purnell, 2021).

of health occurs in the context of everyday lives rather than in the doctor's office or in a hospital. The range of cultural, historical, and social influences on health maintenance and promotion is considerable. Major cultural considerations must be addressed before health maintenance and promotion programs are implemented for culturally diverse groups. To illustrate this, Evidence-Based Practice 11-4 describes a study that sought to understand what matters to Chinese older adults in relation to well-being, quality of life, and life satisfaction. A core theme (Cultural Foundations) emerged that informed the categorical themes and involved participants maintaining some elements of their homeland and traditional culture while facing different challenges in a new country.

Cultural competence in community settings begins with anticipatory planning. In addressing cultural traditions and values, it is important to involve local community leaders and others who are members of the cultural group to promote the acceptance of health promotion programs. Such a leader, for example, might be the pastor of an African American church in the rural south or a member of the tribal council for a Native American tribe. The nurse must also be sensitive to cultural differences in leadership styles. For example, African American pastors may not speak in favor of the health education program from their pulpit, choosing instead to work through more informal networks. Zuniga et al., 2018 found that many African Americans rely on spirituality and/or religious practices when they are ill, and in general, a health program that has the support of the church pastor would be viewed favorably by the church community. In addition to local community and religious leaders, it is important to involve those who are most affected by the specific health problem in the planning process. Those involved in planning and participating in the health program's activities should likewise participate in its evaluation. Forming partnerships and building coalitions is the key to success in community-based health programs (Ervin & Flagg, 2022).

What Matters Most to Older Chinese Adults

Challenges are faced by older Chinese adults as newcomers or immigrants to North America, specifically Canada. Using interpretive description and phenomenology methods, the authors explored the lived experience of older Chinese adults over the age of 70, in two Canadian cities.

The main purpose of this study was to explore what matters to Chinese older adults in relation to well-being, quality of life, and life satisfaction. Eleven participants were interviewed for this study. All self-identified as having Chinese heritage, were age 70 or older, and lived independently in a Canadian city. Interviews were conducted in either Mandarin or Cantonese, questions were presented to the participants in advance, and efforts were undertaken to ensure that the interview's content was correctly interpreted. A core theme and four categorical themes were identified from the data analysis.

Core Theme: Cultural Foundations

Participants identified the importance of their culture and often referred to ways they had lived before immigrating to Canada. Cultural foundations included dietary preferences and lifestyle choices that bring comfort, family values, and general "ways of being" with others. This core theme informs the findings of the study.

Theme One: It's the Little Things That Matter

This theme explains the complexity of Chinese older adults integrating everyday activities into their lives in Canada. The language gap addresses the impact of English as an additional language on a sense of control and confidence in making everyday life decisions. One woman was concerned because the language gap in health needs prevented her from saying the English term for her illness. She wondered how she could discuss her health problem with health professionals because she could not say it.

Having culturally congruent activities in their daily life was important to the participants as they chose activities to participate in and informed where they sought information. One participant played mah-jongg (a traditional Chinese game) every night on her laptop. An older gentleman described how he watched Chinese media to learn the daily news. English-speaking media was used to "learn English." Participants spoke of seeking a balance between Eastern cultural attachments while living in Western living arrangements as the participants lived in their own dwellings away from their grown children. They sought support from their grown children as needed.

Theme Two: Making the Best Out of Life

Participants were resilient in making the best of their circumstances. As their lives unfolded, they made meaning of their circumstances and events through cultural philosophies. The philosophy of the "Five Olds" refers to the importance of having money, a partner/spouse, friends, a home, and health in one's life. This included having an "old partner" so spouses can take care of each other. Old people must have a healthy body and an "old home" or a place to live as well as "old money" and "old friends."

Theme Three: We Take Care of Each Other

This theme shows the participants' appreciation of relationships and social support networks. The strength of the spousal relation was especially valued and having connections with neighbors contributed to a sense of safety, assistance, and support when needed.

Theme Four: The Need to Understand

This theme refers to the desire for knowledge, learning, and growth that provides a foundation for surviving and thriving within a new country. Some participants spoke of how Canada's government helped new immigrants adjust to their new environment. Others related that they had attended seminars to learn how to prepare their taxes and in general took opportunities to learn new things. One woman expressed a desire to "try things that she

What Matters Most to Older Chinese Adults (continued)

had never got to do before: dancing, cooking, and learning English."

Clinical Implications

- Helping older clients maintain some element of their country of origin while facing the difficult challenges in a new country builds a sense of resilience and willingness to face on-going challenges. Listening and asking about their previous experiences is very important to older clients. The strong sense of hope for health, security, and relationships demonstrated a sense of well-being that should be encouraged by health professionals.
- Older clients wish to linguistically understand the new healthcare system and how to maximize and maintain health. Confidence in accessing and using healthcare leads to better quality

outcomes both physically and mentally, thus decreasing morbidities.
- Older clients should be assisted to incorporate a person-centered culturally congruent approach. For example, health information needs to be in the Chinese language and ideally healthcare providers fluent in Mandarin or Cantonese would be available at health facilities.
- Nurses and other healthcare providers should develop an understanding that most immigrants have a desire to integrate into the new society, but they need the culturally familiar tools to assist them to access and use a complex healthcare system.

Reference: Shan Choi, L. L., Jung, P., & Zang, K. (2022). What matters most to older Chinese adults. *Journal of Transcultural Nursing*, *33*(2), 169–177. https://doi.org/10.1177/10436596211053655

Second, family members, churches, employers, and community worksites need to be involved in supporting health promotion/education programs using networks that already exist. For example, a health education program about the importance of having a routine screening such as a mammography can be established at a worksite that employs mostly women. A display could be set up in the cafeteria, dining room, or other accessible site. Women could view the educational material during breaks or after lunch. Providing information about sites where women could obtain a mammography would be an important component of such a program.

Third, health messages are more readily accepted if they do not conflict with existing cultural beliefs. A nurse who plans to talk about prevention of teenage pregnancy to parents and adolescents at a local church, should be sensitive to the group's religious values and norms. The nurse could discuss these plans in advance with some of the parents and the church leaders and ask for

ways to strengthen the church's position, such as the support of abstinence programs. This is the time to be sensitive to the group's religious values.

Fourth, language barriers and cultural differences can present challenges to healthcare providers. For example, in the United States–Mexico border areas, *promotoras* (community health workers) are used to disseminate messages in Spanish and to help organize and present information that is culturally appropriate and understood by community members (Cummins, 2020; McEwen et al., 2015). Many Native American tribes make use of community health representatives to assist individuals to improve their health and/or access care. (Prue-Owens, 2021a, 2021b). The healthcare professional should ask for help and suggestions in finding suitable educational material such as brochures or videos in the appropriate language and with a culturally acceptable message.

Last, **cultural sensitivity**, the ability to be aware of the needs and emotions of others, is essential to meeting health needs. HIV/AIDS is spreading and may be associated with intravenous drug use. Culturally relevant drug treatment programs should be implemented that address both the drug use problems and HIV/AIDS which can be associated with intravenous drug use. However, people seeking treatment programs for cocaine addiction may encounter barriers that seem insurmountable. Treatment programs may not be available in many areas, and childcare facilities may not be provided, even in day-treatment programs. Thus, persons living in a rural area with children may not be able to find a treatment center that meets their needs. If they seek admittance to a residential treatment program, they might have to agree to place their children in foster care.

The Future of Nursing 2020-2030 suggests that promoting health and well-being has been an essential role of nurses—they are bridge builders and collaborators who engage and connect with people, communities, and organizations to ensure people from all backgrounds have what they need to be healthy and well. (*The Future of Nursing 2020-2030: Charting a Path to Achieve Health Equity*).

Family Systems

Because the family is the basic social unit, it provides the context in which health promotion and maintenance are defined and carried out. The nurse can recognize and use the family's role in altering the health status of a family member and in supporting lifestyle changes. This requires an appreciation of the role of the family in healthcare. A family's problem-solving techniques are used to address health issues, including health promotion, and chronic and terminal illness. Immigrant and refugee families also tend to have strong extended ties with their kin, and changes in lifestyle, diet, and other established patterns of daily life that influence health status will need the understanding and support of all family members.

Coping Behaviors

Clients often have distinct, culturally based behaviors to cope with illness as well as to maintain and promote health. These behaviors may be traced to the health–illness paradigms discussed in Chapter 4. Beliefs about hot and cold, yin and yang, and harmony and balance may underlie actions to prevent disease and maintain health. Community nurses must understand their clients' cultural values and beliefs to correctly assess clients' understanding of health and illness. These assessment data serve as the basis for planning health guidance and teaching strategies that incorporate cultural beliefs and practices in the nursing care plan. It seems likely that clients in the process of coping with illness and seeking help may involve a network of persons, ranging from family members and select laypersons, as well as healthcare professionals.

Seeking social support is often a means of coping. Social support varies widely across people, cultural groups, and circumstances. An individual's coping behaviors during a personal or family member illness may differ remarkably over the course of time from diagnosis until resolution depending on intrapersonal, interpersonal, and environmental factors. Nurses working with diverse cultural populations understand how coping styles are used by individuals and family members and how they are often influenced by culture.

Lifestyle Practices

Lifestyle is the typical way of life of an individual, group, or culture. Cultural influences that shape lifestyles have a significant impact on such health-promoting practices as diet, exercise, and stress management. Community health nurses should assess the implications of diet planning and teaching for clients and family members who adhere to culturally prescribed practices concerning foods.

Some cultural groups believe that certain foods maintain or promote health. Specific foods often are restricted or promoted during illness, for example, the proverbial chicken soup. Cultural preferences determine the style of food preparation and consumption, the frequency of eating, the time of eating, and the eating utensils. Milk is not always considered a suitable source of protein for Native Americans, Hispanics, African Americans, and some Asians because of their relatively high incidence of lactose intolerance (Mayo Clinic, 2022).

When working with clients from a different culture, nurses must evaluate patterns of daily living as well as culturally prescribed activities before they suggest forms of physical activity or exercise to clients. Not everyone has access to a tennis court or a gym, and many individuals would not feel comfortable in such surroundings, or in aerobics classes regardless of the setting. Helping clients plan physical activities that are culturally acceptable is an important first step in implementing a program of physical activity for clients in diverse cultures. For example, traditional tribal dancing has become popular on some reservations for Native Americans. Running remains popular for members of the Hopi tribe. Running is deeply rooted in Hopi traditions as a way to carry messages from village to village and is also prominent in Hopi ceremonies. In the past, men of the Hopi tribe were superb distance runners, and the tribe still sponsors running events for its members. Hopi High School located on the Hopi reservation in Arizona has earned 27 consecutive team championships state cross-country titles in a row and is well known throughout the state for its excellent track teams (Perry, 2021).

Another aspect of lifestyle that must be understood for the successful promotion of health and wellness is the manner in which clients manage stress. Stress management is learned from childhood through our parents, our social group, and our cultural group. Smoking, chewing tobacco, and consuming alcoholic beverages and/or drugs, although not healthy habits, are often used to manage stress. Although these practices are not associated with a group's culture *per se*, they are often found in groups

whose members feel that they do not have other options or alternatives based on economic or challenges related to access to appropriate care.

Evidence-Based Practice 11-5 presents a study that describes how homeless individuals have difficulty accessing care and often have poor health outcomes that are compounded by social and economic factors, such as housing insecurity, unemployment, and limited social support. The housing needs of homeless individuals are best contextualized by their health and social needs. Health providers must consider the priorities of homeless individuals to develop culturally congruent services that are appropriate and effective care for this population.

The nurse may find that in some cultural groups, such as Mexican Americans, traditional healers, such as *curanderos*, can be helpful for persons with some emotional or psychological disorders. It has been a tradition for many Mexican Americans to seek care from traditional healers (Zoucha & Zamarripa-Zoucha, 2021). This lifestyle practice or health-seeking behavior seems "appropriate" and the right thing to do, whereas seeking care from a psychiatrist for emotional or psychological disorders would be a highly unlikely behavior. In some aggregate ethnic settings, such as the Chinatown area in San Francisco, there are practitioners of traditional Chinese medicine as well as mainstream U.S. medicine, acupuncturists, neighborhood pharmacies, and herbalists, all of which are available to meet the diverse needs of that particular neighborhood. Lifestyle is about the parts of our lives that make us feel comfortable and "right with the world." It's how we make our homes, relate to our loved ones, raise our children, and manage our health and the well-being of those around us. Feeling comfortable with a healthcare provider's office may depend on the healthcare provider sharing the same ethnic heritage or at least speaking the language of the client as well as having visual materials such as posters, magazines, and videos in languages appropriate for many of their clients.

Experiences of Adult Men Who Are Homeless Accessing Care: A Qualitative Study

This study described the perceptions of individuals experiencing homelessness, related to their health and experiences accessing care. They experienced difficulties accessing care and poor health outcomes compounded by social and economic factors, such as housing insecurity, unemployment, and limited social support. Individuals who are homeless report increased rates of chronic physical and mental health conditions, including cardiovascular disease, mental illness, and substance use disorders. Despite increased morbidity rates, these individuals have difficulty accessing primary and specialty care services and emergency departments are their most accessible source of care. Some authors have argued that homelessness, using transcultural theory, can be viewed as a culture based on the shared beliefs, norms, and patterns of living that exist among homeless populations. Three important themes emerged in this study.

Theme 1: Men Who Are Homeless Experience Bias Throughout Their Healthcare and Interpersonal Relationships

Participants reported that some providers speak down to them and seem to have negative attitudes toward them because they are homeless. They explained that this perceived disrespect dissuades them from seeking care when necessary, even in urgent situations. Participants described inappropriate interactions because they lived in a homeless shelter. This affected their likelihood of seeking care instead opting to self-treat until their symptoms became unmanageable and then they would present at the emergency department.

Theme 2: The Best Care Is Person Centered and Considers Patients' Priorities

Participants wanted person-centered care focusing on their individual needs that increased their function and independence. They wanted the healthcare system to provide care that matched their culture, priorities, and lifestyle. Participants wanted care that addressed their presenting problem and considered issues such as spirituality, family issues, daily activities, and mental well-being. Functionality was one of the most important priorities for the participants in this study. Patients said negative experiences had driven them to seek episodic care at emergency departments.

Theme 3: Care Coordination Resources Are Inadequate

Many participants identified care coordination issues as either a limiting or facilitating factor in their receiving healthcare. They wanted assistance in coordinating care and navigating the healthcare system. Participants with various chronic diseases and conditions including hepatitis C, diabetes, asthma, and cardiac disease. These diseases require care from a multidisciplinary team; but working with such teams was very difficult. They wanted care that was a positive transaction toward their individual goals but reported that they did not receive the care they wanted. A central location was important to those without a stable home location.

"Access to Care is Limited by Insurance Accepted by Providers, Transportation, and Appointment Availability" was also identified as an important sub-theme. Several factors, including health insurance, transportation, and availability of appointments, were identified as barriers to care with health insurance being the most frequently named barrier. Although all individuals in the study had health insurance through a public program, they still had problems finding providers who accepted their insurance coverage.

Transportation was another factor that affected access to care for the participants. Access to public transportation or difficulties of using a van for individuals with disabilities negatively affecting their ability to receive care. A final factor was the availability of an appointment at times that

Experiences of Adult Men Who Are Homeless Accessing Care: A Qualitative Study (continued)

did not affect other appointment times such as case management, employment, or other provider appointments.

Clinical Implications

- Care plans need to be framed in a culturally relevant context and meet individual needs. Such an approach to care provides a framework for addressing the challenges presented by **social determinants of health**.
- Healthcare providers must recognize the complex health and social needs, such as housing insecurity, food insecurity, unemployment, and limited social support experienced by homeless individuals.

- Improving access to care for homeless populations will also require multifaceted changes to care delivery, care coordination, and state and federal health policies. One possible solution might be through community health workers who share demographic similarities with the populations they serve and are specially trained to help clients navigate the complexities of the healthcare system and facilitate care deliveries consistent with the population's values and needs.

Reference: Henderson, M., McCurry, I., Deatrick, J., & Lipman, T. (2022). Experiences of adult men who are homeless accessing care: A qualitative study. *Journal of Transcultural Nursing,* 33(2), 199–207. https://doi.org/10.1177/10436596211057895

Summary

Cultural concepts related to community nursing practice serve as a guide or framework for nurses who work with different cultural groups within a community. Nurses use cultural knowledge in assessing, planning, implementing, and evaluating nursing care. This chapter addressed cultural diversity of clients, families, and communities. Various subcultures, including refugees, asylees, and immigrants, and others were described to help nurses understand and become comfortable working with these groups in community settings.

Cultural concepts as they relate to the community at large will help nurses plan care for individuals, families, and communities. A cultural assessment is an integral component of a community nursing assessment (see Appendix B). Culturally competent nursing interventions ensure health maintenance and health promotion at a community level. Preventive care in the community has been a traditional aspect of

community-based nursing. Community nurses work collaboratively with other team members to address the needs of population groups. New collaborative efforts include disaster preparedness in homes, healthcare facilities, and the workplace.

REVIEW QUESTIONS

1. Describe four cultural concepts and discuss how they can be used to provide transcultural nursing care to families and community aggregates.
2. Describe an example of how cultural factors influence the health of an aggregate group within the community.
3. List the major cultural considerations in implementing preventive programs for culturally diverse groups. How can cultural considerations be used to identify barriers and facilitators for preventive programs?
4. Identify special health considerations in immigrant groups within the community.

5. Describe similarities and differences between folk and scientific healthcare systems. Give an example of each.

CRITICAL THINKING ACTIVITIES

Describe the impact of social determinants of health for a cultural group within your community. Evaluate the access to, availability of, and acceptability of various healthcare services. Is this cultural group at risk? Why?

1. Conduct a community cultural assessment of a group within your community. Critically analyze the cultural knowledge and/or information that should be considered when planning care for the group. Use Appendix B to identify and collect cultural assessment data—family and kinship, social life, political systems, language, worldview, religious behaviors, health beliefs and practices, and health concerns. Compare and contrast the assessment of other groups in your community.

2. Attend religious services at a church, temple, mosque, synagogue, or place of worship to learn about a religion different from your own. How does the church meet the unique needs of its congregation?

3. Identify alternative healthcare practitioners within your community. Which subcultures do they serve? Describe the kinds of care that they offer to community residents.

REFERENCES

Adams-Leander, S. (2022). Transcultural nursing. In C. Rector & M. J. Stanley (Eds.), *Community and public health nursing: Promoting the public's health* (10th ed., pp. 95–119). Wolter Kluwer.

Andrews, M. M., & Boyle, J. S. (Eds.) (2016). *Transcultural concepts in nursing care* (8th ed.). Wolters Kluwer.

Ayón, C. (2018). "Vivimos en Jaula de Oro": The impact of state-level legislation on immigrant Latino families. *Journal of Immigrant & Refugee Studies, 16*(4), 351–371. https://doi.org/10.1080/15562948.2017.1306151

Badakhsh, R., Harville, E., & Banerjee, B. (2010). The childbearing experience during a natural disaster. *Journal of Obstetric, Gynecologic, & Neonatal Nursing, 39*(4), 489–497.

Becenti, A. D. (2022, March 24). *After a 'scary' beginning, Navajo leaders say their COVID-19 response has become a model.* AZ Central. https://www.azcentral.com/story/news/local/arizona/2022/03/24/navajo-nation-leaders-say-their-covid-19-response-has-worked/7123587001

Betancourt, T. S., Newnham, E. A., Birman, D., Lee, R., Ellis, B. H., & Layne, C. M. (2017). Comparing trauma exposure, mental health needs, and service utilization across clinical samples of refugee, immigrant, and U.S.-origin children. *Journal of Traumatic Stress, 30*(3), 209–218. https://doi.org/10.1002/jts.22186

COVID-19 Disproportionate Impact on Navajo National and Tribal Communities. (2020). County Health Rankings & Roadmaps. https://www.countyhealthrankings.org/online-and-on-air/webinars/covid-19-disproportionate-impact-on-navajo-nation-and-tribal-communities#:~:text=The%20Navajo%20Nation%20has%20long,rates%20in%20the%20United%20States

Cummins, D. (2020). Planning, implementing, and evaluating community/public health programs. In C. Rector & M. J. Stanley (Eds.), *Community and public health nursing* (10th ed., pp. 416–422). Wolters Kluwer.

Ellis, T. A., & Purnell, L. D. (2021). People of Guatemalan heritage. In L. D. Purnell & E. Fenkl (Eds.), *Textbook for transcultural health care: a population approach* (5th ed., pp. 445–467). Springer.

Ervin, N. E., & Flagg, L. N. (2022). Community as client. In C. Rector & M. J. Stanley (Eds.), *Community and public health nursing* (10th ed., pp. 416–422). Wolters Kluwer.

The Future of Nursing 2020-2030: Charting a path to achieve health equity. https://www.nap.edu/catalog/12956/the/future/of/nursing-leading-change-advancing-health

Gainsbury, S. M. (2017). Cultural competence in the treatment of addictions: Theory, practice and evidence. *Clinical Psychology & Psychotherapy, 24*(4), 987–1001. https://doi.org/10.1002/cpp.2062

Gaynor, T. (2015, October 23). *UNHCR concerned at reports of sexual violence against refugee women and children.* Retrieved July 20, 2023 from https://www.unhcr.org/us/news/stories/unhcr-concerned-reports-sexual-violence-against-refugee-women-and-children

Golub, N., Seplaki, C., Stockman, D., Thevenet-Morrison, K., Fernandez, D., & Fisher, S. (2018). Impact of length of residence in the United States on risk of diabetes and hypertension in resettled refugees. *Journal of Immigrant and Minority Health, 20*(2), 296–306. https://doi.org/10.1007/s10903-017-0636-y

Heagele, T. (2017). Disaster-related community resilience: A concept analysis and a call to action for nurses. *Public Health Nursing, 34*(3), 295–302.

Heagele, T., & Pacqiao, D. (2018). Disaster vulnerability of elderly and medically frail populations. *Health and Emergency and Disaster Nursing, 6*(1), 50–61. https://doi.org/10.24298/hedn.2016-0009

Healthy People 2000. (1991). *National health promotion and disease prevention objectives.* U.S. Department of Health & Human Services.

Healthy People 2030. (2030). *National health promotion and disease prevention objectives.* Centers for Disease Control and Prevention. https://health.gov>healthypeople

Igielnik, R., & Krogstad, J. (2017, February 3). Where refugees to the U. S. come from. *Fact tank news in the numbers.* http://www.pewresearch.org/fact-tank/2017/02/03/where-refugees-to-the-U-S-come-from/

Institute of Medicine. (2011). *The future of nursing: leading change, advancing health.* The National Academic Press. https://www.ncbi.nlm.nih.gov/books/NBK209880

Kleier, J. A., Krause, D., & Ogilby, T. (2018). Hurricane preparedness among elderly residents in South Florida. *Public Health Nursing, 35*(1), 3–9.

Krogstad, J. (2017). *Key facts about refugees to the U.S.* http://www.pewresearch.org/AUTHOR/JRADFORD/

Leininger, M. (1978). *Transcultural nursing: Concepts, theories and practice.* John Wiley & Sons.

Leininger, M. (1991). Leininger's acculturation health care assessment tool for cultural patterns in traditional and non-traditional lifeways. *Journal of Transcultural Nursing, 2*(2), 40–42. https://www.ncbi.nlm.nih.gov/pubmed/2043295

Leininger, M. (1995). *Transcultural nursing: Concepts, theories, research and practice.* McGraw-Hill.

Mayo Clinic. (2022). https://www.mayoclinic.org/diseases-conditions/lactose-intolerance/symptoms-causes/syc-20374232

McEwen, M., Boyle, J., & Hilfinger Messias, D. (2015). Undocumentedness and public policy: The impact on communities, individuals, and families along the Arizona/Sonora border. *Nursing Outlook, 63*(1), 77–85. https://doi.org/10.1016/j.outlook.2014.10.009

McGuire, S. (2014). Borders, centers, and margins: Critical landscapes for migrant health. *Advances in Nursing Science, 37*(3), 197–212.

Meffert, S. M., Shome, S., Neylan, T. C., Musalo, K., Fineberg, H. V., Cooke, M. M., Volberding, P. A., & Goosby, E. P. (2016). Health impact of human rights testimony: Harming the most vulnerable? *BMJ Global Health, 1*(1), e000001. https://doi.org/10.1136/bmjgh-2015-000001

Musalo, K., & Lee, E. (2017). Seeking a rational approach to a regional refugee crisis: Lessons from the summer 2014 "Surge" of Central American women and children at the US-Mexico border. *Journal on Migration and Human Security, 5*(1), 137–179. https://doi.org/10.14240/jmhs.v5i1.78

Office of Disease Prevention and Health Promotion (gov). (n.d.) Retrieved from; https://health.gov/healthypeople/priority-areas

Office of Refugee Resettlement (ORR). (2013, 2022). *Revised medical screening guidelines for newly arriving refugees.* Retrieved July 20, 2023 from https://www.acf.hhs.gov/orr/policy-guidance/revised-medical-screening-guidelines-newly-arriving-refugees

Perry, N. (2021, May 10). *Hopi (Arizona) High School's Baker Builds Cross Country Dynasty.* https://nfhs.org/articles/hopi-arizona-high-school-s-baker-builds-cross-country-dynasty

Prue-Owens, K. (2021a). American Indians and Alaskan Natives. In L. D. Purnell & E. A. Fenkl (Eds.), *Textbook for transcultural health care: A population approach* (5th ed., pp. 151–185). Springer.

Prue-Owens, K. (2021b). Indigenous American Indians and Alaska Natives. In L. D. Purnell & E. Fenkl (Eds.), *Textbook for transcultural health care: A population approach* (5th ed., pp. 151–185). Springer. https://doi.org/10.1007/978-3-030-51399-3

Purnell, L. D., & Fenkl, E. (Eds.) (2021). *Textbook for transcultural health care: A population approach* (5th ed.). Springer. https://doi.org/10.1007/978-3-030-51399-3

Rector, C. (2022). The journey begins. Introduction. In C. Rector & M. J. Stanley (Eds.), *Community and public health nursing: Promoting the public's health* (10th ed., pp. 1–23). Wolter Kluwer.

Rector, C., & Stanley, M. J. (2022). *Community and public health nursing* (10th ed.). Wolter Kluwer.

Shawyer, F., Enticott, J. C., Block, A. A., Cheng, I., & Meadows, G. N. (2017). The mental health status of refugees and asylum seekers attending a refugee health clinic including comparisons with a matched sample of Australian-born residents. *BMC Psychiatry, 17*, 76–87. https://doi.org/10.1186/s12888-017-1239-9

Shoaf, K. I., & Rottman, S. J. (2000). The role of public health in disaster preparedness. *Prehospital Disaster Medicine, 15*(4), 144–146.

Spector, R. E. (2013). *Cultural diversity in health and illness* (8th ed.). Pearson.

U.S. Department of Health and Human Services. Office of Minority Health. (n.d.) https://minorityhealth.hhsgov/

United Nations. (2022). UNHCR: A record 100 million people forcibly displaced worldwide. *UN News: Global Perspective Human Stories.* https://news.un.org/en/story/2022/05/1118772

United Nations High Commissioner for Refugees. (2010). *Convention and protocol relating to the status of refugees.* https://www.unhcr.org/media/convention-and-protocol-relating-status-refugees

Veenema, T. G., Meyer, D., Bell, S., Couig, M., Friese, C., Lavin, R., Stanley, J., Martin, E., Montegue, M., Toner, E., Schoch-Spana, M., Cicero, A., Ingelsby, T., Sauer, L., Watson, M., Biddison, L. D., Cicerno, A., & Inglesby, T. (2020). *Recommendations for improving national nurse preparedness for pandemic response: Early lessons from COVID-19.* Johns Hopkins Bloomberg School of Public Health, Center for Health Security.

Weech-Maldonado, R., Dreachslin, J. L., Epane, J. P., Gail, J., Gupta, S., & Wainio, J. A. (2018). Hospital cultural competency as a systematic organizational intervention: Key findings from the national center for healthcare leadership diversity demonstration project. *Health Care Management Review, 43*(1), 30–41. https://doi.org/10.1097/HMR.0000000000000128

Wong, W. C. W., Cheung, S., Miu, H. Y. H., Chen, J., Loper, K. A., & Holroyd, E. (2017). Mental health of African asylum-seekers and refugees in Hong Kong: Using the social determinants of health framework. *BMC Public Health, 17*(1), 153–161. https://doi.org/10.1186/s12889-016-3953-5

Xin, H. (2020). Addressing mental health stigmas among refugees: a narrative review from a socio-ecological perspective. *Universal Journal of Public Health, 8*(2), 57–64. Retrieved July 20, 2023 from http://www.hrpub.org. DOI: 10.13189/ujph.2020.080202

Zoucha, R., & Zamarripa-Zoucha, C. (2021). People of Mexican heritage. In L. D. Purnell & E. Fenkl (Eds.), *Textbook for transcultural health care: A population approach* (5th ed.). Springer. https://doi.org/10.1007/978-3-030-51399-3

Zuniga, J. A., Wright, C., Fordyce, J., West Ohueri, C., & Garcia, A. A. (2018). Self-management of HIV and diabetes in African American women: A systematic review of qualitative literature. *The Diabetes Educator, 44*(5), 419–434. https://doi.org/10.1177/0145721718794879

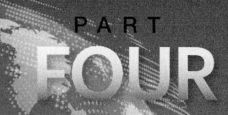

Other Considerations in Culturally Competent Care

Religion, Faith, Culture, and Nursing

• John W. Collins

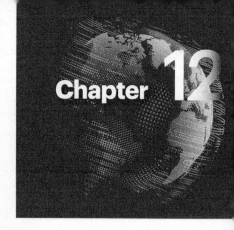

Chapter 19

Key Terms

Allah
Amish
Anointing of the Sick
Bereavement
Brahman
Brit milah
Buddha
Buddhism
Caste system
Catholic
Catholic Charities USA
Christian Science
Church of Jesus Christ of
    Latter-day Saints
Consequential dimension
Enlightenment
Ethnoreligion
Experiential dimension
Faith healing

Fasting
Funeral
Good death
Grief
Hadith
Halal
Health Ministries
Hinduism
Home going
Ideologic dimension
Intellectual dimension
Islam
Jehovah
Jehovah's Witness
Judaism
Karma
Kosher
Mennonites
Mohel
Mourning
Muslim

Nirvana
Ordinances
Pillars of Faith
Principle of totality
Protestantism
Quran (Koran)
Reincarnation
Religion
Ritualistic dimension
Seventh-Day Adventists
Spiritual assessment
Spiritual distress
Spiritual health
Spiritual nursing care
Spirituality
Talmud
Temple garment
Torah
Vedas
Wake
Word of Wisdom

Learning Objectives

1. Explore the meaning of spirituality and religion in the lives of clients across the lifespan.
2. Identify the components of a spiritual needs assessment for clients from diverse cultural backgrounds.
3. Examine the ways in which spiritual and religious beliefs can be incorporated into the nursing care of clients from diverse cultures.
4. Discuss cultural considerations in the nursing care of dying or bereaved clients and families.
5. Describe the health-related beliefs and practices of selected religious groups in North America.

Introduction

As an integral component of culture, religious faith and spiritual beliefs may influence a patient's explanation or understanding of the cause(s) of illness, perception of its severity, decisions about healing interventions, beliefs about healing, and possibly choices about living with chronic or life-limiting (incurable but not eminently terminal) illness. In times of crisis, such as serious illness and impending death, religious faith and spirituality are often a source of hope and inspiration to live each day to its fullest and to enjoy the love of family and friends at a level not previously attained. Faith beliefs and religious traditions also are sources of consolation for the patient and family when a life-limiting or terminal diagnosis is confirmed. A person's faith beliefs and traditions may influence the course of action taken to bring comfort and relational healing, as the patient puts things in order in preparation for death and the afterlife. Acceptance and respect for the patient's and family's values and beliefs will guide culturally appropriate nursing treatment and interventions by the nurse involved in the care of the patient and their family.

The terms faith, religion, religious faith, spiritual beliefs, and spirituality are each unique in definition; however, for the purposes of this chapter, these terms can and will be interchanged for

ease of readability. Definitions and distinctions will be provided where appropriate, while the deeper meanings of these terms will become evident as the reader progresses through the chapter and reflects on their own personal and cultural beliefs of faith, religion, and spirituality.

The first part of this chapter discusses dimensions of religion, religion and spiritual nursing care, religious trends in the United States and Canada, and contributions of religious groups to the healthcare delivery system. The latter half highlights the health-related beliefs and practices of selected religions, which are presented in alphabetical order.

Dimensions of Religion

Religion and spirituality are complex and multifaceted in both form and function. Religious faith and the institutions derived from that faith become a central focus in meeting the human needs of those who believe in the Creator God of Christianity, including Catholicism; EL YHVH (Ye-ho-wah) of Judaism; Allah of Islam; **Brahman** of Hinduism; Brahma of Buddhism, or a non-named Higher Power for those who may believe but not be part of an organized religion. There are many other names for gods of the myriad religious beliefs, sects, and organizations that exist in all parts of the world; this short list is not meant to be comprehensive. The majority of faith traditions address the issues of illness and wellness, disease and healing, and caring and curing (Sorajjakool et al., 2017).

Religious Factors Influencing Human Behavior

First, it is necessary to identify specific religious factors that may influence human behavior. No single religious factor operates in isolation, but rather exists in combination with other religious factors and the person's ethnic, racial, and cultural background. When religion and ethnicity combine to influence a person, the term **ethnoreligion** is sometimes used. Examples of ethnoreligious groups include the Amish; Russian Jewish; Lebanese Muslims; Italian, Irish, and Polish Catholics; Tibetan Buddhists; and so forth.

In their classic work, Faulkner and DeJong (1966) proposed five major dimensions of religion: experiential, ritualistic, ideologic, intellectual, and consequential. The **experiential dimension** recognizes that every religious person will experience religious emotion and/or feeling about their purpose in life and their connection with a higher power. The **ritualistic dimension** refers to religious practices, such as prayer, attending worship services, participating in sacraments, and reading religious literature. The **ideologic dimension** consists of the shared beliefs that members of a religion must adhere to in order to be considered members. The **intellectual dimension**, which is closely related to the ideologic dimension, consists of the cognitive understanding of the basic tenets or beliefs of the religion and its sacred writing or scriptures. Finally, the **consequential dimension** consists of how closely members adhere to the prescribed standards of conduct and/or attitudes as a consequence of belonging to a religion, such as political beliefs, attitudes about sex, and observing holy days.

Religious Dimensions in Relation to Health and Illness

Each religious dimension has a different significance when related to matters of health and illness. Different religious cultures may emphasize one of the five dimensions to the relative exclusion of the others. Similarly, individuals may develop their own priorities related to the dimensions of religion. This affects the nurse providing care to patients with different religious beliefs in several ways.

First, it is the nurse's role to determine from the patient, patient's family, or patient's significant others the dimension or combinations of dimensions that are important so that the patient and nurse can have mutual goals and priorities. Second, it is important to determine what a given member of a specific religious affiliation believes to be important about their faith that is relevant to their health, healing, medical diagnosis, interventions, and nursing care by asking the patient or, if the patient is unable to communicate this information personally, a close family member. Third, the nurse's information must be accurate. Making assumptions about patients' religious belief systems on the basis of their perceived cultural, racial, ethnic, or even religious affiliation is imprudent and may lead to erroneous inferences. For example, Our Lady of Lourdes is a Catholic shrine, yet people from many different Christian and non-Christian faiths visit Lourdes each year seeking peace and healing from illnesses and injuries. Just as nurses do a complete head-to-toe health assessment of patients in the clinical setting to assure complete and comprehensive care is provided, it is just as important for the nurse to also do a cultural and **spiritual assessment** of the patients they are providing care for, to correctly accommodate the patient's religious beliefs and values (McFarland, 2018; McFarland & Wehbe-Alamah, 2019).

Fourth, even when individuals identify with a particular religion, they may accept the "official" beliefs and practices in varying degrees. It is not the nurse's role to judge the religious virtues of patients, but rather to understand those aspects related to religion that are important to the patient and family members. When religious beliefs are translated into practice, they may be manipulated by individuals in certain situations to serve particular ends; that is, traditional beliefs and practices may be altered. Thus, it is possible for a Jewish person to eat pork or for a

Catholic to take contraceptives to prevent pregnancy. Homogeneity among members of any religion cannot be assumed. The nurse should be open to variations in religious beliefs and practices and allow for the possibility of change in an individual's views. Individual choices frequently arise from new situations, changing values and mores, and exposure to new ideas and beliefs. Few people live in total social isolation surrounded by only those with similar religious backgrounds.

Fifth, ideal norms of conduct and actual behavior are not necessarily the same. The nurse is frequently faced with the challenge of understanding and helping patients cope with internal conflict, which can occur when the patient faces differences between their own behaviors and the norms of their religion. Sometimes, conflicting norms are manifested by guilt or by efforts to minimize or rationalize inconsistencies, which may impact their health and desires regarding healthcare.

Sometimes, norms are vaguely formulated and filled with discrepancies that allow for a variety of interpretations. In religions that have a lay organization and structure, moral decision-making may be left to the individual without the assistance of members of a church hierarchy. In religions that have a clerical hierarchy, moral positions may be more clearly formulated and articulated for members. Individuals retain their right to choose, regardless of official church-related guidelines, suggestions, or laws; however, the individual who chooses to violate the norms may experience the consequences of that violation, including social ostracism, public removal from membership rolls, or other forms of censure. Social ostracism is especially problematic for those patients experiencing mental illness who may experience greater difficulty in adhering to the norms of conduct and behavior associated with certain religious traditions. Nurses must be aware of these social norms associated with spiritual beliefs and be able to offer encouragement and resources to patients struggling to align their religious beliefs and practices to minimize social ostracism and to maximize the physical and social benefits of faith and spiritual beliefs (Barbosa et al., 2018).

Religion and Spiritual Nursing Care

For many years, nursing has emphasized a holistic approach to care in which the needs of the total person are recognized. Most nursing textbooks emphasize the physical and psychosocial needs of patients but address little regarding the spiritual needs of the patient (Scammell, 2017). Recently, more has been written about guidelines for providing spiritual care to patients from diverse cultural backgrounds (King & Cayley, 2021; Siritsky, 2020). Because nurses endeavor to provide holistic healthcare, addressing spiritual needs becomes essential.

Religious concerns evolve from and respond to the mysteries of life and death, good and evil, and pain and suffering. Although the religions of the world offer various interpretations of these phenomena, most people seek a personal understanding and interpretation at some time in their lives. Often, serious health concerns, life-limiting diagnoses, and traumatic events heighten personal reflection and interest in such enigmas. These concerns are often heightened in the lives of the patients and their families during the times they are under the care of nurses. Ultimately, this personal search becomes a pursuit to discover a Supreme Being, God, gods, or some unifying truth that will give meaning, purpose, and integrity to existence (Fig. 12-1).

While religion and spirituality have similarities and overlapping concepts, they are separate and distinct from one another (Sorajjakool et al., 2017). In general, religion addresses questions related to what is true and right and helps individuals determine where they belong in the scheme of their life's journey. **Spirituality** emphasizes the pursuit of meaning, purpose, direction, and values.

In 1978, the Third National Conference on the Classification of Nursing Diagnoses recognized the importance of spirituality by including "spiritual concerns," "spiritual distress," and "spiritual despair" in the list of approved diagnoses. Because of practical difficulties, these three categories were combined at the 1980 National Conference into one category, **spiritual distress**,

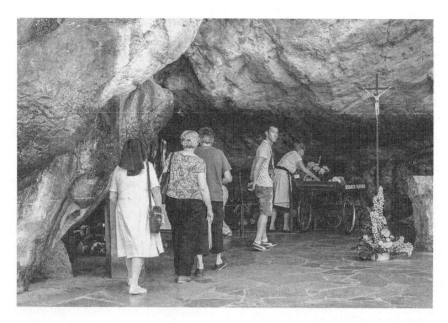

Figure 12-1. Our Lady of Lourdes shrine is in Lourdes, France, and commemorates the site of a Marian apparition in 1858. Our Lady of Lourdes is a Catholic shrine, yet people from many different Christian and non-Christian faiths visit Lourdes annually. Four to six million people visit the shrine each year, seeking peace and healing from physical and mental afflictions. (From Pierre-Olivier/Shutterstock.com.)

which is defined as disruption in the life principle that pervades a person's entire being and that integrates and transcends the person's biologic and psychosocial nature. Pattison (2013) acknowledges the multidimensional nature of spiritual concerns and defines them as the human need to deal with sociocultural deprivations, anxieties and fears, death and dying, personality integration, self-image, personal dignity, social alienation, and philosophy of life.

Spiritual Nursing Care

In 2001, The Joint Commission included an accreditation standard that required a brief spiritual assessment be conducted with all patients in healthcare settings. This standard was revised in 2008 and again in 2022. It is nonprescriptive but states that each organization will define what spiritual assessment means for them and how it will be evaluated. Suggestions include such items as "who or what provides the patient/client with strength and hope, how does the patient express their spirituality, what kind of religious/spiritual support does the patient desire, etc." ("Spiritual beliefs and preferences—Evaluating a patient's spiritual needs," 2022). Given that pastoral services may be limited, obtaining this brief assessment of the patient's spiritual needs and perspective most often is the nurse's responsibility. This assessment is the beginning of providing **spiritual nursing care**. The nurse must be prepared to listen, encourage, and offer hope to patients and their families as they ask questions and express anxiety, fear, or disbelief in times of physical and emotional despair. The nurse can anticipate and prepare themselves for these times by having genuine heart-felt encouragement in the form of scripture, poems, or a personal story of faith to offer patients and families. Nurses who feel comfortable doing so may consider offering prayers for their patients when asked.

Spiritual nursing care promotes clients' physical and emotional health as well as their **spiritual health**. When providing care, the nurse must remember that the goal of spiritual intervention is not, and should not be, to impose their own religious beliefs and convictions on the client (Scammell, 2017).

Although spiritual needs are recognized by many nurses, spiritual care is often neglected. There are many reasons why nurses fail to provide spiritual care, including the following:

1. They view religious and spiritual needs as a private matter concerning only an individual and the individual's Creator.
2. They are uncomfortable about their own religious beliefs or deny having spiritual needs.
3. They lack knowledge about spirituality and the religious beliefs of others.
4. They mistake spiritual needs for psychosocial needs.
5. They view meeting the spiritual needs of clients as a family or pastoral responsibility, not a nursing responsibility.

Spiritual assessment and intervention are as appropriate as any other form of nursing intervention and recognize that the balance of physical, psychosocial, and spiritual aspects of life is essential to overall good health. Nursing is an intimate profession, and nurses routinely inquire without hesitation about very personal matters such as hygiene and sexual habits. The spiritual realm also requires a personal, intimate type of nursing intervention (Bone et al., 2018; Rahmawati et al., 2018).

Assessment of Ethnoreligious and Spiritual Issues

Cultural assessment includes assessment of religious and spiritual issues as they relate to the healthcare status of patients. In the integration of healthcare interventions, medication adherence, and life change decisions as they relate to religious and spiritual beliefs, the focus of nursing intervention is to help the patient maintain their own beliefs in the face of a serious health challenge or crisis and to use those beliefs to strengthen the patient's coping patterns. Situations surrounding the phenomena of life, death, good, evil, pain, and suffering are foundational to the concept that nursing is a *calling* as well as a *career choice*. Nurses deal with patients and families at times when these questions become salient, possibly more salient than at any other time in their lives. Nurses are called upon to offer encouragement and support to individuals regarding these difficult questions. Therefore, they must plan what they might say and how they might say it beforehand. Having previously completed a *Cultural and Spiritual Assessment* of the patient will help inform the nurse of how best to approach these topics (McFarland & Wehbe-Alamah, 2019). Box 12-1 includes guidelines for assessing spiritual needs in patients from diverse cultural backgrounds.

Spiritual Nursing Care for Ill Children and Their Families

Any hospitalization or serious illness can be viewed as stressful and, therefore, has the potential to develop into a crisis. Religion may play an especially significant role when a child is seriously ill and in circumstances that include life-limiting illness, death, or bereavement.

Illness during childhood may be a particularly difficult clinical situation. Children have spiritual needs that vary according to their developmental level and the relative importance of religion and spirituality in the lives of their parents, extended family members, and other primary providers of care. Parental perceptions about the illness of their child may be partially influenced by religious beliefs. For example, some parents may believe that a transgression against a religious teaching, belief, or law has caused an illness, traumatic event, or congenital anomaly in their offspring. Other parents may delay seeking medical care because they believe prayers for healing should be tried first, but may seek traditional medical treatment later if healing has not happened.

BOX 12-1	Assessing Spiritual Needs in Patients From Various Ethnoreligious Backgrounds

What Do You Notice About the Patient's Surroundings?

- Does the patient have religious objects, such as the Quran (Koran), Bible, prayer book, devotional literature, religious medals, cross jewelry, rosary or other type of beads, photographs of historic religious persons or contemporary religious leaders (e.g., Jesus, Catholic Pope, Dalai Lama, or image of another religious figure), paintings of religious events or persons, religious sculptures, crucifixes, objects of religious significance at entrances to rooms (e.g., holy water founts, a mezuzah, or small parchment scroll inscribed with an excerpt from scripture), candles of religious significance (e.g., Paschal candle, menorah), shrine, or other items?
- Does the patient wear clothing that has religious significance (e.g., head covering, undergarment, uniform)? Does the hairstyle connote affiliation with a certain ethnoreligious group, for example, earlocks worn by Hasidic Jewish men?
- Do "Get Well" greeting cards the patient has received depict religious events, scenes, verses, or poems, and are they from a representative of the patient's church, mosque, temple, synagogue, or other religious congregations?

How Does the Patient Act?

- Does the patient appear to pray at certain times of the day or before meals?
- Does the patient make special dietary requests (e.g., kosher diet, vegetarian diet, or refrain from caffeine, pork or pork derivatives such as gelatin or marshmallows, shellfish, or other specific food items)?
- Does the patient read religious magazines or books?

What Does the Patient Say?

- Does the patient talk about God, Allah, Buddha, Yahweh, Jehovah, prayer, faith, or other religious topics?
- Does the patient ask for a visit by a clergy member or other religious representatives?
- Does the patient express anxiety or fear about pain, suffering, dying, or death?

How Does the Patient Relate to Others?

- Who visits? How does the patient respond to visitors?
- Does a priest, rabbi, minister, elder, or other religious representatives visit?
- Does the patient ask the nursing staff to pray for or with them?
- Does the patient prefer to interact with others or to remain alone?

The nurse should be respectful of parents' preferences regarding the care of their child. Religion and spirituality may be a source of consolation and support to parents, especially those facing the unanswerable questions associated with life-threatening illness in their children. If the nurse determines that parental beliefs or practices threaten the child's well-being and health, the nurse is obligated to discuss the matter with the parents. Using caring spiritual assessment techniques, it may be possible to reach a compromise in which parental beliefs are respected and necessary care is provided. Nursing theorist Madeleine Leininger's Culture Care Theory addresses how the nurse can assess the patient's or family's current care wishes, then, using the three major culture care action modes (preservation and/or maintenance, accommodation and/or negotiation, and repatterning and/or restructuring), can assist the patient and family in making optimal healthcare decisions (Leininger, 2002; McFarland, 2018; McFarland & Wehbe-Alamah, 2019).

Spiritual Nursing Care for the Dying or Bereaved Patient and Family

While all people mourn, all people do not mourn alike. **Mourning** is a cultural behavior, and it is manifested in a multicultural society. Mourning customs help people cope with the loss of loved ones. Nurses inevitably focus on restoring health or on fostering environments in which the patient returns to a previous state of health or adapts to physical, psychological, or emotional changes. However, one aspect of nursing care that is often avoided or ignored, although it is every bit as crucial to patients and their families, is dying, death, and the grieving processes.

Death is indeed a universal experience, but one that is highly individual and personal. Although each person must ultimately face death alone, rarely does a person's death fail to affect others. There are many rituals serving many purposes that people use to help them cope with death. These rituals are often determined by cultural and religious orientation. In her seminal work on death, dying, and the stages of grief, Kubler-Ross posited that situational factors, competing demands, and individual differences are also important in determining the dying, bereavement, and grieving behaviors that are considered socially acceptable (Kubler-Ross, 1969).

The role of the nurse in dealing with dying patients and their families varies according to the needs and preferences of both the nurse and patient as well as the clinical setting in which the interaction occurs. By understanding some of the cultural and religious variations related to death, dying, and bereavement, the nurse can individualize the care given to patients and their families (Ohr et al., 2021).

Nurses are often with the patient through various stages of the dying process and at the actual moment of death, particularly when death occurs in a hospital, nursing home, extended care facility, or hospice. The nurse frequently determines when and whom to call as the impending death draws near. Knowing the religious, cultural, and familial heritage of a particular patient, as well as the patient's devotion to the associated traditions and practices, may help the nurse determine whom to call when the need arises.

Death Practices

Universally, people want to die with dignity. Historically, this was not a problem when individuals died at home in the presence of their friends and families. Now, when more and more people are dying in institutions (hospitals, hospices, and extended care facilities), with a variety of technological advances available that may prolong life but decrease dignity, ensuring dignity throughout the dying process is more complex (Madan, 1992; Mixer, 2018). When death is seen as a problem requiring professional management, instead of a natural process, the hospital displaces the home, and specialists with different kinds and degrees of expertise take over for the family, while home-based end-of-life care improves patient satisfaction and quality of life for some patients (Shepperd et al., 2021; Sherwen, 2014).

Preparation of the Body

A nurse may or may not actually participate in the rituals following death. When people die in the United States and Canada, they are usually transported to a mortuary, where the preparation for burial occurs.

In many cultural groups, preparation of the body has traditionally been very important. Whereas members of many cultural groups have now adopted the practice of letting the mortician prepare the body, there are some who want to retain their native and/or religious customs. For Jewish, Muslim, and some immigrants of certain Asian religions, it remains an important ritual for families and friends of the same sex to wash and prepare the body for burial. In other situations, the family or religious representatives may coordinate with the funeral home in preparation of the body for burial and by dressing the person in special religious clothing. If a person dies in an institution, it is common for the nursing staff to "prepare" the body according to the institution's policy and procedure. Depending on the ethnoreligious practices of the family, this may be objectionable, as the family members could view this washing as an infringement on a special task that belongs to them alone. If the family is present, it is important to ask family members about their preference. If ritual washings will eventually take place at the mortuary, it may be necessary to carry out the routine procedures of the institution and reassure the family that the mortician will comply with their requests, if that has in fact been verified (Wehbe-Alamah et al., 2021).

Funeral Practices

By their very nature, people are social beings who have social attachments that are impacted by the death of a loved one. Family members have deep and often multigenerational relationships and memories with the deceased. Cultural traditions often come into play at the time of death, in the values, beliefs, and practices that families employ when a loved one's death occurs. Human social attachments are broken by death; thus, people seek to reconcile and bring closure to the relationships. The **funeral**, a formal commemoration of the person's life, and the **wake**/viewing are appropriate and socially acceptable times for the expression of sorrow and grief. Whether it is called a wake, viewing, or **home going**, it serves the same function: allowing the survivors to mourn together, comfort each other, and say a last goodbye.

Customs for disposal of the body after death vary widely. Burial clothes and other religious or cultural symbols may be important items for the funeral ritual. As part of their lifelong preparation for death, Amish women sew white burial garments for themselves and for their family members ("Countryfarm lifestyles," 2023). For the viewing and burial, faithful Mormons are dressed in white temple garments ("A guide to Mormon burial practices and funeral etiquette," 2022). Among followers of many Christian denominations, the dead are typically prepared by the mortician at the funeral home, and through the restorative art of the profession, the corpse is made to look just as if they were asleep. The refrigerated body may be kept up to 3 to 4 weeks if necessary to allow family to travel and make arrangements, or due to other delays in scheduling the funeral ("How long can you delay a funeral after death?," 2023).

Funeral arrangements vary from short, simple rituals to long, elaborate displays. Among the Amish, family members, neighbors, and friends assist with a short, quiet ceremony ("Countryfarm lifestyles," 2023). Many Jewish families use unadorned coffins, stress simplicity in burial services, do not use embalming, and usually intern the body within 24 hours of death. In traditional Judaism, cosmetic restoration is discouraged, as is any attempt to hasten or retard decomposition by artificial means. Some Jews fly the body to Jerusalem for burial in ground considered to be holy ("Traditional Jewish ritual and mourning practices," 2023). Muslim dead are typically touched only by same-gender Muslim relatives in preparation for the funeral. The body is shrouded in a white garb resembling a sheet, which covers the entire body and face. Embalming is forbidden in Islam and the body is buried in a Muslim cemetery within 24 hours (Wehbe-Alamah et al., 2021).

Taboos Related to Death

In some cultures, people believe that particular omens, such as the appearance of an owl or a message in a dream, warn of approaching death. Breaking a taboo, for example, removing an object believed to have healing powers, is also believed by some to cause death. Nurses should take care to avoid moving or removing any objects of religious or spiritual significance without first consulting the patient or family members. This emphasizes the importance of prior cultural and spiritual assessment in providing nursing care for patients and families that meets with the values, beliefs, and practices of their cultures (McFarland & Wehbe-Alamah, 2019; Mixer, 2018).

Unexpected Death and Death by Suicide

Acceptance of unexpected death or death by suicide is difficult for family members in most societies. For example, suicide is strictly forbidden under Islamic law. In the Filipino culture, suicide brings shame to the individual and to the entire family. Many Christian religions teach against suicide and some may impose sanctions even after death for the "sin." For example, a Roman Catholic who dies by suicide may be denied burial in blessed ground or in a Catholic cemetery (Doyle, 2022). In some religions, a church funeral is not permitted for a person who has died by suicide, requiring the family to make alternative arrangements. This imposition of religious law can further add to the grief of surviving family members and friends. However, many Christian churches in the 21st century teach that suicide is a result of the human condition resultant of the fall into sin by the human ancestors of all mankind, Adam and Eve, in the garden of Eden (Mohler Jr., 2018). Further, suicide or ideation of suicide is understood not as mortal nor unforgivable sin, but it may be considered or carried out at a time "of vulnerability for someone who may be in a moment of spiritual or mental crisis" (Mohler Jr., 2018). Nurses must treat this situation with upmost care to allow individuals and families to express their cultural and familial beliefs surrounding suicide, while offering individuals hope and healing in each encounter.

Deaths resulting from nonviolent but untimely causes can be equally difficult for the patient, family, and friends. Cancers and chronic diseases may give the patient and family time to "prepare" for the death, but the impending illness and subsequent death require skilled nurses to provide empathy and understanding as the patient and family process the reality and the changes in store. Following a terminal diagnosis, there is typically time for individuals and family members to "put things in order" and discuss patients' desired funeral and burial wishes, care of loved ones, especially underage dependents after the patient's death and other pertinent family issues. Often, patients will ask the nurse about their prognosis, amount of "good days and bad days," and an estimate of the time of death. While nurses are usually very positive and encouraging, this communication should be informed and as realistic as possible and may require the nurse to seek hospice resources to assist the patient and family. Some cultures use the terms "**good death**" for this time leading up to and before death actually occurs. An example of *good death* to the older Japanese American often means to not have been a burden to others (Mori et al., 2018).

The Death of a Child

Although a great deal has been written about children's conceptions of death, few cross-cultural studies have yet been reported. Children develop a concept of death through innate cognitive development, which has significant cultural variations, and through acquired notions conveyed by the family, which vary according to the family's cultural beliefs. Thus, it is unsafe to assume that all children, regardless of family culture, will develop parallel concepts of and reactions to death (Vázquez-Sánchez et al., 2019; Wass, 2018).

Most children's initial experiences with death occur with the loss of a pet rather than a person. Because of reduced childhood mortality and delayed adult mortality, children in the United States and Canada are now much less exposed to death in family than they used to be, and they tend to be sheltered from the experience. The current lack of direct exposure of children to death is both a class phenomenon and a cultural phenomenon.

In many Western societies, children are considered precious, valued, and vulnerable; they are protected and often the first to be saved in emergencies. In resource-limited societies, by contrast, parents are less likely to see most of their children grow into adulthood because of high infant mortality rates. As a result, a child's life may be viewed as less valued and precious than an adult's, although the child is still viewed as valuable to the parents and other loved ones. Regardless of the sociocultural situation, each society has a special view of the significance of children and their death as it affects the bereaved family. Nurses caring for a culturally diverse population will recognize and validate familial practices and beliefs related to the death of a child, even when those practices and beliefs vary from the nurse's personally held values.

Bereavement, Grief, and Mourning

Bereavement is a sociologic term indicating the status and role of the survivors of a death. **Grief** is an affective response to a loss, whereas mourning is the culturally patterned behavioral response to a death. What differs between cultural groups is not so much the feelings of grief but their forms of expression or mourning (Heilman, 2018; Markin & Zilcha-Mano, 2018).

Different family systems may alleviate or intensify the pain experienced by bereaved persons. In the typical nuclear American family, the death of a member sometimes leaves a great void, because that individual may have been the only family member who oversaw or completed certain tasks in the family structure. In African American culture, it is often the maternal grandmother who assists with healthcare decisions for the entire family, and her death leaves a void not easily filled. By contrast, cultural groups in which several generations and extended family members commonly reside within a household may find that the acute trauma of bereavement is softened by the fact that the familial role of the deceased is easily filled by multiple other relatives. It should be noted, however, that the loss of a loved one is experienced and mourned irrespective of the person's cultural background, but cultural distinctives do play an important role in how the remaining family members grieve, process, and move forward after a death.

Although nurses frequently encourage patients and their families to express their grief openly, many people are reluctant to do so in the institutional setting. The nurse often sees family members when they are still in shock over the death and are responding to the situation as a crisis rather than expressing their grief. When asked who would be sought for comfort and support in a time of bereavement, most frequently named were a family member or a member of the clergy. In an institutional setting, a nurse who has been with the patient and family throughout the dying process may be surprised at the time of death when the grieving persons turn to other family, and the nurse is "left out" (Anderson et al., 2019).

Contemporary bereavement practices of various cultural and religious groups demonstrate the wide range of expressions of bereavement. Each group reflects practices that best meet its members' needs. The nurse can help promote a culturally appropriate grieving process; hindering or interfering with practices that the patient and family find meaningful can disrupt the grieving process. Bereaved people can experience physical and psychological symptoms, and they may succumb to serious physical illnesses, leading even to death. Although bereavement is regarded as a universal stressor, the magnitude of the stress and its meaning to the individual vary significantly cross-culturally. For example, one Western misconception is that it is universally more stressful to mourn the death of a child than the death of an older or more distant relative. Yet, cross-cultural studies show that emotional attachments to relatives vary significantly and are not based on Western concepts of kinship (Montgomery & Owen-Pugh, 2018).

Although traditional funeral and postfuneral rituals have benefited both bereaved persons and their social groups in their original settings, the influence of the contemporary Western urban setting is unknown. It is likely that in North America, most individuals have assimilated United States and Canadian practices in varying degrees. The role of the nurse is to obtain information from individual patients in a caring manner, explaining that the nurse wishes to provide culturally appropriate nursing care (Wehbe-Alamah et al., 2021).

Religious Trends in the United States and Canada

The United States and Canada are cosmopolitan nations to which all of the major and many of the minor faiths of Europe and other parts of the globe have been transplanted. Figure 12-2 illustrates the diversity of religions present in the world. Religious identification among people from different racial

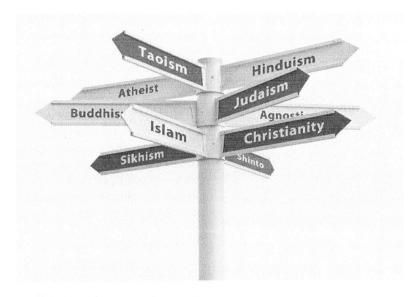

Figure 12-2. Multiple religions are present in all societies, and this diversity enhances opportunities for nurses to encounter multiple belief systems and to adjust their care accordingly. (From Ryan DeBerardinis/Shutterstock.com.)

Table 12-1	Major Religious Affiliations of the United States and Canada (%)		
	United States	**Canada**	**World**
Christianity	70.6	67.3	31.2
Atheism, Agnosticism, no affiliation	22.8	23.9	16
Judaism	1.9	1.0	0.22
Islam	0.9	3.2	24.1
Buddhism	0.7	1.1	6.9
Hinduism	0.7	1.5	15.1
Major Christian Faith Groups			
Roman Catholic	20.8	38.7	32.3
Protestant	49.8	19.2	9.2

Source: *Religious Landscape Study.* (2017). Retrieved February 10, 2023, from https://www.pewresearch.org/religion/religious-landscape-study/

and ethnic groups is important because religion and culture are interwoven. Table 12-1 details the statistical breakdown of major religious affiliations of the United States and Canada.

As discussed, a wide range of beliefs frequently exists within religions, a factor that adds complexity. Some religions have a designated spokesperson or leader who articulates, interprets, and applies theological tenets to daily life experiences, including those of health and illness. These leaders include, but are not limited to, Jewish rabbis, Catholic priests, Protestant ministers, and Muslim imams. The nurse should consider the patient's spiritual leaders (clergy and lay members) as part of the inter-professional healthcare team and encourage patients and families to involve religious leaders in provision of spiritual encouragement and care (Andrews & Boyle, 2019). Some religions rely more heavily on individual conscience, whereas others entrust decisions to individuals or to groups vested with ultimate authority within their religious tradition. Due to the wide variation of beliefs between and within denominations, the nurse should incorporate a cultural assessment of the patient within the history and physical or head-to-toe assessment to identify individual care preferences, dietary restrictions, and religious distinctives that impact delivery of nursing care (McFarland, 2018; Wehbe-Alamah et al., 2021).

Contributions of Religious Groups to the Healthcare Delivery System

In the United States and Canada, many denominations own and operate healthcare institutions and make significant fiscal contributions that help control healthcare costs. For example, the Roman Catholic Church, the largest single denomination in the United States, is also a major stakeholder in the healthcare field. In the United States, there are more than 600 Catholic hospitals, 1,600 long-term care facilities in all 50 states, which treat 5.4 million people annually. This means that more than one in seven patients are cared for in a Catholic hospital ("Catholic Health Care in the United States," 2023). **Catholic Charities USA**, an umbrella agency that oversees nonhospital work, reports that its agencies serve more than 1,046 million people each year, often functioning as a centralized referral source for patients ultimately treated in non-Catholic agencies ("Catholic Charities USA," 2023).

Similarly, there are many Jewish hospitals, day care centers, extended care facilities, and organizations to meet the healthcare needs of Jewish and non-Jewish persons in need. For example, the National Jewish Center for Immunology and Respiratory Medicine is a research and treatment center for respiratory, immunologic, allergic, and infectious diseases, and the Council for Jewish Elderly provides a full range of social and healthcare services for older adults, including adult day care, care/case management, counseling, transportation, and advocacy ("Who We Are," 2023).

According to the Pew Forum on Religion and Public Policy, many other denominations, including the Lutheran, Baptist, Mennonite, Methodist, Muslim, and Seventh-Day Adventist groups, also own and operate hospitals and healthcare organizations ("Health Care," 2023).

In Canada, hospital care, outpatient care, extended care, and medical services have been publicly funded and administered since the Medical Care Act of 1966. However, before the Medical Care Act and into the present, religious organizations have made important contributions to the health and well-being of Canadians at individual, community, and societal levels. For example, countless church-run agencies, charities, and facilities offer care and social support to individuals and families coping with such conditions as chronic illness, disability, poverty, and homelessness. At the national level, church-run organizations, such as the Catholic Health Association of Canada, are committed to addressing social justice issues that affect the health system and offer leadership through research and policy development regarding healthcare ethics, spiritual and religious care, and social justice ("Catholic health alliance of Canada," 2023).

Health-Related Beliefs and Practices of Selected Religions

Health-related beliefs and practices of select religions are important to understand, especially considering the diverse religious groups in the United States and Canada. Evidence-Based Practice 12-1 provides information regarding other research done on this topic. A brief overview of selected religious groups and their health-related beliefs and practices follows.

Two Studies on Religion and Healthcare Practices

The Adventist Health Study-2 studied the relationship of vegan, lacto-ovo vegetarian, pesco-vegetarian, semivegetarian, and nonvegetarian dietary patterns of 97,000 members of the Seventh-Day Adventist church exploring the relationship of those dietary patterns to health outcomes, specifically obesity, metabolic syndrome, hypertension, type 2 diabetes mellitus, osteoporosis, cancer, and mortality. While the data regarding cancer have yet to be analyzed in depth, the data showed that "vegetarian diets in the AHS-2 population studied are associated with lower BMI values, lower prevalence of hypertension & metabolic syndrome and lower prevalence and incidence of type 2 diabetes as well as lower all-cause mortality" (p. 357S). While there has long been a concern that vegetarian diets put the person at risk for osteoporosis, it appears from this study that when plant sources of protein are consumed, the risk is decreased.

In the second study, the researchers explored whether Hispanics in general, and Catholic Hispanics in particular, follow a "cultural belief" called "fatalism," which precludes the person from participating in cancer screening practices. Sixty-seven participants (33 men, 34 women) attended one of eight focus groups with 8 to 10 participants per group. Men and women attended separate groups. The intent was to explore the "participants' cultural explanatory models of cancer, including their cultural beliefs, attitudes, personal life experiences and their understanding of both biomedical and population explanations of health and illness" (p. 841). Contrary to the stereotype of "fatalism," this group "expressed few fatalistic beliefs with regard to cancer" and instead indicated a general belief that cancer was preventable if caught early. This group reported that their religion supported them in their search for health, including cancer screening. They also indicated that there is a role for faith and calling upon God and saints in the face of illness.

Clinical Implications

- What questions might you consider after thinking about the evidence provided in these studies?
- How might this information impact your care of patients who are not from any of the ethnic backgrounds found in these studies?
- What other evidence might you want to explore to seek answers to clinical questions that you have faced?

References: Leyva, B., Allen, J. D., Tom, L. S., Ospino, H., Torres, M. I., & Abraido-Lanza, A. F. (2014). Religion, fatalism, and cancer control: A qualitative study among Hispanic Catholics. *American Journal of Health Behavior*, *38*(6), 839–849; Orlich, M. J., & Fraser, G. E. (2014). Vegetarian diets in the Adventist Health Study 2: A review of initial published findings. *The American Journal of Clinical Nutrition*, *100*(suppl_1), 353S–358S.

Amish

The term **Amish** refers to members of several ethnoreligious Christian groups who choose to live separately from the modern world through manner of dress, language, family life, and selective use of technology. There are four major orders or affiliating groups of Amish ("Amish population profile, 2022," 2022; Purnell & Fenkl, 2019):

1. *Old Order Amish*, the largest group, whose name is often used synonymously with "the Amish"

2. The ultraconservative *Swartzentruber* and *Andy Weaver Amish*, both more conservative than the Old Order Amish in their restrictive use of technology and shunning of members who have dropped out or committed serious violations of the faith

3. The less conservative *New Order Amish*, which emerged in the 1960s with more liberal views of technology but with an emphasis on high moral standards in restricting alcohol and tobacco use and in courtship practices

4. The *Liberal Beachy Amish*, more commonly known as **Mennonites**, who maintain many of the same features as the more conservative Amish, but allow electricity and use of automobiles

The total population of Amish is estimated at approximately 370,000 in 2022 and is spread throughout more than 2,800 districts (congregations) in 32 states and four Canadian provinces ("Amish population profile, 2022," 2022). Each congregation or district represents about 20 to 40 families with a minimal hierarchy of church leaders (a bishop, deacon, and two ministers). The bishop is the spiritual head; the deacon assists the bishop and is responsible for donations to help members with medical bills and other expenses; and the ministers help the bishop with preaching at church services and providing spiritual direction for the church district and its members ("Amish Studies," 2022; Anderson & Potts, 2020).

Substance Use

Once an Amish person is baptized, they are forbidden from using alcoholic beverages and drugs unless prescribed by a physician. Teenagers and unmarried young adults may experiment with cigarettes, alcohol, and sometimes other chemical substances during *Rumspringa*, a rite of passage during adolescence where Amish youth face fewer behavioral restrictions and may venture out of the Amish community ("Amish Studies," 2022; Anderson & Potts, 2020). It is important to assess persons in this age group for signs of substance use disorder.

Healthcare Practices

Illness is seen as the inability to perform daily chores by the Amish, and Amish are often uninterested in health screenings and preventative care. Healthcare practices within the Amish culture are varied and include complementary and alternative medicine incorporating folk, herbal, and homeopathic remedies. Unlike the use of complementary and alternatives medicine, preventive medicine may be seen as against God's will. The use of the mainstream healthcare system is largely episodic and crisis-oriented. If traditional medicine fails, there is no hesitancy in visiting an herb doctor, braucher (a practitioner of folk and faith healing), or a chiropractor. Folk, professional, and alternative care are often used simultaneously (Anderson & Potts, 2020). Cost, access, transportation, and advice from family and friends are the major factors that influence healing choices. The Amish are at risk for a variety of genetic diseases due to frequent intermarriage among close relatives ("Amish population profile, 2022," 2022). Farming accidents are also a common reason for seeking healthcare service (Purnell & Fenkl, 2019).

Medical and Surgical Interventions

The use of narcotic drugs is prohibited among the Amish. There are no restrictions against the use of blood or blood products, if advised by healthcare providers. Vaccinations are acceptable, especially for children, but may not be accepted for adults or older adult individuals ("Amish population profile, 2022," 2022; Anderson & Potts, 2020).

Practices Related to Reproduction

The Amish believe that the fundamental purpose of marriage is procreation, and couples are encouraged to have large families. Children are an economic asset to the family because they assist their parents with housework, farm chores, gardening, and family business. Women are expected to have children until menopause. If situations arise that justify sterilization (e.g., removal of cancerous reproductive organs), those called upon to make the decisions would rely on the best medical advice available and the council of the church leaders. Although the Amish family structure is patriarchal, the grandmother is often a key decision maker concerning reproductive and other health-related issues. Abortion, artificial insemination, genetics, eugenics, stem cell research, and in vitro fertilization are inconsistent with Amish values and beliefs (Purnell & Fenkl, 2019).

Religious Support System for the Sick

Individual members of local and surrounding Amish communities assist and provide social support to one another in times of need. From birth to death, individuals and families know they will be cared for by those in the community, providing informal support, emotional and financial assistance, and advice. The extended family consists of aunts, uncles, cousins, and grandparents, who usually live only a few miles away and can be counted on to assist in times of illness.

The Amish do not use religious titles. Therefore, a nurse may refer to Amish visitors using nonreligious titles such as Mr. or Mrs. When the nurse is providing care, physical touch should be limited except for direct care and physical distance at hand-shaking distance should be maintained. When an Amish person is hospitalized, social support is very evident and there will likely be many visitors. Parents of hospitalized children will likely stay with the child at the hospital, and home healthcare when appropriate is preferred and welcomed. While most Amish are fluent in both English and Pennsylvania Dutch, in times of stress, they may revert to their Pennsylvania Dutch dialect and interpreters may be necessary (Anderson & Potts, 2020; Purnell & Fenkl, 2019).

Practices Related to End of Life

Because of Amish views of God's sovereignty and God's will, advance directives are uncommon and there may be resistance to extensive procedures, tests, and life-prolonging interventions (Anderson & Potts, 2020). Decisions are made on a family-by-family basis. When death is imminent, the bishop may perform an anointing; for the in-clinic patient, space and privacy need to be provided. Autopsy is acceptable in the case of medical necessity but is seldom performed on the Amish. The Amish usually prefer to bury the intact body and generally do not donate body parts for medical research. Bodies are buried in small cemeteries in Amish communities on private property. Cremation is not acceptable ("Amish Studies," 2022).

Buddhist Churches of America

Buddhism is a general term that indicates a belief in **Buddha** and encompasses many individual churches. The Buddhist Churches of America is the largest Buddhist organization in mainland United States. There are numerous Buddhist sects in the United States and Canada, including Indian, Sri Lankan, Vietnamese, Thai, Chinese, Japanese, and Tibetan. There are approximately 3 to 4 million Buddhists in the United States and Canada, and the worldwide membership is greater than 400 million ("Buddhists," 2023; "Population of Christians, Hindus, Muslims and non-religious in Canada according to 2021 census," 2022; "Spread of Buddhism," 2023).

General Beliefs and Religious Practices

Nirvana or **Enlightenment**, a state of greater inner freedom and spontaneity, is the goal of all existence for Buddhists. When one achieves Nirvana, the mind has supreme tranquility, purity, and stability. Buddhists do not believe in healing through a faith or through faith itself. However, Buddhists do believe that spiritual peace and liberation from anxiety by adherence to and achievement of awakening to Buddha's wisdom can be important factors in promoting healing and recovery. Buddhism is not a dogmatic religion, nor does it dictate any specific practices. Individual differences are expected, acknowledged, and respected. Individuals are responsible for finding their own answers through awareness of the total situation. Prayer beads and images of Shakyamuni Buddha and other Buddhist deities may be utilized for specific prayer or meditation practices (Sorajjakool et al., 2017). Figure 12-3 shows Buddhist monks creating a sand mandala, a spiritual and ritual symbol representing the universe.

Holy Days, Rites, and Rituals

The major Buddhist holy day is Saga Dawa (or Vesak), the observance of Shakyamuni Buddha's birth, Enlightenment, and Parinirvana. This holiday falls during the months of May or June and therefore the actual date varies from year to year. Although there is no religious restriction for

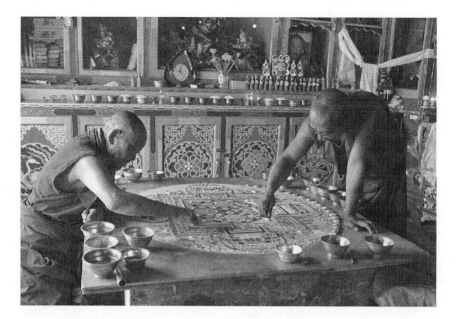

Figure 12-3. Buddhist monks making a sand mandala. The mandala is a spiritual and ritual symbol in both Hinduism and Buddhism, representing the universe. (From Vladimir Melnik/Shutterstock.com.)

therapy on this day, it can be highly emotional, and a Buddhist patient should be consulted about their desires for medical or surgical intervention. Some Buddhists may fast for all or part of this day. Buddhism does not have any sacraments that need to be taken into consideration for a hospitalized member of the Buddhist faith (Swihart et al., 2022).

Healthcare Practices

Moderation in diet is encouraged. Any specific dietary practices are usually interconnected with ethnic practices of the individual, rather than Buddhism. However, it is important for the nurse to inquire about the patient's preferences. There are no restrictions in Buddhism for nutritional therapies, medications, vaccines, and other therapeutic interventions, but some individuals may refrain from alcohol, stimulants, and other drugs that adversely affect mental clarity. Treatments such as amputations, organ transplants, biopsies, and other procedures that may prolong life and allow the individual to attain Enlightenment are encouraged (Swihart et al., 2022).

Practices Related to Reproduction

Buddhism does not condone the taking of a life. Life in all forms is to be respected. Birth control that prevents conception is acceptable, however, contraception that stops the development of a fertilized egg should not be used. Artificial insemination is also acceptable ("Buddhism and contraception," 2009; Swihart et al., 2022).

Practices Related to End of Life

If there is hope for recovery and continuation of the pursuit of Enlightenment, all available means of support are encouraged. If the donation of a body part will help another continue the quest for Enlightenment, it might be considered an act of mercy and is encouraged. The body is considered a shell; therefore, autopsy and disposal of the body are matters of individual practice rather than of religious prescription. Burials are usually a brief graveside service after a funeral at the temple. Cremations are common ("The complete guide to Buddhist burial practices and rituals," 2022).

Catholicism According to the Roman Rite

Roman **Catholic** membership in the United States and Canada includes approximately 73 million people (61.9 million in the United States and 10.8 million in Canada); worldwide membership is more than 1.3 billion (McKeown, 2023; *Profile table, Census Profile, 2021 Census of Population – Canada*, 2022).

General Beliefs, Rites, and Rituals

The Roman Catholic Church traces its beginnings to about 30 A.D., when Jesus Christ is believed to have founded the church. The Roman Catholic Church recognizes seven sacraments: Baptism, Reconciliation (Penance or Confession), Holy Communion (the Eucharist; Fig. 12-4), Confirmation, Matrimony, Holy Orders, and Anointing of the Sick (Extreme Unction). The major principle is that Sunday is a day of rest; therefore, unnecessary servile work is prohibited.

The holy days of obligation are also considered days of rest, although many persons must engage in routine work-related activities on some of these days ("Sacraments and Sacramentals," 2023).

Religious Objects

Rosaries, prayer books, and holy cards are often present and may be of great comfort to the patient and their family. Nurses need to recognize the importance of these objects and ensure they are left in place and within the reach of the patient whenever possible.

Diet and Substance Use

Catholics believe that the goods of the world have been given for use and benefit. The primary obligation people have toward food and beverages is to use them in moderation and in such a way that they are not injurious to health. **Fasting** in moderation is recommended as a valued discipline for healthy persons between the ages of 18 and 59. Additionally, Catholics have an obligation to fast

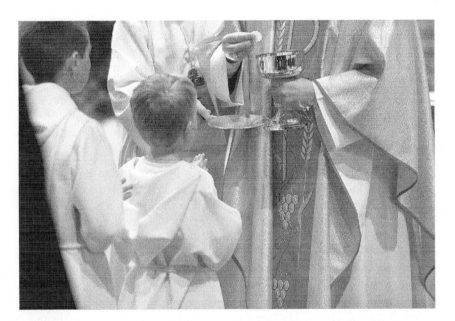

Figure 12-4. In the Roman Catholic tradition, when children reach the age of reason (7 years), they continue the ongoing initiation into their religion by making their First Communion, usually during second grade. In addition to the religious ritual, there are sometimes cultural traditions surrounding this event, many of which involve a family celebration after the religious services have concluded. (From Wideonet/Shutterstock.com.)

on Ash Wednesday and Good Friday. Abstinence from meat is also required on these days and on all of the Fridays of Lent. The sick are never bound by this prescription of the law (Swihart et al., 2022). Alcohol and tobacco are not considered evil per se, but they are to be used in moderation and not in a way that would be injurious to one's health or that of another party. The misuse of any substance is believed to be not only harmful to the body but also sinful.

Healthcare Practices

In time of illness, the basic rite is the sacrament of **Anointing of the Sick**, which is performed by a priest and includes reading of scriptures, prayers, communion if possible, and anointing with oil.

Medical and Surgical Interventions

As long as the benefits outweigh the risk to the individuals, judicious use of medications is permissible and morally acceptable in Catholicism. The Church has traditionally cited the **principle of totality**, which states that medications are allowed as long as they are used for the good of the whole person. Blood, blood products, and amputations are acceptable if consistent with the principle of totality. The transplantation of organs from living donors is morally permissible provided that the loss of such an organ does not deprive the donor of life itself or of the functional integrity of their body. Biopsies and circumcision are also permissible (*Ethical and religious directives for Catholic health care services*, 2020).

Practices Related to Reproduction

In Catholicism, the basic principle is that the conjugal act should be one that is love-giving and potentially life-giving. Only natural means of contraception, such as abstinence, the temperature method, and the ovulation method, are acceptable. Ordinarily, artificial aids and procedures for permanent sterilization are forbidden. Birth control (anovulants) may be used therapeutically to assist in regulating the menstrual cycle ("Natural Family Planning," 2023).

Amniocentesis in and of itself is not objectionable. However, it is morally objectionable if the findings of the amniocentesis are used to lead the couple to decide on termination of the pregnancy or if the procedure injures the fetus. Direct abortion is always considered morally wrong in Catholicism. Indirect abortion may be morally justified by some circumstances (e.g., treatment of a cancerous uterus in a pregnant woman). Abortion on demand is prohibited. The Roman Catholic Church teaches the sanctity of all human life from the time of conception ("Abortion," 2023).

Research in the fields of eugenics and genetics is objectionable. Catholics believe this violates the moral right of the individual to be free from experimentation and also interferes with God's right as the master of life and human beings' stewardship of their lives. Some genetic investigations to help determine genetic diseases may be used, depending on their ends and means. There is support for research using adult stem cells, but opposition to the use of embryonic stem cells ("Natural Family Planning," 2023).

Religious Support System for the Sick

Hispanic Catholic patients may have large numbers of family members visit to show support for their loved one, although this may be more a cultural practice than a religious distinctive (Zoucha & Zamarripa-Zoucha, 2021). Typically, a priest, deacon, or lay minister usually visits a sick person alone, although the family or other visitors may be invited to join in prayer. The priest, deacon, or lay minister will usually bring the necessary supplies for administration of the Eucharist or Anointing of the Sick. The nursing staff can facilitate these rites by ensuring an atmosphere of prayer and quiet and by having a glass of water on hand (in case the patient is unable to swallow the communion wafer). Consecrated wine can be made available but is usually not given in the hospital or home. The nurse may wish to join in the prayer. While real candles would not be allowed in the hospital, the use of electric candles may be used to simulate the solemnity of the occasion. The priest, deacon, or lay minister will usually appreciate any information pertaining to the patient's ability to swallow; however, most other patient information must be kept private due to HIPAA regulations. Privacy is most conducive to prayer and the administration of the sacraments. In emergencies, such as cardiac or respiratory arrest, medical personnel will need to be present. The priest will use an abbreviated form of the rite and will not interfere with the activities of the healthcare team ("Sacraments and Sacramentals," 2023).

Practices Related to End of Life

The Catholic Church endorses the use of advanced directives and recommends that its members prepare these documents and review them periodically. Members are obligated to take ordinary means of preserving life (e.g., intravenous medication) but are not obligated to take extraordinary means. Direct action to end the life of patients is not permitted. Extraordinary means may be withheld, allowing the patient to die of natural causes.

Advance Directives and *Durable Power of Attorney for Health Care* documents assist family members when their loved one is unable to communicate their healthcare wishes and in end-of-life situations. Faith in God often brings comfort to family members during traumatic and emotional situations surrounding end-of-life (Collins et al., 2021).

Autopsy is permissible as long as the corpse is shown proper respect and there is sufficient reason for doing the autopsy. Ordinarily, bodies are buried. Cremation is acceptable in certain circumstances, such as to avoid spreading a contagious disease. Because life is considered sacred, the body should be treated with respect. Any disposal of the body should be done in a respectful and honorable way ("End of Life," 2023).

Christian Science

Christian Science accepts physical and moral healing as a natural part of the Christian experience. Members believe that God acts through universal, immutable, spiritual law. They hold that genuine spiritual or Christian healing through prayer differs radically from the use of suggestion, willpower, and all forms of psychotherapy, which are based on the use of the human mind as a curative agent. In emphasizing the practical importance of a fuller understanding of Jesus' works and teachings, Christian Science believes healing to be a natural result of drawing closer to God in one's thinking and living (Eddy, 1875). The church does not keep specific membership data; however, membership has been declining from a high point in the 1930s. It is estimated that there are about 400,000 members worldwide and around 100,000 adherents in the United States as of 2008 ("Christian Science healing," 2008).

General Beliefs and Religious Practices

Christian Science beliefs and practices rely on the individual's faith and a reliance on prayer to achieve health when disease is present. Christian Science is based on the teachings of Jesus, who said, "He who believes in me, the works that I do he will also do" John 14:12 (*The Holy Bible: New King James Version*, 1769/1982). Mary Baker Eddy, the founder of Christian Science, said, "these mighty works are not supernatural, but supremely natural..." (Eddy, 1875, p. xi). This can mean resolving difficult challenges with health, relationships, employment, and other personal and global issues through prayer. People who practice Christian Science are free to make their own choices about what to think and do in each situation, including healthcare ("Christian Science-beliefs and teaching," 2023).

Social Activities and Substance Use

Members are encouraged to be honest, truthful, and moral in their behavior. Although every effort is made to preserve marriages, divorce is recognized. Members abstain from alcohol and tobacco; some abstain from tea and coffee ("Christian Science-beliefs and teaching," 2023).

Healthcare Practices

Viewed as a byproduct of drawing closer to God, healing is considered proof of God's care and one element in the full salvation at which Christianity aims. Christian Science teaches that faith must rest not on blind belief but on an understanding of the present perfection of God's spiritual creation. The practice of Christian Science healing starts from the Biblical basis that God created the universe and human beings "and made them perfect." Christian Science holds that human imperfection, including physical illness and sin, reflects a fundamental misunderstanding of creation and is therefore subject to healing through prayer and spiritual regeneration (Eddy, 1875).

An individual who is seeking healing may turn to Christian Science practitioners, members of the denomination who devote their full time to the healing ministry in the broadest sense. In cases requiring continued care, nurses grounded in the Christian Science faith provide care in facilities accredited by the mother church, the First Church of Christ, Scientist, in Boston, Massachusetts. Individuals may also receive such care in their own homes. Christian Science nurses are trained to perform the practical duties a patient may need while also providing an atmosphere of warmth and love that supports the healing process. No medication is given, and physical application is limited to the normal measures associated with hygiene. The *Christian Science Journal* contains a directory of qualified Christian Science practitioners and nurses throughout the world ("Christian Science-Christian Science Nursing," 2023).

Christian Scientists are not necessarily opposed to doctors. They are always free to make their own decisions regarding treatment in any given situation. They generally choose to rely on spiritual healing because they have seen its effectiveness in the experience of their own families and fellow church members— experience that goes back over 100 years and in many families for three or four generations. Where medical treatment for minor children is required by law, Christian Scientists strictly adhere to the requirement. At the same time, they maintain that their substantial healing record needs to be seriously considered in determining the rights of Christian Scientists

to rely on spiritual healing for themselves and their children. They do not ignore or neglect disease, but they seek to heal it by the means they believe to be most effective ("Christian Science-How can I be healed?," 2023).

Medical and Surgical Interventions

Christian Scientists ordinarily do not use medications. Immunizations and vaccines are acceptable only when required by law. Ordinarily, members do not use blood or blood products. A Christian Scientist who has lost a limb might seek to have it replaced with a prosthesis. Christian Scientists are unlikely to seek transplants and are unlikely to act as donors. Christian Scientists do not normally seek biopsies or any sort of physical examination. Circumcision is considered an individual matter ("Christian Science-How can I be healed?," 2023).

Practices Related to Reproduction

Matters of family planning (i.e., birth control) are left to individual judgment. Because abortion involves medication and surgical intervention, it is normally considered incompatible with Christian Science. Artificial insemination is unusual among Christian Scientists. Christian Scientists are opposed to programs in the field of eugenics and genetics.

Practices Related to End of Life

A Christian Science family is unlikely to seek medical means to prolong life indefinitely. Family members pray earnestly for the recovery of a person as long as the person remains alive. Euthanasia is contrary to the teachings of Christian Science. Disposal of the body is left to the individual family to decide. The individual family decides the form of burial and burial service (Swihart et al., 2022).

The Church of Jesus Christ of Latter-day Saints

The **Church of Jesus Christ of Latter-day Saints** is a Christian religion established in the United States in the early 1800s. The title of

"Church of Jesus Christ of Latter-day Saints" and "Members" are preferred over the more commonly known names of "Mormonism" and "Mormons." Membership in the United States and Canada is approximately 7 million ("The Church of Jesus Christ of Latter-day Saints-Fact and Statistics," 2023).

General Beliefs and Religious Practices

Members of the Church of Jesus Christ of Latter-day Saints believe in Christianity as preached by Jesus Christ. They believe that the church was lost shortly after the death of Christ and was restored in the early 1800s by Joseph Smith. Consequently, Latter-day Saints hold that God the Father is an embodied being, yet the roles Latter-day Saints ascribe to members of the Godhead largely correspond with the views of others in the Christian world. Latter-day Saints believe that God is omnipotent, omniscient, and all-loving, and they pray to Him in the name of Jesus Christ. They acknowledge the Father as the ultimate object of their worship, the Son as Lord and Redeemer, and the Holy Spirit as the messenger and revealer of the Father and the Son. For members, Sunday is the day observed as the Sabbath in the United States (Swihart et al., 2022).

Religious Objects, Rites, and Rituals

Copies of scriptures are often found at the bedside of members of this church. Reading these scriptures often brings comfort during times of illness. Scriptures sacred to members of the Church of Jesus Christ of Latter-day Saints include the Bible (Old and New Testament), the Book of Mormon, Doctrine and Covenants, and the book *The Pearl of Great Price*, part of the canonical standard works of the Mormon Church. Further, an adult member of the Church of Jesus Christ of Latter-day Saints may wear a special type of underclothing, called a **temple garment**. In a healthcare setting, the garment may be removed to facilitate care. As soon as the individual is well, they are likely to want to wear the garment again. The temple garment has special significance to the person,

symbolizing covenants or promises the person has made to God ("What is the temple garment?," 2023).

Diet and Substance Use

Members have a strict dietary code called the **Word of Wisdom**. Alcohol (including beer and wine), caffeinated beverages such as tea, coffee, and soda, and tobacco are forbidden, while herbal teas are allowed. In recent years, "recreational drugs" and non–medically indicated sedatives and narcotics have also been considered forbidden substances (Swihart et al., 2022). Fasting to a member means no food or drink (including water), usually for 24 hours. Fasting is required once a month on the designated fast Sunday. Those who are pregnant, very young, very old, and ill are not required to fast. The purpose of fasting is to bring oneself closer to God by controlling physical needs. The person is expected to donate the price of what has not been eaten to the church to be used to care for people experiencing poverty (Swihart et al., 2022).

Healthcare Practices

The members of the Church of Jesus Christ of Latter-day Saints believe that the power of God can be exercised on their behalf to bring about healing at the time of illness. The ritual of blessing the sick consists of one member (male Elder) of the priesthood anointing the ill person with oil and a second Elder "sealing the anointing with a prayer and a blessing." Commonly, both Elders place their hands on the individual's head. Faith in Jesus Christ and in the power of the priesthood to heal, requisite to the healing use of priesthood, does not preclude medical intervention but is seen as an adjunct to it. Members believe that medical intervention is one of God's ways of using humans in the healing process (Swihart et al., 2022).

Medical and Surgical Interventions

There is no restriction on the use of medications or vaccines in the Church of Jesus Christ of Latter-day Saints. It is not uncommon to find many members using herbal folk remedies, and it is wise for the nurse to explore in detail what an individual may already have done or taken. There is no restriction on the use of blood or blood components. Surgical intervention is a matter of individual decision in cases of amputations, transplants, and organ donations (both donor and recipient). Biopsies and resultant surgical procedures are also a matter of individual choice. The circumcision of infants is viewed as a medical health promotion measure and is not a religious ritual.

Practices Related to Reproduction

According to church doctrine, one of the major purposes of life is procreation; therefore, any form of prevention of the birth of children is contrary to church teachings. Exceptions to this policy include ill health of the mother or father and genetic conditions that could be passed on to offspring. "The decision of how many children to have and when to have them is extremely intimate and private, and the position of the church is that it should be left between the couple and the Lord" (Swihart et al., 2022); however, all measures that can be taken to promote having children are acceptable. Artificial insemination is acceptable if the semen is from the husband.

Amniocentesis is a matter of individual choice. However, even if the fetus is found to have a physical deformity, abortion is not an option unless the mother's life is in danger. Abortion is forbidden in all cases except when the mother's life is in danger or when a competent physician determines that the fetus has severe conditions that will not allow the baby to survive birth. Abortion on demand is strictly forbidden (Swihart et al., 2022).

Religious Support System for the Sick

The Church of Jesus Christ of Latter-day Saints has a highly organized network, and many church representatives are likely to visit a hospitalized member, including the bishop (pastor), and two counselors (leaders of the local congregation). Two men are usually assigned to men and two women to other women. Various titles are used for members of this church's hierarchy. For men,

the term *Elder* is generally acceptable, regardless of the man's position; the term Sister is acceptable for women, as are the traditional titles of Mr., Mrs., or Ms. (Swihart et al., 2022).

Practices Related to End of Life

Whenever possible, medical science and **faith healing** are used to reverse conditions that threaten life. When death is inevitable, the effort is to promote a peaceful and dignified death. The church teaches that life continues beyond death and that the dead are reunited with loved ones; death is another step in eternal progression. Euthanasia is not acceptable because the church teaches that life and death are in the hands of God, and humans must not interfere in any way. Autopsy is permitted with the consent of the next of kin and within local laws. Organ donation is permitted; it is an individual decision. Cremation is discouraged but not forbidden; burial is customary (Swihart et al., 2022).

Hinduism

There are approximately 1.1 billion Hindus worldwide, with approximately 2.5 million members in the United States and over 828,000 members in Canada ("Population of Christians, Hindus, Muslims and non-religious in Canada according to 2021 census," 2022; "World population review," 2023).

General Beliefs and Religious Practices

Hindus may be monotheistic, polytheistic, or atheistic; the basis of Hindu belief is the unity of everything. The major distinguishing characteristic is the social **caste system** that exists in the social structure and religious status. **Hinduism** is founded on sacred writings called the **Vedas** dating back to between 2300 B.C. and 1500 B.C. **Reincarnation** is a central belief in Hinduism. The law of **karma** determines life. According to karma, rebirth is dependent on moral behavior in a previous stage of existence. Life on earth is transient and a burden. Buddhism is similar to Hinduism, although Buddhism rejects the priests of Hinduism and the caste system, while both sects seek Nirvana, a state of extinction of passion, or the liberation from the cycle of rebirth and redeath. The practice of Hinduism consists of roles and ceremonies performed within the framework of the caste system, a social order determined by birth. These rituals focus on the main ethnoreligious events of birth, marriage, and death ("Hinduism," 2022).

Social Activities, Diet, and Substance Use

Social activities are strictly limited by the caste system. Many Hindus are vegetarians, and most do not eat beef or pork. At different stages of one's life, one may change one's dietary habits. For instance, in old age, a person who has been vegetarian may begin to eat fish or chicken. Substance use is not restricted (*Health care providers' handbook on Hindu patients*, 2011).

Religious Objects

A small picture of a deity may be found at the bedside. Prayer is often accompanied by the use of a "mala" (prayer beads) and a mantra (sacred utterance). Facing North or East during prayer is preferable, but not required.

Medical and Surgical Interventions

The use of medications, blood, and blood components is acceptable. Organ transplantations are acceptable for both donors and recipients. Female patients may prefer to be examined by a female healthcare practitioner. All patients may retain their own clothes underneath a hospital gown.

Practices Related to Reproduction

All types of birth control are acceptable. Amniocentesis is acceptable, although not often available. Abortion, except for medical reasons, is discouraged. Artificial insemination is not restricted, but it is not often practiced. Noting the exact time of a baby's birth is very important because it is used to determine the baby's horoscope. Males are not circumcised. Breastfeeding is expected. The infant is traditionally given a name on the 10th day following the birth, although in American hospitals, the child is sometimes named at birth (*Health care providers' handbook on Hindu patients*, 2011).

Practices Related to End of Life

No religious customs or restrictions related to the prolongation of life exist. Life is seen as a perpetual cycle, and death is considered as just one more step toward Nirvana. Euthanasia is not practiced. Autopsy is acceptable. The donation of body or parts is also acceptable. Cremation is the most common form of body disposal. Ashes are collected and disposed of in holy rivers (*Health care providers' handbook on Hindu patients*, 2011).

Islam

Islam is a monotheistic religion founded between 610 and 632 A.D. by the prophet Muhammad. Derived from an Arabic word meaning "submission," Islam literally translated means "submission to the will of God." Muhammad, revered as the prophet of **Allah** (God), is seen as succeeding and completing both Judaism and Christianity. Good deeds will be rewarded at the last judgment, whereas evil deeds will be punished in hell. Followers of Islam are called **Muslims**, which means "one who submits." In 2020, there were approximately 4.45 million Muslims in the United States, with a worldwide membership of approximately 1.9 billion ("Religious Information Data Explorer, Global Religious Futures," 2023).

General Beliefs and Religious Practices

The sources of the Islamic faith are the **Quran (Koran)**, which is regarded as the uncreated and eternal Word of God, and **Hadith** (tradition), regarded as sayings and deeds of the prophet Muhammad. All Muslims recognize the existence of the sharia, the divine counsel that Muslims follow for moral living and to grow close to God, and the five categories into which it divides human conduct: required, encouraged, permissible, discouraged, and prohibited.

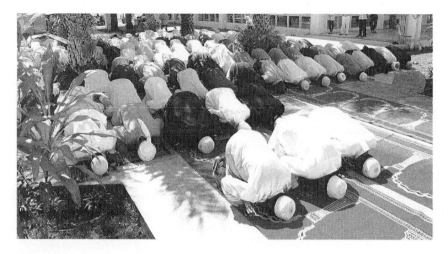

Figure 12-5. Pilgrims praying in the historic Pattani Masjid Mosque. (From Titima Ongkantong/Shutterstock.com.)

Various sects of Islam have developed, following Muhammad's death, including the *Sunni*, who adhere to the belief that the caliphs, or successors of Muhammad, should be chosen as Arab chiefs, customarily by election. The other group, the *Shia* or *Shiite*, maintain that Muhammad chose his cousin and son-in-law, Ali, as his spiritual and secular heir and that succession should be through his bloodline. The Shia and the Sunni are the two major branches of Muslims; the Sunni constitute about 85% of the total number of Muslims. The Sunni are found primarily in Lebanon, the West Bank, Jordan, and throughout Africa; the Shia are primarily in Iran and Iraq (Swihart et al., 2022).

Islam has five essential practices, or **Pillars of Faith** (Attum et al., 2022). These are as follows:

1. The profession of faith (Shahada), which requires bearing witness and complete submission to God and acknowledging Muhammad as His messenger
2. Ritual prayer five times daily for Sunni, and three times daily for Shia—facing Mecca, Saudi Arabia, Islam's holiest city (salat)
3. Almsgiving (zakat) to the needy, reflecting the Quran's admonition to share what one has with those less fortunate, including widows, orphans, people who are homeless, and people experiencing poverty

4. Month-long fast (sawm) of food, drink, and sexual intercourse during daylight hours (dawn until sunset) throughout Ramadan, the 9th month of the Islamic lunar calendar
5. Making a pilgrimage to Mecca at least once during one's lifetime (Hajj); see Figure 12-5 (Swihart et al., 2022)

Holy Days, Diet, and Substance Use

Days of observance in Islam are not "holy" days but days of celebration or observance. The Muslims follow a lunar calendar, so the days of observance change yearly. Eating pork, shellfish, and drinking alcoholic beverages are prohibited. Some Muslims only consume meat that has been ritually slaughtered by the process called **halal**, which means "the lawful or that which is permitted by Allah." A patient may inquire if the food received is "halal." If it is not, the patient may request that food be brought from home by family or friends.

As mentioned previously, fasting during the month of Ramadan is one of the pillars of Islam. Children (boys 7 years and older, girls 9 years and older) and adults are required to fast. Fasting means to abstain from food and drink from dawn until dusk. Those who are pregnant or nursing, older adults, and anyone whose physician has recommended not fasting due to a physical condition are exempt from fasting but are expected to fast later in the year or to feed a person in need to make up for the unfasted Ramadan days (Attum et al., 2022; Swihart et al., 2022).

Religious Objects

A prayer rug and the Quran are often present with a Muslim patient and should not be handled or touched by anyone who is ritually unclean. If the nurse needs to touch or move the prayer rug or the Quran, it is best to ask the patient or a family member for their assistance, unless an immediate emergency necessitates these items be moved.

Healthcare Practices

Female Muslim patients prefer to have female physicians and healthcare providers, while male Muslim patients prefer male physicians and healthcare providers. Vaccinations are encouraged. Touching between different sexes is discouraged, another reason why healthcare providers of the same sex are preferred.

Medical and Surgical Interventions

There are no restrictions on medications. Even items normally forbidden (e.g., pork derivatives) are permitted if prescribed as medicine, although some Muslims will request medications that do not have a pork derivative, such as insulin. The left hand is considered unclean, therefore medication administration, assistance with feeding, and handing objects to patients should be done with the right hand. The use of blood and blood components is not restricted. Amputations are not restricted. Organ transplantations are acceptable for both donor and recipient. Biopsies are acceptable. No age limit is fixed, but circumcision is practiced on boys at an early age (Attum et al., 2022; Swihart et al., 2022).

Practices Related to Reproduction

All types of birth control are generally acceptable in accordance with the law of "what is harmful to the body is prohibited." The family physician's advice on method of contraception is required.

Amniocentesis, if available, is used only to determine the status of the fetus, not the sex of the child; this is left in the hands of God. There is a strong religious objection to abortion, which is based on Muhammad's condemnation of the ancient Arabian practice of burying unwanted newborn girls alive. If in vitro fertilization takes place, the destruction of fertilized eggs would be considered an abortion and not allowed (Attum et al., 2022; Swihart et al., 2022).

Religious Support System for the Sick

In Islam, formal, organized support systems to assist the sick do not exist; family and friends provide emotional and financial support.

Practices Related to End of Life

The right to die is not recognized in Islam. Any attempt to shorten one's life or terminate it (suicide or euthanasia) is prohibited. Autopsy is permitted only for medical and legal purposes. The donation of body parts or body is acceptable, without restrictions. Withholding of life-sustaining care is acceptable to both Sunni and Shia Muslims; however, withdrawal of care is not acceptable from the Shia perspective. Maintaining a patient with a terminal condition on artificial life support is not encouraged in the Sunni tradition but is encouraged in the Shia tradition.

Burial of the dead, including fetuses, is compulsory. It is important in Islam to follow prescribed burial procedures. Rinsing and washing of the dead body according to Muslim tradition must be adhered to. Muslim women cleanse a woman's body and Muslim men a man's body. At the time of death, the person's eyes are closed, the limbs straightened, and the entire body is covered with a sheet of cloth. The body should be prepared and buried as soon as possible. This must occur within 24 hours of the death. Cremation and embalming are prohibited. The body should always be buried so that the head faces toward Mecca. Before a gestational age of 130 days, a fetus is treated like any other discarded tissue. After 130 days, the fetus is considered a fully developed human being and must be treated as such (Attum et al., 2022).

Jehovah's Witnesses

The exact number of membership in the **Jehovah's Witness** faith is difficult to ascertain. A member who fulfills their monthly obligation in proselytizing is known as a "publisher," while those who attend the yearly Memorial service are counted as members only and membership data are reported differently, which confounds the statistics. Membership is estimated at 1.2 million in the United States and 118,000 in Canada, totaling about 1.3 million in North America. Worldwide membership is approximately 8.4 million ("Jehovah's Witnesses," 2023).

General Beliefs and Religious Practices

Jehovah's Witnesses are Christians and derived their name from the Hebrew name for God (**Jehovah**), according to the King James Bible (*The Holy Bible: New King James Version*, 1769/1982). Thus, Jehovah's Witness is a descriptive name, indicating that members profess to bear witness concerning Jehovah, His Godship, and His purposes. Jehovah's Witnesses are opposed to saluting the flag, serving in the armed forces, voting in civil elections, and holding public office. This practice is related to the belief that Jesus Christ is King and Priest and that there is no need to hold citizenship in more than one kingdom. Members also refrain from gambling ("Jehovah's Witnesses," 2023).

Holy Days

Although Witnesses do not celebrate Christmas, Easter, or other traditional Christian holy days, a special annual observance of the Lord's Supper is held. Witnesses and others may attend this important meeting, but only those numbered among the 144,000 chosen members (Revelation 7:4) may partake of the bread and wine as a symbol of the death of Christ and the dedication to God. These elite members will be raised with spiritual bodies (without flesh, bones, or blood) and will assist Christ in ruling the universe. Others who benefit from Christ's ransom will be resurrected with healthy, perfected physical bodies (bodies of flesh, bones, and blood) and will inhabit this earth after the world has been restored to a paradisiacal state ("Jehovah's Witnesses," 2023; Swihart et al., 2022).

Social Activities and Substance Use

Youth are encouraged to socialize with members of their own religious background. Members abstain from the use of tobacco and hold that drunkenness is a serious sin. Alcohol used in moderation is acceptable.

Healthcare Practices

The practice of faith healing is forbidden. However, it is believed that reading the scriptures can comfort the individual and lead to mental and spiritual healing. Vaccinations are encouraged and use of vaccinations is an individual's choice. To the extent that they are necessary, medications are acceptable.

Medical and Surgical Interventions

Blood in any form and agents in which blood is an ingredient are not acceptable. Blood volume expanders are acceptable if they are not derivatives of blood. Mechanical devices for circulating the blood are acceptable as long as they are not primed with blood initially. Although surgical procedures are not in and of themselves opposed, the administration of blood during surgery is strictly prohibited. There is no church rule pertaining to the loss of limbs or the amputation of body parts. If they are a violation of the principle opposing bodily mutilation, transplants are forbidden. However, this is usually an individual decision. Biopsies are acceptable. Circumcision is an individual decision ("Jehovah's Witnesses," 2023; Swihart et al., 2022).

Practices Related to Reproduction

Sterilization is prohibited because it is viewed as a form of bodily mutilation. Other forms of birth control are left to the individual. Amniocentesis is acceptable. Both therapeutic and on-demand abortions are forbidden. Sterility testing is an individual decision. Artificial insemination is forbidden both for donors and for recipients. Jehovah's Witnesses do not condone any activities in the areas of eugenics and genetics; they are considered to interfere with nature and therefore are unacceptable.

Religious Support System for the Sick

Individual members of a congregation, including elders, visit the ill. Visitors pray with the sick person and read scriptures. Male religious representatives are referred to as "Mr." or "Elder" and females as "Ms." or "Mrs." Religious titles are not generally used. Individuals and members of the congregation look after the needs of the sick.

Practices Related to End of Life

The right to die or the use of extraordinary methods to prolong life is a matter of individual conscience. Euthanasia is forbidden. An autopsy is acceptable only if it is required by law. No parts are to be removed from the body. Jehovah's Witnesses believe that the human spirit and the body are never separated. The donation of a body is forbidden. Disposal of the body is a matter of individual preference. Burial practices are determined by local custom. Cremation is permitted if the individual chooses it (Swihart et al., 2022).

Judaism

Judaism is an Old Testament religion that dates back to the time of the prophet Abraham. Worldwide, there are approximately 15.2 million Jewish people. Membership includes approximately 6.0 million members in the United States, and 393,500 members in Canada (DellaPergola, 2022).

General Beliefs and Religious Practices

Judaism is a monotheistic religion. Jewish life historically has been based on interpretation of the laws of God communicated in the Ten Commandments given to Moses on Mount Sanai, as contained in the **Torah** and explained in the **Talmud** and in oral tradition. Ancient Jewish law prescribed most of the daily actions of the people. Diet, clothing, activities, occupation, and ceremonial activities throughout the life cycle are all part of Jewish daily life (Moses, 1611/1967). Today, there are at least three schools of theological thought and social practice in Judaism. The three main divisions include Orthodox, Conservative, and Reform. Any person born of a Jewish mother or anyone converted to Judaism are considered Jewish (Swihart et al., 2022).

Holy Days

The Sabbath is the holiest of all holy days. The Sabbath begins each Friday 18 minutes before sunset and ends on Saturday, 42 minutes after sunset, or when three stars can be seen in the sky with the naked eye.

Other holy days include the following:

1. Rosh Hashanah (Jewish New Year)
2. Yom Kippur (Day of Atonement, a fast day)
3. Chanukah (Festival of Lights, or Rededication of the Temple in Jerusalem)
4. Asara B'Tevet (Fast of the 10th of Tevet; not observed by liberal or Reform Jews)
5. Purim: Preceded by Fast of Esther holiday (no eating or drinking)
6. Passover
7. Shavuot (Festival of the Giving of the Torah)
8. Fast of the 17th of Tammuz
9. Fast of the 9th of Ave (Commemoration of the Destruction of the Temple)

Holy days are very special to practicing Jewish people. If a condition is not life-threatening, medical and surgical procedures should not be performed on the Sabbath or on holy days. Preservation of life is of greatest priority and is the major criterion for determining activity on holy days and the Sabbath. If a Jewish patient is hesitant to receive urgent and necessary treatment because of religious restrictions, the patient or their family should be encouraged to contact their rabbi for consultation (Swihart et al., 2022).

Rites and Rituals

Brit milah, the covenant of circumcision, is performed on all Jewish male children on the 8th day after birth. Although circumcision is a surgical procedure, for members of the Jewish faith, it is a fundamental religious obligation. Circumcision is usually performed by a **mohel**, usually a pious Jewish person with special training or by the child's father. Because the severing of the foreskin constitutes the essence of the ritual, the practice of having a non-Jewish or non-Observant physician perform the circumcision (even in the presence of a rabbi or other person who pronounces the blessing) is not acceptable according to Jewish law. Circumcision may be delayed if medically contraindicated. In Reform and Conservative traditions, a girl marks the 8th day of life with a dedication ceremony in which prayers and blessings are invoked on her behalf.

The *bar mitzvah* (meaning "son of the commandment") is a confirmation ceremony for boys at age 13 that has been preceded by extensive religious study, including mastery of key Torah passages in Hebrew (Fig. 12-6). In Reform and Conservative traditions, the *bas* (or *bat*) *mitzvah* (meaning "daughter of the commandment") is the equivalent ceremony for girls (Eisenberg, 2020).

Diet

The dietary laws of Judaism are very strict; the degree to which they are observed varies according to the individual. Strictly Observant Jewish people never eat pork or predatory fowl and never mix milk dishes and meat dishes. Only fish with fins and scales are permissible; shellfish and other water creatures are prohibited (Moses, 1611/1967).

The word **kosher** comes from a Hebrew word *kashrut* that means "proper." More colloquially, many people think that "kosher" refers to a type of food. If a patient asks for kosher food, it is important to determine what they mean.

Religious and Social Practices

On the Sabbath and on holidays, it is customary to light two candles in candleholders. Many Jewish men and some women wear *kippot* or *yarmulkes* (small head coverings) and *tallit* (prayer shawls) when praying. A *siddur* (prayer book) may also be present. Social activities that might

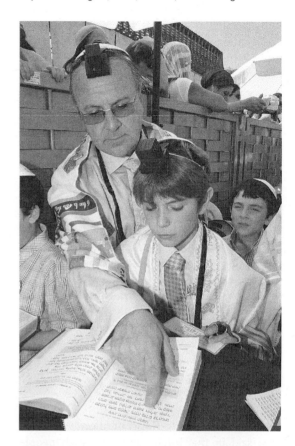

Figure 12-6 Bar Mitzvah ritual at the Wailing Wall in Jerusalem. When a boy becomes bar mitzvah at around the age of 13, he is morally and ethically responsible for his decisions and actions. (From Chameleons Eye/Shutterstock.com.)

lead to marriage outside the faith are discouraged. However, it is recognized that a significant number of individuals in Jewish society will seek partners outside of the Jewish faith. When this occurs, every effort is made to bring the non-Jewish partner into Judaism and to keep the Jewish partner a member and part of Jewish society (Eisenberg, 2020).

Substance Use

The Jewish guideline for substance use is moderation. Wine is a part of religious observance and used as such. Historically, Jewish people are well connected with their faith, with wine as an integral part of religious ceremonies. Further, drunkenness is discouraged in the Jewish scriptures, resulting in a low incidence of alcohol use disorder.

Healthcare Practices

Medical care from a physician in the case of illness is expected according to Jewish law. There are many prayers for the sick in Jewish liturgy. Such prayers and hope for recovery are encouraged.

Medical and Surgical Interventions

There are no restrictions when medications are used as part of a therapeutic process. There is a prohibition in Judaism against ingesting blood (e.g., blood sausage, raw meat). This does not apply to receiving blood transfusions. Beliefs and practices related to body mutilation (e.g., organ transplantation, amputations) vary widely in Judaism. Individual beliefs should be explored with the patient before any procedure that involves anything that could be considered body mutilation (Eisenberg, 2020; Swihart et al., 2022).

Practices Related to Reproduction

It is said in the Torah that the Jewish people should be fruitful and multiply; therefore, it is a *mitzvah* (a good deed) to have at least two children (Moses, 1611/1967). It is permissible to practice birth control in traditional and liberal homes. In the past, contraception was limited to female partners; vasectomy was prohibited. Currently, Judaism permits contraception by either partner, although Hasidic and Orthodox Jewish people rarely use vasectomy. Sterility testing is permissible when the goal is to enable the couple to have children. Artificial insemination is permitted under certain circumstances. A rabbi should be consulted in each individual case (Swihart et al., 2022).

Although therapeutic abortion is always permitted if the health of the mother is jeopardized, traditional Judaism regards the killing of an unborn child to be a serious moral offense; liberal Judaism permits it with strong moral admonitions

(i.e., it is not to be used as a means of birth control). The fetus, although not considered to be imbued with the full sanctity of life, is a potential human being and is acknowledged as such. The Jewish belief in the sanctity of life is a guiding factor in rabbinical counseling (Eisenberg, 2020).

Religious Support System for the Sick

The most likely visitors will be family and friends from the synagogue. To visit the sick is a mitzvah of service (an obligation, a responsibility, and a blessing). The formal religious representative from a synagogue is the rabbi. A visit from the rabbi may be spent talking, or the rabbi may pray with the person. If the patient is male and strictly observant, he may wish to have a prayer shawl (*tallit*), a cap (*kippah*), and *tefillin* (special symbols tied onto the arms and forehead). Prayers are often chanted. If possible, privacy should be provided (Eisenberg, 2020).

Practices Related to End of Life

A person has the right to die with dignity according to the Jewish faith. If a physician sees that death is inevitable, no new therapeutic measures that would artificially extend life need to be initiated; however, the amelioration of pain is paramount. It is important to know the precise time of death for the purpose of honoring the deceased after the first year has passed. Euthanasia is prohibited under any circumstances. It is regarded as murder.

Any unjustified alteration of a corpse is considered a desecration of the dead, to be avoided in normal circumstances. When postmortem examinations are justified, they must be limited to essential organs or systems. Needle biopsy is preferred. All body parts must be returned for burial. Jewish family members may ask to consult with a rabbinical authority before signing an autopsy consent form. Donation of body parts is a complex matter according to Jewish law. If it seems necessary, consultation with a rabbi should be encouraged (Eisenberg, 2020).

The body is ritually washed at a funeral home after death, by members of the Chevra

Kadisha (Ritual Burial Society) if possible. The body is then clothed in a simple white burial shroud. Embalming and cosmetic treatment of the body are forbidden. Public viewing of the body is considered a humiliation of the dead. Relatives are forbidden to touch or embrace the deceased, except when involved in preparation for interment. The exact time of burial is significant for *sitting Shiva*, the mourning period. After death in an institution, a nurse may wash the body for transport to the funeral home. Ritual washing then occurs later. Human remains, including a fetus at any stage of gestation, are to be buried as soon as possible. Cremation is not in keeping with Jewish law (Eisenberg, 2020; Swihart et al., 2022).

Native American and Indigenous People's Churches

There are an estimated 6.6 million Native Americans in the United States, who comprise approximately 573 Native American nations legally recognized by the Bureau of Indian Affairs ("Bureau of Indian Affairs," 2023). First Nations is a term used to describe the 3.1 million Aboriginal People in Canada who are not *Métis* or *Inuit* and self-identify as being of First Nations heritage. Native American and First Nations people have a wide range of group-specific, health-related spiritual, and religious beliefs and practices. Healers are known by a wide array of names, and their scope of practice varies widely from group to group, often encompassing herbal remedies and traditional healing rituals. Traditional healing practices may be used concurrently with contemporary biomedical interventions. In Canada, similar native people, i.e., the Metis and Inuit, are referred to as Indigenous people (Swihart et al., 2022).

General Beliefs and Religious Practices

In both the United States and Canada, Native Americans and Indigenous Canadians may adopt both a Christian tradition with its accompanying health beliefs and practices, as well as traditional healing practices. When trying to support a Native American in physical or psychological crisis, the nurse needs to remember several important items:

1. The Native North American belief about disease is not necessarily based on symptoms. Disease may be attributed to intrusive objects, soul loss, spirit intrusion, breach of taboo, or sorcery. Disease may also be attributed to natural or supernatural causes.
2. Native North Americans may embrace an organized (usually Christian) religion and still be a member of their nations and their religions.
3. Native North Americans also balance "modern theories of disease" with long-standing tribal beliefs or customs. Therefore, during illness and particularly hospitalization, Native Americans may ask to see a priest or minister in addition to their nation's healer. Visits from these people will likely be spiritually supportive, although the form of the support may vary greatly ("What are the religious/spiritual beliefs of Native Americans?," 2023).

Healthcare Practices

The spiritual basis for much of Native North American belief and action is symbolized by the number four. This number is seen in the extended hand, which means life, unity, equality, and eternity. The clasped hand symbolizes unity, the spiritual law that binds the universe. It is this unity on which decisions should be made. Questions about abortion, the use of drugs, giving and receiving blood, the right to life, euthanasia, and so on do not have dogmatic "yes" or "no" answers; rather, answers are based on the situation and the ultimate unity or disunity that a decision would produce.

In concert with the belief in the interconnectedness of all things, natural remedies in the form of herbal medicine are often used. Native

American folk medicine and herbal remedies provided the forerunners of many of today's pharmaceutical remedies. Herbal treatments are still used today and may be requested by Native North American patients. A nurse caring for a Native American patient should obtain a careful and complete history, including a list of whatever folk remedies have been tried. The patient may not know the names of herbs used in the treatment, and the tribal medicine man or woman may need to be consulted.

Respecting the concept that religion, medicine, and healing are inseparable to Native Americans, one must be sensitive to the fact that asking for the names of native medicines or descriptions of healing practices tried in an attempt to cure the person is not just simply obtaining a history but also entering into the realm of what is not only private but also very sacred. The nurse must use care and sensitivity and show deep respect for the information received ("What are the religious/spiritual beliefs of Native Americans?," 2023).

Protestantism

In its broadest meaning, **Protestantism** denotes the whole movement within Christianity that originated in the 16th century with Martin Luther and the Protestant Reformation. Historically and traditionally, the chief characteristics of Protestantism are the acceptance of the Bible as the only source of infallible revealed truth, the belief in the universal priesthood of believers, and the doctrine that Christians are justified in their relationship to God by faith alone, not by good works or dispensations of the church (Fortosis & Atkinson, 2022; *The Holy Bible: New King James Version*, 1769/1982).

General Beliefs and Religious Practices

It is difficult to accurately categorize Protestant churches and impossible to mention them all; there are more than 30,000 different denominations, and approximately 900 million adherents worldwide. Protestantism can be divided into four major forms: Lutheran, Anglican, Reformed, and independent churches. Among independent churches are Baptists, Adventists, Congregationalists, Churches of Christ, Mennonites, Amish, and Anabaptists.

Lutheranism is the oldest and third largest Protestant religion. Lutheranism began in 1517 with Martin Luther's split from the Roman Catholic Church. Lutherans emphasize theological doctrine and spirituality. There are approximately 77 million Lutherans worldwide and more that 5 million in the United States (Fortosis & Atkinson, 2022; "The Lutheran World Federation," 2023).

Anglicanism is represented by the established Church of England, the Episcopal Church in the United States, and similar churches. Methodist churches have their roots in the Anglican church and were established by followers of John Wesley, an 18th-century Anglican who sought to bring reform to the Church of England. Wesley's movement spread to the United States and Canada in the 18th century. There are approximately 91 million Anglicans worldwide and more than 1.8 million in the United States ("WorldData.info," 2023).

The *Reformed denominations* include Presbyterianism and are based on the teachings of John Calvin and his followers. These churches are distinguished from Lutheranism and Anglicanism, which maintain symbolic and sacramental traditions that originated before the Protestant Reformation. There are approximately 75 million people who practice one of the reformed denominations ("WorldData.info," 2023).

Independent churches, including Baptists, Adventists, Congregationalists, Churches of Christ, Mennonites, Amish, and Anabaptists, exercise congregational government. Each local denomination is an independent autonomous unit, and there is no official doctrine. With 37.5 million members of the Baptist faith in the United States and more than 100 million worldwide, the Baptist church makes up more than 11% of the population of the United States ("WorldData.info," 2023).

Healthcare Practices

Given the wide diversity that exists within Protestant denominations, it is beyond the scope of this text to identify health-related beliefs and practices for each group.

Seventh-Day Adventists

Membership of **Seventh-Day Adventists** in United States and Canada is approaching 1.2 million, with worldwide membership of 22 million. Doctrinally, Seventh-Day Adventists are heirs of the interfaith Millerite movement of the late 1840s, although the movement officially adopted the name Seventh-Day Adventist in 1863 ("Office of archives, statistics, and research," 2023).

General Beliefs and Religious Practices

Seventh-Day Adventists accept the Bible as their only creed and hold certain fundamental beliefs to be the teaching of the Holy Scriptures. There are official statements by the General Conference concerning the scriptures, the trinity, creation, nature of man, the great controversy (Christ vs. Satan), life, death, resurrection, and other topics.

Holy Days, Rites, and Rituals
The seventh day of the week, Saturday, is observed as the Sabbath—from Friday sundown to Saturday sundown. The Sabbath is the day that God blessed and sanctified and is a sacred day of worship and rest; worship services are held on Saturday. There are three church **ordinances**: (1) baptism by immersion, (2) the Ordinance of Humility, and (3) the Lord's Supper or Communion. There are no rituals at the time of birth. There is no requirement for a final sacrament at death. If requested by the individual or family member, the dying person might be anointed with oil ("Official Beliefs of the Seventh-day Adventist Church," 2023).

Diet and Substance Use
Seventh-Day Adventists believe that because the body is the temple of God, it is appropriate to abstain from any food or beverage that could prove harmful to the body. Because the first human diet consisted of fruits and grains, the Church encourages a vegetarian diet. Nevertheless, some members choose to eat beef and poultry. Based on a passage in Leviticus 11:3, nonvegetarian members refrain from eating foods derived from any animal that both does not have a cloven hoof and chews its cud or is considered unclean based on the Leviticus passage (e.g., meat derived from pigs, rabbits, or similar animals). Although fish with fins and scales are acceptable (e.g., salmon), shellfish are prohibited. Consumption of common poultry such as chicken and turkey are acceptable. Fasting is practiced, but only when members of a specific church elect to do so. Practiced in degrees, fasting may involve abstention from food or liquids. Fasting is not encouraged if it is likely to have adverse effects on the individual. Fermented beverages are prohibited. Members should abstain from the use of tobacco products ("Official Beliefs of the Seventh-day Adventist Church," 2023).

Healthcare Practices

The church believes in divine healing and practices anointing with oil and prayer. This is in addition to healing brought about by medical intervention. Since 1865, the church has maintained chaplains and physicians as inseparable in its institutions. There are eight principles that guide decisions/actions related to health: nutrition, divine power, exercise, rest, abstemiousness, fresh air, water, and sunlight ("Official Beliefs of the Seventh-day Adventist Church," 2023).

Medical and Surgical Interventions
Adventists operate one of the world's largest religiously operated health systems, including a medical school. Seventh Day Adventist's **Health Ministries** include more than 200 hospitals and sanitariums worldwide, with 77 in the United States. Worldwide, there are also 16 nursing home and rehabilitation sites and 27 senior living centers ("Office of archives, statistics, and

research," 2023). Worldwide, there are many clinics and dispensaries, orphanages, and children's homes, as well as a number of airplanes and medical launches. Physical medicine and rehabilitation are emphasized and recommended, along with therapeutic diets. There are no restrictions on the use of vaccines. Similarly, there are no restrictions on the use of blood and blood products, organ transplants, amputations, donation of organs, biopsies, and circumcisions (Swihart et al., 2022).

Practices Related to Reproduction

The use of birth control is an individual decision; the church prohibits sexual intercourse except between husband and wife. There are no restrictions on amniocentesis. Therapeutic abortion is acceptable if the mother's life is in danger and in cases of rape and incest. On-demand abortion is unacceptable because Adventists believe in the sanctity of life. Artificial insemination between husband and wife is acceptable. Although the church views practices in the fields of eugenics and genetics as an individual decision (elective abortion of unborn children with disabilities), it upholds the principle of responsibility in dealing with children (Swihart et al., 2022).

Religious Support System for the Sick

At the request of the sick person or the family, the pastor and elders of the church will come together to pray and anoint the sick person with oil. The religious representative is referred to as Doctor, Pastor, or Elder.

Practices Related to End of Life

Although there is no official position, the church has traditionally followed the medical ethics of prolonging life and prohibiting euthanasia. Autopsy and the donation of the entire body or parts are acceptable. No directives or recommendations exist regarding disposal of the body. No specific directives concerning burial exist; this is an individual decision (Swihart et al., 2022).

Summary

Religious and cultural beliefs are interwoven and influence a patient's understanding of illness and healthcare practices. In times of serious illness and impending death, religion may be a source of consolation for the patient. The culturally competent nurse will complete a cultural assessment to evaluate the patient's spiritual and religious beliefs, practices, and traditions, to be well informed of these important issues. The goal of spiritual nursing care is to assist patients in integrating their personal spiritual and religious beliefs into the plan of care, and with interventions that are congruent with those beliefs. Health-related beliefs and practices related to spirituality and religious traditions are important to understand, especially considering the broad diversity in religious beliefs in the United States and Canada.

REVIEW QUESTIONS

1. When assessing the spiritual needs of patients from diverse cultural backgrounds, what key components should you consider?
2. In providing nursing care for the dying or bereaved patient and family, what cultural considerations should the nurse include in the plan?
3. Compare and contrast the religious beliefs and practices concerning diet, medications, and procedures for five of the religious groups discussed in this chapter.
4. Analyze the contributions of religious organizations to the United States and/or Canadian healthcare delivery system. What effect do healthcare facilities that are owned and operated by religious groups have on the overall cost and quality of healthcare in the United States and Canada? Critically analyze concerns about these religiously operated facilities in terms of philosophical, ethical, and legal aspects pertaining to types of services offered to patients.

5. What religious rituals mark significant developmental milestones for children and adolescents? Identify the ritual or ceremony, the approximate age at which the child or adolescent participates in it, and the name of the religion(s) associated with it.

CRITICAL THINKING ACTIVITIES

1. Visit a church or worship center not of your own belief system and interview a member of the clergy or an official representative about the health-related beliefs of that religion. Discuss with them the implications of those beliefs for someone hospitalized for an acute or chronic illness. Inquire about the ways in which nurses can be of most help to hospitalized members of this religion.

2. Interview members of various religions concerning their beliefs about health and illness. Compare these interviews with the published beliefs or official statements from these religions. Discuss the implications of the differences (if any) that you found.

3. Interview fellow students, classmates, or coworkers about what they know of the health beliefs of various religions, especially those religions most often encountered among the patients with whom you work. Make a poster or prepare a presentation comparing the results of your interviews with the official beliefs of those religions. Share this information with your classmates.

4. Interview four or more members of the same religious group who are of various ages (i.e., children, teenagers, young adults, middle aged, or older adults). Ask them about their religious beliefs and how they affect their healthcare choices. Compare the results, commenting on similarities and differences.

5. If you have thought about the above exercises in terms of physical health, consider each of the activities from the perspective of mental health and spiritual health.

REFERENCES

Abortion. (2023). *Pro-life activities.* https://www.usccb.org/prolife/abortion

Amish population profile, 2022. (2022). https://groups.etown.edu/amishstudies/statistics/amish-population-profile-2022/

Amish Studies. (2022). https://groups.etown.edu/amishstudies/religion/beliefs/

Anderson, C., & Potts, L. (2020). The Amish health culture and culturally sensitive health services: An exhaustive narrative review. *Social Science and Medicine, 265,* 113466. https://doi.org/10.1016/j.socscimed.2020.113466

Anderson, R. J., Bloch, S., Armstrong, M., Stone, P. C., & Low, J. T. (2019). Communication between healthcare professionals and relatives of patients approaching the end-of-life: A systematic review of qualitative evidence. *Palliative Medicine, 33*(8), 926–941.

Andrews, M. M., & Boyle, J. S. (2019). The Andrews/Boyle transcultural interprofessional practice (TIP) model. *Journal of Transcultural Nursing, 30*(4), 323–330. https://doi.org/10.1177/1043659619849475

Attum, B., Hafiz, S., Malik, A., & Shamoon, Z. (2022). *Cultural competence in the care of Muslim patients and their families.* StatPearls Publishing.

Barbosa, D. J., Tosoli, A. M. G., De Oliveira Fleury, M. L., Dib, R. V., De Oliveira Fleury, L. F., & da Silva, A. N. (2018). Social representations of mental disorders. *The Journal of Nursing, 12*(6), 1813–1816. https://doi.org/10.5205/1981-8963-V126a235018p1813-1816

Bone, N., Swinton, M., Hoad, N., Toledo, F., & Cook, D. (2018). Critical care nurses' experiences with spiritual care: The SPIRIT study. *American Journal of Critical Care, 27*(3), 212–219.

Buddhism and contraception. (2009, November 23). https://www.bbc.co.uk/religion/religions/buddhism/buddhistethics/contraception.shtml

Buddhists. (2023). *Religious landscape study.* https://www.pewresearch.org/religion/religious-landscape-study/religious-tradition/buddhist/

Bureau of Indian Affairs. (2023). https://www.bia.gov/

Catholic Charities USA. (2023). *Our ministry.* https://www.catholiccharitiesusa.org/our-vision-and-ministry/

Catholic Health Alliance of Canada. (2023). https://www.chac.ca/en/

Catholic Health Care in the United States. (2023). *Facts—Statistics*. https://www.chausa.org/about/about/facts-statistics

Christian Science-Beliefs and teaching. (2023). *Christian science*. https://www.christianscience.com/what-is-christian-science/beliefs-and-teachings

Christian Science-Christian Science Nursing. (2023). https://www.christianscience.com/additional-resources/christian-science-nursing-activities

Christian Science healing. (2008). *Religion and ethics*. http://www.pbs.org/wnet/religionandethics/week1148/feature.html

Christian Science-How can I be healed? (2023). *Christian healing today*. https://www.christianscience.com/christian-healing-today/how-can-i-be-healed

The Church of Jesus Christ of Latter-Day Saints-Fact and Statistics. (2023). https://newsroom.churchofjesuschrist.org/facts-and-statistics/country/united-states

Collins, J. W., Zoucha, R., Lockhart, J. S., & Mixer, S. J. (2021). Cultural aspects of end-of-life advance care planning for African Americans: An ethnonursing study. *Journal of Transcultural Nursing*, *32*(5), 558–566. https://doi.org/10.1177/1043659620960788

The complete guide to Buddhist burial practices and rituals. (2022). *Religion*. https://www.betterplaceforests.com/blog/articles/the-complete-guide-to-buddhist-burial-practices-and-rituals

Countryfarm lifestyles. (2023). *Amish customs and culture for funerals and burials, death and dying*. https://www.countryfarm-lifestyles.com/amish-customs_funerals.html#.ZAzSXh_MLct

DellaPergola, S. (2022). World Jewish Population, 2021. In A. Dashefsky & I. M. Sheskin (Eds.), *American Jewish Year Book 2021: The Annual Record of the North American Jewish Communities Since 1899* (pp. 313–412). Springer International Publishing.

Doyle, K. (2022). *Suicide and mortal sin: What is true forgiveness? Catholic review*. https://catholicreview.org/suicide-and-mortal-sin-what-is-true-forgiveness/

Eddy, M. B. (1875). *Science and health with key to the scriptures*.

Eisenberg, R. L. (2020). *Jewish traditions: JPS guide*. U of Nebraska Press.

End of Life. (2023). *Pro-life activities*. https://www.usccb.org/prolife/end-life

Ethical and religious directives for Catholic health care services. (2020, June 2018).

Faulkner, J. E., & DeJong, C. F. (1966). Religiosity in 5D: An empirical analysis. *Social Forces*, *45*, 246–254.

Fortosis, S., & Atkinson, H. T. (2022). *Fallible heroes: Inside the protestant reformation*. Wipf and Stock Publishers.

A guide to Mormon burial practices and funeral etiquette. (2022). *Better place forests*. https://www.betterplaceforests.com/blog/articles/a-guide-to-mormon-burial-practices-and-funeral-etiquette

Health Care. (2023). *Health policy*. https://www.pewresearch.org/topic/religion/

Health care providers' handbook on Hindu patients. (2011). Queensland Health.

Heilman, S. C. (2018). *Death, bereavement, and mourning*. Routledge.

Hinduism. (2022). https://www.history.com/topics/religion/hinduism

The Holy Bible: New King James Version. (1769/1982). Thomas Nelson.

How long can you delay a funeral after death? (2023). https://www.devlinfuneralhome.com/blog/how-long-can-you-delay-a-funeral-after-death/

Jehovah's Witnesses. (2023). https://www.jw.org/en/jehovahs-witnesses/contact/united-states-america/

King, S., & Cayley, W. E. (2021). Choosing faith: The importance of belief in finding purpose in life. *Family Medicine*, *53*(5), 386–387. https://doi.org/10.22454/FamMed.2021.748400

Kubler-Ross, E. (1969). *On death and dying* (Vol. 1). Macmillan.

Leininger, M. M. (2002). The future of transcultural nursing. In M. M. Leininger & M. R. McFarland (Eds.), *Transcultural nursing: Concepts, theories, research, and practice* (3rd ed., pp. 577–595). McGraw-Hill.

Leyva, B., Allen, J. D., Tom, L. S., Ospino, H., Torres, M. I., & Abraido-Lanza, A. F. (2014). Religion, fatalism, and cancer control: A qualitative study among Hispanic Catholics. *American Journal of Health Behavior*, *38*(6), 839–849.

The Lutheran World Federation. (2023). https://www.lutheranworld.org/

Madan, T. N. (1992). Dying with dignity. *Social Science and Medicine*, *35*(4), 425–432.

Markin, R. D., & Zilcha-Mano, S. (2018). Cultural processes in psychotherapy for perinatal loss: Breaking the cultural taboo against perinatal grief. *Psychotherapy*, *55*(1), 20.

McFarland, M. R. (2018). The theory of culture care diversity and universality. In M. R. McFarland & H. Wehbe-Alamah (Eds.), *Leininger's transcultural nursing: Concepts, theories, research, and practice* (4th ed., pp. 39–56). McGraw-Hill.

McFarland, M. R., & Wehbe-Alamah, H. B. (2019). Leininger's theory of culture care diversity and universality: An overview with a historical perspective and a view toward the future. *Journal of Transcultural Nursing*, *30*(6), 540–557. https://doi.org/10.1177/1043659619867134

McKeown, J. (2023). *Where Catholics live in the United States* https://www.catholicnewsagency.com/news/253190/where-catholics-live-in-the-united-states-explained-in-four-charts

Mixer, S. J. (2018). Culturally congruent end-of-life care: A universal health need. *Journal of Transcultural Nursing*, *29*(5), 489–489. https://doi.org/10.1177/1043659618778968

Mohler Jr., R. A. (Writer). (2018). *The briefing, biblical worldview of suicide.* The Southern Baptist Theological Seminary.

Montgomery, L., & Owen-Pugh, V. (2018). Bereavement counselling in Uganda and Northern Ireland: A comparison. *British Journal of Guidance and Counselling, 46*(1), 91–103. https://doi.org/10.1080/03069885.2017.1370691

Mori, M., Kuwama, Y., Ashikaga, T., Parsons, H. A., & Miyashita, M. (2018). Acculturation and perceptions of a good death among Japanese Americans and Japanese living in the US. *Journal of Pain and Symptom Management, 55*(1), 31–38.

Moses. (1611/1967). *King James Bible Gen., Exod., Lev., Num., Deut.* Oxford University Press.

Natural Family Planning. (2023). *Marriage and family life.* https://www.usccb.org/topics/natural-family-planning

Office of archives, statistics, and research. (2023). *Directory.* https://www.adventistdirectory.org/default.aspx?&&pa ge=searchresults&&EntityType=MH&..&PageIndex=4

Official Beliefs of the Seventh-day Adventist Church. (2023). *Seventh Day-Adventist World Church.* https://www. adventist.org/beliefs/

Ohr, S. O., Cleasby, P., Jeong, S. Y.-S., & Barrett, T. (2021). Nurse-led normalised advance care planning service in hospital and community health settings: A qualitative study. *BMC Palliative Care, 20*(1), 139. https://doi.org/10.1186/s12904-021-00835-x

Orlich, M. J., & Fraser, G. E. (2014). Vegetarian diets in the Adventist Health Study 2: A review of initial published findings. *The American Journal of Clinical Nutrition, 100*(suppl_1), 353S–358S.

Pattison, S. (2013). Religion, spirituality and health care: Confusions, tensions, opportunities. *Health Care Analysis, 21*(3), 193–207. https://doi.org/10.1007/s10728-013-0245-4

Population of Christians, Hindus, Muslims and non-religious in Canada according to 2021 census. (2022). https:// www.todocanada.ca/population-of-christians-hindus-muslims-and-non-religious-in-canada-according-to-census-2021/

Profile table, Census Profile, 2021 Census of Population – Canada. (2022). www12.statcan.gc.ca.

Purnell, L. D., & Fenkl, E. A. (2019). *The Amish Handbook for culturally competent care* (pp. 63–71). Springer Nature.

Rahmawati, I., Wihastuti, T. A., Rachmawati, S. D., & Kumboyono, K. (2018). Nursing experience in providing spiritual support to patients with acute coronary syndrome at emergency unit: Phenomenology study. *International Journal of Caring Sciences, 11*(2), 1147–1151.

Religious Information Data Explorer, Global Religious Futures. (2023). www.globalreligiousfutures.org

Religious Landscape Study. (2017). https://www.pewresearch. org/religion/religious-landscape-study/

Sacraments and Sacramentals. (2023). *Prayer and worship.* https://www.usccb.org/prayer-and-worship/sacraments-and-sacramentals

Scammell, J. (2017). Religion, spirituality and belief: Is this the business of nurses? *British Journal of Nursing, 26*(9), 528. https://doi.org/10.12968/bjon.2017.26.9.528

Shepperd, S., Gonçalves-Bradley, D. C., Straus, S. E., & Wee, B. (2021). Hospital at home: Home-based end-of-life care. *Cochrane Database of Systematic Reviews, 3*(3), CD009231. https://doi.org/10.1002/14651858.CD009231.pub3

Sherwen, E. (2014). Improving end of life care for adults. *Nursing Standard, 28*(32).

Siritsky, R. N. (2020). *A Jewish understanding of palliative care: Reclaiming the healing process* (1st ed.). Routledge.

Sorajjakool, S., Carr, M. F., & Bursey, E. J. (2017). *World religions for healthcare professionals* (2nd ed.). Routledge.

Spiritual beliefs and preferences—Evaluating a patient's spiritual needs. (2022, July 19). *Provision of Care Treatment and Services.* https://www.jointcommission.org/standards/standard-faqs/hospital-and-hospital-clinics/provision-of-care-treatment-and-services-pc/000001669/?p=1

Spread of Buddhism. (2023). https://www.worlddata.info/religions/buddhism.php

Swihart, D. L., Yarrarapu, S. N. S., & Martin, R. L. (2022). *Cultural religious competence in clinical practice.* StatPearls Publishing.

Traditional Jewish ritual and mourning practices. (2023). https://www.jcfs.org/our-services/jewish-community-programs/illness-loss-grief/guide-for-the-grieving/traditional-mourning

Vázquez-Sánchez, J. M., Fernández-Alcántara, M., García-Caro, M. P., Cabañero-Martínez, M. J., Martí-García, C., & Montoya-Juárez, R. (2019). The concept of death in children aged from 9 to 11 years: Evidence through inductive and deductive analysis of drawings. *Death Studies, 43*(8), 467–477. https://doi.org/10.1080/07481187.2018.1480545

Wass, H. (2018). Death in the lives of children and adolescents. *Dying: Facing the facts* (pp. 269–301). Taylor & Francis.

Wehbe-Alamah, H., Hammonds, L. S., & Stanley, D. (2021). Culturally congruent care from the perspectives of Judaism, Christianity, and Islam. *Journal of Transcultural Nursing, 32*(2), 119–128.

What are the religious/spiritual beliefs of Native Americans? (2023). *Got questions.* https://www.gotquestions.org/Native-American-beliefs.html

What is the temple garment? (2023). https://www.churchofjesuschrist.org/tools/what-is-the-temple-garment?lang=eng

Who We Are. (2023). https://www.jhf.org/

World population review. (2023). https://worldpopulationreview.com/country-rankings/hindu-countries

WorldData.info. (2023). *Anglicans.* https://www.worlddata. info/religions/anglicans.php

Zoucha, R., & Zamarripa-Zoucha, A. (2021). People of Mexican heritage. In L. D. Purnell & E. A. Fenkl (Eds.), *Textbook for transcultural health care: A population approach: Cultural competence concepts in nursing care* (pp. 613–636). Springer International Publishing.

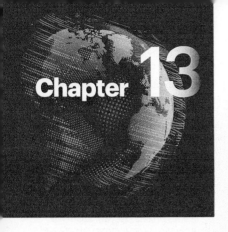

Chapter 13

Health Equity, Social Justice, and Cultural Competence

- Dula F. Pacquiao

Key Terms

Advocacy
Autonomy
Beneficence
Compassion
Cultural preservation,
   accommodation,
   repatterning
Culturally competent care
Culturally congruent care
Deontology

Empathy
Empowerment
Ethic of care
Ethical relativism
Ethical universalism
Fidelity
Health disparities
Health inequity
Human rights
Nonmaleficence
Principlism/Principle-based
   ethics

Population
Population health
Social justice
Social capital
Bonding, bridging, and linking
   social capital
Teleology
Truth telling
Veracity
Vulnerable population

Learning Objectives

1. Differentiate ethical relativism from universalism.
2. Describe how moral philosophies are socially and culturally constituted.
3. Analyze significance of ethics in population health promotion and achievement of health equity.
4. Describe the model of culturally competent ethical decision-making for health equity.
5. Use research findings relevant to ethical decision-making.

Introduction

Nurses are often confronted by ethical dilemmas in their work. Nurses decide on care priorities and allocate human and material resources for their clients. Ethical decisions are complicated by diversity in client populations with different social and cultural backgrounds in healthcare organizations emphasizing common standards of care. Nurses need to negotiate with varying values not only of their clients but also of other care providers and the organization where they work. In addition, there is urgency in addressing health disparities associated with social inequities in local, national, and global societies. Nurses need to be informed of how social inequalities rooted in social determinants of health associated with peoples' life conditions significantly impact their health. Nurses and other health professionals are confronted by the need to develop innovations to promote population health beyond disease-based and individual-focused care. While culturally competent care addresses diversity, ethical practice grounded in social justice and human rights prevents **health inequity**. This chapter aims to give an overview of differing moral assumptions and the need for ethical relativism as well as the growing recognition of ethical universalistic approaches. It presents a model linking cultural competence and ethics to promote health equity.

Ethical Relativism

A moral philosophy consists of beliefs and assumptions about what is right and wrong, which is the basis of ethics that prescribes the proper action to take in a given situation. Morals and philosophical beliefs are constituted within the social, historical, and cultural experiences of a society. These beliefs evolve as normative patterns of assumptions that serve as an implicit framework guiding the actions and thoughts of group members, which may or may not be shared by persons outside of the cultural group.

Ethical relativism holds that morality is relative to the norms of a particular culture; hence, there

are no universal truths in ethics. It emphasizes the need to examine the context of the decision because sociocultural differences influence whether an act is moral. Ethical relativism is unlike universalistic moral philosophies such as **deontology**, which upholds the existence of universal truths and unbreakable moral rules applicable to all situations (Barrow & Khandhar, 2022), and **teleology**, which judges the morality of an act based on its consequence or outcome (The Ethics Centre, 2022). Ethical relativism states that what is right for one group may not be right for another.

Contrasting conceptualizations of human beings exist in Western societies such as the United States and Canada, and non-Western cultures as China and Saudi Arabia. There is a pervasive belief that human beings are endowed with the capacity for reason and action in Western cultures. Reason is assumed to be a universal capacity, and it is through reason that all human beings can be expected to make valid and truthful judgments in any situation. Since the era of Enlightenment, the philosophic traditions of universalism and rationalism have shaped the Western concept of the person as the focus of moral reasoning. The person is the basic unit imbued with a universal capacity for reason and action (Guest, 2017). Ethical conflicts are often attributed to individual differences in cognitive skills, motivation, information, and/or linguistic capacity, and thus, by compensating for these deficits, a person can be expected to make a rational decision that is universally regarded as logical and morally acceptable. However, not all human behaviors can be classified as simply rational or irrational. Culture can be arbitrary, and human beings create their own distinctive, symbolic realities. Many of our ideas and practices are beyond logic and experience.

In some groups, religious and spiritual dimensions highly influence behaviors. Among such ethnoreligious groups as devout Muslims, Hindus, and Jews, religion is embedded in everyday life. Orthodox Jewish people may not accept euthanasia because of their belief in the sanctity of life. Jewish people generally consult their rabbi regarding matters pertaining to life and death decisions

(Wehbe-Alamah et al., 2021), Religion increases the awareness of the power and benevolence of God over humans; hence, earthly decisions are left to God, and the attitude is one of acceptance of fate rather than control over one's destiny. Members of Jehovah's Witness oppose blood transfusion as a lifesaving measure, and Christian Scientists may prefer their own religious and spiritually based practices of healing to those of traditional medicine.

Organ donation may be considered heroic in the biomedical profession and mainstream American culture. Religious, historical, and cultural influences, however, may prevent individuals from becoming organ donors. The legacy of Henrietta Lacks has opened ethico-moral issues that help explain Black Americans' reticence to become organ donors because of past and present experiences that built a collective sense of mistrust of the healthcare system and health professionals (Shah, 2022). Lacks, an African American woman, was the source of the HeLa cell line taken from a biopsy of her cervical tumor at Johns Hopkins Hospital in Baltimore, Maryland in 1951. At that time, no consent was required to culture the cells obtained from her. Lacks and her family were unaware of this development until 1970, when the origins of the immortalized HeLa cell line became known and its continuous use in medical research began. Neither Lacks nor her family were compensated for the extraction or use of the HeLa cells.

Cultural practices such as female genital cutting, body piercing and tattooing, and taking home a newborn's afterbirth may appear illogical and without any scientific basis to those outside the culture. Yet, these practices are supported by value–belief systems that are deeply entrenched in religious, philosophical, and social structure of certain groups. To professional practitioners, resistance to scientifically proven measures belies common sense, but cultural traditions of some groups transcend rationality and logic. Indeed, common sense is not common after all; it is uniquely constructed within the social and cultural life contexts of human groups.

In individualistic cultures, the person is viewed as a self-contained entity, fully integrated and self-motivating, independent of social roles and relationships, and distinct from all others (Guest, 2017). In contrast, among collectivistic cultures, there is greater continuity and mutuality among group members. Collective decisions by the extended family represented by the clan, tribe, or village make major decisions about the distribution of human and material resources to provide care for their members. Members of collective cultures expect to be physically present for family members who are dying or seriously ill. Numbers of family members present generally exceed the norm for visitation in most hospitals. Negotiating with the religious leader and/or group leader can effectively arrange numbers of visitors in one room at the same time with the client.

In cultures that value individualism, the concept of the individual being imbued with rational capacity translates to an expectation that one can make the decision and be responsible for oneself. Respect for autonomy has become the focal context for healthcare decisions in the United States and Canada. Ethical principles are applied to ensure and maximize individual autonomy. The autonomy paradigm, which has been institutionalized in healthcare, underlines interactions with and expectations of clients and families by practitioners. The Patient Self-Determination Act passed by the US Congress in 1991 mandates healthcare practitioners to provide clients with information about advance directives intended to assure their autonomy in situations when they can no longer make a decision. Clients' choices are presumably carried out on their behalf in the event that they cannot consciously and competently represent their own will. Although the intent of advance directives is consistent with an ethos of self-determination that is present in many cultures, other cultures subscribe to the belief that the fate of human beings is beyond their control; thus, discussions of end-of-life issues and advanced directives are taboo (Terpstra et al., 2021).

The US Congress also passed the Health Insurance Portability and Accountability Act (HIPAA) in 1996 that sets national standards for protecting the privacy, confidentiality, and security of individually identifiable health information by covered entities and business associates. HIPAA ensures confidentiality of an individual's health information. Healthcare practitioners are required to seek the client's informed consent before any information is shared with others, including family members. This poses difficulty for collectivistic groups where family members decide which information is shared with the client and other family members (Yiu et al., 2021). The concept of individual autonomy brings an associated expectation of individual responsibility and accountability. This creates a predilection to reward self-care and label those individuals as noncompliant when they do not adhere to prescribed biomedical regimen. Health professionals often ignore social factors that hinder an individual client's ability to act on health teaching and prescribed regimen. Because the focus of care is on individual responsibility and accountability, vulnerable groups tend to avoid seeking medical help unless they are desperately ill or selectively act on parts of the regimen that they have the capacity and resources to implement.

By contrast, collective cultures favor group decisions and role assumptions by individuals based on their status in the established group hierarchy. Family and kinship patterns assign different roles, status, and power among group members. The social hierarchy governs decision-making, interactions, roles, and obligations of members. Conversely, the value of instrumental individualism prizes the ability of individuals to make choices and rely upon themselves to achieve their purpose in life. Although, for example, a Chinese adult who adheres to traditional cultural values relies upon family members and the physician to make decisions, a typical American or Canadian adult expects to be given information to make their own decision.

In some cultures, such as some African and Islamic groups, older men occupy higher status and greater influence in decision-making. They may decide to withhold the truth about hopeless prognosis from the client in order to protect the vulnerable member from the burden of truth and despair. Advance planning to identify potential ethical conflicts should be done so that cultural brokers, such as a community or religious leader respected by the family, can identify an acceptable resolution. Decisions about withdrawal of life support should take into consideration the individual's particular life context (e.g., previous life, current situation, and relationships with significant others). Communitarian ethic of care upholds collective decision-making over individual. In collectivistic groups such as Nigerians, Haitians, and Filipinos, decisions about care of an individual family member are made by the group and may supersede the individual client's decision, regardless of decision-making. In a study of Mexican American families in the US border with Mexico, multiple caregivers including non-kin shared the responsibility for care of the sick at home when the designated family caregiver was not available or incapacitated (Evans et al., 2017). Healthcare providers should make families aware of acceptable legal alternatives to designate a trusted member to communicate decisions on their behalf by executing a healthcare proxy or durable power of attorney. In the United States, the mandate to use a trained interpreter who is not related to the client is another source of potential conflict. Group-oriented cultures tend to trust members of their in-group more than outsiders. In fact, some clients insist that their next of kin is present during their encounter with health professionals and expect their kin to speak on their behalf. Knowing the norms of the groups that the organization serves and working with community members to negotiate between these norms and the legal mandate in healthcare could prevent potential problems. Some hospitals have developed an interpreter program using community volunteers and bilingual staff members.

Feminist theory supports ethical relativism by requiring an examination of the context of the situation before making a decision. Drawn from feminist theories, the **ethic of care** emphasizes the need for healthcare practitioners to develop empathy, compassion, and relationships that promote trust, growth, and the well-being of others (Alacovska, 2020). This relationship is significant in caring for individuals who are unable to advocate for themselves, such as patients with disability or mental illness and victims of abuse.

Principle-based ethics, or **principlism**, attempts to reconcile the divergence between teleological and deontological models. Ethical principles are derived from ethical theories and commonly used to resolve ethical dilemmas because they link moral decision-making to scientific findings rather than universal rules. Principlism is based on the philosophical pragmatism of William James (Beauchamp & Childress, 2019). The principle of **fidelity** is the obligation to remain faithful to one's commitments. Nurses have an obligation to maintain standards of professional practice as a condition of continuing licensure. The principle of **veracity** upholds the virtues of being honest and telling the truth. **Truth telling** is recognized as a prerequisite to a trusting relationship. Informed consent requires veracity of information presented to clients and fidelity of practitioners to professional standards. The principle of **autonomy** upholds the capacity of individuals to act intentionally without controlling influences by others and from personal limitations that prevent meaningful choice. Autonomous persons are allowed to determine their own actions or delegate decision-making to others when they become incapable of making such decisions. Advance directives provide specific directions about the course of treatment to be followed by healthcare providers and caregivers if a client is unable to give informed consent or refuse care because of incapacity. Healthcare providers are obligated to promote patient autonomy and the right to make informed choices (Ubel et al., 2018).

The principles of **nonmaleficence** and **beneficence** require that care providers act in ways that cause no harm and benefit consumers of their care, respectively. Focusing on client safety emphasizes prevention of harm. The goal of using evidence-based practice is to promote the most effective and safe interventions for clients. Beneficence is a much higher-level principle as it not only addresses prevention of harm but also acts to benefit the client. For example, a nurse working with a low-income Vietnamese immigrant family affected by tuberculosis (TB) applies the principle of nonmaleficence by using the services of a culturally appropriate interpreter to explain the care regimen to the client and family. The principle of beneficence is applied when, understanding the high incidence of TB among Vietnamese immigrants, the nurse forms a community collaborative consisting of families, vendors, church leaders, and the local schools to work with the Mayor's Office, Department of Health, and the Visiting Nurses to develop policies and programs for prevention and to control the spread of TB in the community.

Ethical Universalism

Globalization has heightened the awareness of health inequities across population groups in local, national, and global contexts (Labonte' & Ruckert, 2019). The existence of global health inequities calls for health professionals to have a worldwide perspective and commitment to the universalistic ethical principles of advocacy and empowerment. The nursing profession has maintained its advocacy for providing a safe and caring environment that promotes the patient's health and well-being. Nurses have the obligation to advocate for equity and social justice in resource allocation, access to healthcare, and other social and economic services (ICN, 2022). The American Nurses Association (2022) has identified health equity as a key priority stipulating in its Code of Ethics the need for nurses to promote, advocate for, and strive to protect the health, safety, and rights of an individual, family, community, group, or population.

Population Health

The American Association of Colleges of Nursing (2021) has recently emphasized the inclusion of population health, social determinants of health, and health equity in professional nursing curricula. **Population health** is an interdisciplinary, customizable approach and an opportunity for healthcare systems, agencies, and organizations to work together in order to improve the health outcomes of the communities they serve (CDC, 2020). According to the WHO (2022a), a **population** includes all the inhabitants of a country, territory, or geographic area at a specific point of time. Social determinants of health exist across population groups and societies, which result in the social patterning of health vulnerability from differential exposure to life adversities that create cumulative disadvantages in populations. WHO (2022b) has defined social determinants of health as nonmedical factors that influence health outcomes or the conditions in which people are born, grow, work, live, and age, and the wider set of forces and systems shaping the conditions of daily life. These forces and systems include economic policies and systems, development agendas, social norms, social policies, and political systems.

The differential impact of social determinants is evident in health disparities, which are consequences of social inequities. Diseases occur at greater levels among certain population groups more than among others because of social determinants of health. **Health disparities** are differences in the incidence, prevalence, and mortality of a disease and the related adverse health conditions that exist among specific population groups (CDC, 2020). Health disparities are evident in large data sets that allow analysis of social patterning of epidemiological trends across populations. Researchers and educators need to provide the explanatory link between disease patterns with social and environmental inequities.

Vulnerable groups exist across societies because of compounded disadvantages that result in poor physical and mental health. **Vulnerable populations** suffer from multiple, aggravated, compounded or intersecting forms of discrimination based on other related grounds, such as age, sex, language, religion, political or other opinion, social origin, property, disability, birth, or other status. Because of their shared social characteristics they are at a higher risk for [health] risks and a higher distribution of risk exposure than the rest of the population (UN, n.d.) A vulnerable group is a disadvantaged segment of the community requiring utmost considerations because of limited capacity to protect themselves from intended or inherent risks and inability to make informed choices. Vulnerability is created by multiple and cumulative risks experienced through the life course that may not be directly related to health such as low socioeconomic status and discrimination. Exposure to multiple risk factors and a greater number of comorbidities are more frequent in vulnerable populations, for example, persons with low income, the less educated, racial and ethnic minorities, aboriginal peoples, those who experienced discrimination, enslavement, oppression, and violence, etc. Health disparities in access to care affects poor minority groups in the United States. See Box 13-1.

The World Health Organization (WHO, 2018) has identified three strategies to promote health and well-being of individuals and populations:

1. advocacy for health achievement through political, social, economic, environmental, behavioral, and biologic means
2. enablement/empowerment of all people to access opportunities and resources to achieve their fullest health potential and equity in health outcomes
3. mediation of participation by all sectors (public and private organizations, professionals, media, communities, etc.) in health promotion

Targeting socioeconomic, political, and environmental changes to support health goes beyond individual-based care toward actions with high impact on populations and communities. The pursuit of health equity must address the multiple disadvantages of affected populations. The very nature of social determinants requires that approaches toward population health demand interdisciplinary and multisectoral partnerships

BOX 13-1 | Inequity in Emergency Care due to Structural Discrimination

Despite the Emergency Medical Treatment and Labor Act (EMTALA), which requires all hospitals with emergency departments to evaluate and medically stabilize patients, regardless of their ability to pay, disparities in the distribution of emergency services and resources continue to exist in the United States. Minority populations experience 10% longer ambulance response times and are more likely to be diverted to distant care facilities because of closure of nearby hospitals. Once in the emergency room (ER), they are more likely to experience longer wait times and less likely to be given appropriate evidence-based treatment or pain medication. These are attributed to inequitable distribution of ER services and resources in their communities such as

evidence-based emergency resources for acute myocardial infarction.

Structural discrimination, more than individual based discrimination, is the driver of disparities in emergency care because of market-based allocation of emergency services and resources that does not match community needs. Historically underserved populations have disproportionly poor access, treatment, and outcomes. More research is recommended on effects of structural discrimination in healthcare.

Reference: Hsia, R. Y., & Zagorov, S. (2022). Structural discrimination in emergency care: How a sick system, affects us all. *Medicine, 3*, 98–103. https://doi.org/10.1016/j.medj.2022.01.006

and collaboration connecting practice to policy for change to happen locally (CDC, 2020).

Advocacy

The universalistic ethical principle of **advocacy** is rooted in a caring interpersonal relationship and a sense of obligation to care for others. It requires careful attention to the power relationships that influence the individual's or group's well-being, and their affirmation of the responsiveness of care. Advocacy has its roots in the ethics of care emphasizing interpersonal relationships and care or benevolence as central to moral action. Care-based feminism is based on the assumptions that persons have varying degrees of dependence and interdependence on one another; that the vulnerable deserve extra consideration based on their vulnerability; and that there is a need to examine the situational contexts to safeguard and protect the vulnerable (Hall & Asta., 2021).

Advocacy is also founded on the principle of justice and fairness by ensuring that each person is given their due. Justice and fairness are closely related and often used interchangeably. Systemic

inequality and social injustices result in health inequity because of unfair distribution of goods, services, and privileges across populations. Equity refers to justice or fairness in the distribution of goods and services based on people's needs. Needs are not necessarily equal; hence, equal access or equal allocation of resources that ignore differences in needs generally fail to achieve equity of outcomes. According to John Rawls (Brock, 2017), the stability of a society depends upon the extent to which the members feel that they are being treated justly. Lack of fairness and unequal treatment have led to social unrest, disturbances, and strife.

Rights-based care stems from the principles of **human rights**, emphasizing health as a basic right along with access to quality and safe healthcare services for all. The Universal Declaration of Human Rights was influential in creating the movement for advocacy across disciplines and institutions. Health promotion should be grounded in **social justice**, emphasizing a collective societal moral obligation to create equity or fairness in the allocation of risks and rewards to everyone. Social justice must include nondistributive aspects of well-being (Pacquiao, 2018a, 2019), which are affected by the nature of a person's social relationships with others. Unjust relationships impose systemic constraints on the development of well-being. People who are victims of social subordination, violence, discrimination, and stigma often experience lack of respect and lack of attachment and determination, which are essential aspects of well-being.

Protection of basic human rights, particularly of the vulnerable, is a fundamental part of health promotion. Health and well-being are achieved when individuals have the capacity and freedom to exercise their rights. While all individuals have the same basic human rights, social justice ensures the rights of the vulnerable. John Rawls (Brock, 2017) emphasized that a just society exists when the vulnerable are rendered less vulnerable. Health promotion is grounded in the ethical principle of beneficence that aims to make a positive difference in people's lives. Beneficence is actualized through advocacy and empowerment of individuals and populations for health achievement.

The need for advocacy is inherent among humans whose identities, experiences, and life chances are shaped by the social arrangements of power and statuses. Advocacy is needed as one's ability to compete, negotiate, and secure one's "place" in society is differentially structured by the social structural conditions. Patient advocacy has evolved toward health advocacy to protect people who are vulnerable or discriminated against and empower those who need a stronger voice by enabling them to express their needs and make their own decisions (Pacquiao, 2018b). Advocacy for health is a combination of individual and social actions to gain political commitment, policy support, social acceptance, and systems support for a particular health goal or program. Health advocacy encompasses direct service to the individual or family as well as activities that promote health and access to healthcare in communities and the larger public. Advocates support and promote the rights of the patient in healthcare, help build capacity to improve community health, and

enhance health policy initiatives focused on available, safe, and quality care.

The US Supreme Court action on Roe vs. Wade has severely limited access to abortion by women and restricted the care by healthcare providers in some states such as Texas and Florida. Box 13-2 presents some potential health risks and care accommodations at the Emergency Department for women who may perform abortion on their own.

Empowerment

Empowerment is the process through which an individual and groups gain greater control over decisions and actions affecting their health; it is both an individual and a community process (Pacquiao, 2018b). While advocacy tends to be more aligned and driven by others such as health providers or advocates, empowerment is more oriented toward the other's point of view, thus more patient centered. Empowerment is both a process and an outcome; it is considered an outcome of advocacy. Since empowerment involves active engagement and participation by individuals and communities, they achieve greater autonomy, capacity, and self-efficacy in improving their health and well-being. There is greater likelihood for sustainable outcomes through empowerment because it builds individual and community capacity for health achievement. Empowerment links individual strengths and competencies, support systems, and proactive behaviors to social policy and social change.

Patient empowerment is a process by which patients understand their role and are given the knowledge and skills by their healthcare provider to perform a task in an environment that recognizes community and cultural differences and encourages patient participation (WHO, 2022c). Patient empowerment is a cognitive process involving the patient's development of awareness of their health status, followed by active engagement in the healthcare process, and gaining control of their health by collaborating in shared decision-making with care providers (Pacquiao, 2018b).

BOX 13-2 | **Ethical Dilemmas During the Post-Roe Era**

The state abortion ban poses multiple ethical dilemmas for healthcare providers. Between 2000 and 2020, one third of at least 61 instances of people being arrested or criminally self-managing an abortion or helping someone else to do so were brought to law enforcement by healthcare providers. The post-Roe era will aggravate health inequity as 75% of patients who have an abortion in the United States are living below the federal poverty threshold or have low-income status, and 62% are members of marginalized racial or ethnic groups. In restrictive states, only pregnant people who can afford to travel will be able to obtain mainstream care. The abortion ban runs counter to the provisions of EMTALA, HIPAA, and professional confidentiality. It violates the ethics of caring, compassion, respect, and social justice.

Healthcare professionals are likely to encounter patients because of bleeding from use of abortion medications or complications from mechanical abortion methods used. Healthcare providers should be familiar with the laws on abortion in the state where they practice and seek experts on the topic. Taking a harm-reduction approach would help clinicians provide ethical care in a punitive legal environment. The first step is to assure patients that they will be cared for the medical problems they are experiencing and will receive the same confidentiality as other patients. Clinicians should be careful about the information that should be included in the patient's record. They should refer patients to helplines.

Reference: Watson, K., Paul, M., Yanow, S., & Baruch, J. (2022). Supporting, not reporting – Emergency Department Ethics in a post-Roe era. *New England Journal of Medicine, 387*(10):861-863. https://doi.org/10.1056/NEJMp2209312

WHO (2022c) emphasizes community empowerment because it is a social-action process that occurs in the social context of human relationships at home and in communities and institutions. Community empowerment is both a process and an outcome in which individuals and groups act to gain mastery over their lives by changing their social and political environment. Institutions and communities are transformed as people who participate in changing them become transformed. Community empowerment is a basis for healthcare reform as individuals are connected and engaged with others in the community to identify common problems, goals, and strategies for personal and social capacity building to transform their lives. The Ottawa Charter for Health Promotion (WHO, 2018) recognizes the significance of patient and community empowerment in transforming health of individuals and populations.

According to Lieberman (2019), Pierre Bourdieu's theory of social capital is instructive in building community empowerment of vulnerable populations who are disadvantaged by poverty (lack of economic capital) and low educational achievement (lack of cultural capital). **Social capital** refers to the social resources that exist in relationships between individuals and groups and are available to members of a given group or the social network. Social interactions can increase social ties among individuals, enhance trust and reciprocity, affect community participation, and, consequently, impact health and social outcomes. **Bonding** social capital can be strengthened through mutual trusting relationships among members of the group through kinship, close friendships, and daily interactions. **Bridging** social capital is enhanced by building connections and reciprocity across different communities with mutual needs and goals. **Linking** social capital is fostered by connecting communities with individuals and groups with expertise and access to policy making and governance, science and technology, and other resources not available within their own networks. Linking capital is built through interdisciplinary and multisectoral collaboration with vulnerable communities.

In summary, social actions to eliminate population health disparities are grounded in the ethical principles of advocacy, empowerment, human rights, and justice. Social justice mandates public policies and programs aimed to reallocate material and nonmaterial resources, such as goodwill, to remove social determinants of health that increase health risks in certain groups more than others. Social actions for health equity transpire in multisectoral and interdisciplinary engagement with vulnerable communities to transform their life conditions in a way that supports positive health outcomes. Population health approaches go beyond individual and disease-based care. Population health focuses on everyone within the targeted community, as health equity is only achieved when the social and physical environmental aspects of their lives are improved. While population health approaches focus on any group or community, eliminating health disparities necessitates prioritizing those groups and communities with shared social characteristics rendering them vulnerable to multiple health risks.

Model for Culturally Competent Practice for Health Equity

Leininger first articulated the central purpose of nursing as caring that is grounded in the knowledge of culturally constituted values, beliefs, and practices of the people (McFarland & Wehbe-Alamah, 2019). Transcultural nursing aims to identify the differences and similarities across cultural groups and between professional caregivers and their clients. Leininger defined **culturally congruent care** as care that is meaningful, supportive, and beneficial from the lens of the people who experience the care. Culturally congruent action modes include cultural preservation, accommodation, and repatterning.

One or all three modes of action may be used simultaneously or in a continuum of actions. **Cultural preservation** means maintaining the core values, beliefs, and practices significant to the individual or group. **Cultural accommodation** involves negotiating with existing cultural differences in order to find a meaningful coexistence of one's cultural lifeways with those of others. **Cultural repatterning** means attempting to help individuals and groups change their way of life to achieve a healthy, safe, and meaningful existence (McFarland & Wehbe-Alamah, 2019). Cultural repatterning enables health practitioners and organizations to promote preservation and accommodate cultural differences. Leininger's culturally congruent decision modes promote bridging of differences applicable with individuals, organizations, and communities. These are significant approaches in bridging cultural differences and finding a common ground among different groups, which are critical in building multisectoral collaboration and partnerships.

Relevant knowledge, skills, and attitudes of cultural competence can be measured, observed, and validated at any given point using more objective criteria. **Culturally competent care** is ethical care that is built upon the delicate balance between ethical relativism and universalism. While culturally competent care promotes meaningful, supportive, and beneficial care by respectful accommodation of cultural differences, its ultimate aim is achievement of health equity built on an awareness of self and others, valuing diversity and having the capacity to transform differences toward a common, beneficial purpose. Health equity through protection of human rights and promotion of social justice is achieved through culturally competent advocacy and empowerment that integrates diversity within the common aim of health equity and alleviation of vulnerability (see Fig. 13-1).

Culturally competent professionals have a global perspective, meaning they view themselves within their own values and beliefs and identify themselves as part of an emerging and interlocking world community (Gorman & Womack,

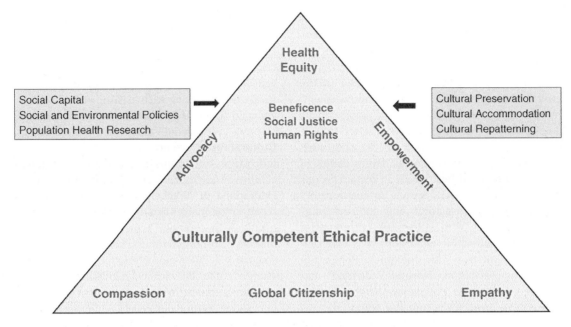

Figure 13-1. The model for Culturally Competent Ethical Practice shows the foundational values at the base of the triangle that motivates one to engage in culturally competent actions to achieve health equity and its undergirding ethical principles.

2017). Because of their genuine concern and commitment to the welfare of others, they have the ability to critically examine their own traditions to determine reasonable support for their personal beliefs rather than accept them as absolute truths As global citizens, culturally competent individuals have the interconnected capacities for **empathy** (a profound understanding of others) and compassion (the emotional understanding of others' experiences).

Alacovska (2020) connected care from individual to the community and cited Nussbaum's concept of **compassion** as the "care-"ful dedication to others; it is the basic social emotion central to bridging between the individual and the community. It is a moral capacity and judgment about what constitutes the well-being of others. The author also cited Heidegger's emphasis on the centrality of care in "being with the world," stating that affective community and neighborhood ties compel us to act "other"-wise when governments and institutions fail to care for us.

In this model, compassion and empathy are the prime movers for culturally competent actions towards health equity. Compassionate understanding of the suffering of others compels one to take action on their behalf through advocacy and empowerment involving an awareness of social inequities, caring for others, social justice, and the responsibility to act.

Culturally competent advocacy and empowerment of vulnerable populations are built on respect and appreciation of differences, natural capacities, and unique lifeways of individuals and groups for health. Achievement of individual and community empowerment requires that culturally competent strategies use multilevel approaches at the individual, organizational/institutional, and community levels. Health equity and elimination of population health disparities are actualized through broad collaborative political action to change policies impacting the vulnerable. Health promotion needs to shift its focus to building healthy communities beyond disease-based care for individuals. Addressing the social determinants of poor health should focus on upstream approaches that transform the capacity of individuals and communities to change their life conditions. As Freire has noted, individual empowerment is sustainable within an empowered community (Pacquiao, 2018b).

There is need for expanding the knowledge and skills of cultural competence at the community level including but not limited to: (1) Population health assessment including social and environmental factors, (2) policy making process, monitoring and evaluation of impact of policies on health of vulnerable populations, (3) local and national governance structure and process, (4) building community social capital by fostering linkages within the community, across other communities and with multilevel stakeholders, (5) secondary analysis of population data sets that complement small qualitative findings to create bigger impact on policy makers, and (6) opportunities for mentorship and service learning in vulnerable communities and influencing policy development.

Model Application

This example was developed from this chapter author's direct observation as a visiting professor at a University in northern Philippines. The Dean of the College of Nursing (a Catholic nun and a nurse) has built a long-standing partnership between the college and the local community. The community is located in a rural *barrio* comprised of low-income families who were engaged in farming and occasional employment in manual labor. For their Community Nursing course, students were affiliated with the rural health clinic and conducted home visits in the barrio. Students used a master list and area map to track the health status of each family member. In the Philippines, higher rates of maternal and infant morbidity and mortality have been reported in low-income isolated rural areas. Hence, the students were focused on maternal and child health promotion and disease prevention and management. While women and

children were generally present during home visits, men were usually away at work. The students scheduled their community visits when men collected their monthly monetary incentives from the barrio center to check on their health status.

The Dean collaborated with the barrio captain to hold a community meeting to find out their priority needs. The men identified their main concern as the lack of a place to dry their *palay* after harvest; palay needs to be dried before it can be processed to rice ready for cooking. Most Filipinos eat rice three meals daily. Palay becomes moldy and fermented if kept moist. Families use bamboo mats to dry their harvest, but the unpaved ground underneath retains moisture. Therefore the families require a few days to completely dry their palay. The Dean collaborated with other disciplines at the university to engage their students in the community. The engineering faculty and students constructed a cement slab at the center of neighborhoods large enough to accommodate several families drying their palay during sunny days. Families developed a rotation schedule to accommodate everyone. The men became more enthusiastic about other projects when their voices were heard. They participated in constructing latrines for residents in collaboration with engineering students. Construction materials used in the project were donated by the city government and businesses; labor was freely donated by the students, their faculty, and male residents. This was significant as the barrio did not have a human waste disposal system.

This project was a nurse-led community initiative involving multisectoral and interdisciplinary collaboration (university, Rural Health Center, barrio captain, and residents). Broad-based collaboration and engagement builds community social capital. It builds bonding capital among the residents, bridging families with local officials and health centers and linking them with different sectors of the community to achieve beneficial changes in their life conditions. The nursing students used a population approach by engaging every resident in the barrio. Partnerships with the barrio captain and the residents revealed different priorities in the community that were not related to medical conditions but essential to their daily existence. Lack of facility to dry their palay and human waste disposal were social determinants of residents' health.

Cultural preservation was used when the Dean sought the collaboration of the barrio captain. Cultural accommodation was used when students scheduled their visits when men were in the barrio. Cultural repatterning was observed when community priorities were generated directly from its residents rather than by health providers. Advocacy for social justice and human rights to health was observed by the Dean's collaborative effort to obtain external funding and free labor for the projects. Her compassion and empathy were the antecedents to her commitment to partner with a vulnerable community and other stakeholders. Population health promotion addressing social determinants required multisectoral and interdisciplinary collaboration with the community, empowering them to identify their own needs and how to best address them.

Summary

Actions that transform life conditions of vulnerable populations begin from compassion and empathy for the least well-off. Culturally competent advocacy and empowerment for social justice and human rights protection are actualized through a multipronged approach at the individual, organizational, and societal level partnership and collaboration. Collaborative partnership with individuals, families, and communities is built on mutual understanding, trust, and reciprocity. Social learning from stories of clients, families, and communities and immersion in their social and environmental contexts can sensitize caregivers to the root cause of health disparities. Immersion in vulnerable communities develops compassionate empathy for their experience of the cumulative impact of social inequities.

Understanding and sensitivity to clients' authentic life experiences at home, at work, and in their neighborhood promotes collaborative assessment of nonmedical factors that may not be evident during individual encounters in care settings. Client encounters in their environments can enhance healthcare professionals' ability in demonstrating attentiveness, genuine concern, presence, warmth, and empathy. Community involvement and immersion in diverse communities create the appropriate context for partnership, collaboration, and compassionate understanding.

Healthcare providers need experience in caring especially for vulnerable populations locally or abroad. Experience with organizations and advocacy groups such as local churches, the Red Cross, homeless shelters, Doctors Without Borders, and other opportunities can build the skills for culturally competent ethical thinking. Awareness of resources locally, nationally, and globally promotes access to and development of more comprehensive services. Building collaborative partnerships with organizations and communities is important, as vulnerable populations have complex, multiple needs that are both simultaneous and evolving.

Partnerships allow sharing of resources, services, and best practices across local, national, and global contexts. Service learning is an excellent opportunity for nursing students to learn about organizations and the communities they serve. Strengthening the community health nursing experience in the curriculum sensitizes students to public health issues and social inequities affecting population health.

REVIEW QUESTIONS

1. Describe ethical dilemmas in achieving health equity for vulnerable populations within the current political milieu in the United States and Canada.
2. Explain how you can promote health for vulnerable populations.
3. Explain the ethical basis for culturally competent care.

CRITICAL THINKING ACTIVITIES

Identify an example of an ethical dilemma that you have encountered at work or in your community. Identify the particulars of the situation:

1. Who are the people involved?
2. What is the setting?
3. How do different individuals or groups perceive the problem?
4. Identify conflicting values and beliefs at the individual, organizational, and societal levels that influence perceptions.
5. What assessment data about the situation are missing?
6. How can additional information be obtained?
7. What culturally congruent strategies do you recommend?

REFERENCES

AACN. (2021). *Essentials of professional nursing education.* https://www.aacnnursing.org/AACN-Essentials.

Alacovska, A. (2020). From passion to compassion: A caring inquiry into creative work as socially engaged art. *Sociology, 54*(4), 727–744. https://doi.org/10.1177/0038038520904716177

ANA. (2022). *ANA brings nurses' voices to health equity.* https://anacapitolbeat.org/2022/09/23/ana-brings-nurses-voices-to-health-equity-priorities/

Barrow, J. M., & Khandhar, P. B. (2022). *Deontology.* Stat Pearls. https://www.ncbi.nlm.nih.gov/books/NBK459296/

Beauchamp, T. L., & Childress, J. F. (2019). *Principles of biomedical ethics.* Oxford University Press.

Brock, D. W. (2017). *John Rawls, A theory of justice.* https://chicagounbound.uchicago.edu/cgi/viewcontent.cgi?article=3767&context=uclrev

CDC. (2020). *Population health training.* https://www.cdc.gov/pophealthtraining/whatis.html

The Ethics Centre. (2022). *Ethics explainer: Teleology.* https://ethics.org.au/teleology/

Evans, B. C., Coon, D. W., Belyea, M. J., & Ume, E. (2017). Collective care: Multiple caregivers and multiple care recipients in Mexican American families. *Journal of Transcultural Nursing, 28*(4), 398–407.

Gorman, D., & Womack, K. (2017). Cultivating humanity with Martha Nussbaum. *Interdisciplinary Literary Studies, 19*, 145–148.

Guest, K. J. (2017). *Essentials of cultural anthropology: A toolkit for global age* (2nd ed.). W.W. Norton & Company.

Hall, K. Q., & Asta. (2021). *The Oxford handbook of feminist philosophy.* Oxford University Press.

Hsia, R. Y., & Zagorov, S. (2022). Structural discrimination in emergency care: How a sick system, affects us all. *Med, 3*, 98–103. https://doi.org/10.1016/j.medj.2022.01.006

ICN. (2022). *ICN strategic priorities.* https://www.icn.ch/nursing-policy/icn-strategic-priorities

Labonte, R., & Ruckert, A. (2019). *Health equity in a globalizing era: Past challenges, future prospects.* Oxford University Press.

Lieberman, E. S. (2019). Building community social capital. In D. Pacquiao & M. Douglas (Eds.), *Social pathways to health vulnerability: Implications for health professionals.* Springer.

McFarland, M. R., & Wehbe-Alamah, H. (2019). Leininger's theory of culture care diversity and universality: An overview with a historical retrospective and a view toward the future. *Journal of Transcultural Nursing, 30*(6), 540–557. https://doi.org/10.1177/1043659619867134

Pacquiao, D. F. (2018a). Conceptual framework for culturally competent care. In M. K. Douglas, D. F. Pacquiao & L. Purnell (Eds.), *Global applications of culturally competent health care: Guidelines for practice* (p. 27). Springer.

Pacquiao, D. F. (2018b). Patient advocacy and empowerment. In M. K. Douglas, D. F. Pacquiao & L. Purnell (Eds.), *Global applications of culturally competent health care: Guidelines for practice* (p. 27). Springer.

Pacquiao, D. F. (2019). Place and health. In I. D. Pacquiao & M. Douglas (Eds.), *Social pathways to health vulnerability: Implications for health professionals.* Springer.

Shah, R. (2022). *Henrietta Lacks: Ethics questions raised by use of HeLa.* https://www.shortform.com/blog/henrietta-lacks-ethics-issues/

Terpstra, J., Lehta, R., & Wyatt, G. (2021). Spirituality, quality of life and end of life among indigenous peoples: A scoping review. *Journal of Transcultural Nursing, 22*(3), 161–172. https://doi.org/10.1177/1043659620952524

Ubel, P. A., Cherr, K. A., & Fagerin, A. (2018). Autonomy: What's shared decision making have to do with it? *American Journal of Bioethics, 18*(2), W11–W12. https://doi.org/10.1080/15265161.2017.1409844

UN. (n.d.). *Fight racism.* https://www.un.org/en/fight-racism/vulnerable-groups

Watson, K., Paul, M., Yanow, S., & Baruch, J. (2022). Supporting, not reporting – Emergency Department Ethics in a post-Roe era. *New England Journal of Medicine, 387*(10), 861–863. https://doi.org/10.1056/NEJMp2209312

Wehbe-Alamah, H., Hammonds, L. S., & Stanley, D. (2021). Culturally-congruent care from the perspectives of Judaism, Christianity and Islam. *Journal of Transcultural Nursing, 32*(2), 119–128. https://doi.org/10.1177/104365961990000

WHO. (2018). *The 1986 Ottawa charter for health promotion.* Retrieved August 20, 2018 from http://www.who.int/healthpromotion/conferences/previous/ottawa/en/

WHO. (2022a). *Population.* https://www.who.int/data/gho/indicator-metadata-registry/imr-details/1121

WHO. (2022b). *Social determinants of health.* https://www.who.int/health-topics/social-determinants-of-health#tab=tab_1

WHO. (2022c). *Community empowerment.* https://www.who.int/teams/health-promotion/enhanced-wellbeing/seventh-global-conference/community-empowerment

Yiu, H. C., Zang, Y., Chew, J. H. S., & Chau, J. P. C. (2021). The influence of Confucianism on the perceptions and process of caring among family caregivers of persons with dementia: A qualitative study. *Journal of Transcultural Nursing, 32*(2), 1513–1160. https://doi.org/10.1177/1043659620905891

Appendix A

Andrews/Boyle Transcultural Nursing Assessment Guide for Individuals and Families

• Joyceen S. Boyle and Margaret M. Andrews

Biocultural Variations and Cultural Aspects of the Incidence of Disease

- Does the client and/or family members relate a health history associated with genetic or acquired conditions that are more prevalent for a specific cultural group (e.g., diabetes, hypertension, cardiovascular disease, sickle cell anemia, Tay-Sachs disease, G-6-PD deficiency, lactose intolerance)? Does the client's family relate such a history?
- Are there socioenvironmental conditions more prevalent among a specific cultural group that can be observed in the client or family members (e.g., lead poisoning, alcohol use disorder, HIV/AIDS, drug use, ear infections, family violence, fetal alcohol spectrum disorder, obesity, respiratory diseases)?
- Are there diseases against which the client has an increased resistance (e.g., skin cancer in individuals with darkly-pigmented skin, malaria for those with sickle cell anemia)?
- Does the client have distinctive features characteristic of a particular ethnic or racial group (e.g., skin color, hair texture)? Does the client's family members have such features? Within the family group, are there variations in anatomy characteristic of a particular ethnic or racial group (e.g., body structure, height, weight, facial shape and structure [nose, eye shape, facial contour], upper and lower extremities)?
- How do anatomic, racial, and ethnic variations affect the physical and mental examination?

Communication

- What language does the client speak at home with family members? In what language would the client prefer to communicate with you? What other languages does the client speak or read? What other languages do the client's family members speak or read?
- What is the fluency level of the client in English—both written and spoken? What is the fluency level of the client's family members?
- Does the client need an interpreter? Do their family members need an interpreter? Does the healthcare setting provide interpreters? Who would the client and their family members prefer to assist with interpretation? Is there anyone whom the client would prefer not to serve as an interpreter (e.g., member of a different sex, person younger or older than the client, member of a rival tribe, ethnic group, or nationality)?
- If the client has a hearing or vision condition, how do they communicate? Are any assistive devices used to foster communication and/or ensure the client's safety?
- What are the rules and style (formal or informal) of communication? If the client has a hearing condition and requires someone who knows sign language, how will arrangements be made? If the client is blind and requires that communications be made available in braille, how will that be accomplished? How much time will it take to provide the resources needed for clients with hearing and vision conditions? How does

the client prefer to be addressed? What do the client's family members prefer? What are the preferred terms for greeting?

- How is it necessary to vary the technique and style of communication during the relationship with the client to accommodate their cultural background (e.g., tempo of conversation, eye contact, sensitivity to topical taboos, norms of confidentiality, and style of explanation)? How do these factors vary with family members, if at all?
- What are the styles of individual and family members' nonverbal communication?
- How does the client's nonverbal communication compare with that of individuals from other cultural groups? How does the client's style of nonverbal communication differ from the healthcare provider's style? How does it affect the client's relationships with you and with other members of the healthcare team? How does communication with the family influence the care environment?
- How do the client and family members feel about healthcare providers who are not of the same cultural or religious background? Does the client prefer to receive care from a nurse of the same cultural background, gender, and/or age? How do family members react to care providers of different cultural backgrounds, ages, and genders?
- If the client and family members are recent migrants from Central America, Mexico, or other countries, do they have a plan in place to deal with the possibility that one or more adults may be detained by immigration officials and not return home after work? To protect family integrity, arrangements should be made in advance for the children's safety.
- Do the client and family members have an "Exit/ Emergency" plan? Such a plan is important for clients and families who live in earthquake or hurricane prone areas. Keeping important papers in a metal box, along with family photos and other souvenirs or valuables that can be stuffed into a backpack at the last minute, is essential. Water and food are also essential if families must evacuate the area. Reviewing the plan with all family members on a routine

basis is necessary for an Exit/Emergency plan to be successful. New immigrants, refugees, or migrants as well as long-time citizens may not be aware of preplanning for a natural disaster.

Cultural Affiliations

- With what cultural group(s) does the client report affiliation (e.g., American, Hispanic, Irish, Black, Navajo, Native American, or combination)? It is becoming increasingly common for Americans to identify with two or more groups, such as Native American and African American. Equally important, to what degree does the client identify with the cultural group (e.g., "we" concept of solidarity or as a fringe member)?
- How do the views of other family members coincide with or differ from those of the client regarding cultural affiliations?
- What is the preferred term that the cultural group chooses for itself? What term does the client choose?
- Where was the client born? Where were their parents born? What are the generational similarities and differences in regard to cultural identification, language, customs, values, and so on?
- Where has the client lived (country, city, or area within a country) and when (during what years of their life)? If the client has recently immigrated to the United States from another country, knowledge of prevalent diseases in their country of origin as well as sociopolitical history may be helpful. If the client is a recent immigrant, did they live in countries of transit or refugee camps? For how long? Current residence? Occupation? Occupation in home country?

Cultural Sanctions and Restrictions

- How does the client's cultural group regard expression of emotion and feelings, spirituality, and religious beliefs? How are feelings related to dying, death, and grieving expressed in a culturally appropriate manner?

- How do different genders express modesty? Are there culturally defined expectations about relationships between different genders, including the nurse–client relationship?
- Does the client or family express any restrictions related to sexuality, exposure of various parts of the body, or certain types of surgery (e.g., vasectomy, hysterectomy, abortion)?
- Are there restrictions against discussion of dead relatives or fears related to the unknown?

Developmental Considerations

- Are there any distinct growth and development characteristics that vary with the cultural background of the client and family (e.g., bone density, psychomotor patterns of development, fat folds)?
- What factors are significant in assessing children of various ages from the newborn period through adolescence (e.g., male circumcision, female genital mutilation, expected growth on standards grid, culturally acceptable age for toilet training, duration of breast-feeding, introduction of various types of foods, gender differences, discipline, and socialization to adult roles)?
- What are the beliefs and practices associated with developmental life events such as pregnancy, birth, puberty, marriage, and death?
- What is the cultural perception of aging (e.g., is youthfulness or the wisdom of old age more valued)?
- How are older adults cared for within the cultural group (e.g., cared for in the home of adult children, placed in institutions for care)? What are culturally accepted roles for older people?

Economics

- Who is the principal wage earner in the family and what is the income level? Is there more than one wage earner? Are there other sources of financial support? (*Note:* These may be potentially sensitive questions.)

- What insurance coverage does the client and their family have? Does the client and/or family members understand the terms/rates/coverage of their health insurance policies?
- What impact does the economic status have on the client and their family's lifestyle and living conditions?
- What has been the client and family's experience with the healthcare system in terms of reimbursement, costs, and insurance coverage?

Educational Background

- What is the client's highest educational level obtained? What values do the family members express regarding educational achievements?
- Does the client's educational level affect their knowledge level concerning their health literacy—how to obtain the needed care, teaching related to or learning about healthcare, and any written material that they are given in the healthcare setting (e.g., insurance forms, educational literature, information about diagnostic procedures and laboratory tests, admissions forms, etc.)? Does the client's educational level affect health behavior? As an example, in the United States, cigarette smoking and obesity have been linked to socioeconomic levels.
- What learning style is most comfortable and familiar? Does the client prefer to learn through written materials, oral explanations, videos, and/or demonstrations?
- Does the client access health information via the internet or use social media as a source of health-related information?
- Do the client and family members prefer intervention settings away from hospitals and other clients, which may have negative connotations for them? Are community sites such as churches, schools, or adult day care centers a good alternate choice for the client and their family, considering they are informal settings that may be more conducive for open discussion, demonstrations, and reinforcement of information and skills? Are the client and family more comfortable in their home setting?

Health-Related Beliefs and Practices

- To what cause does the client attribute illness and disease or what factors influence the acquisition of illness and disease (e.g., divine wrath, imbalance in hot/cold, yin/yang, punishment for moral transgressions, a hex, soul loss, pathogenic organism, past behavior, growing older)? Is there congruence within the family on these beliefs?
- What are the client's cultural beliefs about ideal body size and shape? What is the client's self-image in relation to the ideal?
- How does the client describe their health-related condition? What names or terms are used? How does the client express pain, discomfort, depression, or anxiety? In some cultures, clients may somaticize their emotional feelings, for example, "My heart hurts" rather than say, "I'm feeling sad or depressed about my physical condition."
- What do the client and family members believe promotes health (e.g., eating certain foods, wearing amulets to bring good luck, sleeping, resting, getting good nutrition, reducing stress, exercising, praying, or performing rituals to ancestors, saints, or other deities)?
- What is the client's religious affiliation? How is the client actively involved in the practice of religion? Do other family members have the same religious beliefs and practices? Do the client and/or family members incorporate religious practices, such as healing ceremonies or prayer, into health/illness care?
- Do the client and their family rely on cultural healers (e.g., curandero, shaman, spiritualist, priest, medicine person, minister)? Who determines when the client is sick and when they are healthy? Who influences the choice or type of healer and treatment that should be sought?
- In what types of cultural healing or health-promoting practices does the client engage (e.g., use of herbal remedies, potions, or massage; wearing of talismans, copper bracelets, or chains to discourage evil spirits; healing rituals;

incantations; or prayers)? Do family members share these beliefs and practices?
- How are biomedical healthcare providers perceived? How do the client and their family perceive nurses? What are the expectations of nurses and nursing care workers?
- Who will care for the client at home? What accommodations will family members make to provide caregiving?
- How do the client's family and cultural group view mental disorders? Are there differences in acceptable behaviors for physical versus psychological illnesses?
- Are the client and their family members up-to-date with current vaccines available to adults and children? What are the cultural beliefs and practices that guide divergent cultural views and values systems about vaccines? Are there religious beliefs that influence vaccine objections?

Kinship and Social Networks

- What is the composition of a "typical family" within the kinship network? What is the composition of the client's family?
- Who makes up the client's social network (family, friends, peers, neighbors)? How do they influence the client's health or illness status?
- How do members of the client's social support network define caring or caregiving? What is the role of various family members during health and illness episodes? Who makes decisions about health and healthcare?
- How does the client's family participate in the promotion of health (e.g., lifestyle changes in diet, activity level, etc.) and nursing care (e.g., bathing, feeding, touching, being present) of the client?
- Does the cultural family structure influence the client's response to health or illness (e.g., beliefs, strengths, weaknesses, and social class)?
- What influence do ethnic, cultural, and/or religious organizations have on the lifestyle and quality of life of the client (e.g., the National Association for the Advancement of Colored

People, churches, such as African American, Muslim, Jewish, Catholic, and others, that may provide schools, classes, and/or community-based healthcare programs)?

- Are there special gender issues within this cultural group? Do the client and family members conform to traditional roles (e.g., women may be viewed as the caretakers of home and children, while men work outside the home and have primary decision-making responsibilities)?

Nutrition

- What nutritional factors are influenced by the client's cultural background? What is the meaning of food and eating to the client and their family?
- Does the client have any eating or nutritional disorders (e.g., anorexia, bulimia, obesity, lactose intolerance)? Do the client's family members have any similar disorders? How do the client and family view these conditions?
- With whom does the client usually eat? What types of foods are eaten? What is the timing and sequencing of meals? What are the usual meal patterns?
- What does the client define as food? What does the client believe constitutes a "healthy" versus an "unhealthy" diet? Are these beliefs congruent with what the client actually eats?
- Who shops for and chooses food? Where are the foodstuffs purchased? Who prepares the actual meals? How are the family members involved in nutritional choices, values, and choices about food?
- How are the foods prepared at home (type of food preparation, cooking oil[s] used, length of time foods are cooked [especially vegetables], amount and type of seasoning added to various foods during preparation)? Who does the food preparation?
- Has the client chosen a particular nutritional practice such as gluten-free, vegetarianism, or abstinence from red meat or from alcoholic or fermented beverages? Do other family members adhere to these beliefs and practices?

- Do religious beliefs and practices influence the client's or family's diet (e.g., amount, type, preparation, or delineation of acceptable food combinations [e.g., kosher diets])? Does the client or client's family abstain from certain foods at regular intervals, on specific dates determined by the religious calendar, or at other times? Are there other food prohibitions or prescriptions?
- If the client or client's family's religion mandates or encourages fasting, what does the term *fast* mean (e.g., refraining from certain types of foods, eating only during certain times of the day, skipping certain meals)? For what period of time are family members expected to fast? Are there exceptions to fasting (e.g., are pregnant people or children excluded from fasting)?
- Are special utensils used (e.g., chopsticks, cookware, kosher restrictions)?
- Does the client or client's family use home and folk remedies to treat illnesses (e.g., herbal remedies, acupuncture, cupping, or other healing rituals often involving eggs, lemons, candles)? Which over-the-counter medications are used?

Religion and Spirituality

- How does the client or family's religious affiliation affect health and illness (e.g., life events such as death, chronic illness, body image alteration, cause and effect of illness)?
- What is the role of religious beliefs and practices during health and illness? Are there special rites or blessings for those with serious or terminal illnesses?
- Are there healing rituals or practices that the client and family believe can promote well-being or hasten recovery from illness? If so, who performs these? What materials or arrangements are necessary for the nurse to have available for the practice of these rituals?
- What is the role of significant religious representatives during health and illness? Are there recognized religious healers (e.g., Islamic Imams, Christian Scientist practitioners or nurses, Catholic priests, Church of Jesus Christ of Latter-day Saints elders, Buddhist monks)?

Values Orientation

- What are the client's attitudes, values, and beliefs about their health and illness status? Do family members have similar values and beliefs?
- How do these influence behaviors in terms of promotion of health and treatment of disease? What are the client's or family's attitudes, values, and beliefs about healthcare providers?
- Does culture affect the manner in which the client relates to body image change resulting from illness or surgery (e.g., importance of appearance, beauty, strength, and roles in the cultural group)? Is there a cultural stigma associated with the client's illness (i.e., how is the illness or the manner in which it was contracted viewed by the family and larger culture)?

- How do the client and their family view work, leisure, and education?
- How does the client perceive and react to change?
- How do the client and their family perceive changes in lifestyle related to current illness or surgery?
- How do the client and their family view biomedical healthcare (e.g., suspiciously, fearfully, acceptingly, unquestioningly, with awe)?
- How does the client value privacy, courtesy, touch, and relationships with others?
- How does the client relate to persons outside of their cultural group (e.g., withdrawal, suspicion, curiosity, openness)?

Appendix B

Andrews/Boyle Transcultural Nursing Assessment Guide for Families, Groups, and Communities

- Joyceen S. Boyle and Margaret M. Andrews

Family and Kinship Systems

- Are the families nuclear, extended, or blended? Do family members live in close proximity? What is the role and status of individual family members? By age and gender?
- How do the family and/or group members relate to the larger community or groups?
- Are there distinct neighborhoods or areas of the community where distinct cultural, ethnic, or religious groups, refugees, or immigrants live?
- What are the communication patterns within the distinct community groups?
- If working with a refugee community, ask about names of tribes and/or clans.
- What place do the "ancestors" have in the worldview of the group? How is the belief in the power of the ancestors incorporated into the daily life and rituals of the group?
- Is the group now or has it traditionally been matriarchal or patriarchal? Is there a preference for first cousins to marry? Who is permitted to marry whom among those who are related by blood/genetics?

Social Life and Networks

- What are the daily routines of the group? What are the important life cycle events such as birth, marriage, family bearing, family rearing, and death? How are they celebrated or observed?
- How are the educational systems organized? How do schools receive and accept input from the community? How do they assist students and their families who are new immigrants or refugees?
- What are the social/economic problems experienced by the group within the community or by the community itself?
- Are there special concerns with a particular ethnic or cultural group such as misuse of alcohol, fetal alcohol syndrome disorder, gang membership, or polygamy? How does the group view intimate partner violence and corporal punishment?
- Are newly arrived groups, such as immigrants or refugees, included within the local community or isolated? Who are the group's local leaders?
- Are there centers or organizations that reach out to special groups within the community? What activities or opportunities are available to new community members? For example, are General Educational Development courses, English as a second language classes, housing assistance, and/or work training available to newcomers?
- How does the social environment contribute to a sense of belonging? Do all members of the group belong to a distinct religious group? What are the ways that the group practices its religion? What are the dominant religious groups within the community?

- What are the group's social interaction patterns? Do all members of the group speak a common language?
- Are ethnic grocery stores, restaurants, and churches located within the community? What foods do members of the cultural group commonly eat? What foods/substances do they commonly avoid (i.e., alcohol, pork products)?
- Are members of the group comfortable moving away from the larger group?
- Where are ethnic groups, immigrants, or refugees located within the larger community?

Political or Government Systems

- Which factors in the political system influence the ways in which the group perceives its status vis-à-vis the dominant culture, that is, laws, justice, and cultural heroes?
- How does the economic system influence control of resources such as land, water, housing, education and technical training, jobs, and opportunities?
- What is the legal status of the group members? Refugee or immigrant visas? Temporary worker permits? Documented or undocumented?
- How does the local government respond to the ethnic and cultural makeup of the group? What are the ways that the local community "embraces its diversity"?

Language and Traditions

- Are there differences in dialects or languages spoken between healthcare professionals and local groups within the community?
- What is the literacy level of members of the group? Can they read or write in any language(s)?
- Do healthcare facilities provide educational materials in diverse languages?
- In what ways do the major cultural traditions of history, art, drama, and so on, influence the cultural identity of the group?
- How are local cultures or ethnic traditions embraced during holidays or special celebrations?

Worldviews, Value Orientations, and Cultural Norms

- What are the major cultural values about the relationships of cultural groups to nature and to one another? How can the group's ethical beliefs be described?
- What are the norms and standards of behavior (authority, responsibility, dependability, and competition)?
- Is the group communal or individualistic? How different is their worldview from the dominant worldview of the larger society or culture?
- What are the cultural attitudes about time, family, hospitality, family work, and leisure?
- What are the common values of the group, such as education, work, and so on?
- How are the cultural values reflected in factors such as dress? Do the women cover their hair? Do they prefer skirts or dresses over pants or trousers?
- Are there unique cultural practices within the group that might bring wider community censure, such gender roles, discipline of children, and relationships between spouses?

Religious Beliefs and Practices

- What are the major religious beliefs and practices within the community?
- How do they influence daily life? How do they relate to health practices? What are the practices surrounding major life events such as birth, marriage, and death?
- Does the cultural group have particular practices related to grieving or mourning?

Health Beliefs and Practices

- What are the group's attitudes and beliefs regarding health and illness? Does the cultural group seek care from indigenous (folk) practitioners? Are there traditional practitioners (shamans, curanderos, others) within the group?

Where do group members go to seek care? Who makes the decisions about seeking healthcare? Accepting treatments? Are there biologic variations that are important to the health of this group? What are the group's expressed health concerns? Are there cultural or ethnic stores in neighborhoods selling medicinal herbs? What are the primary health concerns and/or illnesses in this population/cultural group (e.g., malaria, HIV/AIDS, female genital mutilation, malnutrition, tuberculosis)? How do the group's concerns align with those of the local and state vhealthcare systems?

Healthcare Systems

- Do community healthcare facilities provide interpreters? Do physician offices and other healthcare facilities offer educational materials in languages other than English? Are health facilities located in accessible locations, that is, in ethnic neighborhoods? Do healthcare providers incorporate aspects of other healthcare systems, for example, acupuncture and referrals to traditional healers?
- Do members of the group have access to healthcare? Do they have adequate transportation? Are the hours of operation of healthcare facilities and availability of appointment times appropriate for members of the group?

Economic Factors

- Does the group or community own or operate its own clinic, neighborhood health center, child or adult day care center, long-term care facility, or nursing home? How will the group or community pay for healthcare services?
- Is there a group healthcare policy for all members? Will key leaders in the community work with members to collectively pay for healthcare services? For example, although the Amish religious leaders have no health insurance, members pool their resources and often settle a hospital bill in cash at the time of the client's discharge.

Appendix C

Andrews/Boyle Transcultural Nursing Assessment Guide for Healthcare Organizations and Facilities

- Joyceen S. Boyle, Margaret M. Andrews, and Patti Ludwig-Beymer

Environmental Context

- What is the general environment of the community that surrounds the healthcare organization? Where is the facility located in proximity to the population that it serves?
- What is the socioeconomic status of the adjacent community? What are race/ethnicity characteristics of residents? What are the identified health disparities?
- What are the community's views on health and illness?
- Is there appropriate and easy access to the facility? Is the signage to the facility easy to understand and follow? Are there adequate parking facilities? Are bus routes nearby?
- Is there access to social services? Where are residential and business districts located? What are the sources of employment near the facility?
- What is the proximity to other healthcare facilities? What facilities are available for people with disabilities?

Language and Ethnohistory

- What languages are spoken within the institution? By employees? By patients?
- How formal or informal are the lines of communication within the organization?
- Is the organizational governance hierarchical? What communication strategies are used within the organization?

- What is the history of the organization? What was the original mission of the organization? How does the history influence the current organization? How has it traditionally responded to change?

Technology

- How is technology used in the organization? Who uses it?
- Do all workstations have access to computers?
- Do all employees have access to e-mail?
- Are electronic medical records being used?
- Is new technology in place in the emergency department, critical care areas, labor and delivery, laboratory, and x-ray departments?

Religious/Philosophical

- Does the institution have a religious affiliation? How is this shown in the décor of the institution? How does the religious affiliation influence the philosophy, values, and norms of the agency?
- Is the institution public or private? For-profit or not-for-profit?
- Are documents such as The Patient's Bill of Rights prominently displayed within the institution? Are such documents displayed in languages other than English, for example, in Spanish? Are patients/family members provided with documents/explanations related to privacy rights?

Social Factors

- What are the working relationships within nursing? Between nursing and ancillary services? Within each nursing unit? Between physicians and nurses? How closely are staff members aligned throughout the organization?
- Is the environment initially "warm and loving"? How do volunteers or staff members at the information desk behave? Do employees get together outside of work?
- Is there a hierarchal distance between ancillary staff, nurses, and administrators?
- How are family members welcomed (or not welcomed) to the unit? Is the waiting room comfortable? Are there reading materials? Are they appropriate for the visitors?
- Are computers and telephones available for visitors? Vending machines? Dining facilities?
- Is the signage adequate within the institution? Is the signage in languages other than English? Can visitors easily find their way to a specific unit or room?
- What steps has the institution taken to be inclusive to visitors or patients?

Cultural Values

- Are institutional values explicitly stated? What is valued within the institution? What is valued as "good" and "bad"? Is there a gap between stated values and what actually happens on a daily or frequent basis?
- Are interpreter services readily available? Translated medical literature and educational materials available?
- How does the institution value and institutionalize culturally competent care?
- How does the institution recruit and retain staff members from underrepresented groups? How are personnel trained in cultural competencies?
- Is there coordination with traditional healers or use of community health workers?

- How does the organization respond to the community it serves (clinic hours, locations, physical environment, network memberships, and written materials)?
- How does the interior design, décor, and artwork reflect the cultural values of the institution and community at large?

Political/Legal

- Where does the power rest within the institution? With the administration? With the physicians? With the business office? With nursing?
- Is power shared? How is power divided among competing groups?
- Is there an active Board of Directors? What are their responsibilities?
- What types of legal actions have been taken against the institution? On behalf of the institution?
- How do employees or staff have input? How does the institution encourage or value suggestions or contributions from staff?

Economic

- What is the financial viability of the institution? Has this changed over the past 10 years?
- Who makes financial decisions?
- What values are the basis of financial decisions?
- How do the salaries and benefits compare with those of competitors in the immediate environment?

Education

- How is education valued within the institution? What type of assistance (financial, scheduling, flexibility) is provided for staff seeking advanced training or degrees?
- What opportunities are offered to those staff who are earning advanced degrees? Does the institution pay baccalaureate prepared nurses more than associate degree nurses?

- Does the institution provide clinical learning experiences for medicine, nursing, and other health professionals? How does the institution demonstrate that it values students?

- Are advanced practice nurses utilized? What is the educational background of staff nurses? Nurse managers? Nursing leaders? How does this compare with the educational levels of staff in competing institutions?

Appendix D

Baird/Boyle Transcultural Nursing Assessment Guide for Migrants/Refugees

• Joyceen S. Boyle and Martha B. Baird

Migration Experience

According to the UN Refugee Agency (2022), at the end of 2021, "at least 89.3 million people around the world were forced to flee their homes. Among them are nearly 27.1 million refugees, half of whom are under the age of 18." Those who are displaced due to war, persecution, lack of resources, or other circumstances that threaten safety and ability to survive are referred to as migrants, asylees, refugees, or parolees. For the purposes of this assessment guide, the term "migrant/refugee" will include all those displaced from their country of origin who have migrated to another country. Despite the legal status, there are millions of stateless people who have been denied a nationality and lack access to basic rights such as education, healthcare, employment, and freedom of movement.

Migrants/refugees arrive to a host or resettlement country from a variety of cultures and backgrounds. Some may be highly educated and held positions of influence in their home country, whereas others arrive from resource-constrained environments and may have little or no formal education. Therefore, it is important to conduct an individual assessment of each individual arriving in a new country.

Displaced individuals may experience symptoms of mental health distress due to circumstances that led to being forced out of their country of origin, in addition to the stressors associated with their migration journey. There are a number of mental health assessments that have

been found to be reliable and valid in a variety of cultural groups and languages adapted for use in different refugee groups (Davidson et al., 2010; Magwood et al., 2022).

Many refugees have spent time (often years) in so-called transit countries, those countries that they first flee to when they leave their country of origin. For example, Greece and Kenya are examples of transit countries for persons fleeing violence in Syria and Somali.

- Ask your client how to pronounce their name; find out what name they wish to be called. Be sure you're clear on what is the first and last name, as in many cultural groups the children do not share the same surname as their parents. How do they wish to be greeted?
- Ask about the client's primary language and assess their ability to communicate in English in both written and oral forms. What other languages does the client speak and write?
- Ask the clients in which language they prefer to receive written healthcare information.
- How long has your client been in this country? Have they lived in other U.S. cities? How did the client travel here from the home country? How many years did the client spend in the diaspora (or the time from leaving the country of origin to the present day)? What other countries has the client lived in? What were those circumstances like?
- Did the client come to this country with family members? With others from the same village or from the same clan?

- Can the client describe the migration experience? Ask about the events that happened to the client that they believe are important.
- What precipitated the client's leaving their country?
- Did the client have any major health events prior to arrival in the host country? If so, what? And did the client receive treatment? If so, where, and what were the outcomes?

The U.S. Healthcare System

- What were the client's experiences like when seeking healthcare in the United States? Has the client ever experienced discrimination? What was that experience like for their family members?
- What barriers might exist to using the U.S. healthcare system, such as language difficulties, lack of financial resources, and transportation?
- What provisions, if any, are made for refugee healthcare within your community?
- Are bilingual healthcare workers readily available? Is there distrust, suspicion, or unfamiliarity of healthcare workers and biomedicine? Is there eye contact with the healthcare professional?
- Are healthcare professionals genuinely interested in learning about the refugees?
- Does your client or others in the refugee community strongly prefer same-sex providers?
- What are the difficulties of accessing health and social services for refugees? Who is available in the sponsoring refugee agency to assist with health education, referrals, and continuity of care?

Language and Traditions

- What are the differences in dialects or languages spoken by healthcare professionals and the refugees? Can some of the problems be identified prior to a healthcare visit?
- What is the literacy level of members of the refugee group? Can they read and write in any language? This may vary within specific refugee groups depending on educational level and social status within home country.
- Do the healthcare facilities provide educational materials in appropriate languages?
- Are there appropriate numbers and appropriate ages and genders of translators and interpreters available in healthcare agencies? Are the interpreters/translators trained and/or certified?
- Is there adequate outreach to individual homes and families?

Traditional Beliefs and Practices of Healing

- What is the client's understanding of their health problem? The understanding of how a client views their condition is extremely helpful information. It facilitates the healthcare provider's understanding of the social and cultural construction of illness. This information helps us understand the client's beliefs and behavior, facilitates further discussion of an ailment, and guides the course of treatment. It is always helpful to begin this discussion with a statement of respect such as: *"I know different people have very different ways of understanding illness... help me understand how you see things."*
- The following nine questions from Kleinman (1980) can be a useful way to gain the client's perspective about the illness or health condition:

  1. What do you think has caused your problems?
  2. What do you call the problem or illness?
  3. Why do you think it started when it did?
  4. What do you think your sickness does to you?
  5. How severe is your sickness? Will it have a long or short course?
  6. What kind of treatment do you think you should receive?
  7. What are the most important results you hope to receive from this treatment?
  8. What are the chief problems your sickness has caused for you?
  9. What do you fear most about your sickness?

- How do religious beliefs and practices relate to health and illness?
- Do members of the refugee group seek care from indigenous healers and/or folk practitioners? Do they use traditional herbs or medicines? Are there cultural or ethnic stores in the neighborhood that sell herbs and traditional medicines? Does the individual purchase any medicines, herbs, or vitamins from their home country?
- What contemporary healthcare is available for this refugee group? What immunizations has the client received? When? What insurance or payment mechanisms are provided? For how long? Does the client understand how to access care?
- Which individuals in the family and/or in the refugee group make decisions about seeking healthcare? About the treatment options?
- What are the primary health concerns and/or illnesses in this refugee group (e.g., female genital mutilation [FGM], malnutrition, mental health/trauma issues)? How do the refugees' concerns align with those of the local and state healthcare systems? For example, FGM can be a significant concern during labor and delivery. In addition, if the procedure is carried out in the United States by relatives of the female child/adolescent, healthcare providers have ethical and legal reporting obligations.

Family and Kinship Systems

- Are the families extended or nuclear or other? Has the structure of the family changed during or since migration? Do family members live in close proximity? Do they visit often? Where are the members of your client's family?
- What is the role and stature of individual family members? How do family members relate to each other? How have family roles changed since coming to this country?
- Ask if there are tribes and/or clans in the refugee group.
- Do the parents and/or others make arrangements for marriages? Is there a preference for first cousins to marry?

- What is the role of "elders" or "leaders" in this refugee group? How do they function within the community?
- Did the client leave family members behind or lose family members from death in the home country?

Social Life and Networks

- What are the daily routines of this group? How do the routines vary by gender? How have family roles changed? Is the refugee group integrated into the community or fairly isolated? Who are the group's leaders?
- How does the refugee group observe important life cycle events?
- What are the educational aspirations of individual/family refugees? What are the educational experiences of the children?
- Are there special concerns such as abuse of alcohol, domestic violence, gang membership, polygamy, and child marriage? How does this refugee group view these issues?

Religious Beliefs and Practices

- What are the major religious beliefs and practices within the refugee community? Does your client adhere to the predominant beliefs? Is there a special church associated with the refugees? (Churches often serve as a site for social life of the refugee community and are comfortable and acceptable places for health educational programs and other forms of outreach.) How is social life integrated within the church membership?
- How do the religious beliefs and practices influence everyday life? How are they expressed in everyday life?
- Are there special beliefs and practices surrounding major life events such as birth, marriage, and death?
- Are there special "cultural" occasions, such as circumcision rites and *quince años* parties?
- Are there specific beliefs about gender roles? Are these beliefs tied to religious beliefs?

All refugees resettled to the United States receive a comprehensive physical examination and mental health screening within their first 30 days of their arrival. This is usually conducted in a public health clinic or primary care setting. There are several mental health assessment tools that have been translated and culturally adapted for use with different refugee groups. If a refugee has a positive mental health screening, they should be referred to a mental healthcare provider for further assessment.

The Refugee Health Screener-15 (RHS-15) is commonly used to assess newly arrived refugees in host countries. The RHS-15 has been translated into 15 languages and is used to measure indicators of mental health symptoms and distress including depression, anxiety, and coping (Pathways to Wellness, 2013).

The Hopkins Symptoms Checklist-25 measures symptoms of anxiety and depression, and the Harvard Trauma Questionnaire is a checklist that inquiries about a variety of traumatic events as well as the emotional symptoms considered to be uniquely associated with trauma and torture (Mollica et al., 2004).

REFERENCES

Davidson, G. R., Murray, K. E., & Schweitzer, R. D. (2010). Review of refugee mental health assessment: Best practices and recommendations. *Journal of Pacific Rim Psychology*, 4(1), 72–85. https://doi.org/10.1375/prp.4.1.72

Kleinman, A. (1980). *Patients and healers in the context of culture: An exploration of the borderland between anthropology, medicine and psychiatry*. University of California Press.

Magwood, O., Kassam, A., Mavedatnia, D., Mendonca, O., Saad, A., Hasan, H., Madana, M., Ranger, D., Tan, Y., & Pottie, K. (2022). Mental health screening approaches for resettling refugees and asylum seekers: A scoping review. *International Journal of Environmental Research and Public Health*, 19, 3549. https://doi.org/10.3390/ijerph19063549

Mollica, R. F., McDonald, L. S., Massagli, M. P., & Silove, D. M. (2004). *Measuring trauma, measuring torture: Instructions and guidance on the utilization of the Harvard program in refugee trauma version of the Hopkins Symptom Checklist-25 (HSCL-25) & The Harvard Trauma Questionnaire (HTQ)*. Harvard Program in Refugee Trauma.

Pathways to Wellness. (2013). *Refugee health screener-15 (Measurement instrument)*. http://refugeehealthta.org/wpcontent/uploads/2012/09/RHS15_Packet_PathwaysToWellness-1/pdf

The UN Refugee Agency. (2022, June 16). UNHCR *global trends: Figures at a glance*. Retrieved October 6, 2022, from unhcr.org/en-us/figures-at-a-glance.html

United Nations High Commissioner for Refugees (UNHCR) The UN Refugee Agency. (1992). *Handbook on procedures and criteria for determining refugee status under the 1951 convention and the 1967 protocol relating to the status of refugees*. http://www.unhcr.org/cgi-bin/texis/vtx/search?page=search=&docid=3d58el3b4query=definition%20of%20refugee

Index

Note: Page numbers followed by *b* refers to material located in a box; *c* refers to a case study; *e* refers to evidence-based practice; *f* refers to a figure; *t* refers to a table.